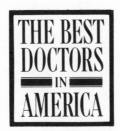

CENTRAL
REGION

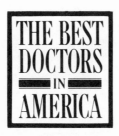

CENTRAL REGION

STEVEN NAIFEH
AND
GREGORY WHITE SMITH

Lucienne Potterfield Stec
MANAGING EDITOR

Kathryn R. Madden
SUPERVISING EDITOR

Suzanne Flowers Arnold • Christopher James Greame
Jonathan Otis Jackson • Susan Quinn Sand
Deanna M. Tremlin • Beverly Jackson Veasey
Melissa A. Westerdahl • Leigh Anne Zalants
SENIOR EDITORS

1996-1997

WOODWARD / WHITE
Aiken, South Carolina

The Best Doctors in America ® is an exclusive trademark and servicemark of Woodward/White, Inc.

Copyright © 1996 by Woodward/White, Inc.
129 First Avenue, SW, Aiken, SC 29801
All rights reserved. This book, or parts thereof, must not be reproduced in any form without permission.

Library of Congress Cataloging-in-Publication Data

Naifeh, Steven W., 1952–
    The best doctors in America: central region, 1996–1997 / Steven Naifeh and Gregory White Smith.
        p.   cm.
    Includes index.
    ISBN 0-913391-15-8
    ISSN 1088-8667
    1. Physicians—North America—Directories.   I. Smith, Gregory
White.   II. Stec, Lucienne Potterfield.   III. Title.

PRINTED IN THE UNITED STATES OF AMERICA

We would like to acknowledge our debt to the thousands of doctors who gave of their time and expertise in the process of compiling these lists.

INTRODUCTION

We are proud to present *The Best Doctors in America: Central Region, 1996-1997*. This new regional guide is designed to accompany our national publication, *The Best Doctors in America,* now in its second edition and widely regarded as the preeminent referral guide to the medical profession. *Best Doctors* has been featured on "The Today Show," on CNN's "Headline News" and on CNBC's "Pozner/Donahue," as well as in a number of papers and magazines (*USA Today, The New York Times, The Los Angeles Times, The Washington Post, Family Circle*). Most recently, it was excerpted in the February and March issues of *Town & Country*.

Unlike the national edition of *Best Doctors,* this new Central regional guide is intended to recognize doctors in communities of all sizes throughout the Central area whose superior clinical abilities may or may not have drawn national attention. It also includes, for the first time, primary care physicians. When used in conjunction with the national guide, the result is a referral list that is both more thorough in its representation of the full range of medical specialties and more geographically balanced—a list, we hope, that will be eminently useful in the search for superior medical care from Alaska to Arizona.

The Best Doctors in America: Central Region is based on an exhaustive survey in which more than five thousand doctors in the Central area were asked to rate the clinical abilities of their peers. The quality of our lists has always been the backbone of both *The Best Doctors in America* and our longstanding publication *The Best Lawyers in America,* and, more than ever before, we have bent every effort to ensure that the lists in our new regional guide to the best doctors in the Central area are reliable, accurate, and current.

COMPILING THE REGIONAL GUIDE

We began the selection process with the doctors from the Central area listed in the national *Best Doctors*. (A detailed description of the methodology used in that publication is included in its introduction.) We called virtually every one of the approximately 1,000 doctors listed in the 1994-1995 edition, asking them to vote on the other listed doctors in their areas of expertise and to nominate doctors not previously listed. We also asked them to nominate and vote on doctors who have extraordinary clinical expertise but who may not have attracted national attention because they do not engage in research or publish as much as other doctors in the field. Also, for the first time, we asked the doctors to nominate and vote on doctors in primary care: Family Medicine, General Internal Medicine, and General Pediatrics.

As in the past, we did not attempt to articulate the criteria for judging professional excellence; we left that to the individual doctor. We did, however, routinely couch our inquiry in the following terms: "If you had a close friend or loved one who needed a neurological surgeon (for example), and you couldn't perform the operation yourself, for whatever reason, to whom would you refer them?" All comments, we promised, would remain confidential.

The rate of response was remarkable. Very few of the doctors we contacted refused to cooperate. Many of the respondents called back and shared their views at great length. Many asked if they could take some time to consider the question and get back to us. Others called later with additional nominations. Although we did not seek official sanction from any national, local, general, or specialized medical associations, individual association officials were among our most cooperative respondents.

We then called the newly nominated doctors—more than 6,000 men and women—who received the most positive votes from the doctors in the national book. We continued to call new nominees, registering positive and negative votes, until a consensus emerged. Many names received unanimous praise. Others earned mixed assessments. In the latter instance, final decisions were made on a case-by-case basis after additional calls. No name was ever removed from the list on the basis of a single negative vote, nor was any name added on the basis of a single nomination.

The vast majority of the doctors listed in the most recent edition of our national *Best Doctors* who practice in the Central area are also included in this regional guide. We did, however, delete some names. Some, of course, died; others retired or moved into private industry or government service. Still others had devoted themselves so completely to research or had curtailed their activities so completely that it was no longer appropriate to include them on what is essentially a referral list. But a few simply did not receive the necessary number of affirmative votes to be included on the list. We attribute this to the fact that, far more than in the polling for the national edition, the voting doctors knew the doctors they were voting on because of their clinical abilities rather than their research abilities.

The quality of the doctors on these lists may not be uniform. While no doctor is listed unless his or her skills have earned the respect of the medical community, those skills were judged relative to those of others practicing in the same community. And while some of the best doctors in the country may practice in small communities far away from the major teaching hospitals, medical talent does tend to gravitate towards the major teaching hospitals in big cities.

Yet the need for first class medical care knows no geographical boundaries. There are times, of course, when a medical emergency won't permit a patient the luxury of travelling to a teaching hospital in another state. On the other hand, there are times when a medical problem can be happily resolved closer to home, or else the medical problem has not yet been diagnosed and the patient does not yet know whether to seek out a doctor with greater expertise. Whatever the reason, there is a need for a list of the best doctors in every major metropolitan area, whether or not those doctors have a national reputation. And it is that need which this book is intended to fulfill.

HOW THIS BOOK IS ORGANIZED

The Best Doctors in America: Central Region is organized alphabetically by state, then by field of expertise. Within each field, the entries are arranged alphabetically, first by city, then by the doctor's last name. Each entry includes the doctor's name; areas of specialization; clinical affiliations; principal address; and telephone number.

It should be noted that the doctors in this book have been categorized according to the field of expertise in which they were nominated. The doctors themselves may or may not think of themselves as principally engaged in the field of medicine under which they are listed. However, we did provide each doctor with an opportunity to inform us of their own fields of expertise as they viewed them, and, to distinguish these from the areas specified by the doctors who nominated them, these fields have been listed within parentheses.

Similarly, while many of the doctors are board certified in their listed areas of expertise (where such certification is available), some are not. Anyone interested in the certification of a particular doctor should check with that doctor or the appropriate certifying body.

THE EDITORS

The Best Doctors in America: Central Region was edited by Steven Naifeh and Gregory White Smith, both graduates of the Harvard Law School and, between them, authors of sixteen books, including four national bestsellers. *Jackson Pollock: An American Saga* was a nonfiction finalist for the 1990 National Book Award and winner of the 1990 Pulitzer Prize for biography.

The senior editors on the book were Lucienne Potterfield Stec, Suzanne Flowers Arnold, Christopher J. Greame, Jonathan O. Jackson, Kathryn Madden, Susan Quinn Sand, Deanna Tremlin, Beverly Veasey, Melissa Westerdahl, and Leigh Anne Zalants. They were assisted by Michael Goldston, Jennifer Heckman, Gabriel Mangiante, Doria Patterson, and Tiffany Rush.

WOODWARD/WHITE REFERRAL SERVICE

In addition to publishing the referral guides, *The Best Doctors in America*, *The Best Lawyers in America*, and *The Best Lawyers in America: Directory of Experts*, Woodward/White, Inc., undertakes specialized searches for doctors and lawyers using our unique access to sources of information on the best professionals in medicine and law. Prospective patients or clients who require a doctor or lawyer in a particular area of expertise or locale not covered in our books, or who wish assistance in refining the list of candidates, are welcome to write us at Woodward/White, Inc., 129 First Avenue, SW, Aiken, SC 29801, call 803-648-0300, or fax 803-641-1709.

Woodward/White can also be contacted by E-Mail at woodward.white@groupz.net. Additional information about Woodward/White products and services is available on the World Wide Web at http://www.bestdoctors.com.

PLEASE NOTE

If you are a patient using this book to find a specialist, we recommend that you ask your personal physician to make the initial contact. The specialists in this book are extremely busy and may have questions about your case that only your personal physician can answer.

CONTENTS

ARKANSAS

ALLERGY & IMMUNOLOGY

Little Rock

A. Wesley Burks, Jr. · General Allergy & Immunology (Allergy) · Arkansas Children's Hospital · Arkansas Children's Hospital, 800 Marshall Street, Mail Slot 512, Little Rock, AR 72202-3591 · 501-320-1060

P. Martin Fiser · General Allergy & Immunology · Arkansas Allergy Clinic, 10310 West Markham Street, Suite 222, P.O. Box 5675, Little Rock, AR 72215 · 501-227-5210

John James · General Allergy & Immunology (General Pediatrics) · Arkansas Children's Hospital · Arkansas Children's Hospital, 800 Marshall Street, Mail Slot 512, Little Rock, AR 72202-3591 · 501-320-1060

Stacie Jones · General Allergy & Immunology (Immunodeficiency, Rheumatology) · Arkansas Children's Hospital · Arkansas Children's Hospital, 800 Marshall Street, Mail Slot 512, Little Rock, AR 72202-3591 · 501-320-1060

Kevin R. Keller · General Allergy & Immunology · Arkansas Allergy Clinic, 10310 West Markham Street, Suite 222, P.O. Box 5675, Little Rock, AR 72215 · 501-227-5210

J. Gary Wheeler · General Allergy & Immunology (Drug Allergy, Pediatric Infectious Disease) · Arkansas Children's Hospital, University Hospital of Arkansas Arkansas Children's Hospital, 800 Marshall Street, Mail Slot 512, Little Rock, AR 72202-3591 · 501-320-1060

ANESTHESIOLOGY

Little Rock

Frank E. Block, Jr. · General Anesthesiology (Engineering, Monitoring of the Anesthetic Patient) · University of Arkansas for Medical Sciences, Department of Anesthesiology, 4301 West Markham Street, Mail Slot 515, Little Rock, AR 72205-7199 · 501-686-6114

Raeford E. Brown · Pediatric Anesthesiology (Pain Management, Malignant Hyperthermia) · Arkansas Children's Hospital, Department of Anesthesia, 800 Marshall Street, Mail Slot 700, Little Rock, AR 72202-3591 · 501-320-2934

H. Jerrel Fontenot · Neuroanesthesia (Neuromuscular Blocking Agents, Anesthetic Pharmacology) · University of Arkansas for Medical Sciences, Department of Anesthesiology, 4301 West Markham Street, Mail Slot 515, Little Rock, AR 72205 · 501-686-6114

E. F. Klein, Jr. · Critical Care Medicine (Respiratory Physiology, Mechanical Ventilation Modalities, Complications of Anesthesia) · University Hospital of Arkansas, Arkansas Children's Hospital, VA Medical Center-Little Rock Division · University of Arkansas for Medical Sciences, Department of Anesthesiology, 4301 West Markham Street, Mail Slot 515, Little Rock, AR 72205-7199 · 501-686-6114

Timothy W. Martin · Pediatric Anesthesiology · Arkansas Children's Hospital · Arkansas Children's Hospital, Division of Pediatric Anesthesia, 800 Marshall Street, Mail Slot 700, Little Rock, AR 72202-3591 · 501-320-1329

Raymond R. Schultetus · Obstetric Anesthesia · University of Arkansas for Medical Sciences, Department of Anesthesiology, 4301 West Markham Street, Mail Slot 515, Little Rock, AR 72205 · 501-686-6114

Astride B. Seifen · Cardiothoracic Anesthesiology (Pharmacology of Anesthetic Drugs, Adult Cardiovascular, Pediatric Anesthesiology) · University of Arkansas for Medical Sciences, Department of Anesthesiology, 4301 West Markham Street, Mail Slot 515, Little Rock, AR 72205-7199 · 501-686-6114

J. Michael Vollers · Pediatric Anesthesiology (Cardiac Anesthesiology, Critical Care Medicine, Pediatric Cardiovascular) · Arkansas Children's Hospital, Department of Anesthesia, 800 Marshall Street, Mail Slot 700, Little Rock, AR 72202-3591 · 501-320-1329

CARDIOVASCULAR DISEASE

Little Rock

Joseph K. Bissett · General Cardiovascular Disease (Coronary Artery Disease, Cardiac Arrhythmias) · University of Arkansas for Medical Sciences, Division of Cardiology, 4301 West Markham Street, Mail Slot 532, Little Rock, AR 72205 · 501-686-5243

Ha Dinh · General Cardiovascular Disease · University of Arkansas for Medical Sciences, Division of Cardiology, 4301 West Markham Street, Mail Slot 532, Little Rock, AR 72205 · 501-686-5243

Jon P. Lindermann · General Cardiovascular Disease · University of Arkansas for Medical Sciences, Division of Cardiology, 4301 West Markham Street, Mail Slot 532, Little Rock, AR 72205 · 501-686-5243

CLINICAL PHARMACOLOGY

Little Rock

Henry C. Farrar III · Arkansas Children's Hospital · Arkansas Children's Hospital, 800 Marshall Street, Little Rock, AR 72202 · 501-320-1418

Henry F. Simmons · (Toxicology, Acute Management of Chemical Exposures & Drug Overdoses, Forensic) · University of Arkansas for Medical Sciences, Department of Emergency Medicine, 4301 West Markham Street, Mail Slot 584, Little Rock, AR 72212 · 800-3-POISON

COLON & RECTAL SURGERY

Little Rock

J. Ralph Broadwater · General Colon & Rectal Surgery (Gastrointestinal Cancer, Colon & Rectal Cancer) · University of Arkansas for Medical Sciences · University of Arkansas for Medical Sciences, Department of Surgery, 4301 West Markham Street, Mail Slot 725, Little Rock, AR 72205-7101 · 501-686-5547

DERMATOLOGY

Blytheville

Lawrence Jack Abramson · Clinical Dermatology (Skin Cancer Surgery & Reconstruction) · 1104 Medical Drive, Blytheville, AR 72315 · 501-763-3330

Fort Smith

Kevin St. Clair · Clinical Dermatology (Skin Cancer Surgery) · Sparks Regional Medical Center · Holt Krock Clinic, 1500 Dodson Avenue, P.O. Box 2418, Fort Smith, AR 72902-2418 · 501-788-4000

Hot Springs

D. Bluford Stough III · Aesthetic Surgery (Hair Transplantation) · St. Joseph's Regional Health Center · Stough Medical Associates, One Mercy Lane, Suite 203, Hot Springs, AR 71913 · 501-624-0673

Little Rock

Rene Edward Bressinick · Clinical Dermatology · Medical Towers Building One, Suite 690, 9601 Lile Drive, Little Rock, AR 72205 · 501-227-8422

Scott M. Dinehart · Skin Cancer Surgery & Reconstruction (Mohs Microsurgery) University of Arkansas for Medical Sciences, Department of Dermatology, 4301 West Markham Street, Mail Slot 580, Little Rock, AR 72205 · 501-686-6389

Gunnar H. Gibson · Clinical Dermatology (Skin Cancer Surgery & Reconstruction, Aging Skin) · Baptist Medical Center · Medical Towers Building One, Suite 690, 9601 Lile Drive, Little Rock, AR 72205 · 501-227-8422

Jere D. Guin · Contact Dermatitis · University Hospital of Arkansas, John L. McClellan Memorial Veterans Hospital · University of Arkansas for Medical Sciences, Department of Dermatology, 4301 West Markham Street, Mail Slot 576, Little Rock, AR 72205 · 501-686-5110

Jay Kincannon · Pediatric Dermatology · Arkansas Children's Hospital · Arkansas Children's Hospital, Department of Pediatric Dermatology, 800 Marshall Street, Little Rock, AR 72202-3591 · 501-320-1144

ENDOCRINOLOGY & METABOLISM

Little Rock

Lawson Glover · General Endocrinology & Metabolism · Little Rock Diagnostic Clinic, 10001 Lile Drive, Little Rock, AR 72205-6299 · 501-227-8000

FAMILY MEDICINE

Fort Smith

Gordon Parham · 1120 Lexington Avenue, Fort Smith, AR 72901 · 501-782-6081

Little Rock

Geoffrey Goldsmith · University of Arkansas for Medical Sciences, Department of Family and Community Medicine, 4301 West Markham Street, Mail Slot 530, Little Rock, AR 72205 · 501-686-6602

Forrest Miller · Columbia Family Clinic, 4202 South University Avenue, Little Rock, AR 72204 · 501-562-4838

Steven W. Strode · University Hospital of Arkansas, Arkansas Children's Hospital · University of Arkansas for Medical Sciences, 4301 West Markham Street, Mail Slot 599-A, Little Rock, AR 72205 · 501-686-2590

GASTROENTEROLOGY

Little Rock

Glenn Raymond Davis · Gastrointestinal Motility (General Gastroenterology) · St. Vincent Infirmary Medical Center, Baptist Medical Center, Columbia Doctor's Hospital · 417 North University Avenue, Little Rock, AR 72205 · 501-666-0249

GERIATRIC MEDICINE

Little Rock

David A. Lipschitz · (Hematology, Oncology, Nutrition) · John L. McClellan Memorial Veterans Hospital, University of Arkansas for Medical Sciences · John L. McClellan Memorial Veterans Hospital, Geriatric Research and Education Clinical Center (GRECC), 4300 West Seventh Street, Mail Code 182, Little Rock, AR 72205 · 501-660-2031

North Little Rock

William J. Carter · (Age-Related Muscle Wasting, Anabolic Hormones, Thyroid Disease, Diabetes, General Endocrinology & Metabolism, General Geriatric Medicine) · VA Medical Center-North Little Rock Division, University Hospital of Arkansas (Little Rock), University of Arkansas for Medical Sciences (Little Rock) · VA Medical Center, 2200 Fort Roots Drive, North Little Rock, AR 72114 501-661-1202

Pham Liem · (Alzheimer's Disease & Other Dementias) · John L. McClellan Memorial Veterans Hospital (Little Rock), University Hospital of Arkansas (Little Rock) · VA Medical Center, 2200 Fort Roots Drive, North Little Rock, AR 72114 501-661-1202 x4689

HAND SURGERY

Little Rock

G. Thomas Frazier, Jr. · General Hand Surgery · Arkansas Hand Center, 600 South McKinley Street, Suite 200, Little Rock, AR 72205 · 501-664-4088

Michael Moore · General Hand Surgery · Arkansas Hand Center, 600 South McKinley Street, Suite 200, Little Rock, AR 72205 · 501-664-4088

INFECTIOUS DISEASE

Little Rock

Robert Shields Abernathy · General Infectious Disease · University of Arkansas for Medical Sciences, Division of Infectious Disease, 4301 West Markham Street, Mail Slot 639, Little Rock, AR 72205 · 501-686-5585

Robert W. Bradsher · General Infectious Disease (Fungal Infections, Respiratory Infections) · University of Arkansas for Medical Sciences, Division of Infectious Disease, 4301 West Markham Street, Mail Slot 639, Little Rock, AR 72205-7199 501-686-5585

Rebecca B. Martin · General Infectious Disease · University of Arkansas for Medical Sciences, Division of Infectious Disease, 4301 West Markham Street, Mail Slot 639, Little Rock, AR 72205 · 501-686-5585

Richard McDonnell · General Infectious Disease · University of Arkansas for Medical Sciences, Division of Infectious Disease, 4301 West Markham Street, Mail Slot 639, Little Rock, AR 72205 · 501-686-5585

Thomas P. Monson · General Infectious Disease · University of Arkansas for Medical Sciences, Division of Infectious Disease, 4301 West Markham Street, Mail Slot 639, Little Rock, AR 72205 · 501-686-5585

INTERNAL MEDICINE (GENERAL)

Fort Smith

Steven A. Edmondson · Fort Smith Internal Medicine, 708 Lexington Avenue, Fort Smith, AR 72901 · 501-782-4470

Lance L. Hamilton · Holt Krock Clinic, 1500 Dodson Avenue, Fort Smith, AR 72901 · 501-782-2071

J. David Staggs · Sparks Regional Medical Center, St. Edward Mercy Medical Center · Fort Smith Internal Medicine, 708 Lexington Avenue, Fort Smith, AR 72901 · 501-782-4470

Jerry Rowland Stewart · Cooper Clinic, 6801 Rogers Avenue, P.O. Box 3528, Fort Smith, AR 72903 · 501-452-2077

Little Rock

Robert T. Cheek · University of Arkansas for Medical Sciences, University Private Medical Group Clinic, 4301 West Markham Street, Mail Slot 547, Little Rock, AR 72205 · 501-686-5545

Jeanne K. Heard · University of Arkansas for Medical Sciences, University Private Medical Group Clinic, 4301 West Markham Street, Mail Slot 547, Little Rock, AR 72205 · 501-686-5545

Roberta Monson · (General Infectious Diseases, Case Management) · University of Arkansas for Medical Sciences, Ambulatory Care Center, 4301 West Markham Street, Mail Slot 547, Little Rock, AR 72205 · 501-686-6957

Robert B. Moore · Five St. Vincent Circle, Little Rock, AR 72205 · 501-666-7041

Jack Wagoner, Jr. · Little Rock Internal Medicine Clinic, 5918 Lee Avenue, Little Rock, AR 72205 · 501-664-2500

MEDICAL ONCOLOGY & HEMATOLOGY

Fort Smith

John D. Wells · General Medical Oncology & Hematology · St. Edward Mercy Medical Center · Cooper Clinic, 6801 Rogers Avenue, P.O. Box 3528, Fort Smith, AR 72903 · 501-452-2077

Little Rock

Bart Barlogie · Myeloma (Bone Marrow Transplantation & Biologicals, Multiple Myeloma) · Arkansas Cancer Research Center, University Hospital of Arkansas · University of Arkansas for Medical Sciences, Arkansas Cancer Research Center, 4301 West Markham Street, Mail Slot 508, Little Rock, AR 72205-9985 · 501-686-5222

Arthur Haut · General Medical Oncology & Hematology (Internal Medicine) · University of Arkansas for Medical Sciences, Arkansas Cancer Research Center, 4301 West Markham Street, Mail Slot 508, Little Rock, AR 72205-9985 · 501-686-8530

Laura F. Hutchins · General Medical Oncology & Hematology · University of Arkansas for Medical Sciences, Department of Hematology & Oncology, 4301 West Markham Street, Mail Slot 721, Little Rock, AR 72205 · 501-686-5222

Sundar Jagannath · Bone Marrow Transplantation (Multiple Myeloma) · University of Arkansas for Medical Sciences, Arkansas Cancer Research Center, 4301 West Markham Street, Mail Slot 508, Little Rock, AR 72205-9985 · 501-686-5222

Ann-Marie E. Maddox · General Medical Oncology & Hematology · University of Arkansas for Medical Sciences, Arkansas Cancer Research Center, 4301 West Markham Street, Mail Slot 508, Little Rock, AR 72205-9985 · 501-686-8530

S. William Ross · General Medical Oncology & Hematology · John L. McClellan Memorial Veterans Hospital, 4300 West Seventh Street, Mail Slot 111-K, Little Rock, AR 72205 · 501-661-3192

Billy Lynn Tranum · General Medical Oncology & Hematology · Arkansas Oncology Clinic, Medical Towers Building Two, Suite 700, 9501 Lile Drive, Little Rock, AR 72205 · 501-223-8003

Guido Tricot · (Bone Marrow Transplantation, Multiple Myeloma, Leukemia) · University of Arkansas for Medical Sciences, Arkansas Cancer Research Center, 4301 West Markham Street, Mail Slot 508, Little Rock, AR 72205-9985 · 501-686-5222

Sue Tsuda · General Medical Oncology & Hematology · St. Vincent Infirmary Medical Center, Baptist Medical Center · Little Rock Hematology-Oncology Associates, One St. Vincent Circle, Suite 450, Little Rock, AR 72205 · 501-664-4820

David H. Vesole · (Bone Marrow Transplantation, Multiple Myeloma) · University of Arkansas for Medical Sciences, Arkansas Cancer Research Center, 4301 West Markham Street, Mail Slot 508, Little Rock, AR 72205-9985 · 501-686-8230

NEPHROLOGY

Hot Springs

Robert F. McCrary, Jr. · General Nephrology (Dialysis, Kidney Disease) · National Park Medical Center, St. Joseph's Regional Health Center · Hot Springs Diagnostic Associates, 1900 Malvern Avenue, Suite 102, Hot Springs, AR 71901 501-321-9803

Little Rock

Martin Bunke · Kidney Transplantation (Dialysis) · University Hospital of Arkansas · University of Arkansas for Medical Sciences, Division of Nephrology, 4301 West Markham Street, Mail Slot 501, Little Rock, AR 72205-9985 · 501-686-5295

Thomas Alan Golper · Dialysis (Hemodialysis) · University Hospital of Arkansas University of Arkansas for Medical Sciences, Department of Nephrology, 4301 West Markham Street, Mail Slot 501, Little Rock, AR 72205 · 501-686-5295

Ronald Dallas Hughes · General Nephrology · Renal Associates, 500 South University Avenue, Suite 219, Little Rock, AR 72205 · 501-664-9881

NEUROLOGICAL SURGERY

Little Rock

Ossama Al-Mefty · Tumor Surgery (Skull-Base Surgery, Vascular Neurological Surgery) · University Hospital of Arkansas, John L. McClellan Memorial Veterans Hospital, Arkansas Children's Hospital · University of Arkansas for Medical Sciences, Department of Neurosurgery, 4301 West Markham Street, Mail Slot 507, Little Rock, AR 72205-7199 · 501-686-8757

Frederick Boop · Pediatric Neurological Surgery (Epilepsy Surgery, Selective Dorsal Rhizotomy, Endoscopic Surgery) · Arkansas Children's Hospital, Department of Neurosurgery, 800 Marshall Street, Little Rock, AR 72202-3591 · 501-320-1448

NEUROLOGY

Little Rock

Robert Leroy Archer · General Neurology · University of Arkansas for Medical Sciences, 4301 West Markham Street, Mail Slot 547, Little Rock, AR 72205 · 501-686-5838

Michael Z. Chesser · General Neurology · John L. McClellan Memorial Veterans Hospital, Department of Neurology, 4300 West Seventh Street, Little Rock, AR 72205 · 501-660-2070

Sami I. Harik · Movement Disorders, Neuro-Oncology · University Hospital of Arkansas · University of Arkansas for Medical Sciences, 4301 West Markham Street, Mail Slot 500, Little Rock, AR 72205-7199 · 501-686-7236

George Morrison Henry · General Neurology · Baptist Medical Center, Columbia Doctor's Hospital, St. Vincent Infirmary Medical Center · Neurology Associates, 8924 Kanis Road, Little Rock, AR 72205 · 501-227-4750

Dennis D. Lucy, Jr. · General Neurology (Electromyography, Neuromuscular Disease) · University of Arkansas for Medical Sciences Medical Center · University of Arkansas for Medical Sciences, 4301 West Markham Street, Mail Slot 500, Little Rock, AR 72205 · 501-686-5135

Sarkis M. Nazarian · General Neurology · John L. McClellan Memorial Veterans Hospital, Department of Neurology, 4300 West Seventh Street, Little Rock, AR 72205 · 501-660-2070

North Little Rock

W. Steven Metzer · General Neurology (Movement Disorders) · Baptist Memorial Medical Center · Arkansas Headache & Neurology Clinic, 1013 Wildwood Avenue, North Little Rock, AR 72120 · 501-835-4525

NEUROLOGY, CHILD

Little Rock

Stephen R. Bates · General Child Neurology (Epilepsy) · Arkansas Children's Hospital · Arkansas Children's Hospital, Department of Pediatric Neurology, 800 Marshall Street, Mail Slot 512, Little Rock, AR 72202-3591 · 501-320-1850

May Louyse Griebel · General Child Neurology (Pediatric Epilepsy, Pediatric Sleep Disorders) · Arkansas Children's Hospital · Arkansas Children's Hospital, Department of Pediatric Neurology, 800 Marshall Street, Mail Slot 512, Little Rock, AR 72202-3591 · 501-320-1850

Bernadette Lange · General Child Neurology · Arkansas Children's Hospital, Department of Pediatric Neurology, 800 Marshall Street, Mail Slot 512, Little Rock, AR 72202 · 501-320-1850

Gregory B. Sharp · General Child Neurology (Epilepsy, Electroencephalography) · Arkansas Children's Hospital · Arkansas Children's Hospital, Department of Pediatric Neurology, 800 Marshall Street, Mail Slot 512, Little Rock, AR 72202 501-320-1850

NUCLEAR MEDICINE

Little Rock

Charles Marion Boyd · General Nuclear Medicine (Ultrasound) · Baptist Medical Center · Radiology Consultants, Medical Towers Building, Suite 1100, Little Rock, AR 72205 · 501-227-5240

W. Turner Harris · General Nuclear Medicine (Nuclear Cardiology, Positron Emission Tomography, Oncology) · St. Vincent Infirmary Medical Center · Radiology Associates, 500 South University Avenue, Suite 101, Little Rock, AR 72205-5399 · 501-664-3914

Jerry L. Prather · General Nuclear Medicine · Radiology Associates, 500 South University Avenue, Suite 101, Little Rock, AR 72205-5303 · 501-664-3914

Gary L. Purnell · General Nuclear Medicine · John L. McClellan Memorial Veterans Hospital, 4300 West Seventh Street, Little Rock, AR 72205 · 501-660-2027

David W. Weiss · General Nuclear Medicine · Radiology Associates, 500 South University Avenue, Suite 108, Little Rock, AR 72205 · 501-664-3914

OBSTETRICS & GYNECOLOGY

Fayetteville

George R. Cole, Jr. · General Obstetrics & Gynecology · Parkhill Clinic for Women, 3336 North Futrall Drive, Fayetteville, AR 72703 · 501-521-4433

Little Rock

David L. Barclay · Gynecologic Cancer · 500 South University Avenue, Suite 614, Little Rock, AR 72205 · 501-664-8502

Cynthia Neal Frazier · General Obstetrics & Gynecology · A Clinic For Women, 5600 West Markham Street, Little Rock, AR 72205 · 501-663-5055

Groesbeck P. Parham · Gynecologic Cancer · University of Arkansas for Medical Sciences, Department of Obstetrics & Gynecology, 4301 West Markham Street, Mail Slot 518, Little Rock, AR 72205 · 501-686-7158

J. Gerald Quirk, Jr. · Maternal & Fetal Medicine · University Hospital of Arkansas · University of Arkansas for Medical Sciences, Department of Obstetrics & Gynecology, 4301 West Markham Street, Mail Slot 518, Little Rock, AR 72205 · 501-686-5380

Juan Roman · General Obstetrics & Gynecology · One St. Vincent Circle, Suite 360, Little Rock, AR 72205 · 501-661-0596

Glenn A. Weitzman · Reproductive Endocrinology · University of Arkansas for Medical Sciences, Department of Obstetrics & Gynecology, 4301 West Markham Street, Mail Slot 508, Little Rock, AR 72205 · 501-686-7160

OPHTHALMOLOGY

Little Rock

James Landers · Vitreo-Retinal Surgery · Five St. Vincent Circle, Little Rock, AR 72205 · 501-663-1700

Pine Bluff

Michael S. McFarland · Anterior Segment—Cataract & Refractive · McFarland Eye Surgery Center · McFarland Eye Surgery Center, 3805 West 28th Avenue, Pine Bluff, AR 71603 · 501-536-4100; 800-451-6686

ORTHOPAEDIC SURGERY

Little Rock

Samuel G. Agnew · Trauma · University Hospital of Arkansas · University of Arkansas for Medical Sciences, Department of Orthopaedic Surgery, 4301 West Markham Street, Mail Slot 531, Little Rock, AR 72205 · 501-686-5595

Carl L. Nelson, Jr. · General Orthopaedic Surgery · University of Arkansas for Medical Sciences, Department of Orthopaedic Surgery, 4301 West Markham Street, Mail Slot 531, Little Rock, AR 72205 · 501-686-5505

Richard W. Nicholas, Jr. · General Orthopaedic Surgery · University of Arkansas for Medical Sciences, Department of Orthopaedic Surgery, 4301 West Markham Street, Mail Slot 531, Little Rock, AR 72205 · 501-686-7816

John L. VanderSchilden · General Orthopaedic Surgery (Sports Medicine/Arthroscopy, Orthopaedic Trauma) · University Hospital of Arkansas · University of Arkansas for Medical Sciences, Department of Orthopaedic Surgery, 4301 West Markham Street, Mail Slot 531, Little Rock, AR 72205-7199 · 501-686-7823

OTOLARYNGOLOGY

Fort Smith

Michael Marsh · Otology/Neurotology (Skull-Base Surgery) · Holt Krock Clinic, 1500 Dodson Avenue, P.O. Box 2418, Fort Smith, AR 72902-2418 · 501-788-4000

Paul I. Wills · Head & Neck Surgery · Sparks Regional Medical Center, St. Edward Mercy Medical Center · West Arkansas Ear, Nose & Throat Clinic, 600 South 16th Street, Fort Smith, AR 72901 · 501-782-6022

Hot Springs

Robert Borg · General Otolaryngology (Facial Plastic Surgery, Head & Neck Surgery, Laryngology, Otology, Sinus & Nasal Surgery) · St. Joseph's Regional Health Center, National Park Medical Center · Hot Springs Clinic of Otolaryngology, 100 Ridgeway Place, Suite Two, Hot Springs, AR 71901-7199 · 501-624-5422

Jim Griffin · General Otolaryngology (General Allergy & Immunology) · St. Joseph's Regional Health Center, National Park Medical Center · 100 Ridgeway Place, Hot Springs, AR 71901 · 501-624-5422

Edwin Leeth Harper · General Otolaryngology · 100 Ridgeway Place, Suite Two, Hot Springs, AR 71901 · 501-624-5422

Little Rock

Jeff Barber · General Otolaryngology · Arkansas Otolaryngology Center, Medical Towers Building, Suite 1200, 9601 Lile Drive, Little Rock, AR 72205-6358 · 501-227-5050

Charles Michael Bower · Pediatric Otolaryngology · Arkansas Children's Hospital Arkansas Children's Hospital, Department of Pediatric Otolaryngology, 800 Marshall Street, Little Rock, AR 72202-3591 · 501-320-1047

Joe Colclasure · General Otolaryngology · Arkansas Otolaryngology Center, Medical Towers Building, Suite 1200, 9601 Lile Drive, Little Rock, AR 72205-6358 · 501-227-5050

John Roddey Edwards Dickins · Otology/ Neurotology · St. Vincent Infirmary Medical Center, Baptist Medical Center, Arkansas Children's Hospital · Arkansas Otolaryngology Center, Medical Towers Building, Suite 1200, 9601 Lile Drive, Little Rock, AR 72205-6358 · 501-227-5050

Guy S. Gardner · General Otolaryngology · 9600 Lile Drive, Suite 220, Little Rock, AR 72205 · 501-221-0086

J. Michael Key · Facial Plastic Surgery (Facial Trauma, Plastic Surgery, Reconstructive Facial Surgery, Laser Surgery & Birthmarks, General Otolaryngology) · University of Arkansas for Medical Sciences, Arkansas Children's Hospital, John L. McClellan Memorial Veterans Hospital · University of Arkansas for Medical Sciences, Department of Otolaryngology, 4301 West Markham Street, Mail Slot 543, Little Rock, AR 72205-7199 · 501-686-5011

Barbara Morris · General Otolaryngology · Arkansas Children's Hospital, Baptist Medical Center, St. Vincent Infirmary Medical Center · Arkansas Otolaryngology Center, Medical Towers Building, Suite 1200, 9601 Lile Drive, Little Rock, AR 72205-6358 · 501-227-5050

James J. Pappas · Otology · Baptist Medical Center · Arkansas Otolaryngology Center, Medical Towers Building, Suite 1200, 9601 Lile Drive, Little Rock, AR 72205-6358 · 501-227-5050

Robert W. Seibert · Pediatric Otolaryngology (Cleft Surgery) · Arkansas Children's Hospital · Arkansas Children's Hospital, Department of Pediatric Otolaryngology, 800 Marshall Street, Little Rock, AR 72202-3591 · 501-320-1047

Scott J. Stern · Head & Neck Surgery (Oncology) · University Hospital of Arkansas, Arkansas Children's Hospital, John L. McClellan Memorial Veterans Hospital · University of Arkansas for Medical Sciences, Department of Otolaryngology, 4301 West Markham Street, Mail Slot 543, Little Rock, AR 72205-7199 · 501-686-5141

James Y. Suen · Head & Neck Surgery (Head & Neck Oncology, Vascular Tumors of the Head & Neck, Voice Disorders, Laryngology, Skull-Base Surgery) · Arkansas Cancer Research Center, University Hospital of Arkansas, Arkansas Children's Hospital · University of Arkansas for Medical Sciences, Department of Otolaryngology, 4301 West Markham Street, Mail Slot 543, Little Rock, AR 72205-7199 · 501-686-5140

Milton Waner · Head & Neck Surgery (Vascular Lesions in Children, Laser Surgery & Birthmarks) · University Hospital of Arkansas, Arkansas Children's Hospital, John L. McClellan Memorial Veterans Hospital · University of Arkansas for Medical Sciences, Department of Otolaryngology, 4301 West Markham Street, Mail Slot 543, Little Rock, AR 72205 · 501-686-5140

Rogers

Michael Reese · General Otolaryngology (Thyroid, Sinus & Nasal Surgery) · Northwest Arkansas Ear, Nose & Throat Clinic, 1110 West Elm Street, Rogers, AR 72756 · 501-636-0110

PEDIATRICS

Fort Smith

Louay K. Nassri · Pediatric Pulmonology · Holt Krock Clinic, 2901 South 74th Street, Fort Smith, AR 72903 · 501-452-7500

Little Rock

Phillip Lee Berry · Pediatric Nephrology (General Pediatrics) · Arkansas Children's Hospital · Arkansas Children's Hospital, 800 Marshall Street, Little Rock, AR 72202-3591 · 501-320-1847

Debra H. Fiser · Pediatric Critical Care (Outcomes Research) · Arkansas Children's Hospital · Arkansas Children's Hospital, Department of Critical Care Medicine, 800 Marshall Street, Little Rock, AR 72202-3591 · 501-320-1442

Elizabeth Frazier · Pediatric Cardiology · Arkansas Children's Hospital, Department of Pediatric Cardiology, 800 Marshall Street, Mail Slot 512, Little Rock, AR 72202-3591 · 501-320-1479

Richard F. Jacobs · Pediatric Infectious Disease (Tuberculosis, Antibiotics, Tick-Borne Infections, Bone Infections, Fungal Infections, Herpes Virus Infections, Respiratory Infections) · Arkansas Children's Hospital, University of Arkansas for Medical Sciences · Arkansas Children's Hospital, Department of Infectious Disease, 800 Marshall Street, Mail Slot 512, Little Rock, AR 72202-3591 · 501-320-1416

Stephen F. Kemp · Pediatric Endocrinology (Growth Disorders) · Arkansas Children's Hospital · Arkansas Children's Hospital, Department of Endocrinology, 800 Marshall Street, Mail Slot 512, Little Rock, AR 72202-3591 · 501-320-1430

Betty Ann Lowe · Pediatric Rheumatology · Arkansas Children's Hospital, 800 Marshall Street, Little Rock, AR 72202 · 501-320-1401

M. Michele Moss · Pediatric Critical Care (Pediatric Cardiology, Pediatric Critical Care Transport) · Arkansas Children's Hospital · Arkansas Children's Hospital, Department of Pediatric Cardiology, 800 Marshall Street, Mail Slot 512, Little Rock, AR 72202-3591 · 501-320-1479

J. B. Norton, Jr. · Pediatric Cardiology (General Pediatrics) · Arkansas Children's Hospital · Arkansas Children's Hospital, Department of Pediatric Cardiology, 800 Marshall Street, Mail Slot 512, Little Rock, AR 72202-3591 · 501-320-1479

Gordon E. Schutze · Pediatric Infectious Disease (Food-Borne Illnesses, Clinical Microbiology, Travel Medicine) · Arkansas Children's Hospital, Department of Infectious Disease, 800 Marshall Street, Mail Slot 512, Little Rock, AR 72202-3591 · 501-320-1416

Terry Yamauchi · Pediatric Infectious Disease · Arkansas Children's Hospital · Arkansas Children's Hospital, Department of Infectious Disease, 800 Marshall Street, Mail Slot 512, Little Rock, AR 72202 · 501-320-1417

PEDIATRICS (GENERAL)

Arkadelphia

Carl Wesley Kluck, Jr. · Arkadelphia Clinic for Children and Young Adults, 2850 Twin Rivers Drive, Arkadelphia, AR 71923 · 501-246-8036

Fayetteville

Charles S. Ball · Washington Regional Medical Center, Northwest Medical Center (Springdale) · Northwest Arkansas Pediatric Clinic, 1792 Joyce Street, Fayetteville, AR 72703 · 501-442-7322

Charles David Jackson · Northwest Arkansas Pediatric Clinic, 1792 Joyce Street, Fayetteville, AR 72703 · 501-442-7322

Terry S. Payton · Northwest Arkansas Pediatric Clinic, 1792 Joyce Street, Fayetteville, AR 72703 · 501-442-7322

Joe T. Robinson · Northwest Arkansas Pediatric Clinic, 1792 Joyce Street, Fayetteville, AR 72703 · 501-442-7322

Forrest City

William C. Patton · (Pediatric Otology, Developmental Pediatrics, Attention Deficit Hyperactive Disorder) · Baptist Memorial Hospital-Forrest City · East Arkansas Children's Clinic, 901 Holiday Drive, Forrest City, AR 72335 · 501-633-0880

Fort Smith

Richard R. Aclin · (Neonatology, Pediatric Hematology) · Sparks Regional Medical Center, St. Edward Mercy Medical Center · Holt Krock Clinic, 2901 South 74th Street, Fort Smith, AR 72903 · 501-452-7500

Hannah Beene · Cooper Clinic Pediatrics, 6801 Rogers Avenue, Fort Smith, AR 72903 · 501-783-3165

Federico C. DeMiranda · Waldron Place Pediatrics, 1501 South Waldron Road, Suite 202, Fort Smith, AR 72903 · 501-452-8311

Jon R. Hendrickson · Holt Krock Clinic, 2901 South 74th Street, Fort Smith, AR 72903 · 501-452-7500

Thomas C. Jefferson · AHEC Family Medical Center, 612 South 12th Street, Fort Smith, AR 72901 · 501-785-2431

Hope

R. Craig Davis · (General Pediatrics, Pediatric Infectious Disease) · Medical Park Hospital · The Clinic for Children, Youth and Young Adults, 114 Medical Park Drive, Hope, AR 71801 · 501-777-7581

Jonesboro

Warren A. Skaug · (Developmental Disabilities) · St. Bernard's Regional Medical Center · The Children's Clinic, 800 South Church Street, Suite 202, Jonesboro, AR 72401 · 501-935-6012

Little Rock

Dale W. Dildy, Jr. · (Attention Deficit Disorder, Medical Management) · Arkansas Children's Hospital · Arkansas Children's Hospital, Department of Pediatrics, 800 Marshall Street, Mail Slot 700, Little Rock, AR 72202 · 501-320-4362

Joseph Elser · Arkansas Children's Hospital, 800 Marshall Street, Little Rock, AR 72202 · 501-320-4361

R. Wayne Herbert · Little Rock Children's Clinic, 11215 Hermitage Road, Little Rock, AR 72215 · 501-227-6727

Susan A. Keathley · Little Rock Children's Clinic, 11215 Hermitage Road, Little Rock, AR 72215 · 501-227-6727

Alan Lucas · Arkansas Children's Hospital, Department of Pediatrics, 800 Marshall Street, Mail Slot 700, Little Rock, AR 72202 · 501-320-4362

Virginia Melhorn · Arkansas Children's Hospital · Arkansas Children's Hospital, Department of Pediatrics, 800 Marshall Street, Mail Slot 700, Little Rock, AR 72202-3591 · 501-320-4362

A. Larry Simmons · (Pediatric Asthma, Attention Deficit Hyperactive Disorder & Related School Problems, Pediatric Primary Care Education) · Arkansas Children's Hospital · Arkansas Children's Hospital, Department of Pediatrics, 800 Marshall Street, Mail Slot 700, Little Rock, AR 72202 · 501-320-4362

Christopher E. Smith · (School Health, Pediatric Education, Child Advocacy) · Arkansas Children's Hospital · Arkansas Children's Hospital, House Staff Office, 800 Marshall Street, Mail Slot 512, Little Rock, AR 72202-3591 · 501-320-1874

Pine Bluff

Thomas Edward Townsend · (Developmental Pediatrics, Adolescent Medicine) Jefferson Regional Medical Center · The Children's Clinic, 1420 West 43rd Street, Pine Bluff, AR 71603-7095 · 501-534-6210

West Memphis

David H. James, Jr. · 228 West Tyler Street, Suite 105, West Memphis, AR 72301 501-732-1191

PHYSICAL MEDICINE & REHABILITATION

Little Rock

F. Patrick Maloney · General Physical Medicine & Rehabilitation (Medical Management) · University of Arkansas for Medical Sciences, Department of Physical Medicine & Rehabilitation, Medical Towers II, Suite 195, 9501 Lile Drive, Little Rock, AR 72205 · 501-221-1311

North Little Rock

Kevin M. Means · General Physical Medicine & Rehabilitation (Geriatric Rehabilitation, Rehabilitation of Balance Disorders & Falls) · VA Medical Center-North Little Rock Division · VA Medical Center, 2200 Fort Roots Drive, North Little Rock, AR 72114 · 501-688-1619

PLASTIC SURGERY

Fort Smith

R. Cole Goodman, Jr. · General Plastic Surgery · Plastic Surgery Specialists, 2717 South 74th Street, Fort Smith, AR 72903 · 501-452-9080

Little Rock

Thomas R. Moffett · General Plastic Surgery · 600 South McKinley, 310 Doctors Plaza, Little Rock, AR 72205 · 501-663-4100

Kris B. Shewmake · General Plastic Surgery (Facial Aesthetic Surgery, Craniomaxillofacial Surgery) · University Hospital of Arkansas, Arkansas Children's Hospital, Columbia Doctor's Hospital, Baptist Medical Center · University of Arkansas for Medical Sciences, Department of Surgery, Division of Plastic Surgery, 4301 West Markham Street, Mail Slot 720, Little Rock, AR 72205-7199 · 501-686-5737; 501-666-7600

James C. Yuen · General Plastic Surgery (Microsurgery, Hand Surgery) · University of Arkansas for Medical Sciences, Arkansas Children's Hospital, Columbia Doctor's Hospital, John L. McClellan Memorial Veterans Hospital · University of Arkansas for Medical Sciences, Division of Plastic and Reconstructive Surgery, 4301 West Markham Street, Mail Slot 720, Little Rock, AR 72205-7199 · 501-686-8711

PSYCHIATRY

Little Rock

James Clardy · General Psychiatry (Psychopharmacology, Outcomes Research) · University of Arkansas for Medical Sciences, Department of Psychiatry, 4301 West Markham Street, Mail Slot 589, Little Rock, AR 72205 · 501-686-6196

Frederick G. Guggenheim · Addiction Psychiatry (General Psychiatry, Mood & Anxiety Disorders) · University Hospital of Arkansas · University of Arkansas for Medical Sciences, Department of Psychiatry, 4301 West Markham Street, Mail Slot 554, Little Rock, AR 72205 · 501-686-5480

Gregory S. Krulin · General Psychiatry (Mood & Anxiety Disorders, Sleep Medicine) · One St. Vincent Circle, Suite 340, Little Rock, AR 72205 · 501-664-1400

Robin L. Ross · General Psychiatry (Mood & Anxiety Disorders) · University Hospital of Arkansas · University of Arkansas for Medical Sciences, Department of Psychiatry, 4301 West Markham Street, Mail Slot 554, Little Rock, AR 72205 · 501-686-5900

G. Richard Smith · General Psychiatry (Consultation/Liaison Psychiatry) · University of Arkansas for Medical Sciences, Department of Psychiatry, 4301 West Markham Street, Mail Slot 554, Little Rock, AR 72205 · 501-686-5600

North Little Rock

Jeffrey L. Clothier · Neuropsychiatry (Mood & Anxiety Disorders, Psychopharmacology) · John L. McClellan Memorial Veterans Hospital (Little Rock) · VA Medical Center, Neuropsychiatry Research Lab (116A1/NLR), Building 58, 2200 Fort Roots Drive, North Little Rock, AR 72114 · 501-370-6629; 501-686-6195

T. Stuart Harris · General Psychiatry (Psychotherapy of Personality Disorders, Psychopharmacology) · Bridgeway Hospital · Arkansas Psychiatric Clinic, 21 Bridgeway Road, North Little Rock, AR 72113 · 501-771-4570

Craig N. Karson · Schizophrenia (Neuropsychiatry, Molecular Psychiatry) · John L. McClellan Memorial Veterans Hospital (Little Rock) · VA Medical Center, Psychiatry Service (116A/NLR), Building 170, 2200 Fort Roots Drive, North Little Rock, AR 72114-1706 · 501-370-6629

Richard R. Owen · Schizophrenia (Psychopharmacology) · Veterans Affairs Medical Center, Neuropsychiatry Research Lab (116A1/NLR), Building 58, 2200 Fort Roots Drive, North Little Rock, AR 72114 · 501-661-1417

PULMONARY & CRITICAL CARE MEDICINE

Fort Smith

David R. Nichols · General Pulmonary & Critical Care Medicine · Holt Krock Clinic, 1500 Dodson Avenue, Fort Smith, AR 72901 · 501-782-2071

Little Rock

Joseph H. Bates · General Pulmonary & Critical Care Medicine (Tuberculosis, Fungal Infections, General Infectious Disease, Hospital-Acquired Infections, Respiratory Infections, General Internal Medicine) · John L. McClellan Memorial Veterans Hospital, University Hospital of Arkansas · John L. McClellan Memorial Veterans Hospital, 4300 West Seventh Street, Mail Slot 111J/LR, Little Rock, AR 72205 · 501-660-2029

RADIATION ONCOLOGY

Little Rock

W. Ducote Haynes · General Radiation Oncology · Central Arkansas Radiation Therapy Institute, Markham Street at University Avenue, P. O. Box 5210, Little Rock, AR 72215 · 501-664-8573

Robert Landgren · General Radiation Oncology (Brachytherapy, Genito-Urinary Cancer) · St. Vincent Infirmary Medical Center · Central Arkansas Radiation Therapy Institute, Markham Street at University Avenue, P. O. Box 5210, Little Rock, AR 72215 · 501-664-8573

Alvah J. Nelson III · General Radiation Oncology · St. Vincent Infirmary Medical Center · Central Arkansas Radiation Therapy Institute, Markham Street at University Avenue, P. O. Box 5210, Little Rock, AR 72215 · 501-664-8573

Cynthia S. Ross · General Radiation Oncology · Central Arkansas Radiation Therapy Institute, Markham Street at University Avenue, P. O. Box 5210, Little Rock, AR 72215 · 501-664-8573

Michael Talbert · General Radiation Oncology (Head & Neck Cancer, Breast Cancer) · Central Arkansas Radiation Therapy Institute, Markham Street at University Avenue, P. O. Box 5210, Little Rock, AR 72215 · 501-664-8573

RADIOLOGY

Fort Smith

Neil E. Crow, Jr. · General Radiology · Holt Krock Clinic, 1500 Dodson Avenue, Fort Smith, AR 72901-5193 · 501-782-2071

Little Rock

Harry Howard Cockrell, Jr. · General Radiology · Radiology Associates, 5800 West 10th Street, Little Rock, AR 72204-1793 · 501-661-1210

Ernest J. Ferris · General Radiology (Vascular & Interventional Radiology, Cardiovascular Radiology, Chest) · University Hospital of Arkansas, John L. McClellan Memorial Veterans Hospital, Arkansas Children's Hospital · University of Arkansas for Medical Sciences, Department of Radiology, 4301 West Markham Street, Mail Slot 556, Little Rock, AR 72205 · 501-686-5747

Jerry C. Holton · General Radiology · Radiology Associates, 500 South University Avenue, Suite 101, Little Rock, AR 72205-5303 · 501-664-3914

Terrence A. Oddson · General Radiology · Radiology Associates, 500 South University Avenue, Suite 101, Little Rock, AR 72205-5303 · 501-664-3914

Joanna J. Seibert · Pediatric Radiology · Arkansas Children's Hospital, Department of Radiology, 800 Marshall Street, Little Rock, AR 72202 · 501-320-1175

RHEUMATOLOGY

Fayetteville

Thomas R. Dykman · General Rheumatology · Fayetteville Diagnostic Clinic, 3344 North Futrall Drive, Fayetteville, AR 72703 · 501-521-8200

Fort Smith

James Deneke · General Rheumatology · St. Edward Mercy Medical Center · Cooper Clinic, 6801 Rogers Avenue, P.O. Box 3528, Fort Smith, AR 72903 · 501-452-2077

Hot Springs

P. Ross Bandy · General Rheumatology (Lupus, Rheumatoid Arthritis, Osteoporosis, Vasculitis) · St. Joseph's Regional Health Center, National Park Medical Center, Levi Hospital · Levi Hospital, 300 Prospect Avenue, P.O. Box 850, Hot Springs, AR 71901 · 501-624-1281 x574

Little Rock

Steven Dacosta Holt · General Rheumatology · Little Rock Diagnostic Clinic, 10001 Lile Drive, Little Rock, AR 72205-6299 · 501-227-8000

Richard W. Houk · General Rheumatology · Little Rock Diagnostic Clinic, 10001 Lile Drive, Little Rock, AR 72205-6299 · 501-227-8000

Hugo E. Jasin · General Rheumatology · University of Arkansas for Medical Sciences · University of Arkansas for Medical Sciences, 4301 West Markham Street, Mail Slot 509, Little Rock, AR 72205-7199 · 501-686-6770

S. Michael Jones · General Rheumatology · Little Rock Diagnostic Clinic, 10001 Lile Drive, Little Rock, AR 72205-6299 · 501-227-8000

Thomas M. Kovaleski · General Rheumatology · Five St. Vincent Circle, Suite 410, Little Rock, AR 72205 · 501-663-6766

Robert L. Lewis · General Rheumatology · John L. McClellan Memorial Veterans Hospital, 4300 West Seventh Street, Mail Slot 111J/LR, Little Rock, AR 72205 · 501-661-1202 x2792

Eleanor Lipsmeyer · General Rheumatology · University of Arkansas for Medical Sciences, Department of Rheumatology, 4301 West Markham Street, Mail Slot 509, Little Rock, AR 72205 · 501-686-5586

James W. Logan · General Rheumatology (Rheumatoid Arthritis, Lupus, Vasculitis) · University of Arkansas for Medical Sciences, John L. McClellan Memorial

Veterans Hospital · University of Arkansas for Medical Sciences, 4301 West Markham Street, Mail Slot 509, Little Rock, AR 72205-7199 · 501-686-5586

Rogers

Ann Miller · General Rheumatology · Rogers Diagnostic Clinic, 1019 West Cypress Street, Rogers, AR 72756 · 501-636-6551

SURGERY

Fort Smith

Robert H. Janes, Jr. · General Surgery · Holt Krock Clinic, 1500 Dodson Avenue, Fort Smith, AR 72901 · 501-782-2071

Samuel E. Landrum · General Surgery · Holt Krock Clinic, 1500 Dodson Avenue, Fort Smith, AR 72901 · 501-782-2071

Little Rock

Robert W. Barnes · General Vascular Surgery (Non-Invasive Testing) · University Hospital of Arkansas, VA Medical Center-Little Rock Division · University of Arkansas for Medical Sciences, Department of Surgery, 4301 West Markham Street, Mail Slot 520, Little Rock, AR 72205 · 501-686-5610

Gary W. Barone · General Vascular Surgery (General Surgery, Surgical Critical Care, Transplantation) · University Hospital of Arkansas, John L. McClellan Memorial Veterans Hospital · University of Arkansas for Medical Sciences, Department of Surgery, 4301 West Markham Street, Mail Slot 520, Little Rock, AR 72205-7199 · 501-686-6644

Lon G. Bitzer · Trauma · University of Arkansas for Medical Sciences, Department of Surgery, 4301 West Markham Street, Mail Slot 520, Little Rock, AR 72205-7199 · 501-686-8753

Hugh F. Burnett · General Surgery · The Surgical Clinic, 9501 Lile Drive, Suite 900, Little Rock, AR 72205 · 501-227-9080

John B. Cone · General Surgery (Trauma, Surgical Critical Care) · University Hospital of Arkansas · University of Arkansas for Medical Sciences, Department of Surgery, 4301 West Markham Street, Mail Slot 520, Little Rock, AR 72205-7199 501-686-6648

John F. Eidt · General Vascular Surgery (Surgical Critical Care, General Surgery) University of Arkansas for Medical Sciences, Department of Surgery, 4301 West Markham Street, Mail Slot 520, Little Rock, AR 72205 · 501-686-6176

Richard J. Jackson · Pediatric Surgery (Surgical Critical Care) · Arkansas Children's Hospital · University of Arkansas for Medical Sciences, Department of Surgery, 4301 West Markham Street, Mail Slot 520, Little Rock, AR 72205-7199 501-320-1446

Beverly L. Ketel · Transplantation · University of Arkansas for Medical Sciences, Department of Surgery, 4301 West Markham Street, Mail Slot 520, Little Rock, AR 72205-7199 · 501-686-6644

Nicholas P. Lang · General Surgery · University of Arkansas for Medical Sciences, Department of Surgery, 4301 West Markham Street, Mail Slot 725, Little Rock, AR 72205 · 501-686-6186

Samuel D. Smith · Pediatric Surgery (Surgical Critical Care) · Arkansas Children's Hospital · Arkansas Children's Hospital, Department of Pediatric Surgery, 800 Marshall Street, Little Rock, AR 72202-3591 · 501-320-1446

Charles W. Wagner · Pediatric Surgery (Pediatric Transplantation Surgery) · Arkansas Children's Hospital · University of Arkansas for Medical Sciences, Department of Surgery, 4301 West Markham Street, Mail Slot 520, Little Rock, AR 72205-7199 · 501-320-1446

West Memphis

Glenn P. Schoettle · General Surgery · 308 South Rhodes, West Memphis, AR 72301 · 501-735-3664

SURGICAL ONCOLOGY

Little Rock

J. Ralph Broadwater · General Surgical Oncology (Breast Surgery, Melanoma) · University of Arkansas for Medical Sciences, Department of Surgery, 4301 West Markham Street, Mail Slot 725, Little Rock, AR 72205-7199 · 501-686-5547

Martin Hauer-Jensen · General Surgical Oncology · University of Arkansas for Medical Sciences, Department of Surgery, 4301 West Markham Street, Mail Slot 520, Little Rock, AR 72205-7199 · 501-686-6505

V. Suzanne Klimberg · Breast Cancer · University of Arkansas for Medical Sciences · University of Arkansas for Medical Sciences, Department of Surgery, 4301 West Markham Street, Mail Slot 725, Little Rock, AR 72205-7199 · 501-686-6503

Nicholas P. Lang · General Surgical Oncology (Endoscopy, Gastrointestinal Cancer) · University Hospital of Arkansas, John L. McClellan Memorial Veterans Hospital · University of Arkansas for Medical Sciences, Department of Surgery, 4301 West Markham Street, Mail Slot 725, Little Rock, AR 72205-7199 · 501-686-6505; 501-660-2038

Richard W. Nicholas · General Surgical Oncology (Orthopaedic Oncology) · University of Arkansas for Medical Sciences, Department of Orthopaedic Surgery, 4301 West Markham Street, Mail Slot 531, Little Rock, AR 72205 · 501-686-7816

Kent C. Westbrook · General Surgical Oncology (Melanoma, Breast Disease, Breast Surgery, Endocrine Surgery, General Surgery) · University Hospital of Arkansas · University of Arkansas for Medical Sciences, Department of Surgery, 4301 West Markham Street, Mail Slot 623, Little Rock, AR 72205-7199 · 501-686-5987

THORACIC SURGERY

Little Rock

Stephen H. Van Devanter · Adult Cardiothoracic Surgery (Pediatric Cardiac Surgery) · University of Arkansas for Medical Sciences, Department of Surgery, 4301 West Markham Street, Mail Slot 520, Little Rock, AR 72205-7199 · 501-320-1809

UROLOGY

Little Rock

Scott Mac Diarmid · General Urology (Neuro-Urology & Voiding Dysfunction, Reconstructive Urology) · University of Arkansas for Medical Sciences · University of Arkansas for Medical Sciences, Department of Urology, 4301 West Markham Street, Mail Slot 540, Little Rock, AR 72205 · 501-686-5242

John F. Redman · (Pediatric Urology) · Arkansas Children's Hospital · Arkansas Children's Hospital, 800 Marshall Street, Little Rock, AR 72202 · 501-320-2632

Michael J. Schutz · General Urology · University of Arkansas for Medical Sciences, Department of Urology, 4301 West Markham Street, Mail Slot 540, Little Rock, AR 72205 · 501-686-6386

COLORADO

ALLERGY & IMMUNOLOGY

Aurora

Sanford E. Avner · General Allergy & Immunology (Allergy) · Colorado Allergy & Asthma Clinic · Colorado Allergy & Asthma Clinic, 1450 South Havana Street, Suite 500, Aurora, CO 80012 · 303-755-5070

David S. Pearlman · General Allergy & Immunology (Allergy, Asthma) · Colorado Allergy & Asthma Clinic · Colorado Allergy & Asthma Clinic, 1450 South Havana Street, Suite 500, Aurora, CO 80012 · 303-755-5070

Boulder

S. Allan Bock · General Allergy & Immunology (Food Allergy, Asthma [especially Pediatric]) · National Jewish Center for Immunology & Respiratory Medicine (Denver), Boulder Community Hospital, Avista Hospital (Louisville) · Boulder Valley Asthma & Allergy Clinics, 3950 Broadway, Boulder, CO 80304-1199 · 303-444-5991

Colorado Springs

William W. Storms · General Allergy & Immunology (Asthma, Nasal Allergies, Exercise Asthma) · Penrose-St. Francis Healthcare System, Memorial Hospital · 2709 North Tejon Street, Colorado Springs, CO 80907 · 719-473-0872

Denver

Erwin W. Gelfand · Immunodeficiency (General Allergy & Immunology) · National Jewish Center for Immunology & Respiratory Medicine · National Jewish Center for Immunology & Respiratory Medicine, 1400 Jackson Street, Room K-801, Denver, CO 80206 · 303-398-1196

James Fly Jones · General Allergy & Immunology (Epstein-Barr Virus) · National Jewish Center for Immunology & Respiratory Medicine, 1400 Jackson Street, Room K-926, Denver, CO 80206-1911 · 303-398-1195

Donald Y. M. Leung · General Allergy & Immunology (Allergy, Kawasaki Disease, Atopic Dermatitis) · National Jewish Center for Immunology & Respiratory Medicine · National Jewish Center for Immunology & Respiratory Medicine, 1400 Jackson Street, Room K-926, Denver, CO 80206-1997 · 303-398-1379

Harold S. Nelson · General Allergy & Immunology (Asthma) · National Jewish Center for Immunology & Respiratory Medicine · National Jewish Center for Immunology & Respiratory Medicine, 1400 Jackson Street, Denver, CO 80206 · 303-398-1562

Lanny J. Rosenwasser · General Allergy & Immunology (Asthma, Vasculitis) · National Jewish Center for Immunology & Respiratory Medicine · National Jewish Center for Immunology & Respiratory Medicine, 1400 Jackson Street, Suite 621, Denver, CO 80206 · 303-398-1656

John C. Selner · General Allergy & Immunology · Allergy Respiratory Institute of Colorado · Allergy Respiratory Institute of Colorado, 5800 East Evans Avenue, Garden Level, Denver, CO 80222 · 303-756-3614

Stanley J. Szefler · General Allergy & Immunology (General Clinical Pharmacology, General Pediatrics, Pediatric Asthma) · National Jewish Center for Immunology & Respiratory Medicine · National Jewish Center for Immunology & Respiratory Medicine, 1400 Jackson Street, Room K-926, Denver, CO 80206 · 303-398-1379

Richard W. Weber · General Allergy & Immunology · National Jewish Center for Immunology & Respiratory Medicine, University Hospital · National Jewish Center for Immunology & Respiratory Medicine, Department of Medicine, 1400 Jackson Street, Room 103A, Denver, CO 80206 · 303-388-4461

Grand Junction

William A. Scott · General Allergy & Immunology · 1120 Wellington Avenue, Grand Junction, CO 81501 · 970-241-0170

Littleton

Allen D. Adinoff · General Allergy & Immunology · 7720 South Broadway, Suite 110, Littleton, CO 80122 · 303-795-8177

Loveland

William G. Culver · General Allergy & Immunology (Asthma, Sinusitis) · McKee Medical Center, Poudre Valley Hospital (Fort Collins) · Aspen Medical Center, 1808 Boise Avenue, Loveland, CO 80538 · 970-669-6660; 970-498-9226

ANESTHESIOLOGY

Colorado Springs

John A. Marta · General Anesthesiology · 308 West Fillmore Avenue, Suite 101, Colorado Springs, CO 80907 · 719-635-0526

Denver

Charles P. Gibbs · Obstetric Anesthesia (Aspiration, Maternal Mortality) · University Hospital · University of Colorado Health Sciences Center, Department of Anesthesiology, 4200 East Ninth Avenue, Campus Box B113, Denver, CO 80262 303-270-4093

Wayne P. Halfer · General Anesthesiology · 44 Cook Street, Suite 203, Denver, CO 80206 · 303-377-6825

Charles H. Lockhart · Pediatric Anesthesiology · Children's Hospital · The Children's Hospital, Department of Anesthesia, 1056 East 19th Avenue, Denver, CO 80218 · 303-861-6226

James Sederberg · General Anesthesiology · 44 Cook Street, Suite 203, Denver, CO 80206 · 303-377-6825

Englewood

Bruce R. Brookens · General Anesthesiology · PorterCare Hospital, PorterCare Hospital-Littleton (Littleton), Swedish Medical Center · 333 West Hampden Avenue, Suite 600, Englewood, CO 80110 · 303-761-5646

Fort Collins

Thomas Boylan · General Anesthesiology · Poudre Valley Hospital, 1024 South Lane, Fort Collins, CO 80524 · 970-224-1677

Grand Junction

Ives P. Murray · General Anesthesiology (Cardiovascular Anesthesiology, Intensive Care Medicine) · 1120 Wellington Avenue, Suite 206, Grand Junction, CO 81501-8157 · 970-243-7245

CARDIOVASCULAR DISEASE

Colorado Springs

John P. Kleiner · General Cardiovascular Disease · Colorado Springs Cardiologists, 25 East Jackson Street, Suite 301, Colorado Springs, CO 80907 · 719-634-6671

Bert Y. Wong · General Cardiovascular Disease (Interventional Cardiology) · Memorial Hospital, Penrose-St. Francis Healthcare System · 455 East Pike's Peak Avenue, Suite 102, Colorado Springs, CO 80903 · 719-471-1775

Denver

Michael R. Bristow · Heart Failure (Cardiac Transplantation) · University Hospital · University of Colorado Health Sciences Center, Division of Cardiology, 4200 East Ninth Avenue, Campus Box B130, Denver, CO 80262 · 303-270-4398

Ira Dauber · General Cardiovascular Disease (Cardiac Catheterization, Heart Failure) · PorterCare Hospital, Swedish Medical Center (Englewood), PorterCare Hospital-Littleton (Littleton) · 950 East Harvard Avenue, Suite 100, Denver, CO 80210 · 303-744-1065

Karl E. Hammermeister · General Cardiovascular Disease · University of Colorado Health Sciences Center, 4200 East Ninth Avenue, Campus Box A009-111B, Denver, CO 80262 · 303-270-7761

William R. Hiatt · General Cardiovascular Disease (Vascular Medicine, Cardiac Rehabilitation, Clinical Exercise Testing, Vaso-Spastic Diseases) · University Hospital · University of Colorado Health Sciences Center, 4200 East Ninth Avenue, Campus Box B180, Denver, CO 80262 · 303-372-9085

Joanne Lindenfeld · General Cardiovascular Disease, Transplantation Medicine, Heart Failure · University Hospital · University of Colorado Health Sciences Center, 4200 East Ninth Avenue, Campus Box B130, Denver, CO 80209 · 303-270-4409

David E. Mann · General Cardiovascular Disease (Cardiac Electrophysiology) · University Hospital · University of Colorado Health Sciences Center, Department of Cardiology, 4200 East Ninth Avenue, Campus Box B130, Denver, CO 80262 · 303-270-5694

Eugene E. Wolfel · General Cardiovascular Disease (Heart Failure, Transplantation Medicine, High Altitude Physiology & Medicine, Cardiac Rehabilitation) · University Hospital · University of Colorado Health Sciences Center, 4200 East Ninth Avenue, Campus Box B130, Denver, CO 80262 · 303-270-8173

Fort Collins

Mark D. Guadagnoli · General Cardiovascular Disease · 1224 East Elizabeth Street, Fort Collins, CO 80524 · 970-224-4434

Grand Junction

Gary L. Snyder · General Cardiovascular Disease · Western Slope Cardiology, 425 Patterson Road, Suite 605, Grand Junction, CO 81506 · 970-245-6965

Greeley

Paul G. Hurst · General Cardiovascular Disease (Valvular Heart Disease) · North Colorado Medical Center · North Colorado Cardiology, 1800 Fifteenth Street, Suite 310, Greeley, CO 80631 · 970-356-8114

Randall C. Marsh · General Cardiovascular Disease · 2525 West 16th Avenue, Suite C, Greeley, CO 80631 · 970-352-8695

CLINICAL PHARMACOLOGY

Denver

Richard C. Dart · (Drug Overdose, Snake Bite, General Clinical Pharmacology) Denver General Hospital, University Hospital · Rocky Mountain Poison & Drug Center, 8802 East Ninth Avenue, Denver, CO 80220-6800 · 303-739-1100

Curt R. Freed · (Parkinson's Disease, Neuro-Transplantation, Neural Regulation of Blood Pressure, General Clinical Pharmacology) · University Hospital · University of Colorado Health Sciences Center, 4200 East Ninth Avenue, Campus Box C237, Denver, CO 80262 · 303-270-8455

John G. Gerber · (Antiviral Therapy) · University Hospital · University of Colorado Health Sciences Center, 4200 East Ninth Avenue, Campus Box C237, Denver, CO 80262 · 303-270-8455

Alan S. Hollister · (Autonomic Dysfunction, Hypertension, Clinical Research, Psychopharmacology, General Clinical Pharmacology, Degenerative Diseases, General Internal Medicine) · University Hospital · University of Colorado Health Sciences Center, Division of Clinical Pharmacology, 4200 East Ninth Avenue, Campus Box C237, Denver, CO 80262 · 303-270-8455

COLON & RECTAL SURGERY

Denver

Robert Khoo · General Colon & Rectal Surgery (Colon & Rectal Cancer, Gastrointestinal Cancer) · Rose Medical Center, Swedish Medical Center (Englewood), St. Joseph Hospital, Provenant St. Anthony Hospital Central, Aurora Regional Medical Center (Aurora), Presbyterian/St. Luke's Medical Center, PorterCare Hospital-Littleton (Littleton) · 4600 Hale Parkway, Denver, CO 80220 303-355-2900

Wheat Ridge

Nelson I. Mozia · General Colon & Rectal Surgery, Colon & Rectal Cancer · 8550 West 38th Avenue, Suite 205, Wheat Ridge, CO 80033-4342 · 303-467-8987

DERMATOLOGY

Colorado Springs

Gerard G. Koehn · Clinical Dermatology · 3208 North Academy Boulevard, Colorado Springs, CO 80917 · 719-574-0310

Barton L. Lewis · Clinical Dermatology (Aging Skin, Dermatopathology) · 26 East Monument Drive, Colorado Springs, CO 80903 · 719-634-5597

Charles W. Ruggles · Clinical Dermatology · 801 North Cascade Avenue, Suite 12, Colorado Springs, CO 80903 · 719-633-1725

Denver

John L. Aeling · Genital Dermatological Disease · University of Colorado Health Sciences Center, 4200 East Ninth Avenue, Campus Box E153, Denver, CO 80262 303-372-1111

Sylvia Brice · Cutaneous Immunology (Mucous Membrane Diseases) · University Hospital · University of Colorado Health Sciences Center, 4200 East Ninth Avenue, Campus Box E153, Denver, CO 80262 · 303-372-1111

J. Clark Huff · Cutaneous Immunology, Herpes Virus Infections (Blistering Disorders) · University Hospital · University of Colorado Health Sciences Center, 4200 East Ninth Avenue, Campus Box E153, Denver, CO 80262 · 303-372-1140

Richard Imber · Clinical Dermatology (Skin Cancer Surgery & Reconstruction, Aging Skin) · Presbyterian/St. Luke's Medical Center, Rose Medical Center, St. Joseph Hospital · Denver Skin Clinic, 2200 East 18th Avenue, Denver, CO 80206 303-322-7789

J. Ramsey Mellette, Jr. · Skin Cancer Surgery & Reconstruction (Aesthetic Surgery, Aging Skin) · University Hospital · University of Colorado Health Sciences Center, 4200 East Ninth Avenue, Campus Box E153, Denver, CO 80262 · 303-372-1111

Joseph G. Morelli · Pediatric Dermatology (Birthmarks, Laser Surgery) · University Hospital · University of Colorado Health Sciences Center, Department of Dermatology, 4200 East Ninth Avenue, Campus Box B153, Denver, CO 80262 · 303-372-1111

David A. Norris · Cutaneous Immunology, Depigmenting Diseases (Collagen Vascular Disease, Vitiligo, Autoimmune Depigmenting Diseases, Psoriasis) · University Hospital · University of Colorado Health Sciences Center, 4200 East Ninth Avenue, Campus Box E153, Denver, CO 80262 · 303-372-1111

Barbara R. Reed · Clinical Dermatology (Genital Dermatological Disease, Dermatological Drugs in Pregnancy & Lactation) · Denver Skin Clinic, 2200 East 18th Avenue, Denver, CO 80206 · 303-322-7789

William L. Weston · Pediatric Dermatology, Cutaneous Immunology · University Hospital · University of Colorado Health Sciences Center, Department of Dermatology, 4200 East Ninth Avenue, Campus Box B153, Denver, CO 80262 · 303-372-1111

Fort Collins

Paul C. Sayers · Clinical Dermatology · Building G, Suite Two, 1120 East Elizabeth Street, Fort Collins, CO 80524-4023 · 970-484-6303

B. Lynn West · Clinical Dermatology (Skin Cancer Surgery & Reconstruction, Aging Skin, Pediatric Dermatology) · Poudre Valley Hospital · Building Three, Suite 3240, 1136 East Stuart Street, Fort Collins, CO 80525-1197 · 970-221-5795

Grand Junction

Maida L. Burrow · Clinical Dermatology · 790 Wellington Avenue, Suite 103, Grand Junction, CO 81501 · 970-242-0060

Perry Rashleigh · Clinical Dermatology (Dermatopathology) · St. Mary's Hospital & Medical Center, Community Hospital · 790 Wellington Avenue, Grand Junction, CO 81501 · 970-242-7273

Pueblo

Kim Dernovsek · Clinical Dermatology · 1925 East Orman Avenue, Suite A335, Pueblo, CO 81004-3556 · 719-564-4500

EATING DISORDERS

Denver

Robert H. Eckel · Obesity (Lipid Disorders) · University Hospital, Rose Medical Center · University of Colorado Health Sciences Center, 4200 East Ninth Avenue, Campus Box E151, Denver, CO 80262 · 303-372-1435

Loveland

Phil L. Hooper · General Eating Disorders · Aspen Medical Center, 1808 Boise Avenue, Loveland, CO 80538-4220 · 970-669-6660

ENDOCRINOLOGY & METABOLISM

Aurora

Michael T. McDermott · General Endocrinology & Metabolism · Fitzsimmons Army Medical Center, Aurora, CO 80045-5000 · 303-361-8241

Susan Sherman · General Endocrinology & Metabolism (Neuroendocrinology, Thyroid) · Aurora Presbyterian Hospital, Aurora Regional Medical Center, Rose Medical Center (Denver) · Aurora Medical Associates, 750 Potomac Street, Suite L5, Aurora, CO 80011 · 303-341-5751

Boulder

Melvin R. Sternholm · General Endocrinology & Metabolism · 1155 Alpine Avenue, Suite 260, Boulder, CO 80304-3966 · 303-444-4441

Colorado Springs

Larry A. Gold · General Endocrinology & Metabolism (Neuroendocrinology, Thyroid) · Memorial Hospital, Penrose-St. Francis Healthcare System · 325 East Fontanero Street, Suite 103, Colorado Springs, CO 80907-7536 · 719-635-5223

W. A. Munson · General Endocrinology & Metabolism · 325 East Fontanero Street, Suite 101, Colorado Springs, CO 80907 · 719-636-3829

Denver

Boris Draznin · Diabetes (General Endocrinology & Metabolism) · VA Medical Center · VA Medical Center, Section of Endocrinology, 1055 Clermont Street, Box 111H, Denver, CO 80220 · 303-399-8020

Robert H. Eckel · General Endocrinology & Metabolism (Lipid Disorders) · University Hospital, Rose Medical Center · University of Colorado Health Sciences Center, 4200 East Ninth Avenue, Campus Box E151, Denver, CO 80262 · 303-372-1435

Mervyn L. Lifschitz · General Endocrinology & Metabolism (Metabolic Bone Disease, Medical Problems of Pregnancy) · Rose Medical Center · 4545 East Ninth Avenue, Suite 310, Denver, CO 80220 · 303-388-4673

John Merenich · General Endocrinology & Metabolism (Lipid Disorders, Diabetes) · St. Joseph Hospital · Kaiser Permanente Medical Center, 11245 Huron Street, Denver, CO 80234 · 303-457-6150

E. C. Ridgway · Neuroendocrinology, Thyroid · University Hospital · University of Colorado Health Sciences Center, 4200 East Ninth Avenue, Campus Box B151, Denver, CO 80262 · 303-270-8443

Margaret E. Wierman · Neuroendocrinology (Reproductive Endocrinology) · University Hospital · University of Colorado Health Sciences Center, Division of Endocrinology, 4200 East Ninth Avenue, Campus Box B151, Denver, CO 80262 303-270-8443

Grand Junction

Joseph Maruca · General Endocrinology & Metabolism · 1120 Wellington Avenue, Suite 205, Grand Junction, CO 81501 · 970-243-2907

FAMILY MEDICINE

Aurora

Richard A. Patt · 1421 South Potomac Street, Aurora, CO 80012 · 303-750-1920

Colorado Springs

Timothy Hoke · 7015 Tall Oak Drive, Colorado Springs, CO 80918 · 719-598-4588

Denver

Martha Illige-Sauicier · (Doctor-Patient Relationship, Obstetrics) · Rose Medical Center, Presbyterian/St. Luke's Medical Center · Swallow Hill Family Doctors, 1615 Downing Street, Denver, CO 80218 · 303-831-6314

Neil F. Sullivan · 1655 Lafayette Street, Suite 100, Denver, CO 80218 · 303-837-0575

Englewood

Frank M. Reed · Orchard Family Practice, 7180 East Orchard Road, Suite 202, Englewood, CO 80111 · 303-694-7377

Fort Collins

Steve J. Thorson · 1212 East Elizabeth Street, Fort Collins, CO 80524 · 970-482-2791

Grand Junction

David M. West · 729 Bookcliff Avenue, Grand Junction, CO 81501 · 970-245-7573

Greeley

Christopher T. Kennedy · 2010 Sixteenth Street, Greeley, CO 80631 · 970-353-7666

Limon

Mark Olson · (Rural Health Issues, Procedural Primary Care, General Geriatric Medicine) · Lincoln Community Hospital & Nursing Home (Hugo) · Plaines Medical Center, 820 First Street, P.O Box 1120, Limon, CO 80828-1120 · 719-775-2367

Littleton

Kenneth R. Atkinson · 8120 South Holly Street, Suite 200, Littleton, CO 80121 303-741-4400

Wheat Ridge

Mary E. Fairbanks · 3655 Lutheran Parkway, Suite 108, Wheat Ridge, CO 80033 303-425-6012

GASTROENTEROLOGY

Denver

Donald G. Butterfield · General Gastroenterology (Hepatology, Endoscopy) · Presbyterian/St. Luke's Medical Center, St. Joseph Hospital · 1721 East 19th Avenue, Suite 520, Denver, CO 80218-1243 · 303-831-6257

Greg T. Everson · Hepatology (Liver Transplantation, Hepatitis Therapy) · University Hospital · University of Colorado Health Sciences Center, Department of Hepatology, 4200 East Ninth Avenue, Campus Box B158, Denver, CO 80262 · 303-270-7134

Barry W. Frank · General Gastroenterology (Endoscopy, Hepatology) · St. Joseph Hospital, Rose Medical Center · Denver Internal Medicine, 4545 East Ninth Avenue, Suite 480, Denver, CO 80220-3901 · 303-321-7018

John S. Goff · General Gastroenterology, Endoscopy · Consultants in Gastrointestinal Diseases, Poudre Valley Hospital (Fort Collins) · Gastroenterology Associates, 4200 West Conejos Place, Suite 402, Denver, CO 80204 · 303-573-9951

Joel S. Levine · General Gastroenterology (Inflammatory Bowel Disease, Hepatology) · University Hospital · University of Colorado Health Sciences Center, 4200 East Ninth Avenue, Campus Box B158, Denver, CO 80262 · 303-270-4649

Andrew Mallory · General Gastroenterology (Hepatology) · Rose Medical Center, St. Joseph Hospital · Denver Internal Medicine, 4545 East Ninth Avenue, Suite 480, Denver, CO 80220 · 303-321-7018

Sunder J. Mehta · General Gastroenterology · 3005 East 16th Avenue, Suite 430, Denver, CO 80206-1630 · 303-388-6874

John W. Singleton · Inflammatory Bowel Disease (General Gastroenterology) · University Hospital · University of Colorado Health Sciences Center, Division of Gastroenterology & Hepatology, 4200 East Ninth Avenue, Campus Box B158, Denver, CO 80262-0001 · 303-270-7132

Englewood

Pete H. Baker · General Gastroenterology (Colorectal Cancer Screening) · Swedish Medical Center, PorterCare Hospital (Denver), PorterCare Hospital-Littleton (Littleton) · 499 East Hampden Avenue, Suite 420, Englewood, CO 80110 · 303-788-8888

Grand Junction

Bernard R. Pacini · General Gastroenterology · 2530 North Eighth Street, Suite 203, Grand Junction, CO 81501 · 970-243-2479

Peter Walsh · General Gastroenterology · 1120 Wellington Avenue, Grand Junction, CO 81501 · 970-242-6600

Westminster

Steven Ayres · General Gastroenterology (Hepatobiliary Disease, Continuous Quality Improvement, Endoscopy, Inflammatory Bowel Disease) · Provenant St. Anthony Hospital North, Provenant St. Anthony Hospital Central (Denver), North Suburban Medical Center (Thornton) · Gastroenterology Associates, 8406 Clay Street, Westminster, CO 80030 · 303-429-3545

Wheat Ridge

C. Robert Dahl · General Gastroenterology (Peptic Disorders, Hepatology) · Lutheran Medical Center, Provenant St. Anthony Hospital Central (Denver) · Rocky Mountain Gastroenterology, 8550 West 38th Avenue, Suite 300, Wheat Ridge, CO 80033 · 303-425-2800

GERIATRIC MEDICINE

Denver

Dennis W. Jahnigen · (Memory Loss, Healthy Aging, Hospice Care, General Geriatric Medicine, General Internal Medicine) · University Hospital · University of Colorado Health Sciences Center, Center on Aging, 4200 East Ninth Avenue, Campus Box B179, Denver, CO 80262 · 303-270-8668

Nora E. Morgenstern · (Frail Elderly [over 80], Dementia, Exercise Promotion, General Internal Medicine) · University Hospital · University of Colorado Health Sciences Center, Seniors Clinic, 4200 East Ninth Avenue, Campus Box B179, Denver, CO 80260 · 303-270-7851

Laurence J. Robbins · VA Medical Center · VA Medical Center, Department of Geriatrics, 1055 Clermont Street, Box 111D, Denver, CO 80220 · 303-399-8020 x2822

Grand Junction

Mary Clark · (Alzheimer's Disease, Long-Term Care, General Geriatric Medicine, General Internal Medicine) · Community Hospital, St. Mary's Hospital & Medical Center, St. Mary's Rehab Center · Western Medical Associates, 1060 Orchard Avenue, Suite H, Grand Junction, CO 81501 · 970-241-7600

Verne A. Smith · 735 Bookcliff Avenue, Grand Junction, CO 81501 · 970-245-1220

HAND SURGERY

Denver

Charles Hamlin · Paralytic Disorders · Craig Rehabilitation Hospital (Englewood), Hand Surgery Associates · Hand Surgery Associates, 2535 South Downing Street, Suite 500, Denver, CO 80210 · 303-744-7078

Fort Collins

Kenneth H. Duncan · General Hand Surgery · Orthopaedic Center of the Rockies, 2500 East Prospect, Fort Collins, CO 80525 · 970-493-0112

Grand Junction

Chris W. Hauge · General Hand Surgery · 1120 Wellington Avenue, Suite 208, Grand Junction, CO 81501 · 970-243-6200

INFECTIOUS DISEASE

Colorado Springs

Jesse M. Hofflin · General Infectious Disease · Infectious Disease Specialists, 721 North Tejon Street, Colorado Springs, CO 80903 · 719-578-5176

Denver

David L. Cohn · AIDS (Lung Infections, Mycobacterial Diseases, Public Health & Epidemiology, Tuberculosis, Sexually Transmitted Disease) · Denver General Hospital · Denver Health & Hospitals, Denver Public Health, 605 Bannock Street, Room 120, Denver, CO 80204 · 303-436-7200

John M. Douglas, Jr. · Sexually Transmitted Disease, Herpes Virus Infections · Denver Disease Control Service · Denver Disease Control, 605 Bannock Street, Mail Code 2600, Denver, CO 80204 · 303-436-7200

John G. Gerber · General Infectious Disease (AIDS, Herpes Virus Infections) · University Hospital · University of Colorado Health Sciences Center, 4200 East Ninth Avenue, Campus Box C237, Denver, CO 80262 · 303-270-8455

Steven C. Johnson · AIDS · University of Colorado Health Sciences Center, 4200 East Ninth Avenue, Campus Box 163, Denver, CO 80262 · 303-270-3872

Franklyn N. Judson · Sexually Transmitted Disease (AIDS, HIV Infections, General Infectious Disease) · Denver General Hospital · Denver Public Health Department, 605 Bannock Street, Mail Code 2600, Denver, CO 80204 · 303-436-7208

Randall Reves · General Infectious Disease (Tuberculosis, AIDS, HIV) · Denver General Hospital · Denver Disease Control Service, Denver Public Health, 605 Bannock Street, Mail Code 2600, Denver, CO 80204-4507 · 303-436-7200

Robert T. Schooley · Virology, AIDS (Herpes Virus Infections) · University Hospital · University of Colorado Health Sciences Center, Division of Infectious Disease, 4200 East Ninth Avenue, Campus Box B168, Denver, CO 80262 · 303-270-6753

Fort Collins

David Cobb · General Infectious Disease · 1247 Riverside Avenue, Suite One, Fort Collins, CO 80524 · 970-224-0429

Greeley

Judith R. Anderson · General Infectious Disease · 2010 Sixteenth Street, Suite B, Greeley, CO 80631 · 970-330-6034

Palisade

William B. Cobb · General Infectious Disease · Palisade Medical Clinic, P.O. Box 490, Palisade, CO 81526 · 970-464-5611

Wheat Ridge

Susan Mason · General Infectious Disease (HIV) · Lutheran Medical Center, Provenant St. Anthony Hospital Central (Denver) · Western Infectious Disease Consultants, 7760 West 38th Avenue, Suite 290, Wheat Ridge, CO 80033-6151 · 303-425-9245

INTERNAL MEDICINE (GENERAL)

Alamosa

Charles Scott Harrod · (Cardiology, Pulmonary Medicine, General Rheumatology) · San Luis Valley Regional Medical Center · San Luis Valley Medical Clinics, 2115 Stuart Street, Alamosa, CO 81101 · 719-589-3000

Colorado Springs

John D. Hillman · (Preventive Medicine) · Penrose-St. Francis Healthcare System, Memorial Hospital · The Penrose-St. Francis Medical Group, 320 East Fontanero Street, Suite 205, Colorado Springs, CO 80907 · 719-475-9574

John D. Norton · 320 East Fontanero Street, Suite 204, Colorado Springs, CO 80907 · 719-475-9574

Duane R. Spaulding · 3709 Parkmore Village Drive, Suite 100, Colorado Springs, CO 80917-5259 · 719-597-8700

Denver

Richard S. Abrams · (Diabetes, Medical Complications During Pregnancy, Medical Informatics) · Rose Medical Center · Colorado Internal Medicine Center, 4545 East Ninth Avenue, Suite 670, Denver, CO 80220 · 303-320-7744

Linda Barbour · University of Colorado Health Sciences Center, Division of General Internal Medicine, 4200 East Ninth Avenue, Campus Box B180, Denver, CO 80262 · 303-270-7783

Lawrence E. Feinberg · University Hospital · University of Colorado Health Sciences Center, Division of General Internal Medicine, 4200 East Ninth Avenue, Campus Box B180, Denver, CO 80262 · 303-270-7783

Richard Hamilton · 1721 East 19th Avenue, Suite 416, Denver, CO 80218 · 303-863-7575

Gregory A. Ippen · 3535 Cherry Creek North Drive, Suite 406, Denver, CO 80209 · 303-393-7268

Harvey B. Karsh · Colorado Internal Medicine Center, 4545 East Ninth Avenue, Suite 670, Denver, CO 80220-3986 · 303-320-7744

Frederick H. Katz · 3535 Cherry Creek North Drive, Denver, CO 80209 · 303-355-0513

Mervyn L. Lifschitz · (Metabolic Bone Disease, Medical Problems of Pregnancy) Rose Medical Center · 4545 East Ninth Avenue, Suite 310, Denver, CO 80220 · 303-388-4673

Thomas MacKenzie · (Tobacco Control Policy, Adolescent Smoking Prevention, Primary Care Education) · Denver General Hospital · Westside Health Center, 1100 Federal Boulevard, Denver, CO 80204 · 303-436-4202

Philip Mehler · (General Internal Medicine, Addiction Medicine, Eating Disorders) · Denver General Hospital · Denver General Hospital, 777 Bannock Street, Mail Code 0150, Denver, CO 80204 · 303-436-6082

Thomas J. Meyer · (Management of Chronic Pain, Outpatient Medical Education) · VA Medical Center · VA Medical Center, Ambulatory Care, 1055 Clermont Street, Mail Code 118, Denver, CO 80220 · 303-393-2839

Peter Monheit · 3545 South Tamarac, Denver, CO 80237 · 303-771-1647

Nora E. Morgenstern · (Geriatric Medicine, General Internal Medicine) · University Hospital · University of Colorado Health Sciences Center, Seniors Clinic, 4200 East Ninth Avenue, Campus Box B179, Denver, CO 80260 · 303-270-7851

Herbert J. Rothenberg · Rose Medical Center · Denver Internal Medicine, 4545 East Ninth Avenue, Suite 480, Denver, CO 80220 · 303-321-7018

Richard P. Rubenstein · Tower One, Suite 205, 999 Eighteenth Street, Denver, CO 80202 · 303-292-6537

Alan J. Spees · (Hyperbaric Medicine, Wound Care) · Presbyterian/St. Luke's Medical Center, St. Joseph Hospital, Spalding Rehabilitation Hospital (Aurora) · 155 South Madison Street, Suite 210, Denver, CO 80209 · 303-333-5456

David Tanaka · University of Colorado Health Sciences Center, Division of General Internal Medicine, 4200 East Ninth Avenue, Denver, CO 80262 · 303-270-7783

Englewood

James L. Benoist · Front Range Internal Medicine, 499 East Hampden Avenue, Suite 400, Englewood, CO 80110 · 303-788-4250

Carol S. Spies · Front Range Internal Medicine, 499 East Hampden Avenue, Suite 400, Englewood, CO 80110-2780 · 303-788-4250

Fort Collins

Robert C. Homburg · Internal Medicine Clinic of Fort Collins, 1100 Poudre River Drive, Fort Collins, CO 80524 · 970-224-9508

Steven R. Sunderman · Internal Medicine Clinic of Fort Collins, 1100 Poudre River Drive, Fort Collins, CO 80524 · 970-224-9508

Glenwood Springs

Alan E. Saliman · Glenwood Medical, 1905 Blake Avenue, Glenwood Springs, CO 81601 · 970-945-8503

Grand Junction

Barry W. Holcomb · 744 Horizon Court, Suite 301, Grand Junction, CO 81506 · 970-243-3300

Highlands Ranch

William T. Gipson, Jr. · 200 West County Line Road, Suite 380, Highlands Ranch, CO 80126 · 303-791-7540

Montrose

Thomas J. Chamberlain · (Adolescent Medicine, General Internal Medicine) · Montrose Memorial Hospital · 300 South Nevada Avenue, Montrose, CO 81401 · 970-249-7751

Steamboat Springs

Mark E. McCauley · Mountain Medical, 100 Park Avenue, Suite 102, Steamboat Springs, CO 80487 · 970-879-3327

Trinidad

Sally L. Fabec · (Critical Care Medicine, Emergency Care, General Cardiovascular Disease, Diabetes Mellitus) · Mount San Rafael Hospital · 328 Bonaventure Street, Suite Five, Trinidad, CO 81082 · 719-846-4433

Vail

Jack Eck · 181 West Meadow Drive, Suite 500, Vail, CO 81657 · 970-476-7601

MEDICAL ONCOLOGY & HEMATOLOGY

Colorado Springs

Paul N. Anderson · General Medical Oncology & Hematology (General Internal Medicine) · Penrose-St. Francis Healthcare System, Memorial Hospital · Rocky Mountain Cancer Center, 110 East Monroe Street, Suite 200, P.O. Box 7148, Colorado Springs, CO 80933-7148 · 719-577-2555

David H. Huffman · General Medical Oncology & Hematology · Penrose-St. Francis Healthcare System, Memorial Hospital · Rocky Mountain Cancer Center, 110 East Monroe Street, Suite 200, P.O. Box 7148, Colorado Springs, CO 80933-7148 · 719-577-2555

David C. Martz · General Medical Oncology & Hematology · Penrose-St. Francis Healthcare System, Memorial Hospital · Rocky Mountain Cancer Center, 110 East Monroe Street, Suite 200, P.O. Box 7148, Colorado Springs, CO 80933-7148 719-577-2555

Robert Sayer · General Medical Oncology & Hematology · Rocky Mountain Cancer Center, 110 East Monroe Street, Colorado Springs, CO 80933 · 719-577-2555

Charles J. Zinn · General Medical Oncology & Hematology · Rocky Mountain Cancer Center, 110 East Monroe Street, Suite 200, Colorado Springs, CO 80933-7148 · 719-577-2555

Denver

Paul A. Bunn, Jr. · Lung Cancer, Lymphomas · University of Colorado Cancer Center, University Hospital · University of Colorado Cancer Center, 4200 East Ninth Avenue, Campus Box E190, Denver, CO 80262 · 303-270-3007

L. Michael Glode · Solid Tumors, Genito-Urinary Cancer (Prostate, Gene Therapy, Immunotherapy, Cancer Biotherapy, Lymphomas, Myeloma) · University Hospital · University of Colorado Health Sciences Center, 4200 East Ninth Avenue, Campus Box B171, Denver, CO 80262 · 303-270-8801

Roy B. Jones · Bone Marrow Transplantation, Clinical Pharmacology · University Hospital · University of Colorado Health Sciences Center, Bone Marrow Transplant Program, 4200 East Ninth Avenue, Campus Box B190, Denver, CO 80262 303-372-9000

Marilyn J. Manco-Johnson · Disorders of Bleeding, Thrombosis (Hemophilia) · University Hospital, Children's Hospital · University of Colorado Health Sciences Center, 4200 East Ninth Avenue, Campus Box C220, Denver, CO 80262 · 303-372-1753

William A. Robinson · (Malignant Melanoma, Chronic Myeloid Leukemia) · University Hospital · University of Colorado Health Sciences Center, 4200 East Ninth Avenue, Campus Box B171, Denver, CO 80262 · 303-270-8802

Scot M. Sedlacek · General Medical Oncology & Hematology (Breast Cancer) · Rose Medical Center, PorterCare Hospital, Lutheran Medical Center (Wheat Ridge), University Hospital · Colorado Breast Specialists, 4500 East Ninth Avenue, Suite 140, Denver, CO 80220 · 303-321-0302

Elizabeth J. Shpall · Bone Marrow Transplantation · University of Colorado Health Sciences Center, 4200 East Ninth Avenue, Campus Box B190, Denver, CO 80262 · 303-372-9000

Douglass C. Tormey · Breast Cancer · Rose Cancer Center, Eastern Cooperative Oncology Group · University of Colorado Health Sciences Center, AMC Cancer Research Center, 1600 Pierce Street, Denver, CO 80214 · 303-239-3370

Fort Collins

Michael P. Fangman · General Medical Oncology & Hematology (Lymphomas, Breast Cancer, Gynecologic Cancer, Lung Cancer, Myeloma) · Poudre Valley Hospital · 1240 Doctors Lane, Suite 200, Fort Collins, CO 80524 · 970-493-6337

Clinton M. Merrill, Jr. · General Medical Oncology & Hematology · 1240 Doctors Lane, Suite 200, Fort Collins, CO 80524 · 970-493-6337

Grand Junction

Donna L. McFadden · (Medical Oncology, Hospice, Breast Cancer) · St. Mary's Hospital & Medical Center · St. Mary's Hospital & Medical Center, Oncology Clinic, Grand Junction, CO 81502 · 970-244-2457

Joanne F. Virgilio · General Medical Oncology & Hematology · 520 Patterson Road, P.O. Box 1300, Grand Junction, CO 81502 · 970-242-2126

NEPHROLOGY

Boulder

Mark N. Harrison · General Nephrology (Dialysis, Hypertension, Kidney Disease) · Boulder Community Hospital, Avista Hospital (Louisville), Longmont United Hospital (Longmont) · 2880 Folson Street, Suite 104, Boulder, CO 80304 303-443-4200

Colorado Springs

John L. Bengfort · General Nephrology · Penrose-St. Francis Healthcare System, Memorial Hospital · Pike's Peak Nephrology, 2130 East LaSalle Street, Colorado Springs, CO 80909-2281 · 719-632-7641

Milton C. von Minden · General Nephrology · Penrose-St. Francis Healthcare System · Pike's Peak Nephrology, 2130 East LaSalle Street, Colorado Springs, CO 80909 · 719-632-7641

Brad Yuan · General Nephrology · Pike's Peak Nephrology, 2130 East LaSalle Street, Colorado Springs, CO 80909 · 719-632-7641

Denver

Allen C. Alfrey · Dialysis · VA Medical Center, Nephrology Section, 1055 Clermont Street, Denver, CO 80220 · 303-399-8020

Robert J. Anderson · General Nephrology · VA Medical Center, 1055 Clermont Street, Box A009, Denver, CO 80220 · 303-393-2840

Tomas Berl · General Nephrology · University of Colorado Health Sciences Center, 4200 East Ninth Avenue, Campus Box C281, Denver, CO 80262 · 303-270-7203

Laurence Chan · Kidney Transplantation · University of Colorado Health Sciences Center, 4200 East Ninth Avenue, Campus Box C281, Denver, CO 80262 · 303-399-1211

Patricia A. Gabow · Kidney Disease · Denver Health & Hospitals, Denver General Hospital, University Hospital · Denver Department of Health & Hospitals, 777 Bannock Street, Denver, CO 80204-4507 · 303-436-6611

Stuart L. Linas · Hypertension · Denver General Hospital, University Hospital · Denver General Hospital, 777 Bannock Street, Mail Code 4000, Denver, CO 80204-4507 · 303-436-5902

Robert W. Schrier · General Nephrology · University Hospital · University of Colorado Health Sciences Center, 4200 East Ninth Avenue, Campus Box B178, Denver, CO 80262 · 303-270-7765

David M. Spiegel · Dialysis · University Hospital · University of Colorado Health Sciences Center, 4200 East Ninth Avenue, Denver, CO 80262 · 303-270-6734

Grand Junction

Rae Dene Schmidt · General Nephrology · 790 Wellington Avenue, Suite 105, Grand Junction, CO 81501 · 970-245-4810

Lakewood

Paul D. Miller · (Metabolic Bone Diseases) · Colorado Center for Bone Research, 3190 South Wadsworth Boulevard, Suite 250, Lakewood, CO 80227 · 303-980-9985

Pueblo

Constance L. Wehling · General Nephrology (General Internal Medicine, Chronic Dialysis, Hypertension) · St. Mary-Corwin Regional Medical Center, Parkview Episcopal Medical Center · Southern Colorado Nephrology, 41 Montebello Road, Suite D, Pueblo, CO 81001 · 719-543-5000

NEUROLOGICAL SURGERY

Colorado Springs

Roberto Masferr · General Neurological Surgery · 1625 Medical Center Plaza, Colorado Springs, CO 80907 · 719-633-2218

Michael J. McNally · General Neurological Surgery · Memorial Hospital, Penrose-St. Francis Healthcare System · 2125 East LaSalle Street, Colorado Springs, CO 80909 · 719-473-3272

Denver

Robert E. Breeze · Vascular Neurological Surgery · University of Colorado Health Sciences Center, 4200 East Ninth Avenue, Campus Box 307, Denver, CO 80262 303-270-7571

Glenn W. Kindt · General Neurological Surgery · University of Colorado Health Sciences Center, Division of Neurological Surgery, 4200 East Ninth Avenue, Campus Box 3659, Denver, CO 80262 · 303-270-7577

Kevin O. Lillehei · Peripheral Nerve Surgery (Neuro-Oncology, Brain Tumors, Pituitary Tumors (Neuro-Oncology, Brain Tumors, Pituitary Tumors) · University of Colorado Health Sciences Center, 4200 East Ninth Avenue, Campus Box C307, Denver, CO 80262 · 303-270-5651

Ken Winston · Pediatric Neurological Surgery (Stereotactic Radiosurgery, Seizure Surgery, Craniofacial Surgery) · The Children's Hospital, 1950 Ogden Street, Denver, CO 80218 · 303-861-3995

Englewood

Lee E. Krauth · General Neurological Surgery (Aneurysm Surgery, Microvascular Neurosurgery, Skull-Base Neurosurgery) · Swedish Medical Center, PorterCare Hospital (Denver) · 701 East Hampden Avenue, Suite 510, Englewood, CO 80110-2776 · 303-788-4000

Gary Vander Ark · General Neurological Surgery (Neurotology, Cranial Nerve Surgery) · Rocky Mountain Neurosurgical Alliance, 701 East Hampden Avenue, Suite 510, Englewood, CO 80110 · 303-788-4000

Fort Collins

Donn M. Turner · General Neurological Surgery (Brain Surgery, Spinal Surgery, Cranial Nerve Surgery, Peripheral Nerve Surgery, Trauma, Tumor Surgery, General Thoracic Surgery) · Poudre Valley Hospital · Front Range Center For Brain & Spine Surgery, 1313 Riverside Avenue, Fort Collins, CO 80524 · 970-493-1292

Grand Junction

Robert H. Fox · General Neurological Surgery · St. Mary's Hospital & Medical Center · 2530 North Eighth Street, Suite 201, Grand Junction, CO 81501-8856 · 970-241-6990

Larry D. Tice · General Neurological Surgery (Cerebrovascular Surgery, Spinal Surgery) · St. Mary's Hospital & Medical Center · 2530 North Eighth Street, Suite 201, Grand Junction, CO 81501-8856 · 970-241-6990

NEUROLOGY

Boulder

Mark A. Dietz · Infectious & Demyelinating Diseases (General Neurology) · Boulder Community Hospital · 1000 Alpine Avenue, Suite 291, Boulder, CO 80304 · 303-449-3566

George P. Garmany · General Neurology · 1000 Alpine Avenue, Suite 291, Boulder, CO 80304 · 303-449-3566

Colorado Springs

Randall Bjork · General Neurology (Headaches, Rehabilitation) · Penrose-St. Francis Health Care System, Memorial Hospital, Rehabilitation Hospital of Colorado Springs · 2125 East LaSalle Street, Colorado Springs, CO 80909 · 719-473-3272

Denver

Christopher M. Filley · (Behavioral Neurology, Neuropsychiatry, Degenerative Diseases) · University Hospital, VA Medical Center · University of Colorado Health Sciences Center, Department of Neurology, Behavioral Neurology Section, 4200 East Ninth Avenue, Campus Box B183, Denver, CO 80262 · 303-270-6461

Donald H. Gilden · Infectious & Demyelinating Diseases (Degenerative Diseases, Multiple Sclerosis, Infectious Disease) · University Hospital · University of Colorado Health Sciences Center, 4200 East Ninth Avenue, Campus Box B182, Denver, CO 80262 · 303-270-8281

Stanley H. Ginsburg · General Neurology (Headache, Neuro-Rehabilitation) · Rose Medical Center · Neurological Consultants, 4545 East Ninth Avenue, Suite 650, Denver, CO 80220-3985 · 303-451-5165

Jack A. Klapper · Headache (Epilepsy, General Neurology) · St. Joseph Hospital, Presbyterian/St. Luke's Medical Center · 1155 East 18th Avenue, Denver, CO 80218 · 303-839-9900

Steven P. Ringel · Neuro-Rehabilitation, Neuromuscular Disease · University Hospital · University of Colorado Health Sciences Center, 4200 East Ninth Avenue, Campus Box B185, Denver, CO 80262 · 303-270-7221

Marc M. Treihaft · General Neurology (Electromyography, Neuromuscular Disease) · PorterCare Hospital, PorterCare Hospital-Littleton (Littleton), Swedish Medical Center (Englewood) · 2480 South Downing Street, Suite 250, Denver, CO 80210-5843 · 303-777-0400

Englewood

Ronald E. Kramer · Epilepsy (Sleep Medicine, Electroencephalogram, Clinical Neurophysiology) · Swedish Medical Center, PorterCare Hospital (Denver), PorterCare Hospital-Littleton (Littleton) · Colorado Neurology, 799 East Hampden Avenue, Suite 500, Englewood, CO 80110 · 303-788-4210

Neil L. Rosenberg · (Toxicology, Neuromuscular Diseases, Neuroimmunology) · Swedish Medical Center · 450 West Jefferson Avenue, Englewood, CO 80110 · 303-788-1634

Don B. Smith · Strokes · Swedish Medical Center, PorterCare Hospital (Denver), PorterCare Hospital-Littleton (Littleton), Craig Hospital, Spalding Rehabilitation Hospital · 701 East Hampden Avenue, Suite 540, Englewood, CO 80110 · 303-781-4485

Fort Collins

Michael P. Curiel · General Neurology · 1240 Doctors Lane, Suite 210, Fort Collins, CO 80524 · 970-221-1993

Grand Junction

Mitchell D. Burnbaum · General Neurology · 2530 North Eighth Street, Grand Junction, CO 81501 · 970-243-9180

NEUROLOGY, CHILD

Denver

Paul G. Moe · General Child Neurology (Epilepsy, Neuromuscular Disease) · The Children's Hospital, 1056 East 19th Avenue, Box 155, Denver, CO 80218 · 303-861-6895

Alan R. Seay · General Child Neurology · The Children's Hospital, 1056 East 19th Avenue, Box 155, Denver, CO 80218 · 303-861-6896

Englewood

Paul M. Levisohn · General Child Neurology (Epilepsy, Neuro-Oncology) · Swedish Medical Center, PorterCare Hospital (Denver), Children's Hospital (Denver) · Colorado Neurological Institute, 701 East Hampden Avenue, Suite 530, Englewood, CO 80110-2776 · 303-788-5979

NUCLEAR MEDICINE

Denver

James L. Lear · General Nuclear Medicine · University Hospital · University of Colorado Health Sciences Center, 4200 East Ninth Avenue, Campus Box A036, Denver, CO 80262 · 303-270-5274

OBSTETRICS & GYNECOLOGY

Colorado Springs

Robert N. Wolfson · Maternal & Fetal Medicine · Penrose-St. Francis Healthcare System · Perinatal & Genetic Resource Center, 3205 North Academy Boulevard, Colorado Springs, CO 80917 · 719-776-3470

Denver

Bruce H. Albrecht · Reproductive Endocrinology · 4500 East Ninth Avenue, Suite 630S, Denver, CO 80220 · 303-399-6515

Samuel E. Alexander · Reproductive Endocrinology · 3600 East Alameda Avenue, Denver, CO 80209 · 303-321-7115

Harvey M. Cohen · General Obstetrics & Gynecology · Building C, Suite One, 1930 South Federal Boulevard, Denver, CO 80219 · 303-934-5621

Susan A. Davidson · Gynecologic Cancer · University Hospital, Rose Medical Center · University of Colorado Health Sciences Center, 4200 East Ninth Avenue, Campus Box B198, Denver, CO 80262 · 303-270-7897

Karlotta M. Davis · General Obstetrics & Gynecology (Urological Gynecology) · University Hospital · University of Colorado Health Sciences Center, 4200 East Ninth Avenue, Campus Box B198, Denver, CO 80262 · 303-270-7897

William Fuller · General Obstetrics & Gynecology (Obstetrics & Gynecology for the Female Athlete, Gynecological Surgery) · Women's Hospital at Presbyterian/St. Luke's Medical Center · Presbyterian/St. Luke's Medical Center, 1719 East 19th Avenue, Denver, CO 80218 · 303-839-7341

Ronald S. Gibbs · Infectious Disease (Sexually Transmitted Disease, High-Risk Obstetrics, Maternal & Fetal Medicine) · University Hospital · University of Colorado Health Sciences Center, 4200 East Ninth Avenue, Campus Box B198, Denver, CO 80262 · 303-270-7616

Stuart A. Gottesfeld · General Obstetrics & Gynecology (Gynecological Surgery, Genital Dermatological Disease, Infectious Disease, Pediatric & Adolescent Gynecology, Reproductive Surgery) · Rose Medical Center · Denver Women's Clinic, 4500 East Ninth Avenue, Suite 200S, Denver, CO 80220 · 303-399-0055

Michael L. Hall · General Obstetrics & Gynecology (Reproductive Surgery) · St. Joseph Hospital, Presbyterian/St. Luke's Medical Center, Rose Medical Center, Swedish Medical Center (Englewood), PorterCare Hospital · Midtown II, Suite 600, 2005 Franklin Street, Denver, CO 80205 · 303-830-2017

John C. Hobbins · Maternal & Fetal Medicine (Ultrasound, Prenatal Diagnosis) University Hospital · University of Colorado Health Sciences Center, 4200 East Ninth Avenue, Campus Box B198, Denver, CO 80262 · 303-270-8310

Bradley S. Hurst · General Obstetrics & Gynecology (Reproductive Endocrinology, Reproductive Surgery) · University Hospital · University of Colorado Health Sciences Center, 4200 East Ninth Avenue, Campus Box B198, Denver, CO 80262 303-270-7128

Francis J. Major · Gynecologic Cancer · Presbyterian/St. Luke's Medical Center Colorado Gynecologic Oncology Group, 1601 East 19th Avenue, Suite 3000, Denver, CO 80218 · 303-860-0246

James A. McGregor · Infectious Disease · University Hospital · University of Colorado Health Sciences Center, 4200 East Ninth Avenue, Campus Box B198, Denver, CO 80262 · 303-270-7924

Richard P. Porreco · Maternal & Fetal Medicine · Presbyterian/St. Luke's Medical Center · Presbyterian/St. Luke's Medical Center, 1718 East 19th Avenue, Denver, CO 80218 · 303-839-7341

William D. Schlaff · Reproductive Endocrinology (Reproductive Tract Anomalies, Infertility, Reproductive Surgery) · University Hospital · University of Colorado Health Sciences Center, 4200 East Ninth Avenue, Campus Box B198, Denver, CO 80262 · 303-270-7128

Robert E. Wall · General Obstetrics & Gynecology (Preterm Birth Prevention, Menopause) · Rose Medical Center · 4500 East Ninth Avenue, Suite 220S, Denver, CO 80220 · 303-320-2077

Fort Collins

Kelvin F. Kesler · General Obstetrics & Gynecology · Fort Collins Women's Clinic, 1106 East Prospect Street, Fort Collins, CO 80525 · 970-493-7442

Grand Junction

Stephen R. Meacham · General Obstetrics & Gynecology · Women's Health Care of Western Colorado, 2525 North Eighth Street, Suite 202, Grand Junction, CO 81501 · 970-245-1168

Littleton

M. Shannon Burke · Maternal & Fetal Medicine · Swedish Medical Center (Englewood) · 7700 South Broadway, Suite 323, Littleton, CO 80122-2628 · 303-730-5862

Vail

Edward Cohen · General Obstetrics & Gynecology · Vail Valley Medical Center Vail Mountain Medical, 181 West Meadow Drive, Suite 200, Vail, CO 81657 · 970-476-5695

OPHTHALMOLOGY

Boulder

Marylin A. Daugherty · General Ophthalmology · 385 Broadway, Boulder, CO 80303 · 303-449-3770

Colorado Springs

Mark E. Chittum · General Ophthalmology · Retina Consultants, 455 East Pike's Peak Avenue, Suite 309, Colorado Springs, CO 80903 · 719-473-9595

Clarence E. Fogleman · Oculoplastic & Orbital Surgery · 25 East Jackson Street, Suite 30, Colorado Springs, CO 80907 · 719-473-8801

Charles D. McMahon · General Ophthalmology · 1715 North Weber Street, Suite 360, Colorado Springs, CO 80907 · 719-471-4000

Denver

J. Bronwyn Bateman · Ophthalmic Genetics (Pediatric Ophthalmology, Strabismus) · University Hospital · University of Colorado Health Sciences Center, Department of Ophthalmology, 4200 East Ninth Avenue, Campus Box 204, Denver, CO 80262 · 303-270-8635

E. Randy Craven · Glaucoma · PorterCare Hospital, Presbyterian/St. Luke's Medical Center, Aurora Regional Medical Center, St. Joseph Hospital · Glaucoma Associates, 850 East Harvard, Suite 205, Denver, CO 80210 · 303-777-3653

Joel H. Goldstein · General Ophthalmology (Anterior Segment—Cataract & Refractive, Intraocular Lens Implant, Glaucoma) · Rose Medical Center, PorterCare Hospital, Presbyterian/St. Luke's Medical Center, Vail Valley Medical Center (Vail) · Cherry Creek Eye Center, 4999 East Kentucky Avenue, Suite 201, Denver, CO 80222 · 303-691-0505

Michael J. Hawes · (Oculoplastic & Orbital Surgery) · PorterCare Hospital, Swedish Medical Center (Englewood) · 850 East Harvard Avenue, Suite 345, Denver, CO 80210 · 303-698-2424

Kenneth R. Hovland · Vitreo-Retinal Surgery, Ocular Oncology · PorterCare Hospital · 850 East Harvard Avenue, Suite 505, Denver, CO 80210 · 303-778-1910

Stephen T. Petty · (Vitreo-Retinal Surgery, Retinal Diseases) · PorterCare Hospital, Children's Hospital, St. Joseph Hospital · 850 East Harvard Avenue, Suite 505, Denver, CO 80210 · 303-778-1910

John D. Zillis · (Retinal Diseases, Vitreo-Retinal Surgery) · PorterCare Hospital, St. Joseph Hospital, HealthOne Hospitals · 850 East Harvard Avenue, Suite 505, Denver, CO 80210 · 303-778-1910

Fort Collins

William A. Shachtman · General Ophthalmology · 1017 Robertson Street, Fort Collins, CO 80524 · 970-484-5322

Grand Junction

Randy J. Rottman · General Ophthalmology (Anterior Segment—Cataract & Refractive, Pediatric Ophthalmology, Glaucoma) · St. Mary's Hospital & Medical Center · Eye Center of Colorado West, 1120 Wellington Avenue, Grand Junction, CO 81501 · 970-242-8811

Greeley

John R. Welch · General Ophthalmology (Glaucoma, Anterior Segment—Cataract & Refractive) · North Colorado Medical Center · 1616 Fifteenth Street, Greeley, CO 80631-4571 · 970-353-3443

Littleton

S. Lance Forstot · Corneal Diseases & Transplantation (Corneal Transplantation, Refractive Surgery) · Corneal Consultants of Colorado, 8381 South Park Lane, Littleton, CO 80120 · 303-730-0404

ORTHOPAEDIC SURGERY

Aurora

John A. Odom · Spinal Surgery · Colorado Spine Center, 1455 South Potomac Street, Suite 307, Aurora, CO 80012-4504 · 303-696-1234

Colorado Springs

Frederick Feiler · General Orthopaedic Surgery (Total Joints & Revisions, Amputations) · Rustic Hills Orthopaedics, 1633 Medical Center Point, Suite 233, Colorado Springs, CO 80907 · 719-473-3332

Tom Mahony · General Orthopaedic Surgery (Sports Medicine/Arthroscopy) · Penrose-St. Francis Healthcare System, Memorial Hospital · Athletic Orthopaedics of Colorado Springs, 320 East Fontanero Street, Suite 106, Colorado Springs, CO 80907-7535 · 719-635-7378

C. Milton Waldron · Hip Surgery (Knee Surgery, Reconstructive Surgery) · Penrose-St. Francis Healthcare System, Memorial Hospital · Colorado Springs Orthopaedic Group, 801 North Cascade Avenue, Suite 23, Colorado Springs, CO 80903-3288 · 719-635-1525

Denver

Douglas A. Dennis · Hip Surgery (Total Hip Replacement, Total Knee Replacement, Arthroscopic Knee Surgery, Foot & Ankle Surgery) · St. Joseph Hospital, Rose Medical Center, Presbyterian/St. Luke's Medical Center · Denver Orthopedic Specialists, 1601 East 19th Avenue, Suite 5000, Denver, CO 80218 · 303-839-5383

Robert E. Eilert · Pediatric Orthopaedic Surgery · Children's Hospital · The Children's Hospital, Department of Orthopaedic Surgery, 1056 East 19th Avenue, Denver, CO 80218 · 303-861-6615

Donald C. Ferlic · (Hand Surgery) · Denver Orthopedic Specialists, 1601 East 19th Avenue, Suite 5000, Denver, CO 80218 · 303-839-5383

David B. Hahn · Pediatric Orthopaedic Surgery · Denver Orthopedic Specialists, 1601 East 19th Avenue, Suite 5000, Denver, CO 80218 · 303-839-5383

Robert D. Loeffler · Sports Medicine/Arthroscopy · University Hospital · Sports Medicine Clinic, 5250 Leetsdale Drive, Suite 301, Denver, CO 80222 · 303-372-2255

Robert P. Mack · Sports Medicine/Arthroscopy (Knee, Ski Injury) · St. Joseph Hospital, Presbyterian/St. Luke's Medical Center, Rose Medical Center · Denver Orthopedic Specialists, 1601 East 19th Avenue, Suite 5000, Denver, CO 80218 303-839-5383

Morris H. Sussman · Hip Surgery · The Children's Hospital, 1601 East 19th Avenue, Denver, CO 80218 · 303-839-5383

Jerome D. Wiedel · Hip Surgery, Knee Surgery, General Orthopaedic Surgery (Hemophilia, Prosthetic Reconstruction, Shoulder Surgery, Sports Medicine/Arthroscopy) · University Hospital, Rose Medical Center · University of Colorado Health Sciences Center, Department of Orthopaedics, 4701 East Ninth Avenue, Campus Box E203, Denver, CO 80262 · 303-372-1254

Ross M. Wilkins · Tumor Surgery (Orthopaedic Infections, Bone Healing Problems) · Presbyterian/St. Luke's Medical Center, St. Joseph Hospital, Rose Medical Center, Children's Hospital · Denver Orthopedic Specialists, 1601 East 19th Avenue, Suite 5000, Denver, CO 80218 · 303-839-5383

David A. Wong · Spinal Surgery · St. Joseph Hospital, Presbyterian/St. Luke's Medical Center, Rose Medical Center · Denver Orthopedic Specialists, Presbyterian/St. Luke's Professional Plaza West, Suite 5000, 1601 East 19th Avenue, Denver, CO 80218 · 303-839-5383

Glenwood Springs

Robert S. Dertkash · (Hand Surgery) · Orthopaedic Associates, 622 Ninteenth Street, Suite 201, Glenwood Springs, CO 81601 · 970-245-8683

Grand Junction

Jeffery M. Nakano · General Orthopaedic Surgery · St. Mary's Hospital & Medical Center · Rocky Mountain Orthopaedic Associates, 790 Wellington Avenue, Suite 201, Grand Junction, CO 81501 · 970-242-3535

Vail

Richard J. Hawkins · Reconstructive Surgery, Sports Medicine/Arthroscopy (Shoulder Surgery, Knee Surgery, General Orthopaedic Surgery, Surgical Critical Care) · Vail Valley Medical Center · Steadman-Hawkins Clinic, 181 West Meadow Drive, Suite 400, Vail, CO 81657 · 303-476-1100

J. Richard Steadman · Sports Medicine/Arthroscopy (Knee, Ski Injury) · Vail Valley Medical Center · Steadman-Hawkins Clinic, 181 West Meadow Drive, Suite 400, Vail, CO 81657 · 303-476-1100

OTOLARYNGOLOGY

Colorado Springs

David M. Barrs · Otology/Neurotology · Memorial Hospital, Penrose-St. Francis Healthcare System · 2125 East LaSalle Street, Suite 201, Colorado Springs, CO 80909 · 719-442-6984

Barton Knox · General Otolaryngology (Head & Neck Surgery, Sinus & Nasal Surgery) · Penrose-St. Francis Healthcare System, Memorial Hospital · Cascade Ear, Nose & Throat Clinic, 715 North Cascade Avenue, Colorado Springs, CO 80903-3246 · 719-633-3803

J. Christopher Pruitt · General Otolaryngology (Sinus & Nasal Surgery) · Penrose-St. Francis Healthcare System, Memorial Hospital · 3100 North Academy Boulevard, Suite 211, Colorado Springs, CO 80917 · 719-596-1217

Denver

Kenny H. Chan · Pediatric Otolaryngology (General Otolaryngology) · Children's Hospital, University Hospital · The Children's Hospital, 1056 East 19th Avenue, Denver, CO 80218 · 303-764-8520

Bruce W. Jafek · Head & Neck Surgery, Taste & Smell Dysfunction (Sinus & Nasal Surgery) · University Hospital, Rose Medical Center, Children's Hospital · University of Colorado Health Sciences Center, 4200 East Ninth Avenue, Campus Box B205, Denver, CO 80262 · 303-270-7988

Alan Lipkin · Otology/Neurotology · 950 East Harvard Avenue, Suite 500, Denver, CO 80210 · 303-744-1961

Arlen D. Meyers · Head & Neck Surgery, Facial Plastic Surgery (Reconstructive Surgery, General Otolaryngology, Sinus & Nasal Surgery, Skull-Base Surgery, Head & Neck Surgery) · University Hospital · University of Colorado Health Sciences Center, 4200 East Ninth Avenue, Campus Box B205, Denver, CO 80262 303-270-7937

Victor L. Schramm · Skull-Base Surgery, Head & Neck Surgery · Presbyterian/St. Luke's Medical Center, University Hospital · Presbyterian/St. Luke's Medical Center, 1601 East 19th Avenue, Suite 3100, Denver, CO 80218 · 303-839-7980

Marshall E. Smith · Pediatric Otolaryngology (Cleft Palate, Voice, General Otolaryngology) · Children's Hospital · University of Colorado Health Sciences Center, Department of Pediatric Otolaryngology, 4200 East Ninth Avenue, Campus Box B205, Denver, CO 80262 · 303-764-8520

Sylvan E. Stool · (Pediatric Otolaryngology) · Children's Hospital · The Children's Hospital, Department of Pediatric Otolaryngology, 1056 East 19th Avenue, Box B455, Denver, CO 80218 · 303-764-8520

Englewood

Barbara A. Esses · Otology · Swedish Medical Center, University Hospital · Denver Ear Associates, 799 East Hampden Avenue, Suite 510, Englewood, CO 80110 · 303-788-7880

David C. Kelsall · Otology (Otology/Neurotology, Skull-Base Surgery) · Swedish Medical Center, University Hospital · Swedish Medical Center, 799 East Hampden Avenue, Suite 510, Englewood, CO 80110 · 303-788-7880

Richard E. Schaler · General Otolaryngology · 701 East Hampden Avenue, Suite 130, Englewood, CO 80110 · 303-788-6632

Fort Collins

Mark C. Loury · General Otolaryngology (Sinus & Nasal Diseases, Head & Neck Surgery) · Poudre Valley Hospital · 1136 East Stuart Street, Suite 3200, Fort Collins, CO 80525 · 970-493-5334

Grand Junction

Denzel F. Hartshorn · General Otolaryngology (Head & Neck Surgery) · St. Mary's Hospital & Medical Center, Community Hospital, Craig Hospital (Englewood), Delta County Memorial Hospital (Delta), VA Medical Center · Colorado West Otolaryngologists, 425 Patterson Road, Suite 503, Grand Junction, CO 81506 970-245-2400

PATHOLOGY

Colorado Springs

Donald L. Dawson · General Pathology (Blood Banking/Transfusion Medicine, Coagulation, Hematopathology) · Penrose Hospital, Department of Pathology, 2215 North Cascade Avenue, Colorado Springs, CO 80907 · 719-776-5816

Cosimo G. Sciotto · General Pathology (Hematopathology, Coagulation, Immunopathology) · Penrose-St. Francis Healthcare System · Penrose Hospital, Department of Pathology, 2215 North Cascade Avenue, P.O. Box 7021, Colorado Springs, CO 80933 · 719-776-5816

Denver

Mitchell Bitter · (Hematopathology) · University Hospital · University of Colorado Health Sciences Center, Department of Pathology, 4200 East Ninth Avenue, Campus Box B216, Denver, CO 80262 · 303-270-5323

Wilbur A. Franklin · (Surgical Pathology, Molecular Pathology, Lung Cancer) · University of Colorado Health Sciences Center, Department of Pathology, 4200 East Ninth Avenue, Campus Box B216, Denver, CO 80262 · 303-270-7625

Fort Collins

John T. Decker · General Pathology · Fort Collins Consultants in Pathology, Poudre Valley Hospital, 1024 Lemay Avenue, Fort Collins, CO 80524 · 970-495-8740

Grand Junction

Geno Saccomanno · General Pathology (Cytopathology, Neuropathology) · St. Mary's Cancer Research Institute, Department of Pathology, 2635 North Seventh Street, P.O. Box 1628, Grand Junction, CO 81502-1628 · 970-244-2066

PEDIATRICS

Denver

Steven H. Abman · Pediatric Pulmonology (Pediatric Critical Care Medicine, Pulmonary Hypertension) · University Hospital, Children's Hospital · The Children's Hospital, 1056 East 19th Avenue, Box B395, Denver, CO 80218 · 303-837-2522

Frank Joseph Accurso · Pediatric Pulmonology (Cystic Fibrosis) · University Hospital, Children's Hospital · The Children's Hospital, 1056 East 19th Avenue, Box B395, Denver, CO 80218 · 303-837-2522

Trina Mary Menden Anglin · Pediatric & Adolescent Gynecology, Adolescent & Young Adult Medicine · Children's Hospital · The Children's Hospital, 1056 East 19th Avenue, Denver, CO 80218 · 303-861-6131

Bruce Blyth · (Pediatric Urology) · Presbyterian/St. Luke's Medical Center, Children's Hospital, Rose Medical Center · 1601 East 19th Avenue, Suite 3750, Denver, CO 80218 · 303-839-7200

Mark M. Boucek · Pediatric Cardiology (Infant Cardiac Transplant, Interventional Cardiology) · Children's Hospital · The Children's Hospital, 1056 East 19th Avenue, Box B100, Denver, CO 80218-1088 · 303-861-6020

H. Peter Chase · Pediatric Endocrinology (Pediatric Diabetes, Prevention of Type I Diabetes, Prevention of Eye/Kidney Complications of Diabetes) · University Hospital, Children's Hospital, Denver General Hospital · University of Colorado Health Sciences Center, Barbara Davis Center for Childhood Diabetes, 4200 East Ninth Avenue, Campus Box B140, Denver, CO 80262 · 303-270-7451

Roger H. Giller · Pediatric Hematology-Oncology (Pediatric Bone Marrow Transplantation) · Children's Hospital · The Children's Hospital, 1056 East 19th Avenue, Denver, CO 80218 · 303-861-6750

Mary Glode · Pediatric Infectious Disease · The Children's Hospital, 1056 East 19th Avenue, Box B158, Denver, CO 80218 · 303-861-6918

Stephen I. Goodman · Metabolic Diseases (Organic Acidemias) · University Hospital · University of Colorado Health Sciences Center, Department of Pediatrics, 4200 East Ninth Avenue, Campus Box C233, Denver, CO 80262 · 303-270-7301

Carol L. Greene · Metabolic Diseases (Genetics, Newborn Screening) · Children's Hospital · The Children's Hospital, 1056 East 19th Avenue, Box B153, Denver, CO 80218 · 303-861-6847

Daniel Hall · Neonatal-Perinatal Medicine · University Hospital, Aurora Regional Medical Center (Aurora), North Suburban Medical Center (Thornton), Provenant St. Anthony Hospital, Lutheran Medical Center (Wheat Ridge) · The Children's Hospital, Department of Neonatology, 1056 East 19th Avenue, Denver, CO 80218 · 303-861-6868

Taru Hays · Pediatric Hematology-Oncology · The Children's Hospital, 1056 East 19th Avenue, Denver, CO 80218 · 303-861-8888

J. Roger Hollister · Pediatric Rheumatology · The Children's Hospital, 1056 East 19th Avenue, Denver, CO 80218 · 303-861-6132

Carole Jenny · Abused Children · Children's Hospital · The Children's Hospital, 1056 East 19th Avenue, Box B138, Denver, CO 80218 · 303-861-6919

Melvin Douglas Jones, Jr. · Neonatal-Perinatal Medicine · Children's Hospital · The Children's Hospital, 1056 East 19th Avenue, Box B065, Denver, CO 80218 303-837-2766

David W. Kaplan · Adolescent & Young Adult Medicine (Eating Disorders) · Children's Hospital · Children's Hospital Adolescent Medicine Clinic, 1056 East 19th Avenue, Box B025, Denver, CO 80218 · 303-861-6131

Michael Steven Kappy · Pediatric Endocrinology (Disorders of Growth & Pubertal Development, Diabetes) · Children's Hospital · The Children's Hospital, Department of Pediatrics, 1056 East 19th Avenue, Box 256, Denver, CO 80218 · 303-861-6061

Georgeanna Klingensmith · Pediatric Endocrinology (General, Growth Problems, Diabetes) · Children's Hospital · The Children's Hospital, Department of Endocrinology, 1056 East 19th Avenue, Third Floor, Suite B265, Denver, CO 80218 · 303-861-6627

Gary L. Larsen · Pediatric Pulmonology (Asthma) · National Jewish Center for Immunology & Respiratory Medicine · National Jewish Center for Immunology & Respiratory Medicine, 1400 Jackson Street, Room J-112, Denver, CO 80206 · 303-398-1617

Gary M. Lum · Pediatric Nephrology · Children's Hospital Kidney Center, 1056 East 19th Avenue, Box B328, Denver, CO 80218 · 303-861-6263

Michael R. Narkewicz · Pediatric Gastroenterology (Pediatric Hepatology) · Children's Hospital · The Children's Hospital, 1056 East 19th Avenue, Denver, CO 80218 · 303-861-6669

Lorrie Furman Odom · Pediatric Hematology-Oncology (Pediatric Leukemias, Pediatric Solid Tumors, Hereditary Cancers, Supportive Care) · Children's Hospital · The Children's Hospital, 1056 East 19th Avenue, Box B115, Denver, CO 80218 · 303-861-6750

Adam A. Rosenberg · Neonatal-Perinatal Medicine · University Hospital, Children's Hospital · The Children's Hospital, 1056 East 19th Avenue, Denver, CO 80218 · 303-270-5979

Harley Rotbart · Pediatric Infectious Disease · The Children's Hospital, Department of Infectious Disease, 1056 East 19th Avenue, Denver, CO 80218 · 303-861-6981

Ronald Jay Sokol · Pediatric Gastroenterology (Pediatric Hepatology, Vitamin E, Liver Disease, Liver Transplantation, Nutrition) · Children's Hospital, University Hospital · The Children's Hospital, 1056 East 19th Avenue, Box B290, Denver, CO 80218 · 303-861-6669

Judith McConnell Sondheimer · Pediatric Gastroenterology (Gastroesophageal Reflux) · Children's Hospital · The Children's Hospital, 1056 East 19th Avenue, Box B290, Denver, CO 80218 · 303-861-6669

Lynn M. Taussig · Pediatric Pulmonology (Asthma, Cystic Fibrosis) · National Jewish Center for Immunology & Respiratory Medicine · National Jewish Center for Immunology & Respiratory Medicine, 1400 North Jackson Street, Room M-113, Denver, CO 80206 · 303-398-1031

James Kennedy Todd · Pediatric Infectious Disease · Children's Hospital · The Children's Hospital, Department of Epidemiology, 1056 East 19th Avenue, Box B276, Denver, CO 80218 · 303-861-6983

Jeffrey Scott Wagener · Pediatric Pulmonology · University Hospital, Children's Hospital · The Children's Hospital, 1056 East 19th Avenue, Box B395, Denver, CO 80218 · 303-837-2522

Randy Wilkening · Neonatal-Perinatal Medicine · University Hospital, Department of Neonatal Medicine, 4200 East Ninth Avenue, Campus Box 195, Denver, CO 80262 · 303-861-8888

PEDIATRICS (GENERAL)

Aurora

Freeman Ginsburg · (Infectious Disease, Growth, Development, Psychosocial Issues) · The Children's Hospital (Denver), Aurora Regional Medical Center, Aurora Presbyterian Hospital · Aurora Pediatric Associates, 830 Potomac Circle, Suite 105, Aurora, CO 80011 · 303-366-3714

Michael Louis Kurtz · Aurora Pediatric Associates, 830 South Potomac Avenue, Suite 105, Aurora, CO 80011 · 303-366-3714

Colorado Springs

David Hoover · 3207 North Academy Boulevard, Suite 315, Colorado Springs, CO 80917 · 719-597-8704

Denver

Jules Amer · Children's Medical Center, 1625 Marion Street, Denver, CO 80218 303-830-7337

Michael Frank · 2121 South Oneida Street, Suite 200, Denver, CO 80224 · 303-757-6418

Edward Goldson · 1919 Ogdon Street, Denver, CO 80218 · 303-861-6630

Roxanne Headley · Children's Hospital, 1056 East 19th Avenue, Denver, CO 80210 · 303-837-2772

Cecil H. Lashlee · Children's Medical Center, 1625 Marion Street, Denver, CO 80218 · 303-333-5448

Karen Leamer · Children's Medical Center, 1625 Marion Street, Denver, CO 80218 · 303-333-5448

Jay Markson · Children's Medical Center, 1625 Marion Street, Denver, CO 80218 303-830-7337

Jody L. Mathie · 950 South Cherry Street, Suite 100, Denver, CO 80222 · 303-756-0101

Frits Mijer · 2465 South Downing Street, Denver, CO 80210 · 303-744-3579

Stefan Mokrohisky · Kaiser Permanente Medical Center, Department of Pediatrics, 2045 Franklin Street, Denver, CO 80205 · 303-861-2121

John W. Ogle · (Pediatric Infectious Diseases, General Pediatrics) · Denver General Hospital · Denver General Hospital, Department of Pediatrics, 777 Bannock Street, Denver, CO 80204 · 303-436-6690

Mark H. Pearlman · Aurora Pediatric Associates, 830 South Potomac Avenue, Suite 105, Denver, CO 80011 · 303-366-3714

Steven Robert Poole · (Pediatric Diagnostic Dilemmas) · Children's Hospital · The Children's Hospital, 1056 East 19th Avenue, Box 085, Denver, CO 80218 · 303-861-8888

Dean Prina · 919 Jasmine Street, Suite 100, Denver, CO 80220 · 303-388-4256

Barton D. Schmitt · Ambulatory Care Center · The Children's Hospital, 1056 East 19th Avenue, Box 085, Denver, CO 80218 · 303-837-2571

Margaret Sheehan · 4500 East Ninth Avenue, Suite 570, Denver, CO 80220 · 303-321-0880

James Edward Shira · The Children's Hospital, 1056 East 19th Avenue, Box B311, Denver, CO 80218 · 303-861-6182

Lee S. Thompson · Aurora Pediatric Associates, 830 South Potomac Avenue, Suite 105, Denver, CO 80011 · 303-366-3714

Thomas J. Wera · The Children's Hospital, 1056 East 19th Avenue, Denver, CO 80218 · 303-861-8888

Wallace C. White · 5150 East Yale Circle, Suite 101, Denver, CO 80222 · 303-759-2591

Mary Zavadil · Children's Medical Center, 1625 Marion Street, Denver, CO 80218 · 303-830-7337

Englewood

Andrew Bauer · Greenwood Pediatrics, 6065 South Quebec Street, Suite 100, Englewood, CO 80111 · 303-694-3200

Gordon J. Blakeman · Children's Hospital (Denver), Swedish Medical Center, Presbyterian/St. Luke's Medical Center (Denver), PorterCare Hospital (Denver), PorterCare Hospital-Littleton (Littleton), Aurora Regional Medical Center (Aurora), Rose Medical Center (Denver) · Pediatric Pathways, 7850 East Berry Place, Suite Three, Englewood, CO 80111 · 303-694-2323

Daniel J. Feiten · Greenwood Pediatrics, 6065 South Quebec Street, Suite 100, Englewood, CO 80111 · 303-694-3200

Lynne R. Studebaker · (Behavioral Pediatrics, Newborn Problems, Infectious Disease) · Children's Hospital (Denver), Rose Medical Center (Denver), Swedish Medical Center, PorterCare Hospital (Denver) · Village Pediatrics, 7840 East Berry Place, Suite One, Englewood, CO 80111 · 303-850-7337

Evergreen

John P. Moyer · 3528 Evergreen Parkway, Evergreen, CO 80439 · 303-674-6671

Fort Collins

Max A. Elliott · Fort Collins Youth Clinic, 1200 East Elizabeth Street, Fort Collins, CO 80524 · 970-482-2515

James G. Meggins · Fort Collins Youth Clinic, 1200 East Elizabeth Street, Fort Collins, CO 80524 · 970-482-2515

Glenwood Springs

Debra Brown Garcia · 1517 Blake Avenue, Glenwood Springs, CO 81601 · 970-945-8621

Grand Junction

David L. Pacini · (Pediatric Infectious Diseases, General Pediatrics) · St. Mary's Hospital & Medical Center · 2323 North Seventh Street, Grand Junction, CO 81501 · 970-243-5437

Harriett Soper-Porter · 2323 North Seventh Street, Grand Junction, CO 81501 · 970-243-5437

Craig Spoering · 2323 North Seventh Street, Grand Junction, CO 81501 · 970-243-5437

Highlands Ranch

Deborah K. Bublitz · (Newborns/Parents Early Adjustment, Diagnostic Problems, Developmental, Educational, Emotional Problems) · Children's Hospital (Denver), Swedish Medical Center (Englewood), PorterCare Hospital (Denver), PorterCare Hospital-Littleton (Littleton) · Littleton Pediatric Medical Center, 206 West County Line Road, Suite 110, Highlands Ranch, CO 80126 · 303-791-9999

Littleton

Robert D. Mauro · Children's Hospital (Denver), PorterCare Hospital-Littleton 6931 South Pierce Street, Littleton, CO 80123 · 303-730-1135

Louisville

Robert C. Bucknam · (Neonatal Medicine, Parenting, General Pediatrics) · Avista Hospital, Boulder Community Hospital (Boulder) · 90 Health Park Drive, Suite 160, Louisville, CO 80027 · 303-673-9030

Westminster

Susan L. Merrill · Kaiser Permanente Medical Center, 11245 Huron Street, Westminster, CO 80234 · 303-338-4444

Wheat Ridge

Barbara L. Gablehouse · 3555 Lutheran Parkway, Suite 340, Wheat Ridge, CO 80033 · 303-420-0525

Ronald C. Meyer · 8550 West 38th Avenue, Suite 200, Wheat Ridge, CO 80033 303-467-8900

PHYSICAL MEDICINE & REHABILITATION

Colorado Springs

G. Thomas Morgan · General Physical Medicine & Rehabilitation (Pain Management, Non-Operative Spine Care, Sports Medicine, Electromyography) · Penrose-St. Francis Healthcare System, Memorial Hospital, St. Mary-Corwin Regional Medical Center (Pueblo) · Pike's Peak Physical Medicine, 2233 Academy Place, Suite 200, Colorado Springs, CO 80909 · 719-591-0011

Denver

Dennis J. Matthews · General Physical Medicine & Rehabilitation · The Children's Hospital, 1056 East 19th Avenue, Denver, CO 80218 · 303-861-6016

Robert H. Meier III · General Physical Medicine & Rehabilitation (Amputee Rehabilitation, Burn Rehabilitation, Spinal Cord Injury Rehabilitation) · University Hospital · University of Colorado Health Sciences Center, 4200 East Ninth Avenue, Campus Box C279, Denver, CO 80262 · 303-372-5608

Englewood

Elena Draznin · General Physical Medicine & Rehabilitation (Neuro-Rehabilitation, Musculoskeletal Rehabilitation) · Spalding Rehabilitation Hospital (Aurora), Swedish Medical Center · 701 East Hampden Avenue, Suite 320, Englewood, CO 80110 · 303-788-6740

Bart Goldman · General Physical Medicine & Rehabilitation (Pain, Electrodiagnostic Medicine) · Aurora Presbyterian Hospital (Aurora), Aurora Regional Medical Center (Aurora), HealthOne Behavioral Health Services-Bethesda Campus (Denver), North Suburban Medical Center (Thornton), Presbyterian/St. Luke's Medical Center (Denver), Rose Medical Center (Denver), Swedish Medical Center, Spalding Rehabilitation Hospital (Aurora) · The Center for Spine & Orthopaedic Rehabilitation, 125 East Hampden Avenue, Englewood, CO 80150-0101 · 303-788-6356

Daniel P. Lammertse · General Physical Medicine & Rehabilitation (Spinal Cord Injury Rehabilitation, Brain Injury Rehabilitation) · Craig Hospital, Provenant St. Anthony Hospital Central (Denver), Swedish Medical Center · 3425 Clarkson Street, Englewood, CO 80110 · 303-789-8220

Grand Junction

Marge L. Keely · General Physical Medicine & Rehabilitation · 1100 Patterson Road, Grand Junction, CO 81506 · 970-244-6018

PLASTIC SURGERY

Colorado Springs

Alfred C. Speirs · General Plastic Surgery · 1490 West Fillmore Avenue, Colorado Springs, CO 80904 · 719-475-1300

Denver

Thomas J. Arganese · (Surgery of the Hand, Reconstructive Surgery, Microsurgery) · Presbyterian/St. Luke's Medical Center, St. Joseph Hospital, Rose Medical Center, PorterCare Hospital, Swedish Medical Center (Englewood) · 1721 East 19th Avenue, Suite 244, Denver, CO 80218 · 303-831-4263

William C. Brown · General Plastic Surgery (Facial Aesthetic Surgery, Breast Surgery, Body Contouring, Head & Neck Surgery, Pediatric Plastic Surgery, Surgery of the Hand) · St. Joseph Hospital, Children's Hospital, Presbyterian/St. Luke's Medical Center, Rose Medical Center, Swedish Medical Center (Englewood) · Plastic Surgery Clinic, 1578 Humboldt Street, Denver, CO 80218 · 303-830-7200

John A. Grossman · General Plastic Surgery (Body Contouring, Breast Surgery, Facial Aesthetic Surgery, Laser Surgery & Birthmarks, Liposuction) · Rose Medical Center, Presbyterian/St. Luke's Medical Center, Cedars-Sinai Medical Center (Los Angeles, CA), Century City Hospital (Los Angeles, CA) · 310 Steele Street, Denver, CO 80206 · 303-320-5566

Lawrence L. Ketch · Reconstructive Surgery (Pediatric Plastic Surgery, Aesthetic Surgery, General Plastic Surgery) · University Hospital, Children's Hospital · University of Colorado Health Sciences Center, Division of Plastic and Hand Surgery, 4200 East Ninth Avenue, Campus Box C309, Denver, CO 80262-0001 · 303-270-8553

R. Chris Weatherley-White · Reconstructive Surgery (Cleft Lip & Palate Surgery) · Children's Hospital, St. Joseph Hospital · 4500 East Ninth Avenue, Suite 470, Denver, CO 80210 · 303-399-7662

Grand Junction

William D. Merkel · General Plastic Surgery · 2525 North Eighth Street, Suite 203, Grand Junction, CO 81501 · 970-242-9127

PSYCHIATRY

Boulder

Jacob G. Jacobson · Psychoanalysis (Psychotherapy, General Psychiatry) · 1636 Sixteenth Street, Boulder, CO 80302 · 303-443-1337

Richard Warner · Schizophrenia · Boulder Community Hospital, Longmont United Hospital (Longmont), Cedar House-Mental Health Center of Boulder County · Mental Health Center of Boulder County, 1333 Iris Avenue, Boulder, CO 80304 · 303-443-8500

Colorado Springs

Ralph E. Everett · Child & Adolescent Psychiatry · 102 North Cascade Avenue, Suite 210, Colorado Springs, CO 80903 · 719-577-9042

Kenneth R. Gamblin · General Psychiatry · 963 East Colorado Avenue, Colorado Springs, CO 80903 · 719-578-1119

Scott McClure · Addiction Psychiatry · 102 North Cascade Avenue, Suite 210, Colorado Springs, CO 80903 · 719-578-9149

Stephan O. Mueller · General Psychiatry · 2135 Southgate Road, Colorado Springs, CO 80906-2605 · 719-520-0700

Gerald S. Stein · General Psychiatry (Mood & Anxiety Disorders, Neuropsychiatry, Forensic Psychiatry, Psychoanalysis, Psychopharmacology) · 1415 North Cascade Avenue, Colorado Springs, CO 80907 · 719-636-2280

Denver

William Bernstein · Psychoanalysis · 4900 South Cherry Creek Drive, Suite F, Denver, CO 80222 · 303-753-6098

Thomas J. Crowley · Addiction Psychiatry · University Hospital, Colorado Psychiatric Hospital · University of Colorado Health Sciences Center, 4200 East Ninth Avenue, Campus Box C268-35, Denver, CO 80262 · 303-270-7573

Steven L. Dubovsky · Mood & Anxiety Disorders (Neuropsychiatry, Psychopharmacology, Psychosomatics) · University Hospital · University of Colorado Health Sciences Center, 4200 East Ninth Avenue, Campus Box C260, Denver, CO 80262 · 303-270-8481

Robert Newcomb Emde · Psychoanalysis · University of Colorado Health Sciences Center, 4200 East Ninth Avenue, Campus Box C268-69, Denver, CO 80262 303-270-8040

Robert Freedman · Schizophrenia (Psychopharmacology of Schizophrenia) · University of Colorado Health Sciences Center, 4200 East Ninth Avenue, Campus Box C268-71, Denver, CO 80262 · 303-399-1211

Robert J. Harmon · Child & Adolescent Psychiatry (Addiction Psychiatry, General Psychiatry) · Colorado Psychiatric Hospital, University Hospital · University of Colorado Health Sciences Center, Department of Psychiatry, 4200 East Ninth Avenue, Campus Box C268-52, Denver, CO 80262 · 303-270-5505

David M. Hurst · Psychoanalysis (General Psychiatry, Couples Therapy, Mood & Anxiety Disorders) · Denver Institute for Psychoanalysis, University Hospital · 601 Emerson Street, Denver, CO 80218 · 303-832-5024

John F. Kelly · Psychoanalysis · 722 Clarkson Street, Denver, CO 80218 · 303-320-0829

Mary Ann C. Levy · General Psychiatry (Psychoanalysis, Child & Adolescent Psychiatry, Trauma & its Sequelae) · 3955 East Exposition Avenue, Suite 404, Denver, CO 80209 · 303-329-8312

Thomas Luparello · Psychoanalysis · 4900 Cherry Creek South Drive, Denver, CO 80222-2283 · 303-758-5206

Gary C. Martin · Psychoanalysis · 4770 East Iliff Avenue, Suite 226, Denver, CO 80222-6061 · 303-756-6115

Peter Mayerson · Psychoanalysis · Cherry Creek Medical Group, 3955 East Exposition Avenue, Suite 402, Denver, CO 80209 · 303-744-6882

John A. Menninger · Addiction Psychiatry · Colorado Psychiatric Hospital, University North Pavilion, 4455 East 12th Avenue, Campus Box A011-15, Denver, CO 80220 · 303-372-3156

Robert D. Miller · Forensic Psychiatry · University Hospital · University of Colorado Health Sciences Center, Department of Psychiatry, 4200 East Ninth Avenue, Campus Box C249-27, Denver, CO 80262 · 303-270-7613

Frederick W. Mimmack · Psychoanalysis (Psychology of Creativity, Sports Psychology) · 1231 South Parker Road, Suite 103, Denver, CO 80231 · 303-755-7606

Calvern E. Narcisi · Psychoanalysis (Adult & Child Psychoanalysis, Adolescent Psychiatry) · 4900 Cherry Creek South Drive, Denver, CO 80222 · 303-691-0941

Homer Olsen · Psychoanalysis · 722 Clarkson Street, Denver, CO 80218 · 303-861-2345

Joanne H. Ritvo · Eating Disorders (Affective & Anxiety Disorders, Physician Health) · University Hospital, HealthOne Behavioral Health Services-Bethesda Campus, Presbyterian/St. Luke's Medical Center · 501 South Cherry Street, Suite 650, Denver, CO 80222 · 303-329-0139

Ruth M. Ryan · Mental Retardation/Mental Health (Diagnosis & Treatment of Mental Disorders in Individuals with Developmental Disabilities and/or Mental Retardation) · University Hospital · University of Colorado Health Sciences Center, 4200 East Ninth Avenue, Campus Box C249-27, Denver, CO 80262 · 303-270-8313

I. Gene Schwarz · Psychoanalysis · Denver Institute for Psychoanalysis, University Hospital · 4900 Cherry Creek South Drive, Suite Two, Denver, CO 80222 · 303-758-3155

James H. Shore · General Psychiatry · Colorado Psychiatric Hospital · University of Colorado Health Sciences Center, 4200 East Ninth Avenue, Campus Box C249-32, Denver, CO 80262 · 303-270-5248

Richard C. Simons · Psychoanalysis (General Psychiatry) · University Hospital · 4900 Cherry Creek South Drive, Suite One, Denver, CO 80222 · 303-758-4711

Samuel Wagonfeld · Psychoanalysis (Adult & Child Psychoanalysis, Forensic Psychiatry, Adult & Child Psychotherapy) · HealthOne Behavioral Health Services-Bethesda Campus · 240 St. Paul Street, Denver, CO 80206 · 303-321-3275

Grand Junction

Robert A. Sammons, Jr. · General Psychiatry (Forensic Psychiatry, Mood & Anxiety Disorders, Psychopharmacology, Schizophrenia) · Mesa Behavioral Medicine Clinic, 2339 North Seventh Street, Grand Junction, CO 81501 · 970-241-1983

Loveland

John K. Nagel · General Psychiatry · 2216 Hoffman Drive, Suite Two, Loveland, CO 80530 · 970-667-2112

PULMONARY & CRITICAL CARE MEDICINE

Aurora

E. Michael Canham · General Pulmonary & Critical Care Medicine · Aurora Presbyterian Hospital, Aurora Regional Medical Center, Spalding Rehabilitation Hospital · Aurora Pulmonary Consultants, 830 Potomac Circle, Suite 345, Aurora, CO 80011 · 303-363-6208

Joseph M. Forrester · General Pulmonary & Critical Care Medicine (Sarcoidosis) Aurora Regional Medical Center, Aurora Presbyterian Hospital, Rose Medical Center (Denver), St. Joseph Hospital (Denver) · Critical Care & Pulmonary Consultants, 830 Potomac Circle, Suite 225, Aurora, CO 80011 · 303-360-3600

Boulder

Hunter R. Smith · General Pulmonary & Critical Care Medicine · 1000 Alpine Avenue, Suite 254, Boulder, CO 80304 · 303-442-2150

Colorado Springs

Allan B. Davidson · General Pulmonary & Critical Care Medicine · Pulmonary Associates, 1725 East Boulder Street, Suite 204, Colorado Springs, CO 80909 · 719-471-1069

Russell Lee · General Pulmonary & Critical Care Medicine · Colorado Springs Pulmonary Consultants, 25 East Jackson Street, Suite 202, Colorado Springs, CO 80907 · 719-471-7064

Robert Varnum · General Pulmonary & Critical Care Medicine · Colorado Springs Pulmonary Consultants, 25 East Jackson Street, Suite 202, Colorado Springs, CO 80907 · 719-471-7064

Denver

Enrique Fernandez · General Pulmonary & Critical Care Medicine · National Jewish Center for Immunology & Respiratory Medicine, 1400 Jackson Street, Room K-320A, Denver, CO 80206 · 303-388-4461

Michael D. Iseman · Lung Infections (Tuberculosis & Other Mycobacterial Diseases) · National Jewish Center for Immunology & Respiratory Medicine · National Jewish Center for Immunology & Respiratory Medicine, 1400 Jackson Street, Room J-205, Denver, CO 80206 · 303-398-1667

Talmadge E. King, Jr. · General Pulmonary & Critical Care Medicine (Interstitial Lung Disease, Bronchiolitis) · National Jewish Center for Immunology & Respiratory Medicine, University Hospital · National Jewish Center for Immunology & Respiratory Medicine, 1400 Jackson Street, Room B-108, Denver, CO 80206 · 303-398-1333

Richard Jay Martin · Asthma (Nocturnal Asthma, Bronchology, General Pulmonary & Critical Care Medicine) · National Jewish Center for Immunology & Respiratory Medicine · National Jewish Center for Immunology & Respiratory Medicine, 1400 Jackson Street, Room J-116, Denver, CO 80206-2761 · 303-398-1545

Thomas L. Petty · General Pulmonary & Critical Care Medicine, Asthma (Emphysema, Chronic Obstructive Pulmonary Disease) · HealthOne Center for Health Sciences Education · Presbyterian/St. Luke's Medical Center, 1719 East 19th Avenue, Denver, CO 80218 · 303-839-6740

Marvin I. Schwarz · General Pulmonary & Critical Care Medicine (Interstitial Lung Disease) · University Hospital, Denver General Hospital, National Jewish Center for Immunology & Respiratory Medicine · University of Colorado Health Sciences Center, 4200 East Ninth Avenue, Campus Box C272, Denver, CO 80262 303-270-7047

David P. White · General Pulmonary & Critical Care Medicine (Sleep Apnea/Sleep Disorders) · VA Medical Center, National Jewish Center for Immunology & Respiratory Medicine/University of Colorado Sleep Center · VA Medical Center, Department of Respiratory Care, 1055 Clermont Street, Box 111A, Denver, CO 80220 · 303-393-2869

Martin Zamora · General Pulmonary & Critical Care Medicine (Lung Transplantation) · University of Colorado Health Sciences Center, 4200 East Ninth Avenue, Campus Box C272, Denver, CO 80262 · 303-270-7047

Englewood

James T. Good · General Pulmonary & Critical Care Medicine (Sports Medicine) Swedish Medical Center, PorterCare Hospital (Denver), PorterCare Hospital-Littleton (Littleton) · South Denver Pulmonary Associates, 499 East Hampden Avenue, Suite 300, Englewood, CO 80110 · 303-788-8500

Fort Collins

Stanley R. Gunstream · General Pulmonary & Critical Care Medicine (Asthma, Pulmonary Rehabilitation) · Poudre Valley Hospital · 1247 Riverside Avenue, Suite One, Fort Collins, CO 80524 · 970-224-9102

Grand Junction

Joel J. Bechtel · General Pulmonary & Critical Care Medicine · 790 Wellington Avenue, Suite 105, Grand Junction, CO 81501 · 970-245-4810

Loveland

Donald R. Rollins · General Pulmonary & Critical Care Medicine · Aspen Medical Center, 1808 Boise Avenue, Loveland, CO 80538 · 970-669-6660

RADIATION ONCOLOGY

Colorado Springs

Mark Bernard Hazuka · Lung Cancer (Head & Neck Cancer) · Penrose-St. Francis Healthcare System, Memorial Hospital · Memorial Hospital, The Cancer Center, First Floor, 525 North Foote Avenue, Colorado Springs, CO 80909 · 719-475-5800

John E. Schiller · General Radiation Oncology · 110 East Monroe Street, Colorado Springs, CO 80907 · 719-776-5281

Grand Junction

F. Bing Johnson · General Radiation Oncology · St. Mary's Hospital, Department of Radiation Oncology, 2635 North Seventh Street, Grand Junction, CO 81501 · 970-244-2442

Gayle Miller · General Radiation Oncology · St. Mary's Hospital, Department of Radiation Oncology, 2635 North Seventh Street, Grand Junction, CO 81501 · 970-244-2442

Pueblo

Joel D. Ohlsen · General Radiation Oncology · St. Mary-Corwin Regional Medical Center, Department of Radiation Therapy, 1008 Minnequa Avenue, Pueblo, CO 81004 · 719-560-5460

RADIOLOGY

Colorado Springs

James P. Borgstede · General Radiology · 1465 North Union Boulevard, P.O. Box 2989, Colorado Springs, CO 80901 · 719-550-1200

Kathleen Davis · General Radiology (Magnetic Resonance Imaging) · Penrad Imaging, 116 East Monroe Street, Colorado Springs, CO 80907 · 719-630-5406

William F. Rogers · General Radiology · 1465 North Union Boulevard, P.O. Box 2989, Colorado Springs, CO 80901 · 719-471-2132

James P. Sweeney · General Radiology (Neuroradiology, Magnetic Resonance Imaging) · Penrose Hospital, Department of Radiology, 2215 North Cascade Avenue, Colorado Springs, CO 80907 · 719-776-5135

Denver

John Armstrong · Chest · University of Colorado Health Sciences Center, 4200 East Ninth Avenue, Campus Box A30, Denver, CO 80262 · 303-329-3066

David A. Kumpe · Cardiovascular Disease (Interventional Radiology, Liver/Biliary Disease, Neurovascular Disease) · University Hospital · University of Colorado Health Sciences Center, 4200 East Ninth Avenue, Campus Box A030, Denver, CO 80262 · 303-270-8198

David A. Lynch · Chest (Cardiovascular Disease) · University of Colorado Health Sciences Center, Department of Radiology, 4200 East Ninth Avenue, Campus Box A030, Denver, CO 80262 · 303-270-7171

Michael L. Manco-Johnson · General Radiology · University of Colorado Health Sciences Center, 4200 East Ninth Avenue, Campus Box C277, Denver, CO 80262 303-399-1211

Fort Collins

Richard J. Pacini · General Radiology · 1221 East Elizabeth Street, Suite Three, Fort Collins, CO 80524 · 970-484-8914

Grand Junction

Michael E. Holt · General Radiology · St. Mary's Hospital, Department of Radiology, 2635 North Seventh Street, Grand Junction, CO 81501 · 970-244-2556

RHEUMATOLOGY

Colorado Springs

C. Douglas Lain · General Rheumatology · 625 North Cascade Avenue, Suite 210, Colorado Springs, CO 80903 · 719-475-9613

Denver

Walter G. Briney · General Rheumatology, Osteoporosis · Rose Medical Center Denver Arthritis Clinic, 4545 East Ninth Avenue, Suite 510, Denver, CO 80220 303-394-2828

Herbert Kaplan · Rheumatoid Arthritis · Rose Medical Center · Denver Arthritis Clinic, 4545 East Ninth Avenue, Suite 510, Denver, CO 80220-3981 · 303-394-2828

Brian L. Kotzin · Lupus · National Jewish Center for Immunology & Respiratory Medicine · National Jewish Center for Immunology & Respiratory Medicine, 1400 Jackson Street, Room K-1020, Denver, CO 80206 · 303-398-1138

Sterling G. West · General Rheumatology (Lupus) · University Hospital, National Jewish Center for Immunology and Respiratory Medicine · University of Colorado Health Sciences Center, Department of Medicine, Division of Rheumatology, 4200 East Ninth Avenue, Denver, CO 80262 · 303-270-6654; 303-398-1475

Grand Junction

Steven Richard Ecklund · General Rheumatology · Western Slope Rheumatology, 790 Wellington Avenue, Suite 207, Grand Junction, CO 81501 · 970-242-2482

SURGERY

Colorado Springs

James M. LaVanway · General Surgery · Penrose-St. Francis Healthcare System Colorado Springs Surgical Associates, 25 East Jackson Street, Suite 201, Colorado Springs, CO 80907 · 719-635-2501

Paul T. O'Rourke · General Surgery (Breast Surgery, General Surgical Oncology) Penrose-St. Francis Healthcare System · Colorado Springs Surgical Associates, Margery Reed Professional Building, Suite 201, 25 East Jackson Street, Colorado Springs, CO 80907 · 719-635-2501

Amilu S. Rothhammer · General Surgery · 320 East Fontanero Street, Suite 306, Colorado Springs, CO 80907 · 719-635-7501

Denver

Charles O. Brantigan · General Vascular Surgery (Limb Preservation, Chronic Nonhealing Wounds, Reoperative Vascular Surgery, General Surgery, Surgical Critical Care, General Thoracic Surgery) · Presbyterian/St. Luke's Medical Center, St. Joseph Hospital · 2253 Downing Street, Denver, CO 80205 · 303-830-8822

Jack H. Chang · Pediatric Surgery (Neonatal Surgery, Pediatric Endosurgery) · Presbyterian/St. Luke's Medical Center, Rose Medical Center, Swedish Medical Center (Englewood), PorterCare Hospital, PorterCare Hospital-Littleton (Littleton), Children's Hospital · Rocky Mountain Pediatric Surgery, 1601 East 19th Avenue, Suite 5200, Denver, CO 80218 · 303-839-6001

Alden H. Harken · General Surgery (Cardiothoracic Surgery, Electrophysiology) University of Colorado Health Sciences Center, Department of Surgery, 4200 East Ninth Avenue, Campus Box C305, Denver, CO 80262 · 303-270-8055

C. Edward Hartford · General Surgery (Burn Surgery) · University Hospital · University of Colorado Health Sciences Center, 4200 East Ninth Avenue, Campus Box C298, Denver, CO 80262 · 303-270-7062

Igal Kam · General Surgery (Liver Transplantation, Major Liver Surgery, Kidney Transplantation) · University Hospital, Children's Hospital, Presbyterian/St. Luke's Medical Center · University of Colorado Health Sciences Center, 4200 East Ninth Avenue, Campus Box C318, Denver, CO 80262 · 303-270-7916

William C. Krupski · General Vascular Surgery · University of Colorado Health Sciences Center, Section of Vascular Surgery, 4200 East Ninth Avenue, Campus Box C312, Denver, CO 80262 · 303-270-6486

Ernest Eugene Moore · Trauma (Surgical Critical Care, Gastroenterologic Surgery, General Surgery, Liver Surgery) · Denver General Hospital, University Hospital · Denver General Hospital, 777 Bannock Street, Denver, CO 80204-4507 303-436-6558

Lawrence W. Norton · Breast Surgery · University Hospital · University of Colorado Health Sciences Center, 4200 East Ninth Avenue, Campus Box C311, Denver, CO 80220-3706 · 303-270-8671

David B. Roos · General Vascular Surgery (Thoracic Outlet Disorders) · Presbyterian/St. Luke's Medical Center · 1721 East 19th Avenue, Suite 206, Denver, CO 80218-1240 · 303-863-7667

Robert B. Rutherford · General Vascular Surgery (Aortic Surgery, Infrainguinal Bypass Surgery, Peripheral Artery Surgery, Extra-Anatomic Bypass, Carotid Surgery, Varicose Vein) · University Hospital · University of Colorado Health Sciences Center, Department of Vascular Surgery, 4200 East Ninth Avenue, Campus Box C312, Denver, CO 80262 · 303-270-8552

Jon Senkowsky · General Vascular Surgery · Colorado Vascular Institute, 2253 Downing Street, Denver, CO 80205 · 303-830-8822

Everett K. Spees, Jr. · Transplantation (Kidney & Pancreas Transplantation) · University Hospital · 1601 East 19th Avenue, Suite 5200, Denver, CO 80215 · 303-894-0200

Gregory Van Stiegmann · Gastroenterologic Surgery (Hepatobiliary Surgery, Pancreatic Surgery, Gastrointestinal Surgery) · University Hospital · University of Colorado Health Sciences Center, 4200 East Ninth Avenue, Campus Box C313, Denver, CO 80262 · 303-270-5526

Englewood

Glenn L. Kelly · General Vascular Surgery · Swedish Medical Center, PorterCare Hospital (Denver), PorterCare Hospital-Littleton (Littleton) · 601 East Hampden, Suite 320, Englewood, CO 80110 · 303-788-6606

Warren Kortz · General Vascular Surgery (Hepatobiliary Surgery, Pancreatic Surgery, Breast Surgery) · PorterCare Hospital (Denver), Swedish Medical Center, PorterCare Hospital-Littleton (Littleton) · 601 East Hampden, Suite 470, Englewood, CO 80110 · 303-789-1877

Grand Junction

George Shanks · General Surgery · 1001 Wellington Avenue, Grand Junction, CO 81501 · 970-243-0900

Loveland

Earl Baumgartel · General Surgery · McKee Medical Center · Loveland Surgical Associates, 1900 North Boise Avenue, Suite 210, Loveland, CO 80538 · 970-669-3212

SURGICAL ONCOLOGY

Denver

Fredrick L. Grover · General Surgical Oncology (Chest) · University Hospital · University of Colorado Health Sciences Center, Division of Cardiothoracic Surgery, 4200 East Ninth Avenue, Campus Box C310, Denver, CO 80262 · 303-270-8527

Nathaniel W. Pearleman · General Surgical Oncology (Colon & Rectal Cancer, Melanoma) · University Hospital · University of Colorado Health Sciences Center, 4500 East Ninth Avenue, Denver, CO 80262 · 303-270-8671

THORACIC SURGERY

Colorado Springs

James T. Anderson · Cardiothoracic Surgery · 25 East Jackson Street, Suite 104, Colorado Springs, CO 80907 · 719-473-3550

John J. Randono · General Thoracic Surgery · 25 East Jackson Street, Suite 104, Colorado Springs, CO 80907 · 719-473-3550

Denver

David N. Campbell · Adult Cardiothoracic Surgery, Pediatric Cardiac Surgery (Heart & Lung Transplantation, Pediatric Thoracic Surgery, General Thoracic Surgery) · University Hospital, Children's Hospital, VA Medical Center · University of Colorado Health Sciences Center, Division of Cardiothoracic Surgery, 4200 East Ninth Avenue, Campus Box C310, Denver, CO 80262 · 303-270-8527

Fredrick L. Grover · Transplantation, Adult Cardiothoracic Surgery (Heart Transplantation, Lung Transplantation, General Thoracic Surgery) · University Hospital · University of Colorado Health Sciences Center, Division of Cardiothoracic Surgery, 4200 East Ninth Avenue, Campus Box C310, Denver, CO 80262 · 303-270-8527

Marvin Pomerantz · General Thoracic Surgery · University Hospital · University of Colorado Health Sciences Center, 4200 East Ninth Avenue, Campus Box C310, Denver, CO 80262 · 303-270-8527

Grand Junction

Robert S. Brooks · General Thoracic Surgery · Western Cardiothoracic Associates, 425 Patterson Road, Suite 506, Grand Junction, CO 81506 · 970-242-7292

Theodore R. Sadler, Jr. · Adult Cardiothoracic Surgery (General Vascular Surgery, General Thoracic Surgery, Thoracic Oncological Surgery, Bronchology, Endoscopy, Pacemakers) · St. Mary's Hospital & Medical Center, Community Hospital · Western Cardiothoracic Associates, 425 Patterson Road, Suite 506, Grand Junction, CO 81506 · 970-242-7292

UROLOGY

Aurora

Joel M. Kaufman · Impotence · Aurora Urology, 1421 South Potomac Street, Suite 120, Aurora, CO 80012 · 303-695-6106

Colorado Springs

Craig K. Carris · General Urology (Urologic Oncology) · 320 East Fontanero Street, Suite 200, Colorado Springs, CO 80907 · 719-636-3811

Michael M. Crissey · General Urology (Urologic Oncology, Endourology) · Penrose-St. Francis Healthcare System, Memorial Hospital · 320 East Fontanero Street, Suite 200, Colorado Springs, CO 80907 · 719-636-3811

Patrick O. Faricy · General Urology · Penrose-St. Francis Healthcare System, Memorial Hospital · 2170 International Circle, Suite 145, Colorado Springs, CO 80910 · 719-634-1994

Denver

E. David Crawford · Urologic Oncology (Prostate Cancer) · University Hospital · University of Colorado Health Sciences Center, Division of Urology, 4200 East Ninth Avenue, Campus Box C319, Denver, CO 80262 · 303-270-5937

Robert E. Donohue · General Urology (Urologic Oncology, Diagnosis & Management of Acute & Chronic Scrotal Pathology) · University Hospital · University of Colorado Health Sciences Center, Division of Urology, 4200 East Ninth Avenue, Denver, CO 80262 · 303-270-5942

Martin A. Koyle · Pediatric Urology · The Children's Hospital, Department of Urology, 1056 East 19th Avenue, Denver, CO 80218 · 303-861-3926

Richard A. Schmidt · Neuro-Urology & Voiding Dysfunction · University of Colorado Health Sciences Center, 4200 East Ninth Avenue, Denver, CO 80262 · 303-270-6038

Grand Junction

Amir Z. Beshai · General Urology · 790 Wellington Avenue, Suite 202, Grand Junction, CO 81501 · 970-243-3061

Kenneth M. Simons · General Urology · 790 Wellington Avenue, Suite 202, Grand Junction, CO 81501 · 970-243-3061

IOWA

ALLERGY & IMMUNOLOGY

Ames

Edward G. Nassif · General Allergy & Immunology · The McFarland Clinic, Department of Allergy & Immunology, 1215 Duff Avenue, Ames, IA 50010 · 515-239-4404

Davenport

James L. Gillilland · General Allergy & Immunology · 2112 East 38th Street, Davenport, IA 52807 · 319-359-0324

Des Moines

James A. Wille · General Allergy & Immunology · 1212 Pleasant Street, Suite 109, Des Moines, IA 50309 · 515-283-0161

Dubuque

Dennis W. Rajtora · General Allergy & Immunology · Medical Associates Clinic, 1000 Langworthy Street, Dubuque, IA 52001-7313 · 319-589-9920

Iowa City

Richard C. Ahrens · General Allergy & Immunology (Allergy, Asthma) · University of Iowa Hospitals & Clinics · University of Iowa Hospitals & Clinics, Department of Pediatrics, 200 Hawkins Drive, Iowa City, IA 52242 · 319-356-1616

Zuhair K. Ballas · Immunodeficiency (Allergy, Clinical & Laboratory Immunology) · University of Iowa Hospitals & Clinics · University of Iowa Hospitals & Clinics, Department of Internal Medicine, 200 Hawkins Drive, Iowa City, IA 52242-1081 · 319-356-3697

Marta M. Little · General Allergy & Immunology (Asthma) · Mercy Hospital · Mercy Medical Plaza, Suite 305, 540 East Jefferson Street, Iowa City, IA 52245-2468 · 319-339-3850

Barbara Ann Muller · General Allergy & Immunology (General Internal Medicine) · University of Iowa Hospitals & Clinics · University of Iowa Hospitals & Clinics, Clinic B, Room BT1035, 200 Hawkins Drive, Iowa City, IA 52242-1009 319-356-3694

Hal B. Richerson · General Allergy & Immunology (Asthma, Clinical & Laboratory Immunology) · University of Iowa Hospitals & Clinics · University of Iowa Hospitals & Clinics, Department of Internal Medicine, 200 Hawkins Drive, Room SE 630GH, Iowa City, IA 52242-1081 · 319-356-2117

John M. Weiler · General Allergy & Immunology (Allergy, Asthma, Hereditary Angioedema, Sports Medicine) · University of Iowa Hospitals & Clinics · University of Iowa Hospitals & Clinics, Department of Internal Medicine, 200 Hawkins Drive, Iowa City, IA 52242-1081 · 319-356-2114

Miles M. Weinberger · General Allergy & Immunology (Allergy, Pediatric Pulmonology, Pediatric Clinical Pharmacology) · University of Iowa Hospitals & Clinics · University of Iowa Hospitals & Clinics, Department of Internal Medicine, 200 Hawkins Drive, Room 2449 CP, Iowa City, IA 52242-1083 · 319-356-3485

Mason City

Brian Alfred Brennan · General Allergy & Immunology (Pediatric Asthma) · North Iowa Mercy Health Center · Mason City Clinic, 250 South Crescent Drive, Mason City, IA 50401 · 515-421-6760

Sioux City

James D. Oggel · General Allergy & Immunology (Asthma, Clinical & Lab Immunology) · Marian Health Center, St. Luke's Regional Medical Center · Sioux City Allergy & Asthma Associates, 701 Pierce Street, Suite 305, Sioux City, IA 51101-1037 · 712-255-3749

ANESTHESIOLOGY

Des Moines

Vinay Kumar · General Anesthesiology · Iowa Methodist Medical Center · Associated Anesthesiologists, 1215 Pleasant Street, Suite 400, Des Moines, IA 50309 515-283-5722

Iowa City

John H. Tinker · Adult Cardiovascular, Cardiothoracic Anesthesiology, General Anesthesiology · University of Iowa Hospitals & Clinics · University of Iowa Hospitals & Clinics, Department of Anesthesia, 200 Hawkins Drive, Room 6621JCP, Iowa City, IA 52242-1079 · 319-356-2382

Michael M. Todd · Neuroanesthesia · University of Iowa Hospitals & Clinics · University of Iowa Hospitals & Clinics, Department of Anesthesia, 200 Hawkins Drive, Iowa City, IA 52242-1079 · 319-335-8540

Mason City

Patricia M. Hoffman · General Anesthesiology · Mason City Clinic, 250 South Crescent Drive, Mason City, IA 50401 · 515-421-6504

Minh K. Nguyen · General Anesthesiology (Pain Management, Acupuncture) · North Iowa Mercy Health Center · Mason City Clinic, Department of Anesthesiology, 250 South Crescent Drive, Mason City, IA 50401 · 515-421-6690

CARDIOVASCULAR DISEASE

Cedar Rapids

Lawrence J. Cook · General Cardiovascular Disease · 1002 Fourth Avenue, SE, Cedar Rapids, IA 52403 · 319-364-7101

Des Moines

David K. Lemon · General Cardiovascular Disease · The Iowa Clinic Mid-Iowa Heart Institute, 1440 Pleasant Street, Suite 200, Des Moines, IA 50314 · 515-241-5988

Hooshang Soltanzadeh · General Cardiovascular Disease · Cardiothoracic Surgery, 1440 Pleasant Street, Suite 150, Des Moines, IA 50314 · 515-241-5735

Craig Alan Stark · General Cardiovascular Disease · Mid-Iowa Heart Institute, 1440 Pleasant Street, Suite 200, Des Moines, IA 50309 · 515-241-5988

Iowa City

James R. Hopson · Electrophysiology (Pacemakers) · University of Iowa Hospitals & Clinics · University of Iowa Hospitals & Clinics, Cardiovascular Division, 200 Hawkins Drive, Iowa City, IA 52242-1009 · 319-356-2344

Richard E. Kerber · Echocardiography (Defibrillation, Cardiopulmonary Resuscitation) · University of Iowa Hospitals & Clinics · University of Iowa Hospitals & Clinics, Department of Internal Medicine, 200 Hawkins Drive, Room 4207RCP, Iowa City, IA 52242 · 319-356-2739

Michael G. Kienzle · Electrophysiology (Cardiac Catheterization, General Cardiovascular Disease, Heart Failure, Pacemakers) · University of Iowa Hospitals & Clinics · University of Iowa Hospitals & Clinics, 222 C Medicine Administration Building, Iowa City, IA 52242 · 319-353-5639

James D. Rossen · General Cardiovascular Disease · University of Iowa Hospitals & Clinics, Cardiovascular Division, 200 Hawkins Drive, Iowa City, IA 52242 · 319-356-3413

Sara J. Sirna · General Cardiovascular Disease (Cardiac Catheterization) · Mercy Hospital · 2460 Towncrest Drive, Iowa City, IA 52240 · 319-338-7862

David J. Skorton · Echocardiography (Congenital Heart Disease in Adolescents and Adults) · University of Iowa Hospitals & Clinics · University of Iowa Hospitals & Clinics, Department of Internal Medicine, 200 Hawkins Drive, Room E321GH, Iowa City, IA 52242-1081 · 319-335-2132

Byron F. Vandenberg · General Cardiovascular Disease (Echocardiography) · University of Iowa Hospitals & Clinics · University of Iowa Hospitals & Clinics, Department of Cardiovascular Disease, 200 Hawkins Drive, Iowa City, IA 52242-1009 · 319-356-3693

Michael D. Winniford · General Cardiovascular Disease · University of Iowa Hospitals & Clinics, Cardiovascular Division, 200 Hawkins Drive, Iowa City, IA 52242 · 319-356-3175

Mason City

Timothy Thomson · General Cardiovascular Disease · Mason City Clinic, Department of Cardiology, 250 South Crescent Drive, Mason City, IA 50401 · 515-421-6502

CLINICAL PHARMACOLOGY

Iowa City

Howard R. Knapp · (Lipid Disorders, Vascular Disease) · University of Iowa Hospitals & Clinics · University of Iowa Hospitals & Clinics, Department of Internal Medicine, 200 Hawkins Drive, Iowa City, IA 52242 · 319-356-4403

COLON & RECTAL SURGERY

Des Moines

Susan Beckwith · Colon & Rectal Cancer, General Colon & Rectal Surgery · Iowa Clinic Surgery, 1212 Pleasant Street, Des Moines, IA 50309 · 515-283-1541

Iowa City

Amanda M. T. Metcalf · General Colon & Rectal Surgery · University of Iowa Hospitals & Clinics, Department of Surgery, 200 Hawkins Drive, Room 4602JCP, Iowa City, IA 52242 · 319-356-3627

DERMATOLOGY

Cedar Rapids

John H. Wollner · Clinical Dermatology · 716 Fifth Avenue, SE, Cedar Rapids, IA 52401-1916 · 319-363-9936

Davenport

Dan Allen Bovenmyer · Clinical Dermatology · Bovenmyer Dermatology, 3319 Spring Street, Davenport, IA 52807-2125 · 319-359-1671

John A. Bovenmyer · Clinical Dermatology · Bovenmyer Dermatology, 3319 Spring Street, Davenport, IA 52807-2125 · 319-359-1671

Fort Dodge

Carey A. Bligard · Clinical Dermatology · Fort Dodge Medical Center, 804 Kenyon Road, Suite M, Fort Dodge, IA 50501 · 515-573-4141

Iowa City

Kathi C. Madison · Psoriasis (Photobiology, Clinical Dermatology) · University of Iowa Hospitals & Clinics · University of Iowa Hospitals & Clinics, Department of Dermatology, 200 Hawkins Drive, Iowa City, IA 52242 · 319-356-2274

Warren W. Piette · Cutaneous Lymphomas (Clinical Dermatology, Vasculitis) · University of Iowa Hospitals & Clinics · University of Iowa Hospitals & Clinics, Department of Dermatology, 200 Hawkins Drive, Iowa City, IA 52242 · 319-356-2274

Thomas L. Ray · Allergic Reactions of the Skin · University of Iowa Hospitals & Clinics, Department of Dermatology, 200 Hawkins Drive, Iowa City, IA 52242 · 319-356-2274

Mary S. Stone · Clinical Dermatology (Dermatopathology) · University of Iowa Hospitals & Clinics · University of Iowa Hospitals & Clinics, Department of Dermatology, 200 Hawkins Drive, Iowa City, IA 52242-1009 · 319-356-2274

John S. Strauss · Acne (Clinical Dermatology) · University of Iowa Hospitals & Clinics · University of Iowa Hospitals & Clinics, Department of Dermatology, 200 Hawkins Drive, Room BT2045-1, Iowa City, IA 52242-1009 · 319-356-2274

Duane C. Whitaker · Skin Cancer Surgery & Reconstruction (Mohs Micrographic Surgery & Reconstruction) · University of Iowa Hospitals & Clinics · University of Iowa Hospitals & Clinics, Department of Dermatology, 200 Hawkins Drive, Room BT2045-1, Iowa City, IA 52242-1090 · 319-356-2274

Mason City

C. Joseph Plank · Clinical Dermatology (Skin Cancer Surgery & Reconstruction, Laser Surgery) · 1023 Second Street, SW, Mason City, IA 50401-2856 · 515-424-0402

Ottumwa

Richard T. Ameln · Clinical Dermatology · Ottumwa Regional Health Center · Associates in Dermatology, 1005 East Pennsylvania Avenue, Suite 210, Ottumwa, IA 52501-6408 · 515-683-3195

West Des Moines

Roger I. Ceilley · Skin Cancer Surgery & Reconstruction (Mohs Micrographic Surgery & Reconstruction, Dermatopathology, Laser Surgery) · Iowa Methodist Medical Center (Des Moines), University of Iowa Hospitals & Clinics (Iowa City) Dermatology Associates, 6000 University Avenue, Suite 450, West Des Moines, IA 50266 · 515-241-2000

Charles W. Love · Clinical Dermatology (Skin Cancer Surgery & Reconstruction, Laser Surgery) · Iowa Dermatology Clinic, 6000 University Avenue, Suite 350, West Des Moines, IA 50266 · 515-226-8484

ENDOCRINOLOGY & METABOLISM

Ames

Richard P. Carano · General Endocrinology & Metabolism · The McFarland Clinic, Department of Endocrinology, 1215 Duff Avenue, Ames, IA 50010 · 515-239-4400

Cedar Rapids

William A. Davis · General Endocrinology & Metabolism · OBGYN, 855 A Avenue, NE, Cedar Rapids, IA 52402 · 319-368-5500

Davenport

Catherine L. Weideman · General Endocrinology & Metabolism · 1351 West Central Park, Suite 460, Davenport, IA 52804 · 319-328-5660

Des Moines

Edward J. Hertko · Diabetes · Iowa Diabetes and Endocrinology Center, 1601 Northwest 114th Street, Suite 138, Des Moines, IA 50325 · 515-225-2401

Nancy Kane Johnson · General Endocrinology & Metabolism · Iowa Diabetes and Endocrinology Center, 1601 Northwest 114th Street, Suite 138, Des Moines, IA 50325 · 515-225-2401

Diana L. Wright · General Endocrinology & Metabolism · Iowa Diabetes and Endocrinology Center, 1601 Northwest 114th Street, Suite 138, Des Moines, IA 50325 · 515-225-2401

Iowa City

Frederick K. Chapler · (Reproductive Endocrinology, Reproductive Surgery) · University of Iowa Hospitals & Clinics · University of Iowa Hospitals & Clinics, Department of Ob-Gyn, Reproductive Endocrinology, Infertility, 200 Hawkins Drive, Iowa City, IA 52242 · 319-356-1767

John Harper MacIndoe · General Endocrinology & Metabolism (Thyroid, Clinical Diabetes) · University of Iowa Hospitals & Clinics · University of Iowa Hospitals & Clinics, Department of Internal Medicine, 200 Hawkins Drive, Room E421GH, Iowa City, IA 52242 · 319-339-7168

FAMILY MEDICINE

Coralville

Susan M. Goodner · Family Health Centre, 414 Tenth Avenue, Coralville, IA 52241 · 319-351-3196

Ralph H. Knudson · Family Health Centre, 414 Tenth Avenue, Coralville, IA 52241 · 319-351-3196

Des Moines

Robert L. Bender II · Mercy West Clinic, 1601 Northwest 114th Street, Suite 247, Des Moines, IA 50325-7036 · 515-222-7070

Iowa City

George R. Bergus · (General Family Practice, Geriatric Medicine) · Mercy Hospital, University of Iowa Hospitals & Clinics · University of Iowa College of Medicine, Department of Family Practice, 2133 Steindler Building, Iowa City, IA 52242-1097 · 319-335-8456

Richard C. Dobyns · University of Iowa Hospitals & Clinics, Department of Family Practice, 200 Hawkins Drive, Iowa City, IA 52242 · 319-356-1616

Charles E. Driscoll · Iowa City Family Practice, 1011 Arthur Street, Iowa City, IA 52242 · 319-351-6852

John W. Ely · University of Iowa Hospitals & Clinics, Mercy Hospital · University of Iowa Hospitals & Clinics, Department of Family Practice, 200 Hawkins Drive, Iowa City, IA 52242 · 319-356-1616

Evan W. Kligman · (Geriatric Medicine, Clinical Prevention) · University of Iowa Hospitals & Clinics, Mercy Hospital · University of Iowa College of Medicine, Department of Family Practice, 2149 Steindler Building, Iowa City, IA 52242-1097 · 319-335-8454

Barcey T. Levy · (Obstetrical Anesthesia, Infant Feeding) · Mercy Hospital, University of Iowa Hospitals & Clinics · University of Iowa Hospitals & Clinics, Department of Family Practice, 200 Hawkins Drive, Iowa City, IA 52242 · 319-356-1616

Thomas A. Novak · Iowa City Family Practice, 1011 Arthur Street, Iowa City, IA 52240 · 319-351-6852

Mason City

Paul Howard Gordon · Mercy Family Care, 1023 Second Street, SW, Mason City, IA 50401 · 515-424-4191

Muscatine

Rhea J. Allen · Muscatine Health Center, 1514 Mulberry Avenue, Muscatine, IA 52761 · 319-264-3220

GASTROENTEROLOGY

Ames

Jon Lee Fleming · General Gastroenterology · The McFarland Clinic, 1215 Duff Avenue, Ames, IA 50010 · 515-239-4400

Des Moines

James G. Piros · General Gastroenterology · Iowa Clinics Gastroenterology, 1215 Pleasant Street, Suite 200, Des Moines, IA 50309 · 515-241-6102

Iowa City

James Christensen · General Gastroenterology (Gastrointestinal Motility) · University of Iowa Hospitals & Clinics · University of Iowa Hospitals & Clinics, Department of Gastroenterology, 200 Hawkins Drive, Mail Code R4548JCP, Iowa City, IA 52242-1081 · 319-356-2670

F. Jeffrey Field · General Gastroenterology · University of Iowa Hospitals & Clinics, Division of Gastroenterology, 200 Hawkins Drive, Iowa City, IA 52242 · 319-356-2579

Frederick Carl Johlin · General Gastroenterology · University of Iowa Hospitals & Clinics, Department of Internal Medicine, 200 Hawkins Drive, Iowa City, IA 52242 · 319-356-4030

Joseph Murray · General Gastroenterology (Celiac Disease, Esophageal Disease) University of Iowa Hospitals & Clinics · University of Iowa Hospitals & Clinics, Department of Gastroenterology, 200 Hawkins Drive, Iowa City, IA 52242 · 319-356-8246

Robert W. Summers · Gastrointestinal Motility (Inflammatory Bowel Disease, General Gastroenterology) · University of Iowa Hospitals & Clinics · University of Iowa Hospitals & Clinics, Division of Gastroenterology/Hepatology, 200 Hawkins Drive, Iowa City, IA 52242-1081 · 319-356-2130

HAND SURGERY

Iowa City

Curtis M. Steyers · General Hand Surgery (Pediatric Orthopaedic Surgery, Peripheral Nerve Surgery) · University of Iowa Hospitals & Clinics · University of Iowa Hospitals & Clinics, Department of Orthopaedics, 200 Hawkins Drive, Room 01077JPP, Iowa City, IA 52242 · 319-356-3943

West Des Moines

Arnis B. Grundberg · General Hand Surgery · Des Moines Orthopaedic Surgeons, 6001 West Town Parkway, West Des Moines, IA 50266 · 515-224-5204

Douglas Stephen Reagan · General Hand Surgery · Des Moines Orthopaedic Surgeons, 6001 West Town Parkway, West Des Moines, IA 50266 · 515-224-5206

INFECTIOUS DISEASE

Davenport

Louis Mayer Katz · General Infectious Disease · Quad City Regional Virology, 1351 West Central Park, Suite 320, Davenport, IA 52804 · 319-328-5469

Des Moines

Lisa A. Veach · General Infectious Disease (AIDS, Hospital-Acquired Infections) Iowa Methodist Medical Center, Iowa Lutheran Hospital · Integra Health, 1221 Pleasant Street, Suite 300, Des Moines, IA 50309-1417 · 515-241-4200

Iowa City

Richard P. Wenzel · Hospital-Acquired Infections (Assessing Quality Health Care) · University of Iowa Hospitals & Clinics · University of Iowa Hospitals & Clinics, Department of Internal Medicine, 200 Hawkins Drive, Room C-41GH, Iowa City, IA 52242 · 319-356-1838

INTERNAL MEDICINE (GENERAL)

Cedar Rapids

Thomas J. McIntosh · (Clinical Pharmacology) · Mercy Medical Center, St. Luke's Methodist Hospital · 115 Eighth Street, NE, Cedar Rapids, IA 52401-1097 319-363-9954

Davenport

Edwin A. Motto · 1228 East Rusholme Street, Suite 310, Davenport, IA 52803 · 319-326-6273

Douglas E. Vickstrom · 1228 East Rusholme Street, Suite 310, Davenport, IA 52803 · 319-326-6273

Des Moines

Steven R. Craig · (Geriatric Medicine) · Iowa Methodist Medical Center, Iowa Lutheran Hospital · Integra Health, Methodist Medical Plaza III, Suite 200, 1221 Pleasant Street, Des Moines, IA 50309-1425 · 515-241-4000

John Hupp Ghrist II · Iowa Clinic, 1428 Woodland Avenue, Des Moines, IA 50309 · 515-283-1733

Iowa City

Craig M. Champion · Internal Medicine, 2460 Towncrest Drive, Iowa City, IA 52240-6622 · 319-338-7862

Bradley N. Doebbeling · (Hospital-Acquired Infections, General Infectious Diseases) · VA Medical Center · University of Iowa Hospitals & Clinics, Department of Internal Medicine, 200 Hawkins Drive, Iowa City, IA 52242 · 319-356-8556

James R. Flanagan · University of Iowa Hospitals & Clinics, Department of Internal Medicine, 200 Hawkins Drive, Iowa City, IA 52242 · 319-356-1616

William B. Galbraith · University of Iowa Hospitals & Clinics, Department of Internal Medicine, 200 Hawkins Drive, Room BT1036, Iowa City, IA 52242-1009 319-353-8766

Karl Larsen · (Hypertension, Hyperlipidemia) · Mercy Hospital · Internal Medicine, 2460 Towncrest Drive, Iowa City, IA 52240-6622 · 319-338-7862

Thomas Nicknish · 2460 Towncrest Drive, Iowa City, IA 52240-6622 · 319-338-7862

Rodney B. Zeitler · VA Medical Center, Department of Internal Medicine, 22 Warwick Circle, Iowa City, IA 52240-2847 · 319-338-0581

Mason City

Charles R. Caughlan · (Geriatric Medicine) · Mason City Clinic, Department of Internal Medicine, 250 South Crescent Drive, Mason City, IA 50401 · 515-421-6782

Linda Grandgenett Floden · Mason City Clinic, 250 South Crescent Drive, Mason City, IA 50401 · 515-421-6783

Mark C. Johnson · Mason City Clinic, Department of Internal Medicine, 250 South Crescent Drive, Mason City, IA 50401 · 515-421-6785

Mt. Pleasant

John P. Bennett · (Lymphomas, Chronic Leukemia) · Henry County Health Center · Family Medicine of Mt. Pleasant, One Park Plaza, Mt. Pleasant, IA 52641 · 319-385-6710

Muscatine

Robert F. Weis · Muscatine General Hospital · Muscatine Health Center, 1514 Mulberry Avenue, Muscatine, IA 52761-3490 · 319-264-3220

Ottumwa

Peter Joseph Reiter · 1005 East Pennsylvania Avenue, Ottumwa, IA 52501 · 515-682-4594

Sioux City

David W. Lucke · (General Cardiovascular Disease, General Geriatric Medicine, Diabetes) · Marian Health Center, St. Luke's Regional Medical Center · 522 Fourth Street, Suite 100, Sioux City, IA 51101 · 712-255-5001

MEDICAL ONCOLOGY & HEMATOLOGY

Ames

M. Michael Guffy · General Medical Oncology & Hematology · The McFarland Clinic, 1215 Duff Avenue, Ames, IA 50010 · 515-239-4400

Larry A. Otteman · General Medical Oncology & Hematology · The McFarland Clinic, Department of Oncology-Hematology, 1215 Duff Avenue, Ames, IA 50010-5400 · 515-239-4401

Des Moines

Thomas R. Buroker · General Medical Oncology & Hematology · Iowa Clinic, 1221 Pleasant Street, Suite 100, Des Moines, IA 50309 · 515-282-2921

Roscoe F. Morton · General Medical Oncology & Hematology · Iowa Clinic, 1221 Pleasant Street, Suite 100, Des Moines, IA 50309-1414 · 515-282-2921

Iowa City

Gerald H. Clamon · General Medical Oncology & Hematology · University of Iowa Hospitals & Clinics · University of Iowa Hospitals & Clinics, Department of Hematology-Oncology, 200 Hawkins Drive, Iowa City, IA 52242 · 319-356-1932

NEPHROLOGY

Des Moines

Prem K. G. Chandran · Dialysis · Edward Hines, Jr. VA Medical Center (Hines, IL), Iowa Methodist Medical Center, Iowa Lutheran Hospital, Mercy Hospital Medical Center, Des Moines General Hospital, Browdlawns Medical Center, Skiff Medical Center (Newton), Greater Community Hospital (Creston) · 1215 Pleasant Street, Suite 100, Des Moines, IA 50309 · 515-241-5710

Iowa City

Michael J. Flanigan · Dialysis · University of Iowa Hospitals & Clinics · University of Iowa College of Medicine, Department of Internal Medicine, 200 Hawkins Drive, Room W340GH, Iowa City, IA 52242-1009 · 319-356-3500

Lawrence G. Hunsicker · Kidney Transplantation, General Nephrology, Glomerular Diseases · University of Iowa Hospitals & Clinics · University of Iowa Hospitals & Clinics, Nephrology Division, 200 Hawkins Drive, Room E 300-F GH, Iowa City, IA 52242-1081 · 319-356-4763

NEUROLOGICAL SURGERY

Iowa City

Patrick W. T. Hitchon · Spinal Surgery, Stereotactic Radiosurgery · University of Iowa Hospitals & Clinics, Department of Neurosurgery, 200 Hawkins Drive, Iowa City, IA 52242 · 319-356-2775

Christopher M. Loftus · Vascular Neurological Surgery, General Neurological Surgery (Carotid Artery Surgery, Intracranial Aneurysms) · University of Iowa Hospitals & Clinics, VA Medical Center · University of Iowa Hospitals & Clinics, Division of Neurosurgery, 200 Hawkins Drive, Room 1845JPP, Iowa City, IA 52242 · 319-356-3853

Arnold H. Menezes · Pediatric Neurological Surgery (Cranial Cervical Stabilization Problems, Spine, Surgery of the Cranial Vertebral Junction, Transoral Surgery) · University of Iowa Hospitals & Clinics · University of Iowa Hospitals & Clinics, Division of Neurosurgery, 200 Hawkins Drive, Room 1841JPP, Iowa City, IA 52242 · 319-356-2768

Vincent C. Traynelis · Spinal Surgery (Tumor Surgery) · University of Iowa Hospitals & Clinics · University of Iowa Hospitals & Clinics, Department of Neurosurgery, 200 Hawkins Drive, Iowa City, IA 52242 · 319-356-2774

John C. VanGilder · General Neurological Surgery (Pituitary) · University of Iowa Hospitals & Clinics · University of Iowa Hospitals & Clinics, Division of Neurosurgery, 200 Hawkins Drive, Room 1840JPP, Iowa City, IA 52242-1086 · 319-356-2772

NEUROLOGY

Ames

Michael Kitchell · General Neurology · The McFarland Clinic, Department of Neurology, 1215 Duff Avenue, Ames, IA 50010 · 515-239-4435

John McKee · General Neurology (Stroke, Epilepsy) · Mary Greeley Medical Center, Skiff Medical Center (Newton), Marshalltown Medical & Surgical Center (Marshalltown) · The McFarland Clinic, Department of Neurology, 1215 Duff Avenue, Ames, IA 50010 · 515-239-4435

Cedar Rapids

Laurence S. Krain · Neuromuscular Disease (General Neurology) · St. Luke's Methodist Hospital, Mercy Medical Center · Iowa Medical Clinic, 600 Seventh Street, SE, Cedar Rapids, IA 52401-2112 · 319-398-1721

Eric W. Streib · General Neurology · Neurological Associates, 1030 Fifth Avenue, SE, Suite 2600, Cedar Rapids, IA 52403 · 319-366-7990

Clive

Lynn L. Struck · General Neurology · Iowa Physicians Clinic, Department of Neurology, 1221 Pleasant Street, Suite 300, Clive, IA 50309 · 515-241-4200

Iowa City

Harold P. Adams, Jr. · Strokes (Subarachnoid Hemorrhage) · University of Iowa Hospitals & Clinics · University of Iowa Hospitals & Clinics, Department of Neurology, 200 Hawkins Drive, Iowa City, IA 52242 · 319-356-8755

Antonio Damasio · Degenerative Diseases, Behavioral Neurology (Language Disorders, Memory Loss, Visual-Perceptual Disorders, Alzheimer's Disease) · University of Iowa Hospitals & Clinics · University of Iowa Hospitals & Clinics, Department of Neurology, 200 Hawkins Drive, Room 2007RCP, Iowa City, IA 52242-1053 · 319-356-0450

Hanna Damasio · Behavioral Neurology, Degenerative Diseases (Advanced Brain Imaging Techniques) · University of Iowa Hospitals & Clinics · University of Iowa Hospitals & Clinics, Department of Neurology, 200 Hawkins Drive, Iowa City, IA 52242-1053 · 319-356-1616

Richard W. Fincham · General Neurology (Epilepsy) · University of Iowa Hospitals & Clinics · University of Iowa Hospitals & Clinics, Department of Neurology, 200 Hawkins Drive, Iowa City, IA 52242 · 319-356-2571

Betsy Beattie Love · General Neurology (Stroke) · University of Iowa Hospitals & Clinics, Knoxville Area Community Hospital (Knoxville), Madison County Memorial Hospital (Winterset), Grinnell Regional Medical Center (Grinnell) · University of Iowa Hospitals & Clinics, Department of Neurology, 200 Hawkins Drive, Iowa City, IA 52242 · 319-356-1616

Robert L. Rodnitzky · General Neurology (Movement Disorders) · University of Iowa Hospitals & Clinics · University of Iowa Hospitals & Clinics, Department of Neurology, 200 Hawkins Drive, Iowa City, IA 52242 · 319-356-2571

Michael Wall · Neuro-Ophthalmology · University of Iowa Hospitals & Clinics · University of Iowa Hospitals & Clinics, Department of Neurology, 200 Hawkins Drive, Room 2149RCP, Iowa City, IA 52242-1009 · 319-356-2932

Mason City

Sohan F. Hayreh · General Neurology (Vascular Diseases) · Mason City Clinic, Department of Neurology, 250 South Crescent Drive, Mason City, IA 50401-1523 515-421-6760

NEUROLOGY, CHILD

Iowa City

James Franklin Bale, Jr. · General Child Neurology (Congenital Infections, Cytomegalovirus Infections) · University of Iowa Hospitals & Clinics · University of Iowa Hospitals & Clinics, Iowa Children's Health Care Center, 200 Hawkins Drive, Iowa City, IA 52242 · 319-356-7727

William E. Bell · Central Nervous System Infections, General Child Neurology · University of Iowa Hospitals & Clinics · University of Iowa Hospitals & Clinics, Department of Neurology, 200 Hawkins Drive, Room 2506JCP, Iowa City, IA 52242 · 319-356-2833

NUCLEAR MEDICINE

Cedar Rapids

John L. Floyd · General Nuclear Medicine · Cedar Rapids Radiologists, 1948 First Avenue, NE, Cedar Rapids, IA 52402 · 319-364-0121

Iowa City

David L. Bushnell · General Nuclear Medicine (Nuclear Cardiology, Radionuclide Therapy, Oncology) · VA Medical Center, Highway Six West, Iowa City, IA 52246-2208 · 319-338-0581 x6030; 319-356-3380

Maleah Grover-McKay · Nuclear Cardiology (Radiology, Cardiovascular Disease, Cardiovascular Disease in Women) · University of Iowa Hospitals & Clinics · University of Iowa Hospitals & Clinics, Department of Internal Medicine, 200 Hawkins Drive, Iowa City, IA 52242 · 319-356-8248

Daniel Kahn · General Nuclear Medicine · VA Medical Center, Highway Six West, Iowa City, IA 52246 · 319-338-0581 x6030

Peter T. Kirchner · General Nuclear Medicine · University of Iowa Hospitals & Clinics · University of Iowa Hospitals & Clinics, Division of Nuclear Medicine, 200 Hawkins Drive, Iowa City, IA 52242-1077 · 319-356-4302

Karim Rezai · General Nuclear Medicine · University of Iowa Hospitals & Clinics, Nuclear Medicine/Radiology Department, 200 Hawkins Drive, Iowa City, IA 52242 · 319-356-1911

James E. Seabold · General Nuclear Medicine (Radiopharmaceutical Therapy) · University of Iowa Hospitals & Clinics, Department of Radiology, 200 Hawkins Drive, Iowa City, IA 52242 · 319-356-4388

OBSTETRICS & GYNECOLOGY

Des Moines

William Gordon Cross · Gynecologic Cancer · Mid-Iowa OB-GYN, 1212 Pleasant Street, Suite 405, Des Moines, IA 50309 · 515-243-8842

Steven A. Keller · General Obstetrics & Gynecology · Iowa Methodist Medical Center, Mercy Hospital Medical Center · Iowa Physicians Clinic, 1221 Pleasant Street, Suite 400, Des Moines, IA 50309 · 515-241-4161

Rebecca D. Shaw · General Obstetrics & Gynecology · Mid-Iowa OB-GYN, 1212 Pleasant Street, Suite 405, Des Moines, IA 50309-1413 · 515-243-8842

Iowa City

Barrie Anderson · Gynecologic Cancer · University of Iowa Hospitals & Clinics University of Iowa Hospitals & Clinics, Department of Obstetrics & Gynecology, 200 Hawkins Drive, Room 4630JCP, Iowa City, IA 52242 · 319-356-2015

Jennifer R. Niebyl · Maternal & Fetal Medicine · University of Iowa Hospitals & Clinics · University of Iowa Hospitals & Clinics, Department of Obstetrics & Gynecology, 200 Hawkins Drive, Iowa City, IA 52242 · 319-356-1976

Frank J. Zlatnik · Maternal & Fetal Medicine · University of Iowa Hospitals & Clinics, Department of Obstetrics & Gynecology, 200 Hawkins Drive, Iowa City, IA 52242 · 319-356-3617

Mason City

Gene M. Kuehn · General Obstetrics & Gynecology · Associates in Obstetrics & Gynecology, 1023 Second Street, SW, Suite 200, Mason City, IA 50401 · 515-423-3062

OPHTHALMOLOGY

Cedar Falls

Norman F. Woodlief · General Ophthalmology (Anterior Segment—Cataract & Refractive, Vitreo-Retinal Surgery) · Sartori Memorial Hospital, Covenant Medical Center (Waterloo), Waverly Municipal Hospital (Waverly) · Wolfe Eye Clinic, Sartori Professional Building, 516 South Division Street, Cedar Falls, IA 50613-2380 · 319-277-0103

Cedar Rapids

Steven J. Jacobs · General Ophthalmology · Iowa Eye Center, 1650 First Avenue, NE, Cedar Rapids, IA 52402 · 319-362-3937

Alexander G. Smith · General Ophthalmology · Iowa Eye Center, 1650 First Avenue, NE, Cedar Rapids, IA 52402 · 319-362-3937

Davenport

Siv Brit Saetre · General Ophthalmology · Davenport Medical and Surgical Eye Group, 1228 East Rusholme Street, Davenport, IA 52803-2467 · 319-322-0923

Kristen K. Wells · General Ophthalmology · Davenport Medical and Surgical Eye Group, 1228 East Rusholme Street, Davenport, IA 52803-2467 · 319-322-0923

Des Moines

Robert S. Brown · General Ophthalmology · 974 Seventy-Third Street, Suite 33, Des Moines, IA 50312 · 515-225-3546

Fort Dodge

Eric W. Bligard · General Ophthalmology · Wolfe Clinic, 804 South Kenyon Road, Fort Dodge, IA 50501 · 515-576-7777

Iowa City

Wallace L. M. Alward · Glaucoma · University of Iowa Hospitals & Clinics · University of Iowa Hospitals & Clinics, Department of Ophthalmology, 200 Hawkins Drive, Iowa City, IA 52242-1091 · 319-356-2228

H. Culver Boldt · Vitreo-Retinal Surgery, Medical Retinal Diseases (Ocular Oncology) · University of Iowa Hospitals & Clinics · University of Iowa Hospitals & Clinics, Department of Ophthalmology, 200 Hawkins Drive, Iowa City, IA 52242-1091 · 319-353-6112

Keith D. Carter · Oculoplastic & Orbital Surgery · University of Iowa Hospitals & Clinics, Department of Ophthalmology, 200 Hawkins Drive, Iowa City, IA 52242 319-356-7997

James C. Folk · Vitreo-Retinal Surgery (Retinal Diseases) · University of Iowa Hospitals & Clinics, Department of Ophthalmology, 200 Hawkins Drive, Iowa City, IA 52242-1091 · 319-356-2215

Randy H. Kardon · Neuro-Ophthalmology (Pupillography) · University of Iowa Hospitals & Clinics, VA Medical Center · University of Iowa Hospitals & Clinics, Department of Ophthalmology, 200 Hawkins Drive, Iowa City, IA 52242-1091 · 319-356-1951

Ronald V. Keech · Pediatric Ophthalmology (Strabismus, Pediatric Cataracts) · University of Iowa Hospitals & Clinics · University of Iowa Hospitals & Clinics, Department of Ophthalmology, 200 Hawkins Drive, Iowa City, IA 52242-1091 · 319-356-3990

Alan E. Kimura · Medical Retinal Diseases, Vitreo-Retinal Surgery (Electroretinography) · University of Iowa Hospitals & Clinics · University of Iowa Hospitals & Clinics, Department of Ophthalmology, 200 Hawkins Drive, Iowa City, IA 52242-1091 · 319-356-2215

William D. Mathers · Corneal Diseases & Transplantation · University of Iowa Hospitals & Clinics · University of Iowa Hospitals & Clinics, Department of Ophthalmology, 200 Hawkins Drive, Iowa City, IA 52242-1091 · 319-356-2861

Mariannette J. Miller-Meeks · General Ophthalmology (Cataract/Intraocular Lens Implant, Glaucoma) · University of Iowa Hospitals & Clinics · University of Iowa Hospitals & Clinics, Department of Ophthalmology, 200 Hawkins Drive, Iowa City, IA 52242-1091 · 319-356-2215

Jeffrey A. Nerad · Oculoplastic & Orbital Surgery (Reconstructive Surgery, Facial Aesthetic Surgery) · University of Iowa Hospitals & Clinics · University of Iowa Hospitals & Clinics, Department of Ophthalmology, 200 Hawkins Drive, Iowa City, IA 52242-1091 · 319-356-2590

William E. Scott · Pediatric Ophthalmology (Strabismus) · University of Iowa Hospitals & Clinics · University of Iowa Hospitals & Clinics, Department of Ophthalmology, 200 Hawkins Drive, Iowa City, IA 52242-1091 · 319-356-2877

Edwin M. Stone · Ophthalmic Genetics (Retinal Diseases) · University of Iowa Hospitals & Clinics · University of Iowa Hospitals & Clinics, Department of Ophthalmology, 200 Hawkins Drive, Iowa City, IA 52242-1091 · 319-335-8270

Lyse S. Strnad · General Ophthalmology · Mercy Hospital · Eye Physicians And Surgeons, Mercy Medical Plaza, Suite 201, 540 East Jefferson, Iowa City, IA 52245-2464 · 319-338-3623

John E. Sutphin, Jr. · Corneal Diseases & Transplantation (Keratorefractive Surgery) · University of Iowa Hospitals & Clinics · University of Iowa Hospitals & Clinics, Department of Ophthalmology, 200 Hawkins Drive, Iowa City, IA 52242-1091 · 319-356-2861

H. Stanley Thompson · Neuro-Ophthalmology (Pupillary Problems) · University of Iowa Hospitals & Clinics · University of Iowa Hospitals & Clinics, Department of Ophthalmology, 200 Hawkins Drive, Iowa City, IA 52242-1091 · 319-356-2868

Thomas A. Weingeist · Medical Retinal Diseases, Vitreo-Retinal Surgery (Medical & Surgical Retinal Diseases, Ocular Oncology) · University of Iowa Hospitals & Clinics · University of Iowa Hospitals & Clinics, Department of Ophthalmology, Pomerantz Family Pavilion, 200 Hawkins Drive, Iowa City, IA 52242-1091 · 319-356-2867

Marshalltown

James A. Davison · Anterior Segment—Cataract & Refractive · Marshalltown Medical & Surgical Center · Wolfe Clinic, 309 East Church Street, Marshalltown, IA 50158 · 515-754-6200

John M. Graether · General Ophthalmology · Wolfe Clinic, 309 East Church Street, Marshalltown, IA 50158 · 515-752-1565

Mason City

Randall S. Brenton · General Ophthalmology (Corneal Diseases & Transplantation) · North Iowa Mercy Health Center, Floyd County Memorial Hospital (Charles City) · North Iowa Eye Clinic, Highway 18 West, P.O. Box 1877, Mason City, IA 50402-1877 · 515-423-8861

Addison W. Brown · General Ophthalmology (Anterior Segment—Cataract, Vitreo-Retinal Surgery) · North Iowa Eye Clinic, Highway 18 West, P.O. Box 1877, Mason City, IA 50402-1877 · 515-423-8861

Ottumwa

Gregory L. Thorgaard · General Ophthalmology · Ottumwa Regional Health Center · Southeast Iowa Eye Specialists, 1005 East Pennsylvania Avenue, Suite 207, Ottumwa, IA 52501 · 515-682-8571

West Des Moines

Christopher F. Blodi · Vitreo-Retinal Surgery (Retinal Diseases, Ocular Oncology) · Iowa Methodist Medical Center (Des Moines), Mercy Hospital Medical Center (Des Moines), Mercy Hospital (Cedar Rapids) · Iowa Retina Consultants, Regency West Building One, Suite 133, 1501 Fiftieth Street, West Des Moines, IA 50266-5920 · 515-222-6400

Jean B. Spencer · General Ophthalmology · Central Iowa Pediatric Ophthalmology, 6000 University Avenue, Suite 475, West Des Moines, IA 50266 · 515-222-1180

ORTHOPAEDIC SURGERY

Des Moines

Jeffrey Michael Farber · Pediatric Orthopaedic Surgery · Iowa Orthopaedic Center, 411 Laurel Street, Suite 3300, Des Moines, IA 50314-3005 · 515-247-8400

Iowa City

John J. Callaghan · Reconstructive Surgery (Total Joint, Hip & Knee, Sports Medicine/Arthroscopy, Trauma) · University of Iowa Hospitals & Clinics · University of Iowa Hospitals & Clinics, Department of Orthopaedic Surgery, 200 Hawkins Drive, Iowa City, IA 52242-1009 · 319-356-3110

James N. Weinstein · Spinal Surgery · University of Iowa Hospitals & Clinics, Department of Orthopaedic Surgery, 200 Hawkins Drive, Room 01069JPP, Iowa City, IA 52242 · 319-356-1638

Stuart L. Weinstein · Pediatric Orthopaedic Surgery (Hip Surgery, Pediatric Spine Surgery) · University of Iowa Hospitals & Clinics · University of Iowa Hospitals & Clinics, Department of Orthopaedic Surgery, 200 Hawkins Drive, Iowa City, IA 52242-1009 · 319-356-1872

Mason City

Sterling John Laaveg · General Orthopaedic Surgery · 250 South Crescent Drive, Mason City, IA 50401 · 515-421-6630

West Des Moines

Richard C. Johnston · Reconstructive Surgery (Knee Surgery, Hip Surgery) · Iowa Methodist Medical Center (Des Moines) · 6001 Westown Parkway, West Des Moines, IA 50266 · 515-224-1414

OTOLARYNGOLOGY

Des Moines

Peter V. Boesen · General Otolaryngology · 1000 Seventy-Third Street, Suite 18, Des Moines, IA 50311-1321 · 515-267-0691

Richard Boyd Merrick · General Otolaryngology (Facial Aesthetic Surgery, Head & Neck Surgery) · Iowa Clinic, 3901 Ingersoll Avenue, Des Moines, IA 50312 · 515-274-9135

Iowa City

Gerry F. Funk · Head & Neck Surgery (Reconstructive Surgery, Free-Tissue Transfer, Facial Plastic Surgery) · University of Iowa Hospitals & Clinics · University of Iowa Hospitals & Clinics, Department of Otolaryngology, 200 Hawkins Drive, Iowa City, IA 52242-1009 · 319-356-2165

Bruce J. Gantz · Otology/Neurotology, Skull-Base Surgery (Acoustic Neuroma, Cochlear Implants, Skull-Base Tumors) · University of Iowa Hospitals & Clinics University of Iowa Hospitals & Clinics, Department of Otolaryngology-Head & Neck Surgery, 200 Hawkins Drive, Iowa City, IA 52242-1078 · 319-356-2173

Henry T. Hoffman · Head & Neck Surgery, Laryngology · University of Iowa Hospitals & Clinics · University of Iowa Hospitals & Clinics, Department of Otolaryngology, 200 Hawkins Drive, Iowa City, IA 52242-1009 · 319-356-2166

Richard J. H. Smith · Pediatric Otolaryngology (Hereditary Hearing Loss, Airway Anomalies) · University of Iowa Hospitals & Clinics · University of Iowa Hospitals & Clinics, Department of Otolaryngology, 200 Hawkins Drive, Room E230GH, Iowa City, IA 52242-1078 · 319-356-3612

Mason City

Philip C. Lee · General Otolaryngology (Sinus & Nasal Surgery) · Mason City Clinic, Department of Ear, Nose and Throat, 250 South Crescent Drive, Mason City, IA 50401 · 515-421-6600

PATHOLOGY

Iowa City

Fred R. Dick · Hematopathology (Bone Marrow, Lymph Node) · University of Iowa Hospitals & Clinics, Department of Pathology, 200 Hawkins Drive, Iowa City, IA 52242 · 319-356-1616

PEDIATRICS

Ames

Edward G. Nassif · Pediatric Pulmonology · The McFarland Clinic, Department of Pediatrics, 1215 Duff Avenue, Ames, IA 50010 · 515-239-4404

Des Moines

Jennifer S. Cook · Pediatric Endocrinology · Pediatric Specialties, 1200 Pleasant Street, Des Moines, IA 50309-1406 · 515-241-8222

Dee Narawong · (Pediatric Neurology) · Pediatric Specialties, 1200 Pleasant Street, Des Moines, IA 50309-1406 · 515-241-8222

Iowa City

Richard C. Ahrens · Pediatric Pulmonology (Cystic Fibrosis, Asthma) · University of Iowa Hospitals & Clinics · University of Iowa Hospitals & Clinics, Department of Pediatrics, 200 Hawkins Drive, Iowa City, IA 52242 · 319-356-1616

Randell C. Alexander · Abused Children · University of Iowa Hospitals & Clinics University of Iowa Hospitals & Clinics, 209 Hospital School, Iowa City, IA 52242-1011 · 319-353-6136

Dianne L. Atkins · Pediatric Cardiology (Electrophysiology) · University of Iowa Hospitals & Clinics · University of Iowa Hospitals & Clinics, Department of Pediatrics, Division of Pediatric Cardiology, 200 Hawkins Drive, Iowa City, IA 52242-1009 · 319-356-3540

Edward F. Bell · Neonatal-Perinatal Medicine · University of Iowa Hospitals & Clinics · University of Iowa Hospitals & Clinics, Department of Pediatrics, Division of Neonatology, 200 Hawkins Drive, Iowa City, IA 52242-1009 · 319-356-4006

Patricia A. Donohoue · Pediatric Endocrinology · University of Iowa Hospitals & Clinics · University of Iowa Hospitals & Clinics, Division of Pediatric Endocrinology, 200 Hawkins Drive, Second Floor JPP, Iowa City, IA 52242 · 319-356-3164

Charles F. Grose · Pediatric Infectious Disease · University of Iowa Hospitals & Clinics, Department of Pediatrics, 200 Hawkins Drive, Iowa City, IA 52242 · 319-356-2288

Robert P. Hoffman · Pediatric Endocrinology (Pediatric Diabetes) · University of Iowa Hospitals & Clinics · University of Iowa Hospitals & Clinics, Department of Pediatric Endocrinology, 200 Hawkins Drive, Room 2860JPP, Iowa City, IA 52242 · 319-356-4511

Mary M. Jones · (Pediatric Rheumatology) · University of Iowa Hospitals & Clinics, Department of Pediatrics, 200 Hawkins Drive, Iowa City, IA 52242 · 319-356-3484

Robert P. Kelch · Pediatric Endocrinology (Sexual Development) · University of Iowa College of Medicine, 212 C Medicine Administration Building, Iowa City, IA 52242-1101 · 319-335-8064

Jonathan M. Klein · Neonatal-Perinatal Medicine · University of Iowa Hospitals & Clinics · University of Iowa Hospitals & Clinics, Department of Pediatrics, 200 Hawkins Drive, Iowa City, IA 52242-1009 · 319-356-3340

Jennifer Hunder Kyllo · Pediatric Endocrinology · University of Iowa Hospitals & Clinics · University of Iowa Hospitals & Clinics, 200 Hawkins Drive, Iowa City, IA 52242-1009 · 319-356-2838

Ronald M. Lauer · Pediatric Cardiology · University of Iowa Hospitals & Clinics University of Iowa Hospitals & Clinics, Department of Pediatrics, 200 Hawkins Drive, Room 2801JPP, Iowa City, IA 52242-1057 · 319-356-2839

Larry T. Mahoney · Pediatric Cardiology (Preventive Cardiology) · University of Iowa Hospitals & Clinics · University of Iowa Hospitals & Clinics, Division of Pediatric Cardiology, 200 Hawkins Drive, Iowa City, IA 52242-1009 · 319-356-2837

Mary Jeannette Hagan Morriss · Pediatric Cardiology · University of Iowa Hospitals & Clinics · University of Iowa Hospitals & Clinics, 200 Hawkins Drive, Iowa City, IA 52242-1009 · 319-356-4084

Jeffrey C. Murray · (Genetics, Neonatology) · University of Iowa Hospitals & Clinics, Department of Pediatrics, 200 Hawkins Drive, Iowa City, IA 52242 · 319-356-2674

William J. Rhead · Metabolic Diseases (Fatty Acid Oxidation, Organic Acidemias, Inherited Biochemical Disorders) · University of Iowa Hospitals & Clinics University of Iowa Hospitals & Clinics, Department of Pediatrics, Medical Genetics, 200 Hawkins Drive, Room 2606JCP, Iowa City, IA 52242-1057 · 319-356-2674

Jean E. Robillard · Pediatric Nephrology (General Pediatrics) · University of Iowa Hospitals & Clinics · University of Iowa Hospitals & Clinics, Department of Pediatrics, 225 Medical Laboratories, 200 Hawkins Drive, Iowa City, IA 52242 · 319-335-7560

James A. Royall · Pediatric Critical Care (Pediatric Pulmonology) · University of Iowa Hospitals & Clinics · University of Iowa Hospitals & Clinics, Department of Pediatrics, Division of Pediatric Critical Care, 200 Hawkins Drive, Iowa City, IA 52242-1009 · 319-356-1057

Raymond Tannous · Pediatric Hematology-Oncology · University of Iowa Hospitals & Clinics, Department of Pediatrics, 200 Hawkins Drive, Iowa City, IA 52242 · 319-356-1905

Michael E. Trigg · Pediatric Hematology-Oncology (Bone Marrow Transplantation) · University of Iowa Hospitals & Clinics · University of Iowa Hospitals & Clinics, Department of Pediatric Hematology-Oncology, 2526 John Colloton Pavilion, Iowa City, IA 52242 · 319-356-1608

Eva Tsalikian · Pediatric Endocrinology (Diabetes) · University of Iowa Hospitals & Clinics · University of Iowa Hospitals & Clinics, Department of Pediatrics, 200 Newton Road, Room 2JPP, Iowa City, IA 52242 · 319-356-1833

Miles M. Weinberger · Pediatric Pulmonology (Clinical Pharmacology, Pediatric Allergy & Immunology) · University of Iowa Hospitals & Clinics · University of Iowa Hospitals & Clinics, Department of Pediatrics, 200 Hawkins Drive, Room 2449 CP, Iowa City, IA 52242-1083 · 319-356-3485

John A. Widness · Neonatal-Perinatal Medicine · University of Iowa Hospitals & Clinics · University of Iowa Hospitals & Clinics, Department of Pediatrics, 200 Hawkins Drive, Iowa City, IA 52242 · 319-356-8102

Ekhard E. Ziegler · (Nutrition of Normal Infants, Nutrition of Premature Infants, Mineral Metabolism) · University of Iowa Hospitals & Clinics · University of Iowa Hospitals & Clinics, Department of Pediatrics, 200 Hawkins Drive, Iowa City, IA 52242 · 319-356-2836

PEDIATRICS (GENERAL)

Ames

Jack T. Swanson · Mary Greeley Medical Center · McFarland Clinic, Department of Pediatrics, 1215 Duff Avenue, Ames, IA 50010 · 515-239-4404

Burlington

William R. Daws · Burlington Pediatric Association, 610 North Fourth Street, Burlington, IA 52601 · 319-753-5177

Cedar Rapids

Kenneth W. Anderson · Health Source Pediatrics, 855 A Avenue, NE, Suite 100, Cedar Rapids, IA 52402 · 319-368-9301

Julianne H. Thomas · Pediatric Center, 411 Tenth Street, SE, Suite 150, Cedar Rapids, IA 52403 · 319-363-3600

Davenport

Robert F. Anderson, Jr. · Pediatric Group, 4017 Devil's Glen Road, Suite 200, Davenport, IA 52722 · 319-332-6500; 319-328-5109

Barry S. Barudin · 1230 East Rusholme Street, Suite 109, Davenport, IA 52803-2400 · 319-326-2755

Gregory L. Garvin · Genesis Medical Center, Davenport Medical Center · PremierCare, Medical Pavilion, Suite 1100, 1351 West Central Park, Davenport, IA 52804 · 319-383-2581

Dubuque

Keevin J. Franzen · Dubuque Pediatrics, Professional Arts Plaza, Suite 106, 200 Mercy Drive, Dubuque, IA 52001 · 319-557-1711

Donald Harvey Reyerson · Medical Associates Clinic, 1000 Langworthy Street, Dubuque, IA 52001 · 319-589-9700

Iowa City

Carlyn Christensen-Szalanski · Adolescent and Pediatric Health Clinic, 540 East Jefferson Street, Suite 102, Box 146, Iowa City, IA 52244 · 319-337-8467

Claibourne I. Dungy · (General Pediatrics, Infant Feeding, Primary Care Research) · University of Iowa Hospitals & Clinics · University of Iowa Hospitals & Clinics, Department of Pediatrics, 200 Hawkins Drive, Room 2558, Iowa City, IA 52242 · 319-356-3644

Stanley Hackbarth · Pediatric Associates, 605 East Jefferson Street, Iowa City, IA 52245 · 319-351-1448

Mary S. Larew · Pediatric Associates, 605 East Jefferson Street, Iowa City, IA 52245 · 319-351-1448

John R. Maxwell · 611 East Market Street, Iowa City, IA 52245-2634 · 319-338-7821

Jody R. Murph · (Cytomegalovirus Infections, Violence Prevention, General Pediatrics) · University of Iowa Hospitals & Clinics · University of Iowa Hospitals & Clinics, Department of Pediatrics, 200 Hawkins Drive, Iowa City, IA 52242 · 319-356-3986

Mason City

John C. Justin · (Attention Deficit Hyperactivity Disorder) · North Iowa Mercy Health Center · Pediatric and Adolescent Clinic, 1190 Briarstone Drive, Mason City, IA 50401-4638 · 515-424-0640

David L. Little · (Behavior, Asthma, General Pediatrics) · North Iowa Mercy Health Center · Pediatric and Adolescent Clinic, 1190 Briarstone Drive, Mason City, IA 50401 · 515-424-0640

Russell G. Smidt · Forest Park Pediatrics, 1023 Second Street, SW, Suite 240, Mason City, IA 50401 · 515-421-5681

Leah M. Willson · Forest Park Pediatrics, 1023 Second Street, SW, Suite 240, Mason City, IA 50401 · 515-421-5681

Ottumwa

Jay C. Heitsman · Ottumwa Pediatrics, 1005 East Pennsylvania Avenue, Ottumwa, IA 52501-6408 · 515-682-8739

Sioux City

Ray C. Sturdevant · Prairie Pediatrics, 2800 Pierce Street, Suite 207, Sioux City, IA 51104 · 712-255-8901

West Des Moines

William G. Bartlett · Iowa Physicians Clinic, 6000 University Avenue, Suite 100, West Des Moines, IA 50266 · 515-241-2500

Carol R. Rodemyer · Iowa Physicians Clinic, Department of Pediatrics, 6000 University Avenue, Suite 100, West Des Moines, IA 50266 · 515-241-2500

PLASTIC SURGERY

Des Moines

Jeffrey S. Carithers · General Plastic Surgery (Facial Plastic Surgery, Reconstructive Surgery, Rhinoplasty, Facelift) · Iowa Methodist Medical Center, Mercy Hospital Medical Center, Iowa Lutheran Hospital · Carithers Facial Surgery, 535 Fortieth Street, Des Moines, IA 50312 · 515-277-5555

Iowa City

John W. Canady · General Plastic Surgery (Pediatric Plastic Surgery, Craniofacial Surgery) · University of Iowa Hospitals & Clinics · University of Iowa Hospitals & Clinics, Department of Plastic Surgery & Otolaryngology, 200 Hawkins Drive, Iowa City, IA 52242-1009 · 319-356-2168

PSYCHIATRY

Cedar Rapids

Judith H. W. Crossett · Geriatric Psychiatry · St. Luke's Methodist Hospital, Mercy Medical Center · Cedar Center Psychiatric Group, 1730 First Avenue, NE, Cedar Rapids, IA 52402-5433 · 319-365-3993

Des Moines

Richard E. Preston · General Psychiatry · 1221 Center Street, Suite Eight, Des Moines, IA 50309 · 515-283-1221

Iowa City

Arnold E. Andersen · Eating Disorders, General Psychiatry (Anorexia Nervosa, Bulimia Nervosa) · University of Iowa Hospitals & Clinics · University of Iowa Hospitals & Clinics, Department of Psychiatry Administration, 200 Hawkins Drive, Room 2887JPP, Iowa City, IA 52242-1057 · 319-356-1354

Nancy C. Andreasen · Schizophrenia (Behavioral Neurology) · University of Iowa Hospitals & Clinics · University of Iowa Hospitals & Clinics, Mental Health Clinical Research Center, Room 2911JPP, 200 Hawkins Drive, Iowa City, IA 52242-1057 · 319-356-1553

Donald W. Black · General Psychiatry (Obsessive Compulsive Disorders) · University of Iowa Hospitals & Clinics · University of Iowa Hospitals & Clinics, Psychiatry Research, Medical Education Building, 200 Hawkins Drive, Iowa City, IA 52242-1000 · 319-353-4431

James C. N. Brown · General Psychiatry · 432 East Bloomington Street, Iowa City, IA 52245 · 319-338-7941

Remi Jere Cadoret · General Psychiatry (Antisocial Personality, Substance Abuse) · University of Iowa College of Medicine, Psychiatric Research, Medical Education Building, 200 Hawkins Drive, Iowa City, IA 52242-1000 · 319-353-3887

Brian L. Cook · Addiction Psychiatry (Alcoholism, Affective Disorders, Psychopharmacology) · VA Medical Center · VA Medical Center, Psychiatry Service, Highway Six West, Iowa City, IA 52246 · 319-338-0581

William Coryell · Mood & Anxiety Disorders (Depression, Mania, Psychopharmacology) · University of Iowa Hospitals & Clinics · University of Iowa Hospitals & Clinics, Psychiatry Research, Medical Education Building, Iowa City, IA 52242-1000 · 319-353-4434

Raymond R. Crowe · Mood & Anxiety Disorders (Behavior Genetics) · University of Iowa Hospitals & Clinics, Department of Psychiatry, 200 Hawkins Drive, Iowa City, IA 52242 · 319-356-1616

Roger G. Kathol · (Medical Psychiatry, Health Services/Outcomes, General Internal Medicine) · University of Iowa Hospitals & Clinics · University of Iowa Hospitals & Clinics, Department of Psychiatry, 200 Hawkins Drive, Iowa City, IA 52242 · 319-356-3131

Russell Noyes, Jr. · Mood & Anxiety Disorders (Anxiety) · University of Iowa Hospitals & Clinics · University of Iowa Hospitals & Clinics, Psychiatry Research, Medical Education Building, Iowa City, IA 52242-1000 · 319-353-3898

Bruce M. Pfohl · General Psychiatry (Personality Disorders) · University of Iowa Hospitals & Clinics, Department of Psychiatry, 200 Hawkins Drive, Iowa City, IA 52242 · 319-356-1350

Joseph Piven · Child & Adolescent Psychiatry (Neuropsychiatry, Mental Retardation/Mental Health) · University of Iowa Hospitals & Clinics · University of Iowa Hospitals & Clinics, 1875 John Pappajohn Pavilion, 200 Hawkins Drive, Iowa City, IA 52242-1057 · 319-356-2011

Robert G. Robinson · Neuropsychiatry, Mood & Anxiety Disorders (Mood Disorders Related to Depression in Brain Injury, Strokes, Geriatric Psychiatry) · University of Iowa Hospitals & Clinics · University of Iowa Hospitals & Clinics, Department of Psychiatry, 200 Hawkins Drive, Room 2887JPP, Iowa City, IA 52242-1057 · 319-356-4658

George Winokur · Mood & Anxiety Disorders (General Psychiatry, Schizophrenia) · University of Iowa Hospitals & Clinics · University of Iowa Hospitals & Clinics, Psychiatry Research, Medical Education Building, Room 2887JPP, 200 Hawkins Drive, Iowa City, IA 52242-1000 · 319-353-4551

William R. Yates · General Psychiatry (Substance Use Disorders, Mood & Anxiety Disorders, Psychopharmacology) · University of Iowa Hospitals & Clinics · University of Iowa Hospitals & Clinics, Department of Psychiatry, 200 Hawkins Drive, Iowa City, IA 52242 · 319-353-8529

PULMONARY & CRITICAL CARE MEDICINE

Iowa City

William Lister Dull · General Pulmonary & Critical Care Medicine · 321 East Market Street, Suite 106, Iowa City, IA 52245 · 319-351-1860

John Frederick Fieselmann · General Pulmonary & Critical Care Medicine · University of Iowa Hospitals & Clinics · University of Iowa Hospitals & Clinics, 200 Hawkins Drive, Iowa City, IA 52242 · 319-356-8343

Jeffrey Kern · General Pulmonary & Critical Care Medicine (Asthma, Bronchology, Lung Infections, Lung Cancer) · University of Iowa Hospitals & Clinics · University of Iowa Hospitals & Clinics, 200 Hawkins Drive, Iowa City, IA 52242-1081 · 319-356-4186

RADIATION ONCOLOGY

Des Moines

William L. McGinnis · General Radiation Oncology · John Stoddard Cancer Center, 1221 Pleasant Street, Suite A-100, Des Moines, IA 50309 · 515-241-4330

Iowa City

David H. Hussey · General Radiation Oncology, Genito-Urinary Cancer, Head & Neck Cancer · University of Iowa Hospitals & Clinics · University of Iowa Hospitals & Clinics, Division of Radiation Oncology, 200 Hawkins Drive, Room W189Z-GH, Iowa City, IA 52242-1077 · 319-356-2699

RADIOLOGY

Des Moines

Kevin J. Koch · General Radiology · Iowa Methodist Hospital, Radiology Department, 1200 Pleasant Street, Level C, Des Moines, IA 50309 · 515-241-6171

Iowa City

George Y. El-Khoury · (Musculoskeletal Trauma, Spinal Imaging, Musculoskeletal Tumor Imaging) · University of Iowa Hospitals & Clinics · University of Iowa Hospitals & Clinics, Department of Radiology, 200 Hawkins Drive, Iowa City, IA 52242-1009 · 319-356-3654

E. A. Franken, Jr. · Pediatric Radiology · University of Iowa Hospitals & Clinics, Department of Radiology, 200 Hawkins Drive, Iowa City, IA 52242 · 319-356-3391

Wilbur L. Smith, Jr. · Pediatric Radiology · University of Iowa Hospitals & Clinics, Department of Radiology, 200 Hawkins Drive, Iowa City, IA 52240 · 319-356-1956

William Stanford · Cardiovascular Disease (Chest, Magnetic Resonance Imaging) University of Iowa Hospitals & Clinics, Department of Radiology, 200 Hawkins Drive, Iowa City, IA 52242-1077 · 319-356-3393

Mason City

Timothy John Lucas · General Radiology · Radiologists of Mason City, Forest Park Medical Building, Suite 100, 1023 Second Street, SW, Mason City, IA 50401 515-424-4932

RHEUMATOLOGY

Ames

David D. Gerbracht · General Rheumatology · The McFarland Clinic, Department of Rheumatology, 1215 Duff Avenue, Ames, IA 50010 · 515-239-4400

Cedar Rapids

Michael S. Brooks · General Rheumatology (Lupus, Vasculitis) · Iowa Medical Clinic, 600 Seventh Street, SE, Cedar Rapids, IA 52401-2112 · 319-398-1546

Steven Eyanson · General Rheumatology (Lupus, Scleroderma) · Mercy Medical Center, St. Luke's Methodist Hospital · Iowa Medical Clinic, 600 Seventh Street, SE, Cedar Rapids, IA 52401 · 319-398-1546

George Ho, Jr. · Infectious Arthritis · Iowa Medical Clinic, Mercy Medical Center, St. Luke's Methodist Hospital · Iowa Medical Center, 600 Seventh Street, SE, Cedar Rapids, IA 52401 · 319-398-1546

Davenport

Nancy E. Sadler · General Rheumatology (Osteoporosis) · Genesis Medical Center · Orthopaedic Surgery Associates, 1414 West Lombard Street, Davenport, IA 52804-2151 · 319-322-0971

David B. Staub · General Rheumatology · Genesis Medical Center, Genesis Medical Center-West Campus · Orthopaedic Surgery Associates, 1414 West Lombard Street, Davenport, IA 52804-2151 · 319-322-0971

Des Moines

Michael J. Finan · General Rheumatology · Mercy Arthritis Center, 1601 Northwest 114th Street, Suite 151, Des Moines, IA 50325-7046 · 515-222-7400

Nathan Josephson · General Rheumatology · Iowa Methodist Medical Center, The Consortium, 1415 Woodland Avenue, Suite 130, Des Moines, IA 50309 · 515-241-4455

Mary A. Radia · General Rheumatology · Iowa Methodist Medical Center · Iowa Physicians Clinic, 1221 Pleasant Street, Suite 200, Des Moines, IA 50309-1417 · 515-241-4200

Lawrence J. Rettenmaier · General Rheumatology · Mercy Arthritis & Osteoporosis Center, 1601 Northwest 114th Street, Suite 151, Des Moines, IA 50325-7046 · 515-222-7400

Theodore W. Rooney · General Rheumatology (Osteoporosis, Clinical Research) Mercy Hospital Medical Center, Iowa Methodist Medical Center, Iowa Lutheran Hospital, Des Moines General Hospital · Mercy Arthritis & Osteoporosis Center, 1601 Northwest 114th Street, Suite 151, Des Moines, IA 50325-7046 · 515-222-7400

Dubuque

Mark W. Niemer · General Rheumatology · Medical Associates Clinic, 1000 Langworthy Street, Dubuque, IA 52001-7313 · 319-556-1166

Iowa City

Robert F. Ashman · General Rheumatology · University of Iowa Hospitals & Clinics · University of Iowa Hospitals & Clinics, Department of Internal Medicine, Division of Rheumatology, 200 Hawkins Drive, Iowa City, IA 52242-1009 · 319-356-2287

John S. Cowdery, Jr. · General Rheumatology (Vasculitis, Rheumatoid Arthritis) University of Iowa Hospitals & Clinics · University of Iowa Hospitals & Clinics, Department of Rheumatology, 200 Hawkins Drive, Iowa City, IA 52242-1009 · 319-356-4414

Elizabeth H. Field · General Rheumatology · VA Medical Center, Highway Six West, Mail Code 6W33, Iowa City, IA 52246 · 319-338-0581 x6240

George V. Lawry II · General Rheumatology · University of Iowa Hospitals & Clinics, Division of Rheumatology, 200 Hawkins Drive, Room 612GH, Iowa City, IA 52242-1081 · 319-356-1777

Stanley J. Naides · General Rheumatology · University of Iowa Hospitals & Clinics · University of Iowa Hospitals & Clinics, Department of Internal Medicine, Division of Rheumatology, 200 Hawkins Drive, Iowa City, IA 52242 · 319-356-2809

John W. Rachow · General Rheumatology (Geriatric Medicine) · University of Iowa Hospitals & Clinics · University of Iowa Hospitals & Clinics, Department of Internal Medicine, 200 Hawkins Drive, Iowa City, IA 52242 · 319-356-4529

Kenneth G. Saag · General Rheumatology (Rheumatoid Arthritis, Arthritis Epidemiology Research) · University of Iowa Hospitals & Clinics · University of Iowa Hospitals & Clinics, Department of Internal Medicine, Division of Rheumatology, 200 Hawkins Drive, Iowa City, IA 52242-1081 · 319-356-4413

Louise H. Sparks · General Rheumatology (Rheumatoid Arthritis, Seronegative Spondyloarthropathies) · Mercy Hospital · Steindler Orthopedic Clinic, 2403 Towncrest Drive, Iowa City, IA 52240 · 319-338-3606

M. Paul Strottman · General Rheumatology · University of Iowa Hospitals & Clinics, Department of Rheumatology, 200 Hawkins Drive, Iowa City, IA 52242 319-356-2413

Mason City

R. Bruce Trimble · General Rheumatology · Mason City Clinic, Department of Rheumatology, 250 South Crescent Drive, Mason City, IA 50401-1523 · 515-421-6780

SURGERY

Ames

Bruce M. Hardy · General Surgery (Breast Surgery, Gastroenterologic Surgery) · Mary Greeley Medical Center · The McFarland Clinic, Department of Surgery, 1215 Duff Avenue, Ames, IA 50010 · 515-239-4725

Des Moines

Louis D. Rodgers · General Surgery · 1212 Pleasant Street, Suite 211, Des Moines, IA 50309-1411 · 515-283-1541

Iowa City

Gerald Patrick Kealey · General Surgery (Burns, Trauma) · University of Iowa Hospitals & Clinics, Department of Surgery, 200 Hawkins Drive, Room 1504JCP, Iowa City, IA 52242-1086 · 319-356-1616

John Preston Lawrence · Pediatric Surgery · University of Iowa Hospitals & Clinics, 200 Hawkins Drive, Iowa City, IA 52242 · 319-353-8331

Maureen Frances Martin · Transplantation · University of Iowa Hospitals & Clinics · University of Iowa Hospitals & Clinics, 200 Hawkins Drive, Iowa City, IA 52242 · 319-356-1334

Mason City

Steven C. Allgood · General Surgery · North Iowa Mercy Health Center · Mason City Clinic, 250 South Crescent Drive, Mason City, IA 50401 · 515-421-6710

Pablo Rene Recinos-Rivera · General Surgery (General Vascular Surgery, Non-Cardiac Thoracic Surgery) · Mason City Clinic, 250 South Crescent Drive, Mason City, IA 50401 · 515-421-6710

THORACIC SURGERY

Des Moines

Ronald K. Grooters · General Thoracic Surgery · The Iowa Clinic Mid-Iowa Heart Institute, 1440 Pleasant Street, Des Moines, IA 50309 · 515-241-5735

Iowa City

Douglas M. Behrendt · General Thoracic Surgery · University of Iowa Hospitals & Clinics, Department of Surgery, 200 Hawkins Drive, Iowa City, IA 52242-1009 319-356-2761

Wayne E. Richenbacher · Adult Cardiothoracic Surgery (Transplantation, Mechanical Circulatory Support) · University of Iowa Hospitals & Clinics · University of Iowa Hospitals & Clinics, Department of Surgery, Division of Cardiothoracic Surgery, 200 Hawkins Drive, Iowa City, IA 52242 · 319-356-4087

UROLOGY

Cedar Rapids

Dennis L. Boatman · General Urology · Lynn County Urology, 1260 Second Avenue, SE, Cedar Rapids, IA 52403 · 319-363-8171

Davenport

Thomas C. McKay · General Urology · Urology Associates, 3319 Spring Street, Suite 202, Davenport, IA 52807 · 319-359-1641

Des Moines

Harlan K. Rosenberg · General Urology · Iowa Methodist Medical Center · Iowa Clinic, 1212 Pleasant Street, Suite 414, Des Moines, IA 50309-1413 · 515-244-8000

Steven Joel Rosenberg · General Urology (Pediatric Urology, Urologic Oncology) Iowa Methodist Medical Center · Iowa Clinic, 1212 Pleasant Street, Suite 414, Des Moines, IA 50309 · 515-244-8000

Iowa City

Bernard Fallon · Impotence (Endourology, Stones) · University of Iowa Hospitals & Clinics · University of Iowa Hospitals & Clinics, Department of Urology, 200 Hawkins Drive, Iowa City, IA 52242-1089 · 319-356-1616

Charles E. Hawtrey · General Urology (Pediatric Urology) · University of Iowa Hospitals & Clinics, Department of Urology, 200 Hawkins Drive, Iowa City, IA 52242-1009 · 319-356-2273

Karl J. Kreder · Neuro-Urology & Voiding Dysfunction · University of Iowa Hospitals & Clinics, Department of Urology, 200 Hawkins Drive, Iowa City, IA 52242-1089 · 319-356-1616

Richard D. Williams · Urologic Oncology (Immunotherapy, Cancer Biotherapy, Genito-Urinary Cancer) · University of Iowa Hospitals & Clinics · University of Iowa Hospitals & Clinics, Department of Urology, 200 Hawkins Drive, Room 3251RCP, Iowa City, IA 52242 · 319-356-2934

Howard N. Winfield · Endourology (Stone Disease, Ureteroscopy, Percutaneous, Laparoscopic Surgery) · University of Iowa Hospitals & Clinics · University of Iowa Hospitals & Clinics, Department of Urology, 200 Hawkins Drive, Iowa City, IA 52242-1089 · 319-356-1895

Mason City

Paul S. MacGregor · General Urology · North Iowa Mercy Health Center · Mason City Clinic, Department of Urology, 250 South Crescent Drive, Mason City, IA 50401 · 515-421-6700

Kevin Rier · General Urology (Pediatric Urology, Endourology) · North Iowa Mercy Health Center · Mason City Clinic, Department of Urology, 250 South Crescent Drive, Mason City, IA 50401 · 515-421-6700

Steven H. Schurtz · General Urology (Oncology, Impotence) · North Iowa Mercy Health Center, Franklin General Hospital (Hampton), Ellsworth Municipal Hospital (Iowa Falls), Kossuth Regional Health Center (Algona), Mitchell County Regional Health Center (Osage) · Mason City Clinic, Department of Urology, 250 South Crescent Drive, Mason City, IA 50401-2926 · 515-421-6700

KANSAS

ALLERGY & IMMUNOLOGY

Hays

Katheryn Black · General Allergy & Immunology · 2517 Canterbury Road, Hays, KS 67601 · 913-628-1551

Kansas City

Daniel J. Stechschulte · General Allergy & Immunology · University of Kansas Medical Center · University of Kansas Medical Center, 3901 Rainbow Boulevard, Room 4035B, Kansas City, KS 66160-7317 · 913-588-6008

Topeka

Allen F. Kossoy · General Allergy & Immunology · Cotton-O'Neil Clinic, 901 Southwest Garfield Avenue, Topeka, KS 66606 · 913-354-9591 x133

ANESTHESIOLOGY

Hays

Keith W. Green · General Anesthesiology · P.O. Box 821, Hays, KS 67601 · 913-623-2964

Bryce Trump · General Anesthesiology (Pediatric Anesthesiology, Obstetric Anesthesia) · Hays Medical Center · 2220 Canterbury Road, P.O. Box 821, Hays, KS 67601 · 913-623-2964

Leawood

Steven D. Waldman · Pain (Chronic Pain Management) · Headache & Pain Center · Pain Consortium of Greater Kansas City, 11111 Nall Avenue, Suite 202, Leawood, KS 66211 · 913-491-3999

Topeka

Jeffery D. Sellers · General Anesthesiology (Pain Management) · Stormont-Vail Regional Medical Center · Anesthesia Associates, 823 Southwest Mulvane Street, Suite 2A, Topeka, KS 66606 · 913-235-3451

Wichita

Karl E. Becker, Jr. · General Anesthesiology · Wichita Anesthesiology, 1650 Georgetown Street, Suite 200, Wichita, KS 67218 · 316-686-7327

M. Kent Cooper · General Anesthesiology · Wichita Anesthesiology, 1650 Georgetown Street, Suite 200, Wichita, KS 67218 · 316-686-7327

CARDIOVASCULAR DISEASE

Kansas City

Marvin Dunn · General Cardiovascular Disease · University of Kansas Medical School, Department of Cardiology, 3901 Rainbow Boulevard, Kansas City, KS 66160 · 913-588-6015

Topeka

Robert E. Roeder · General Cardiovascular Disease · Cotton-O'Neil Clinic, 901 Southwest Garfield Avenue, Topeka, KS 66606 · 913-354-9591 x360

Patrick Sheehy · General Cardiovascular Disease · 901 Southwest Garfield Avenue, Topeka, KS 66606 · 913-354-9591

Wichita

Gregory F. Duick · General Cardiovascular Disease · Cardiovascular Consultants, 1035 North Emporia Street, Suite 210, Wichita, KS 67214 · 316-265-1308

James C. Mershon · General Cardiovascular Disease · Midtown Cardiology, 933 North Topeka Road, Wichita, KS 67214 · 316-263-5889

Barry L. Murphy · General Cardiovascular Disease (Cardiac Catheterization, Clinical Exercise Testing, Echocardiography, Heart Failure) · Wesley Hospital, Via Christi Regional Medical Center-St. Francis Campus · Crow Tretbar Medical Associates, 818 North Emporia Street, Suite 100, Wichita, KS 67214 · 316-291-4646

COLON & RECTAL SURGERY

Wichita

Jace W. Hyder · General Colon & Rectal Surgery (Gastroenterologic Surgery, Trauma, Colon & Rectal Cancer, General Surgery) · Via Christi Regional Medical Center-St. Joseph Campus, Via Christi Regional Medical Center-St. Francis Campus, Wesley Medical Center · 1431 South Bluffview, Suite 210, Wichita, KS 67218-3089 · 316-687-1090

DERMATOLOGY

Hays

Donald K. Tillman · Clinical Dermatology · Great Plains Dermatology, 2714 Plaza Avenue, Hays, KS 67601 · 913-625-7546

Kansas City

Donald V. Belsito · Contact Dermatitis · University of Kansas Medical Center, Division of Dermatology, 3901 Rainbow Boulevard, Room 4023 Wescoe, Kansas City, KS 66160 · 913-588-3840

Overland Park

Mark A. McCune · Clinical Dermatology · Kansas City Dermatology, 10600 Quivira Road, Suite 430, Overland Park, KS 66215-2317 · 913-541-3230

Topeka

Michael Giessel · Clinical Dermatology · Cotton-O'Neil Clinic, 901 Southwest Garfield Avenue, Topeka, KS 66606 · 913-354-9591

Wichita

Martha L. S. Housholder · Clinical Dermatology · The Dermatology Clinic, 835 North Hillside Drive, Wichita, KS 67214 · 316-685-4395

Marlene Mendiones · Clinical Dermatology · North Building, Room 1700-3, 80100 East 22nd Street, Wichita, KS 67226 · 316-687-5733

Herman Solomon · Clinical Dermatology · The Dermatology Clinic, 835 North Hillside Drive, Wichita, KS 67214 · 316-685-4395

ENDOCRINOLOGY & METABOLISM

Kansas City

Joseph L. Kyner · Diabetes · University of Kansas Medical Center, Division of Endocrinology & Genetics, 3901 Rainbow Boulevard, Room 4023 Wescoe, Kansas City, KS 66160-7318 · 913-588-6048

Barbra Lukert · General Endocrinology & Metabolism · University of Kansas Medical Center, Division of Endocrinology & Genetics, 3901 Rainbow Boulevard, Room 4023 Wescoe, Kansas City, KS 66160-7318 · 913-588-6048

R. Neil Schimke · General Endocrinology & Metabolism · University of Kansas Medical Center, Department of Endocrinology & Metabolism, 3901 Rainbow Boulevard, Kansas City, KS 66160-0001 · 913-588-6043

Shawnee Mission

Bradd Silver · General Endocrinology & Metabolism · Johnson County Medical Group, 7301 Frontage Road, Suite 100, Shawnee Mission, KS 66204 · 913-432-2280

Topeka

Richard S. Fairchild · General Endocrinology & Metabolism · Cotton-O'Neil Clinic, Department of Endocrinology, 901 Southwest Garfield Avenue, Topeka, KS 66606-1695 · 913-354-9591

Wichita

James K. Speed · General Endocrinology & Metabolism (Diabetes, Thyroid) · Via Christi Regional Medical Center-St. Francis Campus, Wesley Medical Center Crow Tretbar Medical Associates, 3243 East Murdock Street, Suite 500, Wichita, KS 67208 · 316-688-7300

FAMILY MEDICINE

Hays

Victor H. Hildyard · Colby Medical and Specialists Center, 175 South Range Road, Hays, KS 67701 · 913-462-3332

Kansas City

Jane L. Murray · University of Kansas Family Practice, Department of Family Medicine, 3901 Rainbow Boulevard, Kansas City, KS 66160 · 913-588-1908

Norton

Roy W. Hartley · (General Family Medicine, General Anesthesiology, General Cardiovascular Disease) · Norton County Hospital · Doctors Clinic, 711 North Norton Avenue, Norton, KS 67654 · 913-877-3305

Plainville

Daniel J. Sanchez · 300 South Colorado Street, P.O. Box 407, Plainville, KS 67663 · 913-434-2622

Quinter

Michael E. Machen · Gove County Medical Center · 501 Garfield Street, P.O. Box 510, Quinter, KS 67752-0510 · 913-754-3333

Smith Center

Ferrill R. Conant · (General Obstetrics & Gynecology) · Smith County Memorial Hospital · Smith County Family Practice, 119 East Parliament Street, Smith Center, KS 66967 · 913-282-6834

Topeka

Michael D. Atwood · Cotton-O'Neil Clinic, 901 Southwest Garfield Avenue, Topeka, KS 66606 · 913-354-0570

Stephen Saylor · Cotton-O'Neil Clinic, 901 Southwest Garfield Avenue, Topeka, KS 66606 · 913-354-0570

Wichita

Ronald Brown · 818 North Carriage Parkway, Wichita, KS 67208 · 316-651-2200

James M. Hartley · Wichita Clinic Family Physicians, 818 North Carriage Parkway, Wichita, KS 67208 · 316-685-8231

James F. Hesse · Lake Point Family Physicians, 9350 East Central Avenue, Suite 100, Wichita, KS 67208 · 316-636-2662

Diane K. Ketterman · St. Francis Regional Medical Center · St. Francis Family Center Practice, 925 North Emporia Street, Wichita, KS 67214 · 316-265-2876

Terry Merrifield · 818 North Carriage Parkway, Wichita, KS 67208 · 316-651-2200

Stanley J. Mosier · Wesley Medical Center, Via Christi Regional Medical Center-St. Joseph Campus · 818 North Carriage Parkway, Wichita, KS 67208 · 316-651-2200

GASTROENTEROLOGY

Kansas City

Norton J. Greenberger · General Gastroenterology · University of Kansas Medical Center, Department of Medicine, 3901 Rainbow Boulevard, Kansas City, KS 66160 · 913-588-6001

Philip B. Miner, Jr. · General Gastroenterology · University of Kansas Medical Center, Division of Gastroenterology, 3901 Rainbow Boulevard, Room 4035 DELP, Kansas City, KS 66160-7350 · 913-588-6003

Olathe

Charles L. Brooks · General Gastroenterology (Hepatology, Endoscopy) · Shawnee Mission Medical Center (Shawnee Mission), Olathe Medical Center, Providence Medical Center (Kansas City), Bethany Medical Center (Kansas City) · Doctors Building II, Suite 170, 20375 West 151st Street, Olathe, KS 66061-5353 913-829-2829

Topeka

Robert Braun · General Gastroenterology · Cotton-O'Neil Clinic, 901 Southwest Garfield Avenue, Topeka, KS 66606 · 913-354-9591

Wichita

James A. Whittaker · General Gastroenterology · Crow Tretbar Medical Associates, 3243 East Murdock Street, Wichita, KS 67208 · 316-688-7300

GERIATRIC MEDICINE

Kansas City

Stephanie A. Studenski · University of Kansas Medical Center · University of Kansas Medical Center, Center on Aging, 3901 Rainbow Boulevard, Kansas City, KS 66160-7117 · 913-588-1265

HAND SURGERY

Hays

Robert L. Bassett · General Hand Surgery (Microsurgery, Reconstructive Surgery) · Hays Medical Center · Hays Orthopaedic Clinic, 2818 North Vine Street, Hays, KS 67601 · 913-628-8221

Olathe

Lynn D. Ketchum · General Hand Surgery · 12301 West 106th Street, Suite 201, Olathe, KS 66215-2292 · 913-451-8567

Wichita

Bruce G. Ferris · General Hand Surgery · Plastic and Reconstructive Surgery, 825 North Hillside Road, Wichita, KS 67214 · 316-688-7500

INFECTIOUS DISEASE

Hays

Jennifer Rupp · General Infectious Disease (General Internal Medicine, AIDS) Hays Medical Center · Hays Internal Medicine, 2501 East 13th Street, Suite 10, Hays, KS 67601 · 913-625-4224

Kansas City

Elliot Goldstein · General Infectious Disease · University of Kansas Medical Center, Department of Infectious Disease, 3901 Rainbow Boulevard, Kansas City, KS 66160-7354 · 913-588-6035

Daniel R. Henthorn · General Infectious Disease · University of Kansas Medical Center, Department of Infectious Disease, 3901 Rainbow Boulevard, Kansas City, KS 66160-7354 · 913-588-6035

Topeka

Lawerence Rumans · General Infectious Disease · Medical Consultants, 31 Horne Street, Suite 420, Topeka, KS 66606 · 913-234-8405

Wichita

Hewitt C. Goodpasture · General Infectious Disease · Infectious Disease Consultants, 1100 North St. Francis Street, Suite 130, Wichita, KS 67214 · 316-264-3505

Jerry D. Peterie · General Infectious Disease (Hospital-Acquired Infections, Transplantation Infections) · Infectious Disease Consultants, 1100 North St. Francis Street, Suite 130, Wichita, KS 67214 · 316-264-3505

INTERNAL MEDICINE (GENERAL)

Hays

Robert C. Albers · Hays Internal Medicine, 2501 East 13th Street, Suite 10, Hays, KS 67601 · 913-625-4224

B. N. Reddy · Graham County Medical Clinic, 114 East Walnut Street, Hays, KS 67642 · 913-674-2191

Dallas L. Richards · Hays Internal Medicine, 2501 East 13th Street, Suite 10, Hays, KS 67601 · 913-625-4224

Kansas City

Bruce E. Johnson · University of Kansas Medical Center, Department of Medicine, 3901 Rainbow Boulevard, Kansas City, KS 66160-7330 · 913-588-6063

Merriam

Charles W. Ragland · 8800 West 75th Street, Suite 300, Merriam, KS 66204 · 913-722-4240

Overland Park

John L. Dunlap · 4860 College Boulevard, Suite 216, Overland Park, KS 66211 913-491-6633

Prairie Village

Ernest A. Cattaneo · Penn Valley Internal Medicine, 7301 Mission Road, Suite 350, Prairie Village, KS 66208-3005 · 913-262-3930

Shawnee Mission

Maureen Dudgeon · Johnson County Medical Group, 7301 Frontage Road, Suite 100, Shawnee Mission, KS 66204 · 913-432-2280

George E. Stamos · Kenyon Clinic, 10600 Quivira Road, Suite 201, Shawnee Mission, KS 66215-2317 · 913-541-3340

Topeka

Robert W. Holmes · (Geriatric Medicine) · Stormont-Vail Regional Medical Center, St. Francis Hospital & Medical Center, Kansas Rehabilitation Hospital · Cotton-O'Neil Clinic, 901 Southwest Garfield Avenue, Topeka, KS 66606 · 913-354-9591

Stanley D. Hornbaker · Cotton-O'Neil Clinic, 901 Southwest Garfield Avenue, Topeka, KS 66606 · 913-354-9591 x136

John D. Rockefeller · (General Internal Medicine, Preventive Health Care) · Stormont-Vail Regional Medical Center, St. Francis Hospital & Medical Center · Cotton-O'Neil Clinic, 901 Southwest Garfield Avenue, Topeka, KS 66606 · 913-354-9591

Wichita

Dean I. Youngberg · 959 North Emporia Street, Suite 201, Wichita, KS 67214 · 316-268-6075

MEDICAL ONCOLOGY & HEMATOLOGY

Hays

Eric Carlson · (Medical Oncology only) · Hays Medical Center · 2220 Canterbury Drive, Hays, KS 67601 · 913-623-5774

Kansas City

Carol J. Fabian · Breast Cancer · University of Kansas Medical Center · University of Kansas Cancer Center, 3901 Rainbow Boulevard, Kansas City, KS 66160 · 913-588-7791

Ronald L. Stephens · General Medical Oncology & Hematology · University of Kansas Medical Center, Department of Clinical Oncology, 3901 Rainbow Boulevard, Room 6F, Kansas City, KS 66160 · 913-588-6029

Olathe

David L. Lee · General Medical Oncology & Hematology · 375 West 151st Street, Suite 403, Olathe, KS 66061 · 913-780-4000

Overland Park

Robert J. Belt · General Medical Oncology & Hematology · Oncology/Hematology Clinic of Kansas City, 2000 West 110th Street, Suite 400, Overland Park, KS 66210 · 913-469-8023

Shawnee Mission

Mark C. Myron · (Medical Oncology only, Palliative Care) · Menorah Medical Center (Kansas City, MO) · Oncology & Hematology Associates, 5701 West 119th Street, Suite 325, Shawnee Mission, KS 66209 · 913-451-7710

Topeka

Stanley J. Vogel · General Medical Oncology & Hematology · Cotton-O'Neil Clinic, Department of Medical Oncology & Hematology, 901 Southwest Garfield Avenue, Topeka, KS 66606-1695 · 913-354-9591

Wichita

David B. Johnson · General Medical Oncology & Hematology · Cancer Center of Kansas, 18 North Emporia Street, Suite 403, Wichita, KS 67214 · 316-262-4467

NEPHROLOGY

Hays

Bradley R. Stuewe · General Nephrology · Murrie Clinic, Box 206, Hays, KS 67402 · 913-827-7261

Kansas City

Arnold M. Chonko · General Nephrology · University of Kansas Medical Center, Division of Nephrology, 3901 Rainbow Boulevard, Kansas City, KS 63160-7382 · 913-588-6074

Dennis A. Diederich · General Nephrology · University of Kansas Medical Center, Division of Nephrology, 3901 Rainbow Boulevard, Kansas City, KS 63160-7382 · 913-588-6075

Jared J. Grantham · Kidney Disease (Polycystic Disease) · University of Kansas Medical Center · University of Kansas Medical Center, Department of Medicine, Division of Nephrology, 3901 Rainbow Boulevard, Kansas City, KS 66160-7382 · 913-588-6074

Wichita

Jerry B. Cohlmia · General Nephrology · Wichita Nephrology Group, 818 North Emporia Street, Suite 310, Wichita, KS 67218 · 316-263-5891

Howard A. Day · General Nephrology · Wichita Nephrology Group, 818 North Emporia Street, Suite 310, Wichita, KS 67218 · 316-263-5891

Linda L. Francisco · General Nephrology · Wichita Nephrology Group, 818 North Emporia Street, Suite 310, Wichita, KS 67218 · 316-263-5891

Michael E. Grant · General Nephrology · Wichita Nephrology Group, 818 North Emporia Street, Suite 310, Wichita, KS 67218 · 316-263-5891

NEUROLOGICAL SURGERY

Kansas City

Paul L. Oboynick · General Neurological Surgery · University of Kansas Medical Center, Department of Neurosurgery, 3901 Rainbow Boulevard, 5045 Sudler, Kansas City, KS 66160 · 913-588-6118

Topeka

K. N. Arjunan · General Neurological Surgery · Neurosurgical Associates, 634 Southwest Mulvane Street, Suite 202, Topeka, KS 66606-1678 · 913-232-3555

John D. Ebeling · General Neurological Surgery · Neurosurgical Associates, 634 Southwest Mulvane Street, Suite 202, Topeka, KS 66606-1678 · 913-232-3555

Craig H. Yorke · General Neurological Surgery · Neurosurgical Associates, 634 Southwest Mulvane Street, Suite 202, Topeka, KS 66606-1678 · 913-232-3555

Wichita

John Hered · General Neurological Surgery (Spinal Surgery, Vascular Neurological Surgery) · Via Christi Regional Medical Center-St. Francis Campus, Via Christi Regional Medical Center-St. Joseph Campus, Wesley Medical Center · Heritage Plaza, Suite 200, 818 North Emporia Street, Wichita, KS 67214 · 316-263-0296

William M. Shapiro · General Neurological Surgery · Wichita Surgical Specialists, 818 North Emporia Street, Wichita, KS 67214 · 316-263-0348

NEUROLOGY

Hays

Barbara-Jean Lewis · General Neurology · 201 East Seventh Street, Third Floor, Hays, KS 67601 · 913-623-5660

Kansas City

William C. Koller · Movement Disorders (Tremor, Parkinson's Disease) · University of Kansas Medical Center · University of Kansas Medical Center, 3901 Rainbow Boulevard, Kansas City, KS 66160-7314 · 913-588-6094

Chi-Wan Lai · Epilepsy · University of Kansas Medical Center, Department of Neurology, 3901 Rainbow Boulevard, Kansas City, KS 66160 · 913-588-7189

Dewey K. Ziegler · Headache · University of Kansas Medical Center · University of Kansas Medical Center, 3901 Rainbow Boulevard, Kansas City, KS 66160-7314 913-588-6970

Topeka

Wade B. Welch · General Neurology · Cotton-O'Neil Clinic, 901 Southwest Garfield Avenue, Topeka, KS 66606 · 913-354-9591 x116

Wichita

Calvin G. Olmstead · General Neurology · 818 North Emporia Street, Suite 67214, Wichita, KS 67218 · 316-268-6856

NEUROLOGY, CHILD

Hays

Barbara-Jean Lewis · General Child Neurology · 201 East Seventh Street, Third Floor, Hays, KS 67601 · 913-623-5660

Wichita

William D. Svobda · Epilepsy · 1035 North Emporia Street, Suite 235, Wichita, KS 67214 · 316-267-5215

NUCLEAR MEDICINE

Kansas City

David F. Preston · General Nuclear Medicine · University of Kansas Medical Center, Department of Diagnostic Radiology, 3901 Rainbow Boulevard, Kansas City, KS 66160 · 913-588-6841

OBSTETRICS & GYNECOLOGY

Hays

Richard D. Bauer · General Obstetrics & Gynecology · 1517 East 27th Street, Hays, KS 67601 · 913-625-0044

Kansas City

Sebastian Faro · Infectious Disease · University of Kansas Medical Center · University of Kansas Medical Center, 3901 Rainbow Boulevard, Kansas City, KS 66160-7316 · 913-588-6200

Overland Park

Tom G. Sullivan · General Obstetrics & Gynecology · Overland Park Regional Medical Center, Saint Joseph Health Center (Kansas City, MO) · Kansas City Women's Clinic, 10600 Quivira Road, Suite 320, Overland Park, KS 66215-2317 · 913-894-8500

Marty Thomas · General Obstetrics & Gynecology · Kansas City Women's Clinic, 10600 Quivira Road, Suite 320, Overland Park, KS 66215 · 913-541-3200

Topeka

Morgan M. Hostetter · General Obstetrics & Gynecology (Adolescent Gynecology, Geriatric Gynecology, Maternal & Fetal Medicine) · Stormont-Vail Regional Medical Center, St. Francis Hospital & Medical Center · Lincoln Center Ob-Gyn, 800 Southwest Lincoln Street, Topeka, KS 66606 · 913-233-5101

David Robinson · General Obstetrics & Gynecology (Urogynecology, Pelvic Reconstruction) · Stormont-Vail Regional Medical Center, St. Francis Hospital & Medical Center · Lincoln Center OBGYN, 2830 Southwest Urish Street, Topeka, KS 66614-5614 · 913-273-4010

Wichita

Carl M. Christman · General Obstetrics & Gynecology · Wesley Medical Center, Via Christi Regional Medical Center-St. Francis Campus, Surgicare of Wichita, Via Christi Regional Medical Center-St. Joseph Campus · Wichita OBGYN Associates, 551 North Hillside Drive, Suite 510, Wichita, KS 67214 · 316-685-0559

Lorna L. Cvetkovich · General Obstetrics & Gynecology · St. Francis Regional Medical Center · 818 North Emporia Street, Suite 415, Wichita, KS 67218 · 316-264-6267

Douglas D. Douthit · General Obstetrics & Gynecology · Wichita OBGYN Associates, 551 North Hillside Drive, Suite 510, Wichita, KS 67214 · 316-685-0559

Douglas V. Horbelt · Gynecologic Cancer · Wesley Medical Center · Wesley Medical Center, 3243 East Murdock Street, Level G, Wichita, KS 67208-3052 · 316-681-0251

Scott Roberts · Maternal & Fetal Medicine (Infectious Disease) · Children's Mercy Hospital (Kansas City, MO) · 3243 East Merda Street, Suite 201, Wichita, KS 67208 · 316-688-7990

OPHTHALMOLOGY

Garden City

Luther L. Fry · Anterior Segment—Cataract & Refractive · Fry Eye Associates, 310 East Walnut Street, Suite 101, Garden City, KS 67846 · 316-275-7248

Hays

Thomas L. McDonald · General Ophthalmology · Eye Specialists, 1010 Downing Avenue, Hays, KS 67601 · 913-628-8218

Hutchinson

S. L. Francis Depenbusch · General Ophthalmology (Anterior Segment—Cataract & Refractive, Glaucoma, Oculoplastic & Orbital Surgery) · Hutchinson Eye Physicians & Surgeons, 1708 East 23rd Street, Hutchinson, KS 67502 · 316-663-7187

Richard T. Falter · General Ophthalmology (Anterior Segment—Cataract & Refractive, Corneal Diseases & Transplantation) · Hutchinson Hospital · Hutchinson Eye Physicians & Surgeons, 1708 East 23rd Street, Hutchinson, KS 67502 · 316-663-7187

Kansas City

Martin A. Mainster · Medical Retinal Diseases (Macular and Retinal Vascular Diseases) · University of Kansas Medical Center · Associates in Ophthalmology, 3901 Rainbow Boulevard, Kansas City, KS 66160-7379 · 913-588-6600

Newton

William R. Beck · General Ophthalmology · Axtell Clinic, 203 East Broadway Street, Newton, KS 67114 · 316-283-2800

Overland Park

Thomas B. Coulter · General Ophthalmology (Retinal Diseases) · Shawnee Mission Medical Center (Shawnee Mission) · Kansas City Eye Clinic, 7504 Antioch Road, Overland Park, KS 66204 · 913-341-3100

Michael E. Headinger · General Ophthalmology · Kansas City Eye Clinic, 7504 Antioch Road, Overland Park, KS 66204-2622 · 913-341-3100

Carl V. Migliazzo · Glaucoma (Laser Surgery, Cataract) · Shawnee Mission Medical Center (Shawnee Mission) · Kansas City Eye Clinic, 7504 Antioch Road, Overland Park, KS 66204-2622 · 913-341-3100

Pittsburg

Roger B. Schlemer · General Ophthalmology · 103 South Broadway, Pittsburg, KS 66762 · 316-231-6380

Shawnee Mission

King Y. Lee · General Ophthalmology · Georgetown Medical Building 8974, 8901 West 74th Street, Suite 385, Shawnee Mission, KS 66204 · 913-362-7800

Topeka

Cindy E. Penzler · General Ophthalmology (Anterior Segment—Cataract & Refractive, Glaucoma) · St. Francis Hospital & Medical Center, Stormont-Vail Regional Medical Center, Geary Community Hospital (Junction City) · Continental Medical Building, Suite 130, 631 Southwest Horne Street, Topeka, KS 66606-1663 · 913-233-0011

Wichita

Samuel W. Amstutz · General Ophthalmology · Eye Clinic of Wichita, 655 North Woodlawn Street, Wichita, KS 67208 · 316-684-5158

David A. Johnson · Pediatric Ophthalmology · Wesley Medical Center, Via Christi Regional Medical Center-St. Francis Campus · Eye Clinic of Wichita, 655 North Woodlawn Street, Wichita, KS 67208-3685 · 316-684-5158

Leslie W. Nesmith · Vitreo-Retinal Surgery (Retinal Diseases) · Wesley Medical Center · Vitreo-Retinal Consultants & Surgeons, 530 North Lorraine Street, Suite 200, Wichita, KS 67214-4837 · 316-683-0044

Michael P. Varenhorst · Vitreo-Retinal Surgery · Vitreo-Retinal Consultants & Surgeons, 530 North Lorraine Street, Wichita, KS 67214 · 316-683-5611

Lowell W. Wilder · Anterior Segment—Cataract & Refractive · Eye Clinic of Wichita, 655 North Woodlawn Street, Wichita, KS 67208 · 316-684-5158

ORTHOPAEDIC SURGERY

Hays

Robert L. Bassett · General Orthopaedic Surgery (Hand Surgery, Shoulder Surgery) · Hays Medical Center · Hays Orthopaedic Clinic, 2818 North Vine Street, Hays, KS 67601 · 913-628-8221

Gregory A. Woods · Sports Medicine/Arthroscopy · Hays Orthopaedic Clinic, 2818 North Vine Street, Hays, KS 67601 · 913-628-8221

Kansas City

Marc A. Asher · General Orthopaedic Surgery · University of Kansas Medical Center, Department of Orthopaedic Surgery, 3901 Rainbow Boulevard, 5012 Eaton, Kansas City, KS 66160 · 913-588-6130

Topeka

Richard Polly · General Orthopaedic Surgery · Orthopaedic Associates, 909 Mulvane Street, Topeka, KS 66606 · 913-357-0301

Wichita

James Joseph · General Orthopaedic Surgery · Advanced Orthopaedic Associates, 2778 North Webb Road, Wichita, KS 67226 · 316-631-1600

David A. McQueen · General Orthopaedic Surgery · Advanced Orthopaedic Associates, 2778 North Webb Road, Wichita, KS 67226 · 316-262-7598

OTOLARYNGOLOGY

Hays

James Black · General Otolaryngology · Ear, Nose & Throat Clinic, 2517 Canterbury Road, Hays, KS 67601 · 913-628-3131

Kansas City

Gregory A. Ator · Otology/Neurotology · University of Kansas Medical School, Ear, Nose and Throat Department, Eaton Building, Third Floor, 3901 Rainbow Boulevard, Kansas City, KS 66160 · 913-588-6700

Leawood

Edwin A. Cortez · Facial Plastic Surgery · Baptist Medical Center (Kansas City, MO), Menorah Medical Center (Kansas City, MO) · 11213 Nall Street, Suite 140, Leawood, KS 66211 · 913-451-7970

Overland Park

Mark J. Maslan · General Otolaryngology · Head & Neck Surgical Associates, 5520 College Boulevard, Room 350, Overland Park, KS 66211 · 913-663-5100

Topeka

Song-Ping Lee · General Otolaryngology · 823 Mulvane Street, Suite 250, Topeka, KS 66605 · 913-233-6001

Wichita

Glen R. Kubina · General Otolaryngology · Mid-Kansas Ear, Nose and Throat, 310 South Hillside Drive, Wichita, KS 67211 · 316-684-2838

Yoram B. Leitner · General Otolaryngology · Wichita Clinic, ENT Clinic, 3311 East Murdock Street, Wichita, KS 67208 · 316-689-9227

George R. Randall · General Otolaryngology (Sinus & Nasal Surgery, Head & Neck Surgery) · Via Christi Regional Medical Center-St. Francis Campus, Via Christi Regional Medical Center-St. Joseph Campus, Wesley Medical Center · Mid-Kansas Ear, Nose and Throat Associates, 310 South Hillside Drive, Wichita, KS 67211 · 316-684-2838

PATHOLOGY

Hays

Ward M. Newcomb · General Pathology · Hays Pathology Laboratories, 1300 East 13th Street, Hays, KS 67601 · 913-625-5646

Kansas City

John J. Kepes · Neuropathology (Brain Tumors) · University of Kansas Medical Center · University of Kansas Medical Center, 39th Street & Rainbow Boulevard, Kansas City, KS 66103 · 913-588-5000

Wichita

Joe J. Lin · General Pathology · 929 North Francis Street, Wichita, KS 67214 · 316-268-5420

PEDIATRICS

Kansas City

Wayne V. Moore · Pediatric Endocrinology (Growth) · University of Kansas Medical Center · University of Kansas Medical Center, Department of Pediatrics, 3901 Rainbow Boulevard, Kansas City, KS 66160-7330 · 913-588-6326

Wichita

Sechin Cho · Metabolic Diseases (Birth Defects, Medical Genetics) · Wesley Medical Center · Wesley Medical Center, 550 North Hillside Drive, Wichita, KS 67214-4976 · 316-688-2362

Richard A. Guthrie · Pediatric Endocrinology (Pediatric & Adult Diabetes, Metabolic Diseases) · Diabetes Treatment Center and Robert L. Jackson Diabetes Institute, Via Christi Regional Medical Center-St. Joseph Campus, Via Christi Regional Medical Center-St. Francis Campus · Mid-America Diabetes Associates, 200 South Hillside Street, Wichita, KS 67211-2127 · 316-687-3100

George H. Khoury · Pediatric Cardiology (Congenital Heart Disease) · 3333 East Central Street, Suite 416, Wichita, KS 67208 · 316-681-2021

F. W. Manfred Menking · Pediatric Endocrinology · Wichita Clinic, Department of Pediatrics, 3311 East Murdock Street, Wichita, KS 67208 · 316-689-9336

David Rosen · Pediatric Hematology-Oncology · Wesley Medical Center, Via Christi Regional Medical Center-St. Francis Campus · 818 North Emporia Street, Suite 307, Wichita, KS 67214 · 316-263-4311

PEDIATRICS (GENERAL)

Chanute

Greta S. McFarland · Neosho Memorial Regional Medical Center · 505 South Plummer Street, Chanute, KS 66720 · 316-431-2500

Hays

Lester B. Horrell · (Neonatal & Perinatal Medicine, Pediatric Pulmonology) · Hays Medical Center · HMC Pediatric Center, 201 East Seventh Street, Hays, KS 67601 · 913-623-5600

Kansas City

Pamela Kay Shaw · University of Kansas Medical Center, Department of Pediatrics, 3901 Rainbow Boulevard, Kansas City, KS 66160-7330 · 913-588-5919

Overland Park

Carolyn T. Davis · (Preventive Medicine, Clinical Dermatology) · Saint Joseph Health Center (Kansas City, MO), Shawnee Mission Medical Center (Shawnee Mission), Overland Park Regional Medical Center · Pediatric Specialists, 4601 West 109th Street, Suite 122, Overland Park, KS 66211 · 913-491-4045

Shawnee Mission

Bryan C. Nelson · Johnson County Pediatrics, 8800 West 75th Street, Suite 220, Shawnee Mission, KS 66204 · 913-384-5500

Mary M. Tyson · Johnson County Pediatrics, 8800 West 75th Street, Suite 220, Shawnee Mission, KS 66204 · 913-384-5500

Topeka

Dennis M. Cooley · Pediatric Associates, 3500 Southwest Sixth Street, Topeka, KS 66606 · 913-235-0335

Wichita

F. W. Manfred Menking · Wichita Clinic, Department of Pediatrics, 3311 East Murdock Street, Wichita, KS 67208 · 316-689-9336

PHYSICAL MEDICINE & REHABILITATION

Hays

Joann Mace · General Physical Medicine & Rehabilitation · 201 East Seventh Street, Hays, KS 67601 · 913-623-5680

Kansas City

George Varghese · General Physical Medicine & Rehabilitation · University of Kansas Medical Center, Department of Rehabilitation Medicine, 3901 Rainbow Boulevard, Kansas City, KS 66160 · 913-588-6944

Wichita

Jane K. Drazek · General Physical Medicine & Rehabilitation · Via Christi Regional Medical Center-St. Francis Campus, Via Christi Regional Medical Center-St. Joseph Campus, Wesley Medical Center · Via Christi Rehabilitation Center, 1151 North Rock Road, Wichita, KS 67206 · 316-634-3500

PLASTIC SURGERY

Olathe

John B. Moore · General Plastic Surgery (Hand Surgery, Microsurgery) · Olathe Medical Center, Shawnee Mission Medical Center (Shawnee Mission), Menorah Medical Center (Kansas City, MO), Overland Park Regional Medical Center (Overland Park) · Plastic, Reconstructive and Hand Surgery Center, 20375 West 151st Street, Suite 370, Olathe, KS 66061 · 913-782-0707

Overland Park

Ted E. Lockwood · Body Contouring (Facial Aesthetic Surgery) · Overland Park Regional Medical Center · 10600 Quivira Road, Suite 470, Overland Park, KS 66215 · 913-894-1070

Wichita

Gerald D. Nelson · General Plastic Surgery (Cleft Lip & Palate, Cosmetic Surgery) · Plastic Surgery Center, 825 North Hillside Drive, Wichita, KS 67214-4998 316-688-7500

PSYCHIATRY

Topeka

Joyce Davidson · Psychopharmacology · The Menninger Clinic · C. F. Menninger Memorial Hospital, 5800 Southwest Sixth Avenue, Box 829, Topeka, KS 66601 · 913-350-5321

Glen O. Gabbard · Psychoanalysis · The Menninger Clinic, Topeka Institute for Psychoanalysis · The Menninger Clinic, 5800 Southwest Sixth Avenue, P.O. Box 829, Topeka, KS 66601-0829 · 913-273-7500 x5529

Wichita

Sheldon Preskorn · Psychopharmacology (Affective Disorders) · University of Kansas School of Medicine/Wichita, Department of Psychiatry, 1010 North Kansas Street, Wichita, KS 67214-3199 · 316-261-2680

PULMONARY & CRITICAL CARE MEDICINE

Kansas City

Gerald R. Kerby · General Pulmonary & Critical Care Medicine · University of Kansas Medical Center, Department of Pulmonary Medicine, 3901 Rainbow Boulevard, Kansas City, KS 66160 · 913-588-6045

Shawn M. Magee · General Pulmonary & Critical Care Medicine · Bethany Medical Center, Providence Medical Center · 6013 Leavenworth Road, Kansas City, KS 66104 · 913-299-2069

Susan K. Pingleton · General Pulmonary & Critical Care Medicine, Asthma (Chronic Obstructive Pulmonary Disease, Nutrition) · University of Kansas Medical Center · University of Kansas Medical Center, 3901 Rainbow Boulevard, Kansas City, KS 66160-7381 · 913-588-6045

RADIATION ONCOLOGY

Kansas City

Richard G. Evans · Pediatric Radiation Oncology · University of Kansas Medical Center, Department of Radiation Oncology, 3901 Rainbow Boulevard, Kansas City, KS 66160-7329 · 913-588-3670

Shankar P. G. Gire · Head & Neck Cancer · University of Kansas Medical Center, Department of Radiation Oncology, 3901 Rainbow Boulevard, Kansas City, KS 66160-0001 · 913-588-3613

Olathe

Stephen R. Smalley · General Radiation Oncology (Gastrointestinal Multimodality Therapy, Genito-Urinary Radiation Oncology) · Olathe Medical Center · Doctors Building, Suite 180, 20375 West 151st Street, Olathe, KS 66061 · 913-768-7200

Overland Park

James R. Coster · General Radiation Oncology (Breast Cancer, Prostate Cancer, Head & Neck Cancer) · Shawnee Mission Medical Center (Shawnee Mission), Saint Joseph Health Center (Kansas City, MO), Overland Park Regional Medical Center, Olathe Medical Center (Olathe) · Radiation Oncology Associates of Kansas City, 12000 West 110th Street, Suite 100, Overland Park, KS 66210 · 913-469-0002

David A. Deer · General Radiation Oncology · Radiation Oncology Associates of Kansas City, 12000 West 110th Street, Suite 100, Overland Park, KS 66210 · 913-469-0002

Topeka

Stephen D. Coon · General Radiation Oncology · Medical Park West, Department of Radiation Oncology, 823 Southwest Mulvane Street, Topeka, KS 66606 913-234-3451

Judith A. Kooser · General Radiation Oncology (Gynecologic Cancer, Lung Cancer) · St. Francis Hospital & Medical Center, Stormont-Vail Regional Medical Center · Medical Park West, 823 Southwest Mulvane Street, Suite One, Topeka, KS 66606 · 913-234-3451

Ralph Reymond · General Radiation Oncology · St. Francis Hospital & Medical Center, Stormont-Vail Regional Medical Center · St. Francis Hospital, Department of Radiation Oncology, 1700 West Seventh Street, Topeka, KS 66606 · 913-295-8008

Terry J. Wall · General Radiation Oncology · Medical Park West, Department of Radiation Oncology, 823 Southwest Mulvane Street, Topeka, KS 66606 · 913-234-3451

Wichita

Paul A. Baumann · General Radiation Oncology (Genito-Urinary Cancer, Gynecologic Cancer, Lung Cancer, Sarcomas) · Wesley Medical Center · Wesley Medical Center, Department of Radiation Therapy, 550 North Hillside Drive, Wichita, KS 67214-4976 · 316-688-2920

Barbara Dewitt · General Radiation Oncology · St. Francis Hospital, St. Francis Radiation Therapy, 929 North St. Francis Street, Wichita, KS 67214 · 316-268-5927

RADIOLOGY

Hays

Michael J. Wright · General Radiology · Radiology Associates, 2501 East 13th Street, P.O. Box 833, Hays, KS 67601 · 913-625-6521

Kansas City

Glendon G. Cox · General Radiology · University of Kansas Medical Center, Department of Radiology, 3901 Rainbow Boulevard, Kansas City, KS 66160-7234 913-588-1842

Donald Eckard · Neuroradiology · University of Kansas Medical Center, Department of Radiology, 3901 Rainbow Boulevard, Kansas City, KS 66160 · 913-588-6886

Topeka

Richard Meidinger · General Radiology · Medical Park West, 823 Southwest Mulvane Street, Suite One, Topeka, KS 66606 · 913-234-3451

Wichita

David Breckbill · General Radiology (Pediatric Radiology) · Wichita Radiology Group, 550 North Hillside Drive, Wichita, KS 67214 · 316-688-2900

Norman T. Pay · Magnetic Resonance Imaging (Neuroradiology) · Via Christi Regional Medical Center-St. Francis Campus · MR Imaging Center, 928 North St. Francis Street, Wichita, KS 67214 · 316-268-6742

RHEUMATOLOGY

Topeka

Doug Gardner · General Rheumatology · Cotton-O'Neil Clinic, 901 Southwest Garfield Avenue, Topeka, KS 66606 · 913-354-9591

Wichita

Teresa A. Reynolds · General Rheumatology · Wichita Clinic, Department of Rheumatology, 3311 East Murdock Street, Wichita, KS 67208 · 316-689-9400

Frederick Wolfe · Rheumatoid Arthritis, Fibromyalgia, General Rheumatology · St. Francis Regional Medical Center · Arthritis Center, 1035 North Emporia Street, Suite 230, Wichita, KS 67214 · 316-263-2125

SURGERY

Hays

A. Christine Kelly · Breast Surgery · Hays Medical Center · 1010 Downing Avenue, Hays, KS 67601 · 913-625-8553

Charles C. Schultz · General Surgery · Surgical Associates of Hays, 2501 East 13th Street, Suite Seven, Hays, KS 67601 · 913-628-3217

Ross E. Stadalman · General Surgery (Endoscopy) · Hays Medical Center · Surgical Associates of Hays, 2501 East 13th Street, Suite Seven, Hays, KS 67601-2732 · 913-628-3217

Kansas City

Laurence Y. Cheung · Gastroenterologic Surgery · University of Kansas Medical Center · University of Kansas Medical Center, 3901 Rainbow Boulevard, Kansas City, KS 66160-7385 · 913-588-6101

Arlo S. Hermreck · General Vascular Surgery · University of Kansas Medical Center, Department of Surgery, 3901 Rainbow Boulevard, Kansas City, KS 66160-7308 · 913-588-7232

Overland Park

Keith W. Ashcraft · Pediatric Surgery (Esophageal Surgery) · Children's Mercy Hospital (Kansas City, MO), University of Missouri, Kansas City School of Medicine · Pediatric Surgical Associates, 5520 College Boulevard, Suite 206, Overland Park, KS 66211 · 913-491-0880

Shawnee Mission

Joseph B. Petelin · Gastroenterologic Surgery (Endoscopy) · 9119 West 74th Street, Suite 255, Shawnee Mission, KS 66204 · 913-432-5420

Topeka

Charles P. Graham · General Surgery · 1501 Southwest Sixth Avenue, Topeka, KS 66606 · 913-354-1484

Nason Lui · General Surgery · 1516 Southwest Sixth Avenue, Suite Two, Topeka, KS 66606 · 913-233-1747

Wichita

R. Larry Beamer · General Surgery · Wichita Surgical Specialists, 818 North Emporia Street, Suite 200, Wichita, KS 67214 · 316-263-0296

Frederic C. Chang · General Surgery (Trauma) · Via Christi Regional Medical Center-St. Francis Campus · Wichita Surgical Specialists, Heritage Plaza, Suite 200, 818 North Emporia Street, Wichita, KS 67214-3788 · 316-263-0296

H. James Farha · General Surgery · Wichita Surgical Specialists, 818 North Emporia Street, Suite 200, Wichita, KS 67214 · 316-263-0296

Paul B. Harrison · General Surgery · Research Medical Center (Kansas City, MO) Kansas Surgical Consultants, 3243 East Murdock Street, Suite 404, Wichita, KS 67208 · 316-685-6222

Marilee F. McBoyle · Breast Surgery · Wichita Surgical Specialists, 818 North Emporia Street, Suite 200, Wichita, KS 67214 · 316-263-0296

Charles F. Shield III · Transplantation · St. Francis Regional Medical Center · Wichita Surgical Specialists, 818 North Emporia Street, Suite 200, Wichita, KS 67214 · 316-263-0296

SURGICAL ONCOLOGY

Kansas City

William R. Jewell · General Surgical Oncology · University of Kansas Medical Center, 3901 Rainbow Boulevard, Kansas City, KS 66160-7308 · 913-588-6112

THORACIC SURGERY

Overland Park

Peter B. Manning · Pediatric Cardiac Surgery (Pediatric Non-Cardiac Thoracic Surgery, General Surgery, Pediatric Surgery, Surgical Critical Care) · Children's Mercy Hospital (Kansas City, MO) · 5520 College Boulevard, Suite 206, Overland Park, KS 66211 · 913-491-0880

Prairie Village

Hamner Hannah III · General Thoracic Surgery (Adult Cardiothoracic Surgery, Thoracic Oncological Surgery, General Vascular Surgery) · Research Medical Center (Kansas City, MO), University of Kansas Medical Center (Kansas City), Baptist Medical Center (Kansas City, MO), Menorah Medical Center (Kansas City, MO), Saint Joseph Health Center (Kansas City, MO) · Thoracic & Vascular Surgeons, 4121 West 83rd Street, Suite 132, Prairie Village, KS 66208 · 913-649-6677

Frederic L. Seligson · General Thoracic Surgery (Adult Cardiothoracic Surgery) Research Medical Center (Kansas City, MO), Baptist Medical Center (Kansas City, MO), Saint Joseph Health Center (Kansas City, MO), Menorah Medical Center (Kansas City, MO), University of Kansas Medical Center (Kansas City) · Thoracic & Vascular Surgeons, 4121 West 83rd Street, Suite 132, Prairie Village, KS 66208 · 913-649-6677

Topeka

Norman W. Thoms · General Thoracic Surgery (Adult Cardiothoracic Surgery, General Vascular Surgery) · Stormont-Vail Regional Medical Center, St. Francis Hospital & Medical Center · Cardiovascular & Thoracic Surgeons, 901 Southwest Garfield Avenue, Topeka, KS 66606 · 913-233-1710

Peter J. Tutuska · General Thoracic Surgery · Cardiovascular & Thoracic Surgeons, 901 Southwest Garfield Avenue, Topeka, KS 66606 · 913-233-1710

Wichita

Thomas H. Estep · Adult Cardiothoracic Surgery (Transplantation) · Wichita Surgical Specialists, 818 North Emporia Street, Suite 200, Wichita, KS 67214 · 316-263-0296

Gyan Khicha · General Thoracic Surgery (Adult Cardiothoracic Surgery) · St. Francis Regional Medical Center, Via Christi Regional Medical Center-St. Joseph Campus, Wesley Medical Center · Wichita Surgical Specialists, 818 North Emporia Street, Suite 200, Wichita, KS 67214-3788 · 316-263-0296

Douglas J. Milfeld · Adult Cardiothoracic Surgery (Peripheral Vascular Surgery, Thoracoscopic Surgery, General Vascular Surgery, Trauma, General Thoracic Surgery, Thoracic Oncological Surgery) · Via Christi Regional Medical Center-St. Francis Campus, Wesley Medical Center, Via Christi Regional Medical Center-St. Joseph Campus · Wichita Surgical Specialists, 818 North Emporia Street, Suite 200, Wichita, KS 67214-3788 · 316-263-0296

UROLOGY

Hays

Kevin R. McDonald · General Urology (Impotence) · Western Kansas Urological Associates, Building One, Suite Three, 2501 East 13th Street, P. O. Box 1176, Hays, KS 67601 · 913-628-6014

Darrell D. Werth · General Urology · Western Kansas Urological Associates, Building One, Suite Three, 2501 East 13th Street, Hays, KS 67601 · 913-628-6014

Kansas City

Winston K. Mebust · General Urology · University of Kansas Medical Center, Section of Urology, 3901 Rainbow Boulevard, Kansas City, KS 66160-7390 · 913-588-6146

John W. Weigel · Urologic Oncology (Incontinence, Sexual Dysfunction) · University of Kansas Medical Center, 3901 Rainbow Boulevard, Kansas City, KS 66160-7390 · 913-588-6147

Overland Park

J. Patrick Murphy · Pediatric Urology (Pediatric Surgery, Surgical Critical Care) Children's Mercy Hospital (Kansas City, MO) · Pediatric Surgical Associates, 5520 College Boulevard, Suite 206, Overland Park, KS 66211 · 913-491-0880

Topeka

Richard N. Isaacson · General Urology (Urologic Oncology, Stone Disease) · Stormont-Vail Regional Medical Center, St. Francis Hospital & Medical Center · 1001 Southwest Garfield Avenue, Topeka, KS 66604 · 913-233-4256

Larry G. Rotert · General Urology · Stormont-Vail Regional Medical Center, St. Francis Hospital & Medical Center · 1001 Southwest Garfield Avenue, Suite 301, Topeka, KS 66604-1368 · 913-233-4256

Wichita

Edward Bass · General Urology · Wichita Urology, 851 North Hillside Drive, Wichita, KS 67213 · 316-685-1371

Richard Steinberger · General Urology · Wichita Urology, 851 North Hillside Drive, Wichita, KS 67213 · 316-685-1371

MINNESOTA

ADDICTION MEDICINE

Minneapolis

Sheila M. Specker · General Addiction Medicine · University of Minnesota Hospital & Clinic · University of Minnesota Hospital & Clinic, Department of Psychiatry, 420 Delaware Street, SE, Box 393, Minneapolis, MN 55455 · 612-626-3698

ALLERGY & IMMUNOLOGY

Duluth

Jay L. Parker · General Allergy & Immunology · Duluth Clinic, Department of Allergy & Immunology, 400 East Third Street, Duluth, MN 55805 · 218-722-8364

Minneapolis

Malcolm N. Blumenthal · General Allergy & Immunology (Genetics of Allergy) University of Minnesota Hospital & Clinic · University of Minnesota Hospital & Clinic, 420 Delaware Street, SE, Box 434, Minneapolis, MN 55455 · 612-624-5456

Alexandra H. Filipovich · Immunodeficiency (Bone Marrow Transplantation) · University of Minnesota Hospital & Clinic · University of Minnesota Hospital & Clinic, 516 Delaware Street, SE, Box 261, Minneapolis, MN 55455 · 612-624-7686

David F. Graft · General Allergy & Immunology (Allergy) · Park Nicollet Clinic, Methodist Hospital · Park Nicollet Clinic, 3800 Park Nicollet Boulevard, Minneapolis, MN 55416-2699 · 612-993-3090

William F. Schoenwetter · General Allergy & Immunology (Allergy, Asthma, Occupational Asthma, Latex Allergy) · Methodist Hospital · Park Nicollet Clinic-Health System Minnesota, Department of Allergy & Immunology, 3800 Park Nicollet Boulevard, Minneapolis, MN 55416-2699 · 612-993-3091

Richard J. Sveum · General Allergy & Immunology (Pediatric & Adult Asthma, Allergic Rhinitis, Chronic Urticaria) · Methodist Hospital · Park Nicollet Clinic-Health System Minnesota, 3800 Park Nicollet Boulevard, Minneapolis, MN 55416-2699 · 612-927-3090

Stephen C. Weisberg · General Allergy & Immunology (Asthma, Clinical & Lab Immunology) · Abbott-Northwestern Hospital · Allergy & Asthma Specialists, Medical Arts Building, Suite 1149, 825 Nicollet Mall Avenue, Minneapolis, MN 55402 · 612-338-3333

Rochester

Edward J. O'Connell · General Allergy & Immunology (Allergy) · Mayo Clinic · Mayo Clinic, 200 First Street, SW, Rochester, MN 55905 · 507-284-2922

John W. Yunginger · General Allergy & Immunology (Pediatrics) · Mayo Clinic Mayo Clinic, 200 First Street, SW, Rochester, MN 55905 · 507-284-2922

ANESTHESIOLOGY

Duluth

John R. Gray · General Anesthesiology · St. Luke's Hospital, Department of Anesthesiology, 915 East First Street, Duluth, MN 55805 · 218-726-555

Thomas J. Losasso · General Anesthesiology (Neuroanesthesia) · Anesthesia Associates Duluth, 407 East Third Street, Duluth, MN 55805 · 218-726-4467

Donald A. Muzzi · General Anesthesiology (Neuroanesthesia) · St. Mary's Medical Center · St. Mary's Medical Center, Department of Anesthesiology, 407 East Third Street, Duluth, MN 55805 · 218-726-4469

Minneapolis

Kumar G. Belani · Pediatric Anesthesiology (Anesthesia for Solid Organ Transplantation, Malignant Hyperthermia, Complications of Anesthesia, General Anesthesiology) · University of Minnesota Hospital & Clinic, Department of Anesthesiology, 420 Delaware Street, SE, Box 294, Minneapolis, MN 55455 · 612-624-9142

Calvin B. Cameron · General Anesthesiology · University of Minnesota Hospital & Clinic, Department of Anesthesiology, 420 Delaware Street, SE, Box 294, Minneapolis, MN 55455 · 612-626-0411

Michael F. Sweeney · Pediatric Anesthesiology (Adult Cardiovascular, Cardiothoracic Anesthesiology, Pediatric Cardiovascular, Pediatric Critical Care, Extracorporeal Membrane Oxygenation) · University of Minnesota Hospital & Clinic · University of Minnesota Hospital & Clinic, Department of Anesthesiology, 420 Delaware Street, SE, Box 294 UMHC, Minneapolis, MN 55455 · 612-624-5605

Rochester

Martin D. Abel · Adult Cardiovascular (Critical Care) · Mayo Clinic · Mayo Clinic, Department of Anesthesiology, 200 First Street, SW, Rochester, MN 55905 · 507-255-4234

David L. Brown · Orthopaedic Procedures, Complications of Anesthesia (Regional Anesthesia, Pain Management) · Mayo Clinic · Mayo Clinic, Department of Anesthesiology, 200 First Street, SW, Rochester, MN 55905 · 507-284-9700

Robert C. Chantigan · Obstetric Anesthesia · Mayo Clinic, Department of Anesthesiology, 200 First Street, SW, Rochester, MN 55905 · 507-284-9697

William L. Lanier · Neuroanesthesia · Mayo Clinic · Mayo Clinic, Department of Anesthesiology, 200 First Street, SW, Rochester, MN 55905 · 507-255-4235

Robert J. Lunn · Pediatric Cardiovascular · Mayo Clinic, Department of Anesthesiology, 200 First Street, SW, Rochester, MN 55905 · 507-255-3298

Joseph M. Messick, Jr. · Pain (Pain Management) · Mayo Clinic · Mayo Clinic, Department of Anesthesiology, 200 First Street, SW, Rochester, MN 55905 · 507-255-4240

Michael J. Murray · Critical Care Medicine · Mayo Clinic, Department of Anesthesiology, 200 First Street, SW, Rochester, MN 55905 · 507-284-6129

Bradley J. Narr · Critical Care Medicine · Mayo Clinic, 200 First Street, SW, Rochester, MN 55905 · 507-285-4240

William C. Oliver, Jr. · Pediatric Cardiovascular · Mayo Clinic, Department of Anesthesiology, 200 First Street, SW, Rochester, MN 55905 · 507-255-5601

Hugo S. Raimundo · Pediatric Cardiovascular · Mayo Clinic · Mayo Clinic, Department of Anesthesiology, 200 First Street, SW, Rochester, MN 55905 · 507-255-4234

David O. Warner · General Anesthesiology · Mayo Clinic, Department of Anesthesiology, 200 First Street, SW, Rochester, MN 55905 · 507-255-4288

Mark A. Warner · General Anesthesiology (Abdominal, Prostate) · Mayo Clinic · Mayo Clinic, Department of Anesthesiology, 200 First Street, SW, Rochester, MN 55905 · 507-255-4236

Denise J. Wedel · Orthopaedic Procedures · Mayo Clinic · Mayo Clinic, Department of Anesthesiology, 200 First Street, SW, Rochester, MN 55905 · 507-284-2511

Roger D. White · Adult Cardiovascular · Mayo Clinic · Mayo Clinic, Department of Anesthesiology, 200 First Street, SW, Rochester, MN 55905 · 507-255-4235

Peter R. Wilson · Pain (Pain Management) · Mayo Clinic, The Pain Clinic, 200 First Street, SW, Rochester, MN 55905 · 507-284-8311

CARDIOVASCULAR DISEASE

Duluth

Glen Albin · General Cardiovascular Disease · Duluth Clinic, Department of Cardiology, 400 East Third Street, Duluth, MN 55805 · 218-722-8364

Carl E. Heltne · General Cardiovascular Disease · Duluth Clinic, Department of Cardiology, 400 East Third Street, Duluth, MN 55805 · 218-722-8364

Gale G. Kerns · General Cardiovascular Disease · Duluth Clinic, Department of Cardiology, 400 East Third Street, Duluth, MN 55805 · 218-722-8364

James Langeger · General Cardiovascular Disease · Duluth Clinic, Department of Cardiology, 400 East Third Street, Duluth, MN 55805 · 218-722-8364

Mark C. Neustel · General Cardiovascular Disease · Duluth Clinic, Department of Cardiology, 400 East Third Street, Duluth, MN 55805 · 218-722-8364

Edward A. Ryan · General Cardiovascular Disease · Duluth Clinic, Department of Cardiology, 400 East Third Street, Duluth, MN 55805 · 218-722-8364

Richard D. Taylor · General Cardiovascular Disease · Duluth Clinic, Department of Cardiology, 400 East Third Street, Duluth, MN 55805 · 218-722-8364

Minneapolis

Adrian K. Almquist · General Cardiovascular Disease · Minneapolis Cardiology, 920 East 28th Street, Suite 300, Minneapolis, MN 55407 · 612-863-3900

David G. Benditt · Electrophysiology · University of Minnesota Hospital & Clinic University of Minnesota Hospital & Clinic, 420 Delaware Street, SE, Box 341, Minneapolis, MN 55455 · 612-625-4401

Jay N. Cohn · Heart Failure (General Cardiovascular Disease) · University of Minnesota Hospital & Clinic · University of Minnesota Hospital & Clinic, Cardiovascular Division, 420 Delaware Street, SE, Box 488, Minneapolis, MN 55455 612-625-5646

Gary S. Francis · Heart Failure · University of Minnesota Hospital & Clinic · University of Minnesota Hospital & Clinic, Department of Cardiology, 420 Delaware Street, SE, Box 508, Minneapolis, MN 55455-0392 · 612-625-7924

Frederick L. Gobel · General Cardiovascular Disease · Minneapolis Cardiology, 920 East 28th Street, Minneapolis, MN 55407-1139 · 612-863-3900

Alan T. Hirsch · General Cardiovascular Disease (Vascular Medicine, Heart Failure, Vaso-Spastic Diseases, General Internal Medicine) · University of Minnesota Hospital & Clinic · University of Minnesota, Cardiovascular Division, 420 Delaware Street, SE, Box 508, Minneapolis, MN 55455 · 612-625-9100

Spencer H. Kubo · Heart Failure · University of Minnesota Hospital & Clinic, Department of Cardiology, 420 Delaware Street, SE, Minneapolis, MN 55455 · 612-626-3000

Marc R. Pritzker · General Cardiovascular Disease · Minneapolis Cardiology Associates, 920 East 28th Street, Suite 300, Minneapolis, MN 55407 · 612-863-3900

Robert A. Van Tassel · General Cardiovascular Disease (Interventional Cardiology, Cardiac Catheterization) · Abbott-Northwestern Hospital · Minneapolis Cardiology Associates, 920 East 28th Street, Suite 300, Minneapolis, MN 55407 · 612-863-3900

Rochester

Mark J. Callahan · General Cardiovascular Disease · Mayo Clinic · Mayo Clinic, 200 First Street, SW, Rochester, MN 55905 · 507-284-0383

Brooks S. Edwards · Transplantation Medicine (Post-Heart Transplantation Care) · Mayo Clinic · Mayo Clinic, Department of Cardiology, 200 First Street, SW, Rochester, MN 55905 · 507-284-4072

Robert L. Frye · General Cardiovascular Disease · Mayo Clinic · Mayo Clinic, 200 First Street, SW, Rochester, MN 55905 · 507-284-3681

Raymond J. Gibbons · Nuclear Cardiology · Mayo Clinic · Mayo Clinic, 200 First Street, SW, Rochester, MN 55905 · 507-284-2541

David L. Hayes · Pacemakers · Mayo Clinic, Department of Cardiology, 200 First Street, SW, Suite E16-A, Rochester, MN 55905 · 507-284-2511

David R. Holmes, Jr. · Cardiac Catheterization (Invasive Cardiology) · Mayo Clinic · Mayo Clinic, Department of Cardiology, 200 First Street, SW, Rochester, MN 55905 · 507-284-3580

Fletcher A. Miller, Jr. · General Cardiovascular Disease · Mayo Clinic · Mayo Clinic, 200 First Street, SW, Rochester, MN 55905 · 507-284-3682

Michael Mock · General Cardiovascular Disease · Mayo Clinic, Department of Cardiology, 200 First Street, SW, Rochester, MN 55905 · 507-284-2511

Rick A. Nishimura · General Cardiovascular Disease · Mayo Clinic · Mayo Clinic, 200 First Street, SW, Rochester, MN 55905 · 507-284-3265

Jae K. Oh · Echocardiography · Mayo Clinic, Department of Cardiology, 200 First Street, SW, Rochester, MN 55905 · 507-284-0783

Thom W. Rooke · General Cardiovascular Disease (Vascular Medicine) · Mayo Clinic, 200 First Street, SW, Rochester, MN 55905 · 507-284-4139

James B. Seward · Echocardiography (Invasive Echocardiography, Pediatric Cardiology) · Mayo Clinic · Mayo Clinic, 200 First Street, SW, Rochester, MN 55905 507-284-3581

Hugh C. Smith · General Cardiovascular Disease · Mayo Clinic · Mayo Clinic, 200 First Street, SW, Rochester, MN 55905 · 507-284-8341

A. Jamil Tajik · Echocardiography · Mayo Clinic · Mayo Clinic, 200 First Street, SW, Rochester, MN 55905 · 507-284-9032

Carole A. Warnes · General Cardiovascular Disease (Adult Congenital Heart Disease) · Mayo Clinic, Department of Cardiovascular Disease, 200 First Street, SW, Rochester, MN 55905 · 507-284-2511

Arnold Weissler · General Cardiovascular Disease · Mayo Clinic, 200 First Street, SW, Rochester, MN 55905 · 507-284-2511

Douglas L. Wood · General Cardiovascular Disease · Mayo Clinic, 200 First Street, SW, Rochester, MN 55905 · 507-284-8341

St. Paul

Margaret A. Beahrs · General Cardiovascular Disease · St. Paul Heart & Lung Center, 255 North Smith Avenue, Suite 100, St. Paul, MN 55102 · 612-292-0616

CLINICAL PHARMACOLOGY

Rochester

James J. Lipsky · Mayo Clinic, Department of Clinical Pharmacology, 200 First Street, SW, Rochester, MN 55905 · 507-284-4456

Richard M. Weinshilboum · (Hypertension) · Mayo Clinic · Mayo Clinic, 200 First Street, SW, Rochester, MN 55905 · 507-284-2790

COLON & RECTAL SURGERY

Duluth

Thomas M. Nelson · General Colon & Rectal Surgery · Northland Gastroenterology & Surgery, 915 East First Street, Third Floor, Duluth, MN 55805 · 218-725-6050

Edina

Ann C. Lowry · General Colon & Rectal Surgery · Colon and Rectal Surgery, 6545 France Avenue, South, Suite 474, Edina, MN 55435 · 612-920-6111

Minneapolis

Charles O. Finne III · General Colon & Rectal Surgery (Colon & Rectal Cancer, Therapeutic & Diagnostic Colonoscopy) · Abbott-Northwestern Hospital, Fairview Ridges Hospital (Burnsville), Fairview-Southdale Hospital (Edina) · Colon & Rectal Surgery Associates, Medical Arts Building, Suite 1731, 825 Nicollet Mall Avenue, Minneapolis, MN 55402 · 612-339-4534

Stanley M. Goldberg · General Colon & Rectal Surgery · University of Minnesota Hospital & Clinic, Fairview-Southdale Hospital (Edina), Abbott-Northwestern Hospital · Colon & Rectal Surgery Associates, Medical Arts Building, Suite 1731, 825 Nicollet Mall Avenue, Minneapolis, MN 55402 · 612-339-4534

Robert D. Madoff · General Colon & Rectal Surgery (Colon & Rectal Cancer, Inflammatory Bowel Disease, Incontinence) · Abbott-Northwestern Hospital, Fairview-Southdale Hospital, Methodist Hospital · Colon & Rectal Surgery Associates, Medical Arts Building, Suite 1731, 825 Nicollet Mall Avenue, Minneapolis, MN 55402 · 612-339-4534

Frederick D. Nemer · General Colon & Rectal Surgery · Colon & Rectal Surgery Associates, Medical Arts Building, Suite 1731, 825 Nicollet Mall Avenue, Minneapolis, MN 55402 · 612-339-4534

David A. Rothenberger · General Colon & Rectal Surgery, Colon & Rectal Cancer · University of Minnesota Hospital & Clinic · University of Minnesota Hospital & Clinic, 420 Delaware Street, SE, Box 450, Minneapolis, MN 55455 · 612-625-3288; 612-291-1151

W. Douglas Wong · General Colon & Rectal Surgery (Colon & Rectal Cancer, Anal Incontinence) · University of Minnesota Hospital & Clinic, Department of Surgery, 516 Delaware Street, SE, Box 450, Minneapolis, MN 55455 · 612-625-5423

Robbinsdale

Brett T. Gemlo · General Colon & Rectal Surgery · Oakdale Medical Building, Suite 605, 3366 Oakdale Avenue, North, Robbinsdale, MN 55422 · 612-786-7130

Michael P. Spencer · General Colon & Rectal Surgery (Colon & Rectal Cancer, Diseases of Colon & Rectum, Inflammatory Bowel Disease) · VA Medical Center (Minneapolis), North Memorial Health Care, Mercy Hospital (Coon Rapids), Unity Hospital (Fridley) · Colon & Rectal Surgical Associates, Oakdale Medical Building, Suite 605, 3366 Oakdale Avenue, North, Robbinsdale, MN 55422 · 612-786-7130

Rochester

Roger R. Dozois · General Colon & Rectal Surgery · Mayo Clinic · Mayo Clinic, Division of Colon & Rectal Surgery, 200 First Street, SW, Rochester, MN 55905 · 507-284-2218

Heidi Nelson · General Colon & Rectal Surgery · Mayo Clinic, Division of Colon & Rectal Surgery, 200 First Street, SW, Rochester, MN 55905 · 507-284-2511

Santhat Nivatvongs · General Colon & Rectal Surgery, Colon & Rectal Cancer · Mayo Clinic · Mayo Clinic, Department of Colon & Rectal Surgery, 200 First Street, SW, Rochester, MN 55905 · 507-284-2622

John H. Pemberton · General Colon & Rectal Surgery · Mayo Clinic, Department of Surgery, 200 First Street, SW, Rochester, MN 55905 · 507-284-2359

Bruce G. Wolff · General Colon & Rectal Surgery · Mayo Clinic, Rochester Methodist Hospital, St. Mary's Hospital of Rochester · Mayo Clinic, Division of Colon & Rectal Surgery, 200 First Street, SW, Rochester, MN 55905 · 507-284-2472

St. Paul

John G. Buls · Colon & Rectal Cancer · United Hospital · 360 Sherman Street, Suite 299, St. Paul, MN 55102 · 612-291-1151

DERMATOLOGY

Duluth

Joel T. M. Bamford · Clinical Dermatology · Duluth Clinic, Department of Dermatology, 400 East Third Street, Duluth, MN 55805 · 218-722-8364

Robert H. Lund · Clinical Dermatology · Duluth Clinic, Department of Dermatology, 400 East Third Street, Duluth, MN 55805 · 218-722-8364

Thomas T. Myers II · Clinical Dermatology · Duluth Clinic, Department of Dermatology, 400 East Third Street, Duluth, MN 55805 · 218-722-8364

Fridley

H. Irving Katz · Hair, Psoriasis · Minnesota Clinical Studies Center · Minnesota Clinical Studies Center, 7205 University Avenue, NE, Fridley, MN 55432 · 612-571-4200

Minneapolis

Thomas H. Alt · Aesthetic Surgery (Cosmetic Surgery, Hair Transplantation, Chemical Peel, Dermabrasion, Face-Lifts, Eyelifts, Liposuction) · Methodist Hospital (St. Louis Park), Unity Hospital (Fridley) · Alt Cosmetic Surgery Center, 4920 Lincoln Drive, Minneapolis, MN 55436 · 612-936-0920

Bruce Bart · Clinical Dermatology · 825 South Eighth Street, Suite 260, Minneapolis, MN 55404 · 612-347-6450

Mark V. Dahl · Clinical Dermatology (Dermatologic Immunology, General Infectious Disease, Eczema/Irritation, General Allergy & Immunology) · University of Minnesota Hospital & Clinic · University of Minnesota Hospital & Clinic, Department of Dermatology, 420 Delaware Street, SE, Box 98, Minneapolis, MN 55455 · 612-625-8625

H. Spencer Holmes · Clinical Dermatology · Park Nicollet Medical Center, 3800 Park Nicollet Boulevard, Minneapolis, MN 55416 · 612-993-3260

Maria K. Hordinsky · Hair (Hair Disorders, Depigmenting Diseases) · University of Minnesota Hospital & Clinic · University of Minnesota Hospital & Clinic, Department of Dermatology, 420 Delaware Street, SE, Box 98, Minneapolis, MN 55455-0392 · 612-625-8625

Rajneesh Madhok · Clinical Dermatology · Skin Specialists, Medical Arts Building, Suite 1002, 825 Nicollet Mall Avenue, Minneapolis, MN 55402 · 612-338-0711

Christopher B. Zachary · Skin Cancer Surgery & Reconstruction (Laser Surgery, Aesthetic Surgery) · University of Minnesota Hospital & Clinic · University of Minnesota, Department of Dermatology, 420 Delaware Street, SE, Box 98, Minneapolis, MN 55455-0392 · 612-626-4454

Brian D. Zelickson · Clinical Dermatology (Cutaneous Laser Surgery) · Abbott-Northwestern Hospital, Fairview-Southdale Hospital, Methodist Hospital · Skin Specialists Downtown, Medical Arts Building, Suite 1002, 825 Nicollet Mall Avenue, Minneapolis, MN 55402 · 612-338-0711

Robbinsdale

Milton Orkin · Clinical Dermatology (Dermatopathology, Scabies) · North Memorial Health Care · Skin Consultants, 3366 Oakdale Avenue, North, Suite 300, Robbinsdale, MN 55422 · 612-529-9181

Rochester

Iftikar Ahmed · Dermatopathology · Mayo Clinic, Department of Dermatology, 200 First Street, SW, Suite E5, Rochester, MN 55905 · 507-284-2511

David G. Brodland · Skin Cancer Surgery & Reconstruction · Mayo Clinic, Department of Dermatology, 200 First Street, SW, Rochester, MN 55905 · 507-284-3579

Charles H. Dicken · Psoriasis, Clinical Dermatology · Mayo Clinic, Department of Dermatology, 200 First Street, SW, Rochester, MN 55905 · 507-284-4157

Lawrence E. Gibson · Clinical Dermatology, Cutaneous Lymphomas · Mayo Clinic, Department of Dermatology, 200 First Street, SW, Rochester, MN 55905 507-284-4672

Kristin M. Leiferman · Atopic Dermatitis, Allergic Reactions of the Skin · Mayo Clinic, Department of Dermatology, 200 First Street, SW, Rochester, MN 55905 507-284-3668

Marian T. McEvoy · Photobiology · Mayo Clinic, Department of Dermatology, 200 First Street, SW, Rochester, MN 55905 · 507-284-3837

Harold Otto Perry · Clinical Dermatology · Mayo Clinic · Mayo Clinic, 200 First Street, SW, Rochester, MN 55905 · 507-284-2522

Mark B. Pittelkow · Wound Healing (Skin Biology) · Mayo Clinic, Department of Dermatology, 200 First Street, SW, Rochester, MN 55905 · 507-284-2555

Randall K. Roenigk · Skin Cancer Surgery & Reconstruction · Mayo Clinic · Mayo Clinic, Department of Dermatology, 200 First Street, SW, Rochester, MN 55905 · 507-284-3579

Roy S. Rogers III · Mucous Membrane Diseases, Clinical Dermatology, Cutaneous Immunology (Mouth Diseases) · Mayo Clinic, St. Mary's Hospital of Rochester, Rochester Methodist Hospital · Mayo Clinic, 200 First Street, SW, Rochester, MN 55905 · 507-284-3837

W. P. Daniel Su · Dermatopathology · Mayo Clinic, Department of Dermatology, 200 First Street, SW, Rochester, MN 55905 · 507-284-3668

EATING DISORDERS

Rochester

Michael D. Jensen · Obesity · Mayo Clinic, 200 First Street, SW, West 18-A, Rochester, MN 55905 · 507-284-2462

ENDOCRINOLOGY & METABOLISM

Duluth

Michael F. Slag · General Endocrinology & Metabolism · Duluth Clinic, 400 East Third Street, Duluth, MN 55805 · 218-722-8364

Minneapolis

John P. Bantle · Diabetes (General Endocrinology) · University of Minnesota Hospital & Clinic · University of Minnesota Hospital & Clinic, 420 Delaware Street, SE, Box 504 UMHC, Minneapolis, MN 55455 · 612-626-0476

Richard M. Bergenstal · Diabetes · Park Nicollet Medical Center · International Diabetes Center, 3800 Park Nicollet Boulevard, Minneapolis, MN 55416 · 612-927-3393

Lisa H. Fish · General Endocrinology & Metabolism (Diabetes, Thyroid) · Methodist Hospital · Park Nicollet Medical Center, 3800 Park Nicollet Boulevard, Minneapolis, MN 55416-2699 · 612-993-3530

Cary N. Mariash · General Endocrinology & Metabolism · University of Minnesota Hospital & Clinic, Mayo Building, 515 Delaware Street, SE, Box 91 UMHC, Minneapolis, MN 55455 · 612-624-5150

R. Paul Robertson · Diabetes · University of Minnesota Hospital & Clinic · University of Minnesota Hospital & Clinic, 516 Delaware Street, SE, Box 101, Minneapolis, MN 55455 · 612-626-1960

Elizabeth R. Seaquist · Diabetes (Pituitary Disease, General Endocrinology & Metabolism, Neuroendocrinology, Thyroid, General Internal Medicine) · University of Minnesota Hospital & Clinic · University of Minnesota Hospital & Clinic, 420 Delaware Street, SE, Box 101, Minneapolis, MN 55455 · 612-626-1960

Rochester

Charles Abboud · General Endocrinology & Metabolism · Mayo Clinic · Mayo Clinic, 200 First Street, SW, Rochester, MN 55905 · 507-284-2617

Michael D. Brennan · General Endocrinology & Metabolism · Mayo Clinic, Department of Endocrinology and Metabolism, 200 First Street, SW, Rochester, MN 55905 · 507-284-2511

Vahab Fatourechi · General Endocrinology & Metabolism · Mayo Clinic, 200 First Street, SW, Rochester, MN 55905 · 507-284-3150

Colum A. Gorman · Thyroid · Mayo Clinic · Mayo Clinic, 200 First Street, SW, Rochester, MN 55905 · 507-284-4738

Ian D. Hay · Thyroid · Mayo Clinic · Mayo Clinic, 200 First Street, SW, Rochester, MN 55905 · 507-284-3915

Frank P. Kennedy · Diabetes (Obesity) · Mayo Clinic, 200 First Street, SW, Rochester, MN 55905 · 507-284-2511

Molly M. McMahon · General Endocrinology & Metabolism (Nutrition) · Mayo Clinic, Department of Endocrinology and Metabolism, 200 First Street, SW, Rochester, MN 55905 · 507-284-2511

Roger Nelson · Diabetes · Mayo Clinic · Mayo Clinic, 200 First Street, SW, Rochester, MN 55905 · 507-284-3707

Tu T. Nguyen · General Endocrinology & Metabolism (Lipids) · Mayo Clinic, Department of Endocrinology and Metabolism, 200 First Street, SW, Rochester, MN 55905 · 507-284-2511

Robert A. Rizza · Diabetes · Mayo Clinic · Mayo Clinic, 200 First Street, SW, Rochester, MN 55905 · 507-284-2784

F. John Service · Diabetes · Mayo Clinic · Mayo Clinic, 200 First Street, SW, Rochester, MN 55905 · 507-284-3964

William F. Young, Jr. · General Endocrinology & Metabolism (Hypertension, Adrenal Gland Disorders) · Mayo Clinic · Mayo Clinic, 200 First Street, SW, Rochester, MN 55905 · 507-284-8712

Bruce R. Zimmerman · Diabetes · Mayo Clinic · Mayo Clinic, 200 First Street, SW, Rochester, MN 55905 · 507-266-4322

St. Cloud

Hans H. Engman · General Endocrinology & Metabolism · Centracare Clinic, 1200 Sixth Avenue, North, St. Cloud, MN 56303-2735 · 612-252-5131 x249

FAMILY MEDICINE

Duluth

Byron J. Crouse · (Immunizations, Disease Prevention, Sports Medicine) · Mercy Hospital & Health Care Center (Moose Lake), St. Mary's Medical Center, St. Luke's Hospital, Miller Dwan Medical Center · University of Minnesota School of

Medicine, Department of Family Medicine, 10 University Drive, Duluth, MN 55812 · 218-726-7916

Stephen C. Harrington · Duluth Clinic West, 4325 Grand Avenue, Duluth, MN 55807 · 218-725-3500

Hermantown

Mark W. Boyce · Duluth Clinic-Hermantown, 4855 West Arrowhead Road, Hermantown, MN 55811 · 218-725-3540

Kasson

David C. Agerter · 411 West Main Street, Kasson, MN 55944 · 507-284-3967

Minneapolis

Michael P. Dukinfield · Park Nicollet Medical Center, 3800 Park Nicollet Boulevard, Minneapolis, MN 55416 · 612-927-3400

Charles E. McCoy · (Diabetes Prevention Medicine) · Methodist Hospital · Park Nicollet Medical Center, 3800 Park Nicollet Boulevard, Minneapolis, MN 55416-2620 · 612-927-3400

Thomas K. Pettus · (Geriatrics) · Integer Clinic, 2545 Chicago Avenue, Minneapolis, MN 55404 · 612-863-3160

Harold C. Seim · (Obesity) · University of Minnesota Hospital & Clinic · University of Minnesota Hospital & Clinic, Department of Family Practice and Community Health, 702 Washington Avenue, SE, Minneapolis, MN 55414 · 612-627-1095

Minnetonka

Timothy David Pryor · (Preventive Medicine, Hypertension, Hyperlipidemia) · Methodist Hospital (St. Louis Park) · Park Nicollet Clinic, Carlson Parkway Office, 15111 Twelve Oaks Center Drive, Minnetonka, MN 55305 · 612-993-4500

Rochester

Steven C. Adamson · Mayo Clinic, 200 First Street, SW, Rochester, MN 55905 507-284-2511

Gregory L. Angstman · Mayo Clinic · Mayo Clinic, Department of Family Medicine, 200 First Street, SW, Rochester, MN 55905 · 507-284-3967

John W. Bachman · Mayo Clinic · Mayo Clinic, Department of Family Medicine, 200 First Street, SW, Rochester, MN 55905 · 507-284-2774

Walter B. Franz III · Mayo Clinic, 200 First Street, SW, Rochester, MN 55905 · 507-284-5307

Thomas R. Harman · Mayo Clinic · Mayo Clinic, Department of Family Medicine, 200 First Street, SW, Rochester, MN 55905 · 507-284-5919

Shoreview

Ross E. Anderson · Family Physicians, 4194 North Lexington Avenue, Shoreview, MN 55126 · 612-483-5461

St. Paul

Nancy J. Baker · Ramsey Family Physicians, 640 Jackson Street, St. Paul, MN 55101 · 612-221-8666

Allen E. McCamy · Maryland Clinic, 911 East Maryland Avenue, St. Paul, MN 55106 · 612-776-2719

GASTROENTEROLOGY

Duluth

Johannes Aas · General Gastroenterology · Duluth Clinic, Department of Gastroenterology, 400 East Third Street, Duluth, MN 55805 · 218-722-8364

Robert V. Erikson · General Gastroenterology · Duluth Clinic, Department of Gastroenterology, 400 East Third Street, Duluth, MN 55805 · 218-722-8364

Daniel P. McKee · General Gastroenterology · St. Luke's Hospital, Department of Gastroenterology, 915 East First Street, Duluth, MN 55805 · 218-725-6050

Minneapolis

John Allen · General Gastroenterology (Gastrointestinal Cancer, Cancer Genetics) · Abbott-Northwestern Hospital · Digestive Healthcare, 2545 Chicago Avenue, South, Minneapolis, MN 55407 · 612-871-1145

John H. Bond · Endoscopy · VA Medical Center · Minneapolis Veterans Affairs Medical Center, Gastroenterology Section, One Veterans Drive, Mail Code 111D, Minneapolis, MN 55417 · 612-725-2000

Cecil H. Chally · General Gastroenterology (Esophageal Disease, Inflammatory Bowel Disease) · Abbott-Northwestern Hospital · Digestive Healthcare, 2545 Chicago Avenue, South, Minneapolis, MN 55407 · 612-871-1145

Robert A. Ganz · General Gastroenterology (Esophageal Disease, Peptic Disorders, Inflammatory Bowel Disease) · Digestive Healthcare, 2545 Chicago Avenue, South, Minneapolis, MN 55407 · 612-871-1145

Arnold P. Kaplan · General Gastroenterology (Colon Cancer, Esophageal Disease, Biliary Disorders) · Abbott-Northwestern Hospital · Digestive Healthcare, 2545 Chicago Avenue, South, Minneapolis, MN 55407 · 612-871-1145

Michael D. Levitt · General Gastroenterology (Gastrointestinal Motility, Pancreatic Disease) · VA Medical Center · VA Medical Center, Research Service, One Veterans Drive, Minneapolis, MN 55417 · 612-725-2033

Robert Mackie · General Gastroenterology · Digestive Healthcare, 2545 Chicago Avenue, South, Minneapolis, MN 55407 · 612-871-1145

Mark J. Schmidt · General Gastroenterology (General Internal Medicine) · Metropolitan Medical Office Building, Suite 1122, 825 South Eighth Street, Minneapolis, MN 55404 · 612-332-3517

Stephen E. Silvis · Endoscopy (Esophageal Disease, Biliary Disease) · VA Medical Center · VA Medical Center, Gastroenterology Section, One Veterans Drive, Mail Code 111D, Minneapolis, MN 55417 · 612-725-2000

Coleman Smith · General Gastroenterology (Hepatology) · Digestive Healthcare, 2545 Chicago Avenue, South, Suite 700, Minneapolis, MN 55404 · 612-871-1145

Ronald D. Soltis · General Gastroenterology · University of Minnesota Hospital & Clinic, Department of Gastroenterology, 516 Delaware Street, SE, Minneapolis, MN 55455 · 612-625-8999

Joseph Tombers · General Gastroenterology (Inflammatory Bowel Disease, Liver Disease) · Fairview-Southdale Hospital (Edina), Abbott-Northwestern Hospital · Digestive Healthcare, 2545 Chicago Avenue, South, P.O. Box 7128, Minneapolis, MN 55407-0128 · 612-871-1145

David I. Weinberg · General Gastroenterology (Inflammatory Bowel Disease, Endoscopy) · Abbott-Northwestern Hospital, North Memorial Health Care (Robbinsdale) · Minnesota Gastroenterology, 2545 Chicago Avenue, South, Suite 700, Minneapolis, MN 55404 · 612-871-1145

Rochester

David A. Ahlquist · General Gastroenterology · Mayo Clinic, Department of Gastroenterology, 200 First Street, SW, Rochester, MN 55905 · 507-284-8700

Michael Camilleri · Gastrointestinal Motility (Colon Motility) · Mayo Clinic · Mayo Clinic, 200 First Street, SW, Rochester, MN 55905 · 507-284-2511

Jonathan E. Clain · General Gastroenterology · Mayo Clinic, Department of Gastroenterology, 200 First Street, SW, Rochester, MN 55905 · 507-284-2478

Albert J. Czaja · Hepatology · Mayo Clinic, Department of Gastroenterology, 200 First Street, SW, Rochester, MN 55905 · 507-284-8118

E. Rolland Dickson · Hepatology (Liver Transplantation) · Mayo Clinic, St. Mary's Hospital of Rochester, Rochester Methodist Hospital · Mayo Clinic, 200 First Street, SW, Rochester, MN 55905 · 507-284-8700

Eugene P. DiMagno · Pancreatic Disease · Mayo Clinic · Mayo Clinic, 200 First Street, SW, Rochester, MN 55905 · 507-255-4303

Christopher J. Gostout · Endoscopy · Mayo Clinic, Department of Gastroenterology, 200 First Street, SW, Rochester, MN 55905 · 507-289-2511

Nicholas F. LaRusso · Hepatology (Cholestatic Liver Disease) · Mayo Clinic, 200 First Street, SW, Rochester, MN 55905 · 507-284-1006

Douglas B. McGill · Hepatology · Mayo Clinic, Department of Gastroenterology, 200 First Street, SW, Rochester, MN 55905 · 507-284-2217

Albert D. Newcomer · General Gastroenterology · Mayo Clinic, Department of Gastroenterology, 200 First Street, SW, Rochester, MN 55905 · 507-284-2467

Sidney Phillips · Functional Gastrointestinal Disorders · Mayo Clinic, St. Mary's Hospital of Rochester · Mayo Clinic, 200 First Street, SW, West 19B, Rochester, MN 55905 · 507-255-6028

William J. Sandborn · General Gastroenterology · Mayo Clinic, Department of Gastroenterology, 200 First Street, SW, Rochester, MN 55905 · 507-284-0083

Johnson Thistle · Hepatology · Mayo Clinic, Department of Gastroenterology, 200 First Street, SW, Rochester, MN 55905 · 507-284-8714

William J. Tremaine · Inflammatory Bowel Disease · Mayo Clinic, Department of Gastroenterology, 200 First Street, SW, Rochester, MN 55905 · 507-284-2469

St. Cloud

Bradley E. Currier · General Gastroenterology (General Internal Medicine, Critical Care Medicine) · Centracare Clinic, 1200 Sixth Avenue, North, St. Cloud, MN 56303-2735 · 612-252-5131

Peter E. Nelson · General Gastroenterology · Centracare Clinic, 1200 Sixth Avenue, North, St. Cloud, MN 56303 · 612-252-5131

St. Paul

Thomas C. Bagnoli · General Gastroenterology · Gastroenterology Consultants, 1959 Sloan Place, Suite 100, St. Paul, MN 55117-2070 · 612-778-9694

Arnold M. Brier · General Gastroenterology · Gastroenterology Consultants, 1959 Sloan Place, Suite 100, St. Paul, MN 55117-2070 · 612-778-9694

GERIATRIC MEDICINE

Minneapolis

Patrick W. Irvine · Hennepin County Medical Center · United Healthcare/Evercare, Mail Route MN08-W211, P.O. Box 59193, Minneapolis, MN 55459-0193 · 612-936-6022

Joseph M. Keenan · (Home Care, Preventive Cardiology) · University of Minnesota Hospital & Clinic · University of Minnesota Hospital & Clinic, Department of Family Practice, 825 Washington Avenue, SE, Suite 201, Minneapolis, MN 55414-3034 · 612-627-4935

John R. Mach · 4001 Stinson Boulevard, Suite 207, Minneapolis, MN 55421 · 612-788-9258

HAND SURGERY

Edina

Allen L. Van Beek · Peripheral Nerve Surgery · North Memorial Health Care (Robbinsdale), Fairview-Southdale Hospital, Abbott-Northwestern Hospital (Minneapolis), Children's Health Care-Minneapolis (Minneapolis) · Plastic Surgery Specialists, 7373 France Avenue, South, Suite 510, Edina, MN 55435 · 612-588-0593; 612-830-1028

Minneapolis

James H. House · Paralytic Disorders, Reconstructive Surgery (Tendon Transfer Reconstruction, Congenital, Pediatric Orthopaedic Surgery) · University of Minnesota Hospital & Clinic · University of Minnesota Hospital & Clinic, Department of Orthopaedic Surgery, 420 Delaware Street, SE, Box 492, Minneapolis, MN 55455 · 612-625-7951

Edward C. McElfresh · General Hand Surgery · University of Minnesota Hospital & Clinic · University of Minnesota Hospital & Clinic, Orthopaedic & Sports Medicine Clinic, 420 Delaware Street, SE, Box 492 UMHC, Minneapolis, MN 55455 · 612-625-1177

Rochester

Peter C. Amadio · General Hand Surgery · Mayo Clinic, St. Mary's Hospital of Rochester · Mayo Clinic, 200 First Street, SW, Rochester, MN 55905 · 507-284-2806

Allen T. Bishop · General Hand Surgery · Mayo Clinic, Department of Hand Surgery, 200 First Street, SW, Rochester, MN 55905 · 507-284-2511

William Patrick Cooney III · General Hand Surgery · Mayo Clinic · Mayo Clinic, 200 First Street, SW, Rochester, MN 55905 · 507-284-2994

Michael B. Wood · Reconstructive Surgery, Microsurgery · Rochester Methodist Hospital · Mayo Clinic, 200 First Street, SW, Rochester, MN 55905 · 507-284-3689; 507-284-2511

Wayzata

Thomas F. Varecka · General Hand Surgery (Shoulder Surgery) · Abbott-Northwestern Hospital (Minneapolis), Hennepin County Medical Center (Minneapolis), Fairview Riverside Medical Center (Minneapolis) · Wayzata Orthopaedics, 250 Central Avenue, North, Suite 303, Wayzata, MN 55391 · 612-337-0415

INFECTIOUS DISEASE

Duluth

Johan S. Bakken · General Infectious Disease · Duluth Clinic, Department of Infectious Disease, 400 East Third Street, Duluth, MN 55805 · 218-722-8364

Mark Eckman · General Infectious Disease · Duluth Clinic, 400 East Third Street, Duluth, MN 55805 · 218-722-8364

Linda L. VanEtta · General Infectious Disease · Duluth Clinic, Department of Infectious Disease, 400 East Third Street, Duluth, MN 55805 · 218-722-8364

Minneapolis

Leslie A. Baken · General Infectious Disease (HIV, Viral Diseases, Sexually Transmitted Diseases, Immunodeficiency) · Methodist Hospital · Park Nicollet Clinic, 3800 Park Nicollet Boulevard, Minneapolis, MN 55416-2699 · 612-993-3131

M. Colin Jordan · General Infectious Disease (AIDS, Herpes Virus Infections) · University of Minnesota Hospital & Clinic, Mayo Medical Building, 516 Delaware Street, SE, Box 250, Minneapolis, MN 55455 · 612-624-9996

Edward L. Kaplan · Endocarditis (Pediatric) · University of Minnesota Hospital & Clinic · University of Minnesota Hospital & Clinic, 420 Delaware Street, SE, Box 296, Minneapolis, MN 55455 · 612-624-1112

Allan C. Kind · General Infectious Disease · Park Nicollet Medical Center, 3800 Park Nicollet Boulevard, Minneapolis, MN 55416-2527 · 612-993-3131

Phillip Keith Peterson · General Infectious Disease (Transplantation Infections, Infections in Immunocompromised Patients) · Hennepin County Medical Center Hennepin County Medical Center, Division of Infectious Diseases, 701 Park Avenue, South, Mail Code 865B, Minneapolis, MN 55415 · 612-347-2705

Frank S. Rhame · Hospital-Acquired Infections, AIDS (Tropical Disease & Travel Medicine, General Infectious Disease) · Abbott-Northwestern Hospital · Abbott-Northwestern Hospital, 800 East 28th Street, Clinic 42, Minneapolis, MN 55407 · 612-863-5336

Dean T. Tsukayama · General Infectious Disease (Musculoskeletal Infections) · Hennepin County Medical Center, Division of Infectious Diseases, 701 Park Avenue, South, Minneapolis, MN 55415-1623 · 612-347-2705

David N. Williams · General Infectious Disease (Travel Medicine, Bone & Joint Infections, Endocarditis) · Hennepin County Medical Center · Hennepin Faculty Associates Internal Medicine, 825 South Eighth Street, Suite 206, Minneapolis, MN 55404 · 612-347-7534

Rochester

Robert E. Van Scoy · General Infectious Disease · Mayo Clinic · Mayo Clinic, 200 First Street, SW, Rochester, MN 55905 · 507-284-3309

Conrad Wilkowske · General Infectious Disease · Mayo Clinic · Mayo Clinic, 200 First Street, SW, Rochester, MN 55905 · 507-284-1903

Walter R. Wilson · Endocarditis · Mayo Clinic · Mayo Clinic, 200 First Street, SW, Rochester, MN 55905 · 507-255-7761

St. Paul

Kent B. Crossley · General Infectious Disease · St. Paul-Ramsey Medical Center, Department of Internal Medicine, 640 Jackson Street, St. Paul, MN 55101 · 612-221-3486

Wayzata

Kathryn R. Love · General Infectious Disease (Transplantation Infections, Hospital-Acquired Infections) · Abbott-Northwestern Hospital (Minneapolis), North Memorial Health Care (Robbinsdale) · Infectious Disease Consultants, 641 East Lake Street, Suite 234, Wayzata, MN 55391 · 612-473-6625

INTERNAL MEDICINE (GENERAL)

Duluth

Michael J. Huska · Duluth Internal Medicine, 324 West Superior Street, Suite 220, Duluth, MN 55802 · 218-727-8585

Alan M. Johns · Duluth Clinic, Department of Internal Medicine, 400 East Third Street, Duluth, MN 55805 · 218-722-8364

Paul B. Sanford · Duluth Clinic, Department of Internal Medicine, 400 East Third Street, Duluth, MN 55805 · 218-722-8364

David N. Sproat · (General Cardiovascular Disease, General Geriatric Medicine) St. Luke's Hospital, St. Mary's Medical Center · Duluth Internal Medicine, 220 Medical Arts Building, 324 West Superior Street, Duluth, MN 55802 · 218-727-8585

Minneapolis

Richard Adair · Abbott-Northwestern Hospital · Medical Arts Building, Suite 300, 825 Nicollet Mall Avenue, Minneapolis, MN 55402 · 612-332-8314

Jeffery Balke · University of Minnesota Hospital & Clinic · University of Minnesota Hospital & Clinic, Department of General & Preventive Medicine, 420 Delaware Street, SE, Minneapolis, MN 55455 · 612-626-1477

Terese M. Collins · University of Minnesota Hospital & Clinic, Department of General & Preventive Medicine, 420 Delaware Street, SE, Minneapolis, MN 55455 · 612-626-1477

Craig L. Davidson · Park Nicollet Medical Center, 5000 West 39th Street, Minneapolis, MN 55416 · 612-927-3333

Thomas F. Ferris · University of Minnesota, Department of Medicine, 516 Delaware Street, Box 194, Minneapolis, MN 55455 · 612-625-4162

Heather Gantzer · Park Nicollet Medical Center, Department of Internal Medicine, 3800 Park Nicollet Boulevard, Minneapolis, MN 55416 · 612-993-3333

Guilford G. Hartley · Hennepin Faculty Associates Internal Medicine, 825 South Eighth Street, Suite 206, Minneapolis, MN 55404 · 612-347-7534

Robert B. Howe · University Minnesota Hospital & Clinic, Harvard Street and East River Parkway, Minneapolis, MN 55455 · 612-625-2981

Nancy J. Jarvis · Park Nicollet Medical Center, 3800 Park Nicollet Boulevard, Minneapolis, MN 55416 · 612-927-3333

Gary McVeigh · (Hypertension, Hypercholesterolemia, Diabetes Mellitus, General Internal Medicine) · University of Minnesota Hospital & Clinic · University of Minnesota Hospital & Clinic, General Internal Medicine, 420 Delaware Street, SE, Box 741, Minneapolis, MN 55455 · 612-626-1477

Charles Moldow · Minneapolis Veterans Affairs Medical Center, Office of the Chief of Staff, One Veterans Drive, Mail Code 11, Minneapolis, MN 55417 · 612-725-2104

Eugene W. Ollila · (Cardiovascular Disease, Diabetes, Outdoor Medicine, General Internal Medicine) · Abbott Clinic, Internists Division, Medical Arts Building, Suite 300, 825 Nicollet Mall Avenue, Minneapolis, MN 55402 · 612-333-8883

R. Charles Petersen · Abbott Clinic, Medical Arts Building, Suite 300, 825 Nicollet Mall Avenue, Minneapolis, MN 55402 · 612-332-8314

Gregory A. Plotnikoff · (Asthma, Chronic Illness, Chronic Pain, General Pediatrics, General Geriatric Medicine, General Internal Medicine) · University of Minnesota Hospital & Clinic · University of Minnesota Hospital & Clinic, 420 Delaware Street, SE, Box 741, Minneapolis, MN 55455 · 612-626-1477

Henry T. Smith · (Hypertension) · Hennepin County Medical Center · Hennepin Faculty Associates Internal Medicine, 825 South Eighth Street, Suite 206, Minneapolis, MN 55404 · 612-347-7534

Scott R. Strickland · (AIDS) · Park Nicollet Medical Center, 3800 Park Nicollet Boulevard, Minneapolis, MN 55416 · 612-927-3267

Paul Sutter · Abbott-Northwestern Hospital · Minneapolis Internal Medicine, 300 Medical Arts Building, Minneapolis, MN 55402 · 612-332-8314

Carl E. Vaurio · Metropolitan Medical Office Building, Suite 1122, 825 South Eighth Street, Minneapolis, MN 55404 · 612-332-3517

Kathleen V. Watson · University of Minnesota Hospital & Clinic, Department of General & Preventive Medicine, 420 Delaware Street, SE, Minneapolis, MN 55455 · 612-626-1477

Kathleen Whitley · Park Nicollet Medical Center, 3800 Park Nicollet Boulevard, Minneapolis, MN 55416 · 612-927-3333

Anthony C. Woolley · (Hypertension, General Nephrology) · Methodist Hospital Park Nicollet Medical Center, Department of Internal Medicine, 3800 Park Nicollet Boulevard, Minneapolis, MN 55416 · 612-927-3333

Minnetonka

Jennifer Olson · Park Nicollet Internal Medicine, 15111 Twelve Oaks Center Drive, Minnetonka, MN 55305 · 612-993-4540

Ridgefield

Bradley Heltemes · (Preventive Cardiology) · Abbott-Northwestern Hospital (Minneapolis) · Woodlake Medical Clinic, 407 West 66th Street, Ridgefield, MN 55423 · 612-798-8800

Rochester

Lawrence R. Bergstrom · Mayo Clinic, Area General Internal Medicine, Bauldwin Building, Suite 4B, 201 Fourth Avenue, SW, Rochester, MN 55905 · 507-284-2511

Kurt W. Carlson · Mayo Clinic, Department of General Internal Medicine, 200 First Street, SW, Rochester, MN 55905 · 507-284-4921

Lowell C. Dale · Mayo Clinic, Department of Community Internal Medicine, 200 First Street, SW, Rochester, MN 55905 · 507-284-5171

Nancy C. Grubbs · Mayo Clinic, Department of Community Internal Medicine, 200 First Street, SW, Rochester, MN 55905 · 507-284-0319

Richard D. Hurt · Mayo Clinic, 200 First Street, SW, Rochester, MN 55905 · 507-284-5171

Charles C. Kennedy · Mayo Clinic, Department of Community Internal Medicine, Bauldwin Building, Suite 6A, 201 Fourth Avenue, SW, Rochester, MN 55905 · 507-284-2511

Malcolm I. Lindsay, Jr. · Mayo Clinic, Department of Community Internal Medicine, 200 First Street, SW, Rochester, MN 55905 · 507-284-5171

David N. Mohr · Mayo Clinic, 200 First Street, SW, Rochester, MN 55905-0002 507-284-2511

Thomas H. Poterucha · Mayo Clinic, Department of Community Internal Medicine, Bauldwin Building, Suite 6B, 201 Fourth Avenue, SW, Rochester, MN 55905 · 507-284-2511

Charles H. Rohren · Mayo Clinic, 200 First Street, SW, Rochester, MN 55905 · 507-284-5171

Henry J. Schultz · Mayo Clinic, 200 First Street, SW, Rochester, MN 55905 · 507-284-5171

Nina M. Schwenk · Mayo Clinic, 200 First Street, SW, Rochester, MN 55905 · 507-284-3977

Douglas M. Zerbe · Mayo Clinic, Department of Community Internal Medicine, 200 First Street, SW, Rochester, MN 55905 · 507-284-5171

St. Paul

Peter B. Arnesen · United Internal Medicine, 280 North Smith Avenue, Suite 750, St. Paul, MN 55102 · 612-220-6383

Stephen J. Kolar · (General Internal Medicine, General Geriatric Medicine) · HealthEast Bethesda Lutheran Hospital & Rehabilitation Center, HealthEast Midway Hospital, HealthEast St. Joseph's Hospital, United Hospital · Minnesota Internal Medicine, 1690 University Avenue, Suite 570, St. Paul, MN 55104-3729 612-232-4800

Thomas R. Smith · (Endocrinology, Diabetes) · United Hospital, HealthEast Midway Hospital, HealthEast St. Joseph's Hospital · Aspen Medical Group, 17 West Exchange Street, Suite 600, St. Paul, MN 55100 · 612-228-7800

MEDICAL ONCOLOGY & HEMATOLOGY

Duluth

James E. Crook · General Medical Oncology & Hematology · Duluth Clinic · Duluth Clinic, Department of Oncology, 400 East Third Street, Duluth, MN 55805-1951 · 218-722-8364

Robert J. Dalton · General Medical Oncology & Hematology · Duluth Clinic · Duluth Clinic, Department of Oncology, 400 East Third Street, Duluth, MN 55805-1951 · 218-722-8364

Ronald J. Kirschling · General Medical Oncology & Hematology · Duluth Clinic, Department of Oncology, 400 East Third Street, Duluth, MN 55805 · 218-722-8364

Robert D. Neidringhaus · General Medical Oncology & Hematology · Duluth Clinic, Department of Oncology-Hematology, 400 East Third Street, Duluth, MN 55805 · 218-722-8364

Minneapolis

Linda J. Burns · General Medical Oncology & Hematology (Bone Marrow Transplantation, Lymphomas) · University of Minnesota Hospital & Clinic, Department of Medicine, Division of Medical Oncology, 420 Delaware Street, SE, Minneapolis, MN 55455 · 612-624-8144

J. Paul Carlson · General Medical Oncology & Hematology · Methodist Hospital Park Nicollet Cancer Center, 3800 Park Nicollet Boulevard, Minneapolis, MN 55416-2527 · 612-927-3248

Helen Enright · Bone Marrow Transplantation (Myelodysplastic Syndromes, General Hematology) · University of Minnesota Hospital & Clinic · University of Minnesota Hospital & Clinic, Department of Medicine, Division of Hematology, 420 Delaware Street, SE, Minneapolis, MN 55455 · 612-625-2654

P. J. Flynn · General Medical Oncology & Hematology · Abbott-Northwestern Hospital · Minnesota Oncology/Hematology, Piper Building, Suite 405, 800 East 28th Street, Minneapolis, MN 55407-3799 · 612-863-8585

B. J. Kennedy · Breast Cancer, Genito-Urinary Cancer (Medical Oncology only, Lymphomas, Cancer & Aging, Chemotherapy, Testicular Cancer) · University of Minnesota Hospital & Clinic · University of Minnesota Hospital & Clinic, 420 Delaware Street, SE, Box 286, Minneapolis, MN 55455 · 612-624-9611

David T. Kiang · Breast Cancer · University of Minnesota Hospital & Clinic · University of Minnesota Hospital & Clinic, 420 Delaware Street, SE, Box 286, Minneapolis, MN 55455 · 612-624-6982

Philip B. McGlave · Bone Marrow Transplantation (Hematologic Malignancies, Immunotherapy, Cancer Biotherapy, Leukemia, Lymphomas, Myeloma) · University of Minnesota Hospital & Clinic · University of Minnesota Hospital & Clinic, Division of Hematology, 420 Delaware Street, SE, Box 480, Minneapolis, MN 55455 · 612-624-5422; 612-624-6409

Jeffrey S. Miller · Bone Marrow Transplantation (Immunotherapy, Cancer Biotherapy, Leukemia, Lymphomas, Myeloma, Hematologic Malignancy) · University of Minnesota Hospital & Clinic · University of Minnesota Hospital & Clinic, Department of Medicine, Division of Hematology, 420 Delaware Street, SE, Minneapolis, MN 55455 · 612-625-7409

Kathleen Ogle · General Medical Oncology & Hematology · Park Nicollet Cancer Center, 3800 Park Nicollet Boulevard, Minneapolis, MN 55416-2527 · 612-927-3248

Martin M. Oken · Lymphomas, Myeloma (Leukemia, Breast Cancer, Gastrointestinal Cancer, General Medical Oncology & Hematology, Lung Cancer) · The Virginia Piper Cancer Institute, Abbott-Northwestern Hospital · Abbott-Northwestern Hospital, Virginia Piper Cancer Institute, 800 East 28th Street, Minneapolis, MN 55407 · 612-863-4633

Bruce A. Peterson · Lymphomas · University of Minnesota Hospital & Clinic · University of Minnesota Hospital & Clinic, Division of Oncology, 420 Delaware Street, Box 286 UMHC, Minneapolis, MN 55455 · 612-624-5631

Douglas J. Raush · General Medical Oncology & Hematology · Methodist Hospital · Park Nicollet Medical Center, 3800 Park Nicollet Boulevard, Minneapolis, MN 55416 · 612-993-3248

Catherine M. Verfeillie · Bone Marrow Transplantation (Leukemia, Lymphoma Therapy, Stem Cell Transplantation) · University of Minnesota Hospital & Clinic, Department of Medicine/Hematology, 420 Delaware Street, SE, Minneapolis, MN 55455 · 612-624-3921

Daniel J. Weisdorf · Bone Marrow Transplantation (Leukemia, Lymphoma Therapy, Stem Cell Transplantation, Myeloma) · University of Minnesota Hospital & Clinic · University of Minnesota Hospital & Clinic, 420 Delaware Street, SE, Box 480, Minneapolis, MN 55455 · 612-624-3101

Rochester

David L. Ahmann · Breast Cancer · Mayo Clinic · Mayo Clinic, 200 First Street, SW, Rochester, MN 55905 · 507-284-2779

Philip R. Greipp · Myeloma · Mayo Clinic · Mayo Clinic, 200 First Street, SW, Rochester, MN 55905 · 507-284-3159

H. Clark Hoagland · General Medical Oncology & Hematology · Mayo Clinic · Mayo Clinic, 200 First Street, SW, Rochester, MN 55905 · 507-284-3151

James N. Ingle · Breast Cancer · Mayo Clinic · Mayo Clinic, 200 First Street, SW, Rochester, MN 55905 · 507-284-2511

Robert A. Kyle · Myeloma (Amyloidosis) · Mayo Clinic · Mayo Clinic, 200 First Street, SW, Rochester, MN 55905 · 507-284-2865

Michael J. O'Connell · Gastrointestinal Cancer · Mayo Clinic · Mayo Clinic, 200 First Street, SW, Rochester, MN 55905 · 507-284-3903

Ronald Lee Richardson · Genito-Urinary Cancer · Mayo Clinic · Mayo Clinic, 200 First Street, SW, Rochester, MN 55905 · 507-284-4430

NEPHROLOGY

Duluth

Richard N. Hellman · General Nephrology · Duluth Clinic, Department of Nephrology, 400 East Third Street, Duluth, MN 55805 · 218-722-8364

Theodore Johnson · General Nephrology · Duluth Clinic, Department of Nephrology, 400 East Third Street, Duluth, MN 55805 · 218-722-8364

Thomas E. Russ · General Nephrology · Duluth Clinic, Department of Nephrology, 400 East Third Street, Duluth, MN 55805 · 218-722-8364

Minneapolis

Allan J. Collins · Dialysis (Hemodialysis) · University of Minnesota Hospital & Clinic · University of Minnesota Hospital & Clinic, 825 South Eighth Street, Suite 400, Minneapolis, MN 55404 · 612-347-5811

Thomas H. Hostetter · Kidney Disease (Diabetic Kidney Disease) · University of Minnesota Hospital & Clinic · University of Minnesota Hospital & Clinic, Department of Nephrology, 420 Delaware Street, SE, Minneapolis, MN 55455 · 612-624-9444

Bertram L. Kasiske · Kidney Transplantation (Kidney Diseases, Glomerular Diseases) · Hennepin County Medical Center · Hennepin County Medical Center, Division of Nephrology, 701 Park Avenue, South, Minneapolis, MN 55415 · 612-347-6088

William F. Keane · General Nephrology · Hennepin County Medical Center · Hennepin County Medical Center, Department of Medicine, 701 Park Avenue, South, Minneapolis, MN 55415-1623 · 612-347-6177

Connie L. Manske · General Nephrology (Renal Transplantation, Diabetic Nephropathy) · University of Minnesota Hospital & Clinic · University of Minnesota Hospital & Clinic, Renal Division, 516 Delaware Street, SE, Box 736, Minneapolis, MN 55455 · 612-624-3126

Karl A. Nath · General Nephrology · University of Minnesota Hospital & Clinic University of Minnesota Hospital & Clinic, Renal Division, 516 Delaware Street, SE, Box 736, Minneapolis, MN 55455 · 612-624-0916

Mark S. Paller · General Nephrology (Dialysis, Kidney Transplantation) · University of Minnesota Hospital & Clinic · University of Minnesota Hospital & Clinic, 420 Delaware Street, SE, Box 736, Minneapolis, MN 55455 · 612-624-9930

Rochester

James V. Donadio · Glomerular Diseases, General Nephrology · Mayo Clinic · Mayo Clinic, 200 First Street, SW, Rochester, MN 55905 · 507-284-3588

Stephen C. Textor · Hypertension · Mayo Clinic · Mayo Clinic, 200 First Street, SW, Rochester, MN 55905 · 507-284-4841

Jorge A. Velosa · Glomerular Diseases, Kidney Transplantation, General Nephrology · Mayo Clinic · Mayo Clinic, 200 First Street, SW, Rochester, MN 55905 507-266-1963

St. Cloud

William L. Cowardin · General Nephrology · Centracare Clinic, 1200 Sixth Avenue, North, St. Cloud, MN 56303-2735 · 612-252-5131

NEUROLOGICAL SURGERY

Duluth

Robert F. Donley · General Neurological Surgery · Duluth Clinic, Department of Neurosurgery, 400 East Third Street, Duluth, MN 55805 · 218-722-8364

Minneapolis

Donald Erickson · General Neurological Surgery (Spinal Surgery) · University of Minnesota Hospital & Clinic, 420 Delaware Street, SE, Box 96, Minneapolis, MN 55455 · 612-624-6666

Stephen J. Haines · General Neurological Surgery (Skull-Base Surgery, Pediatric Neurological Surgery, Cranial Nerve Surgery, Stereotactic Radiosurgery, Tumor Surgery) · University of Minnesota Hospital & Clinic, Children's Health Care— Minneapolis · University of Minnesota Hospital & Clinic, Department of Neurosurgery, 420 Delaware Street, SE, Box 96, Minneapolis, MN 55455-0374 · 612-624-6666

Robert E. Maxwell · Epilepsy Surgery · University of Minnesota Hospital & Clinic · University of Minnesota Hospital & Clinic, Mayo Memorial Building, Suite D429, 420 Delaware Street, SE, Box 96, Minneapolis, MN 55455 · 612-624-1114

Rochester

Michael J. Ebersold · Tumor Surgery (Spine, Skull-Base) · Mayo Clinic · Mayo Clinic, 200 First Street, SW, Rochester, MN 55905 · 507-284-2254

William E. Krauss · Spinal Surgery · Mayo Clinic, Department of Neurosurgery, 200 First Street, SW, Rochester, MN 55905 · 507-284-2816

W. Richard Marsh · General Neurological Surgery · Mayo Clinic, 200 First Street, SW, Rochester, MN 55905 · 507-284-2511

David G. Piepgras · Vascular Neurological Surgery, General Neurological Surgery (Cerebrovascular Neurological Surgery) · St. Mary's Hospital of Rochester, Mayo Clinic · Mayo Clinic, 200 First Street, SW, Rochester, MN 55905 · 507-284-3331

Corey Raffel · Pediatric Neurological Surgery · Mayo Clinic, Department of Neurosurgery, 200 First Street, SW, Rochester, MN 55905 · 507-284-8167

NEUROLOGY

Duluth

Mark L. Young · General Neurology · Duluth Clinic, Department of Neurology, 400 East Third Street, Duluth, MN 55805 · 218-722-8364

Golden Valley

Bruce A. Norback · General Neurology (Stroke, Clinical Neurophysiology) · North Memorial Health Care (Minneapolis) · Minneapolis Clinic of Neurology, 4225 Golden Valley Road, Golden Valley, MN 55422-4215 · 612-588-0661

Paul Silverstein · Movement Disorders · Minneapolis Clinic of Neurology, 4225 Golden Valley Road, Golden Valley, MN 55422-4215 · 612-588-0661

Minneapolis

David C. Anderson · Strokes · University of Minnesota Hospital & Clinic, Hennepin County Medical Center · Hennepin County Medical Center, Department of Neurology, 701 Park Avenue, South, Minneapolis, MN 55415-1829 · 612-347-2595

Gary Birnbaum · Infectious & Demyelinating Diseases (Multiple Sclerosis) · University of Minnesota Hospital & Clinic · University of Minnesota Hospital & Clinic, Department of Neurology, 420 Delaware Street, SE, Box 295, Minneapolis, MN 55455 · 612-625-2633

John W. Day · General Neurology (Neuromuscular Disease, Electromyography) University of Minnesota Hospital & Clinic · University of Minnesota Hospital & Clinic, Department of Neurology, 420 Delaware Street, SE, Box 295, Minneapolis, MN 55455-2545 · 612-625-6180

Robert J. Gumnit · Epilepsy (Adults & Children) · Abbott-Northwestern Hospital, Gillette Children's Hospital (St. Paul), University of Minnesota Hospital & Clinic · Minnesota Comprehensive Epilepsy Program, 5775 Wayzata Boulevard, Suite 255, Minneapolis, MN 55416 · 612-525-2400

Ilo E. Leppik · Epilepsy (Geriatric Neurology) · Abbott-Northwestern Hospital, University of Minnesota Hospital & Clinic · MINCEP Epilepsy Care, 5775 Wayzata Boulevard, Suite 255, Minneapolis, MN 55416 · 612-525-2400

Mark W. Mahowald · General Neurology · Hennepin County Medical Center · Hennepin County Medical Center, Sleep Disorders Center, 701 Park Avenue, South, Minneapolis, MN 55415 · 612-347-6288

Gareth J. G. Parry · General Neurology · University of Minnesota Hospital & Clinic, Department of Neurology, 420 Delaware Street, SE, Box 295, Minneapolis, MN 55455 · 612-626-4107

Richard W. Price · Infectious & Demyelinating Diseases, Neuro-Oncology (AIDS) · University of Minnesota Hospital & Clinic · University of Minnesota Hospital & Clinic, 420 Delaware Street, SE, Box 295, Minneapolis, MN 55455 · 612-625-8983

Randall T. Schapiro · Infectious & Demyelinating Diseases (Multiple Sclerosis, Neuro-Rehabilitation) · Fairview Riverside Medical Center · Fairview Multiple Sclerosis Center, 701 Twenty-Fifth Avenue, South, Suite 200, Minneapolis, MN 55454-1400 · 612-672-6100

Rochester

Allen J. Aksamit, Jr. · General Neurology · Mayo Clinic, 200 First Street, SW, Rochester, MN 55905 · 507-284-2511

J. Keith Campbell · Headache · Mayo Clinic · Mayo Clinic, 200 First Street, SW, Rochester, MN 55905 · 507-284-3334

Gregory D. Cascino · Epilepsy · Mayo Clinic · Mayo Clinic, Department of Neurology, 200 First Street, SW, Rochester, MN 55905 · 507-284-4037

Terrence L. Cascino · Neuro-Oncology (Cancer in the Nervous System) · Mayo Clinic · Mayo Clinic, 200 First Street, SW, Rochester, MN 55905 · 507-284-2511

Jasper R. Daube · Electromyography · Mayo Clinic · Mayo Clinic, 200 First Street, SW, Rochester, MN 55905 · 507-284-2675

Peter J. Dyck · Neuromuscular Disease, Degenerative Diseases (Peripheral Nerve Disorders, Motor-Neuron Disease) · Mayo Clinic · Mayo Clinic, 200 First Street, SW, Rochester, MN 55905 · 507-284-3769

Andrew G. Engel · Neuromuscular Disease · Mayo Clinic · Mayo Clinic, 200 First Street, SW, Rochester, MN 55905 · 507-284-2511

David W. Kimmel · Neuro-Oncology · Mayo Clinic · Mayo Clinic, 200 First Street, SW, Rochester, MN 55905 · 507-284-2120

William J. Litchy · Electromyography · Mayo Clinic · Mayo Clinic, 200 First Street, SW, Rochester, MN 55905 · 507-284-4006

Phillip A. Low · Neuromuscular Disease (Peripheral Nerve Disorders, Autonomic Nervous Systems) · Mayo Clinic · Mayo Clinic, 200 First Street, SW, Rochester, MN 55905 · 507-284-3375

John H. Noseworthy · Infectious & Demyelinating Diseases (Multiple Sclerosis) Mayo Clinic · Mayo Clinic, 200 First Street, SW, Rochester, MN 55905 · 507-284-8533

Ronald C. Petersen · Behavioral Neurology · Mayo Clinic · Mayo Clinic, 200 First Street, SW, Rochester, MN 55905 · 507-284-4006

Moses Rodriguez · Infectious & Demyelinating Diseases (Multiple Sclerosis) · Mayo Clinic · Mayo Clinic, 200 First Street, SW, Rochester, MN 55905 · 507-284-8533

Burton A. Sandok · General Neurology · Mayo Clinic · Mayo Clinic, 200 First Street, SW, Rochester, MN 55905 · 507-284-3334

Franklin W. Sharbrough III · Epilepsy · Mayo Clinic, 200 First Street, SW, Rochester, MN 55905 · 507-284-4349

Brian G. Weinshenker · Infectious & Demyelinating Diseases (Multiple Sclerosis) · Mayo Clinic · Mayo Clinic, 200 First Street, SW, Rochester, MN 55905 · 507-284-4961

Jack P. Whisnant · Strokes · Mayo Clinic · Mayo Clinic, 200 First Street, SW, Rochester, MN 55905 · 507-284-2720

David O. Wiebers · Strokes (Cerebrovascular Disease) · Mayo Clinic · Mayo Clinic, 200 First Street, SW, Rochester, MN 55905 · 507-284-4234

Anthony J. Windebank · Neuromuscular Disease (Peripheral Nerve Disorders) · Mayo Clinic · Mayo Clinic, 200 First Street, SW, Rochester, MN 55905 · 507-284-2511

St. Paul

Terrance D. Capistrant · General Neurology (Stroke, Movement Disorders) · HealthEast St. Joseph's Hospital, United Hospital · Neurological Associates of St. Paul, 280 North Smith Avenue, Suite 550, St. Paul, MN 55102 · 612-221-9051

NEUROLOGY, CHILD

Minneapolis

Kenneth F. Swaiman · Inherited Biochemical Disorders, General Child Neurology (Movement Disorders) · University of Minnesota Hospital & Clinic · University of Minnesota Hospital & Clinic, 420 Delaware Street, SE, Box 486, Minneapolis, MN 55455 · 612-625-7466

Rochester

Mark C. Patterson · General Child Neurology · Mayo Clinic, Department of Neurology, 200 First Street, SW, Rochester, MN 55905 · 507-284-2511

Mary L. Zupanic · General Child Neurology · Mayo Clinic, Department of Neurology, 200 First Street, SW, Rochester, MN 55905 · 507-284-2511

St. Paul

Frank J. Ritter · Epilepsy · Minnesota Epilepsy Group, 310 Smith Avenue, North, Suite 300, St. Paul, MN 55102 · 612-220-5290

NUCLEAR MEDICINE

Minneapolis

Robert J. Boudreau · General Nuclear Medicine · University of Minnesota Hospital & Clinic · University of Minnesota Hospital & Clinic, 420 Delaware Street, SE, Box 292, Minneapolis, MN 55455 · 612-626-5912

Rochester

Lee L. Forstrom · General Nuclear Medicine · Mayo Clinic · Mayo Clinic, 200 First Street, SW, Rochester, MN 55905 · 507-284-3055

Raymond J. Gibbons · Nuclear Cardiology · Mayo Clinic · Mayo Clinic, 200 First Street, SW, Rochester, MN 55905 · 507-284-2541

Mary F. Hauser · General Nuclear Medicine · Mayo Clinic, 200 First Street, SW, Rochester, MN 55905 · 507-284-2511

Brian P. Mullan · General Nuclear Medicine · Mayo Clinic, 200 First Street, SW, Rochester, MN 55905 · 507-284-2511

Gregory A. Wiseman · General Nuclear Medicine · Mayo Clinic, 200 First Street, SW, Rochester, MN 55905 · 507-284-2511

OBSTETRICS & GYNECOLOGY

Duluth

Glen E. Holt · General Obstetrics & Gynecology · Duluth Clinic, Department of Obstetrics & Gynecology, 400 East Third Street, Duluth, MN 55805 · 218-722-8364

Scott W. Johnson · General Obstetrics & Gynecology · Duluth Clinic, Department of Obstetrics & Gynecology, 400 East Third Street, Duluth, MN 55805 · 218-722-8364

James A. Sebastian · General Obstetrics & Gynecology (Infertility, Operative Laparoscopy) · St. Luke's Hospital, St. Mary's Medical Center, Miller Dwan Medical Center · Duluth Ob-Gyn, Northland Medical Center, Suite LL, 1000 East First Street, Duluth, MN 55805 · 218-722-5629

Minneapolis

Linda F. Carson · General Obstetrics & Gynecology (Gynecologic Cancer, Gynecologic Surgery, Urogynecology, Genital Dermatological Disease) · University of Minnesota Hospital & Clinic, Abbott-Northwestern Hospital, United Hospital (St. Paul), Fairview Riverside Medical Center, Methodist Hospital · University of Minnesota Medical School, Department of Obstetrics and Gynecology, 420 Delaware Street, SE, Box 395, Minneapolis, MN 55455 · 612-625-6991

Jeffrey M. Fowler · (Gynecologic Cancer, Pelvic Surgery, Laparoscopy) · University of Minnesota Hospital & Clinic · University of Minnesota Medical School, Department of Obstetrics & Gynecology, 420 Delaware Street, SE, Box 395 UMHC, Minneapolis, MN 55455 · 612-626-4338

G. Eric Knox · Maternal & Fetal Medicine · Abbott-Northwestern Hospital · Abbott-Northwestern Hospital, Perinatal Department, 800 East 28th Street, Minneapolis, MN 55407 · 612-863-5030

Leo B. Twiggs · Gynecologic Cancer (Pelvic Surgery, Women's Cancer Treatment) · University of Minnesota Hospital & Clinic · University of Minnesota Hospital & Clinic, 420 Delaware Street, SE, Box 395, Minneapolis, MN 55455 · 612-626-3111

Minnetonka

John T. Hachiya · General Obstetrics & Gynecology (Endoscopic Surgery, Urogynecology) · Methodist Hospital (St. Louis Park) · Park Nicollet Medical Center, Carlson Office, 15111 Twelve Oaks Center Drive, Minnetonka, MN 55305 · 612-993-4510

Rochester

Raymond A. Lee · Reproductive Surgery (Gynecologic Surgery, Oncologic Surgery) · Mayo Clinic · Mayo Clinic, 200 First Street, SW, Rochester, MN 55905 · 507-284-2511

Karl C. Podratz · Gynecologic Cancer · Mayo Clinic · Mayo Clinic, 200 First Street, SW, Rochester, MN 55905 · 507-266-7712

C. Robert Stanhope · Gynecologic Cancer · Mayo Clinic · Mayo Clinic, Department of Obstetrics & Gynecology, 200 First Street, SW, Rochester, MN 55905 · 507-266-8686

Maurice J. Webb · General Obstetrics & Gynecology · Mayo Clinic, Department of Obstetrics & Gynecology, 200 First Street, SW, Rochester, MN 55905 · 507-266-8683

St. Paul

John William Malo · General Obstetrics & Gynecology · Reproductive Health Associates, 360 Sherman Street, Suite 350, St. Paul, MN 55102-2425 · 612-222-8666

Theodore Nagel · (Reproductive Endocrinology, Infertility, Reproductive Surgery) · United Hospital, University of Minnesota Hospital & Clinic (Minneapolis) Reproductive Health Associates, 360 Sherman Street, Suite 350, St. Paul, MN 55102-2425 · 612-222-8666

OPHTHALMOLOGY

Bloomington

Emmett F. Carpel · General Ophthalmology (Corneal Disease & Transplantation, Anterior Segment—Cataract & Refractive, Glaucoma) · Philips Eye Institute (Minneapolis) · Health Partners Bloomington Clinic, 8600 Nicollet Avenue, South, Bloomington, MN 55420-2824 · 612-887-6633

Duluth

Upali P. Aturaliya · General Ophthalmology · Duluth Clinic, Department of Ophthalmology, 400 East Third Street, Duluth, MN 55805 · 218-722-8364

Peter S. Austin · General Ophthalmology · Medical Arts Building, Suite 800, 324 West Superior Street, Duluth, MN 55802 · 218-722-6655

Kevin W. Treacy · General Ophthalmology · Medical Arts Building, Suite 800, 324 West Superior Street, Duluth, MN 55802 · 218-722-6655

Edina

Eric R. Nelson · (Ophthalmic Plastic & Reconstructive Surgery) · Fairview-Southdale Hospital, Philips Eye Institute (Minneapolis) · Southdale Medical Center, 6545 France Avenue, South, Suite 355, Edina, MN 55435-2131 · 612-925-4161

John A. Nilsen · General Ophthalmology · Fairview-Southdale Hospital · Eye Physicians & Surgeons, 4450 West 76th Street, Edina, MN 55435 · 612-445-5760

Jonathan Edward Pederson · Glaucoma · Philips Eye Institute (Minneapolis), Fairview-Southdale Hospital · 6545 France Avenue, South, Suite 405, Edina, MN 55435 · 612-928-8029

Fridley

Alan E. Sadowsky · General Ophthalmology · Columbia Park Medical Group, 6341 University Avenue, NE, Fridley, MN 55432 · 612-572-5705

Grand Rapids

Timothy C. Bonner · General Ophthalmology · Itasca Medical Center, Northern Itasca Health Care Center (Bigfork), Deer River Health Care System (Deer River) Bonner Eye Clinic, 111 Southeast Third Street, Suite 101, Grand Rapids, MN 55744-3663 · 218-326-3433

Minneapolis

Steven R. Bennett · (Vitreo-Retinal Surgery, Retinal Diseases, Ocular Oncology) Fairview-Southdale Hospital (Edina), Philips Eye Institute, United Hospital (St. Paul) · Vitreo-Retinal Surgery, 6363 France Avenue, South, Suite 570, Minneapolis, MN 55435-2139 · 612-929-1131

Herbert L. Cantrill · Medical Retinal Diseases, Vitreo-Retinal Surgery · Fairview-Southdale Hospital (Edina), United Hospital (St. Paul), Philips Eye Institute · Vitreo-Retinal Surgery, 6363 France Avenue, South, Suite 570, Minneapolis, MN 55435 · 612-929-1131

Daniel K. Day · General Ophthalmology · Northwest Eye Clinic, 3366 Oakdale Avenue, North, Room 402, Minneapolis, MN 55422-2986 · 612-588-0755

Donald J. Doughman · Corneal Diseases & Transplantation, General Ophthalmology (Anterior Segment—Cataract & Refractive, Eximer Laser Refractive Surgery) · University of Minnesota Hospital & Clinic · University of Minnesota Hospital & Clinic, Department of Ophthalmology, 420 Delaware Street, SE, Box 493, Minneapolis, MN 55455-0501 · 612-625-5415

Edward J. Holland · Corneal Diseases & Transplantation · University of Minnesota Hospital & Clinic · University of Minnesota Hospital & Clinic, 420 Delaware Street, SE, Box 493, Minneapolis, MN 55455-0501 · 612-625-6914

Jay H. Krachmer · Corneal Diseases & Transplantation · University of Minnesota Hospital & Clinic · University of Minnesota Hospital & Clinic, Department of Ophthalmology, 420 Delaware Street, SE, Box 493, Minneapolis, MN 55455 · 612-625-4400

Richard L. Lindstrom · Corneal Diseases & Transplantation, Anterior Segment—Cataract & Refractive · Philips Eye Institute, Abbott-Northwestern Hospital, St. Paul-Ramsey Medical Center (St. Paul), United Hospital (St. Paul), University of Minnesota Hospital & Clinic, Fairview-Southdale Hospital (Edina) Lindstrom, Samuelson & Hardten, Ophthalmology Associates, Park Avenue Medical Office Building, Suite 106, 710 East 24th Street, Minneapolis, MN 55404 · 612-336-5493

Theodore R. Pier · Pediatric Ophthalmology (General Ophthalmology) · Minnesota Medical Eye Clinic, 2545 Chicago Avenue, South, Suite 501, Minneapolis, MN 55404 · 612-871-3611

Robert C. Ramsay · Vitreo-Retinal Surgery, Medical Retinal Diseases (Diabetic Retinopathy, Retinal Detachment) · Philips Eye Institute, Fairview-Southdale Hospital · Vitreo-Retinal Surgery, 6363 France Avenue, South, Suite 570, Minneapolis, MN 55435 · 612-929-1131

Thomas W. Samuelson · Glaucoma · Philips Eye Institute, St. Paul-Ramsey Medical Center (St. Paul) · Lindstrom, Samuelson & Hardten Ophthalmology Associates, Park Avenue Medical Office Building, Suite 106, 710 East 24th Street, Minneapolis, MN 55404 · 612-336-5493; 612-221-8745

Jonathan D. Wirtschafter · Neuro-Ophthalmology (Optic Nerve Compressions, Graves Disease, Eyelid Spasms, Oculoplastic & Orbital Surgery) · University of Minnesota Hospital & Clinic · University of Minnesota Hospital & Clinic, 420 Delaware Street, SE, Box 493 UMHC, Minneapolis, MN 55455-0501 · 612-625-4400

Martha M. Wright · Glaucoma · University of Minnesota Hospital & Clinic, 420 Delaware Street, SE, Box 493, Minneapolis, MN 55455-0501 · 612-625-4400

Todd A. Zwickey · Anterior Segment—Cataract & Refractive · Ophthalmology, Downtown, Medical Arts Building, Suite 2000, 825 Nicollet Mall Avenue, Minneapolis, MN 55402 · 612-339-5511

Owatonna

Grant D. Heslep · General Ophthalmology (Anterior Segment—Cataract & Refractive, Optics & Refraction) · Owatonna Hospital · Owatonna Clinic, 134 Southview Street, Owatonna, MN 55060 · 507-451-1120

Rochester

William M. Bourne · Corneal Diseases & Transplantation · Mayo Clinic · Mayo Clinic, 200 First Street, SW, Rochester, MN 55905 · 507-284-3614

Richard Brubaker · Glaucoma · Mayo Clinic · Mayo Clinic, 200 First Street, SW, Rochester, MN 55905 · 507-284-3760

James A. Garrity · Oculoplastic & Orbital Surgery, Neuro-Ophthalmology · Mayo Clinic · Mayo Clinic, 200 First Street, SW, Rochester, MN 55905 · 507-284-4946

David C. Herman · Uveitis · Mayo Clinic · Mayo Clinic, 200 First Street, SW, Rochester, MN 55905 · 507-284-4152

Leo J. Maguire · Corneal Diseases & Transplantation (Refractive Surgery) · Mayo Clinic · Mayo Clinic, 200 First Street, SW, Rochester, MN 55905 · 507-284-4152

Dennis M. Robertson · Medical Retinal Diseases, Vitreo-Retinal Surgery (Diabetic Retinopathy, Macular Degeneration, Vascular Occlusions, Laser Surgery) · Mayo Clinic · Mayo Clinic, 200 First Street, SW, Rochester, MN 55905 · 507-284-3721

Brian R. Younge · Neuro-Ophthalmology · Mayo Clinic · Mayo Clinic, 200 First Street, SW, Rochester, MN 55905 · 507-284-4152

St. Paul

Richard P. Carroll · Oculoplastic & Orbital Surgery (Eyelid, Lacrimal, Orbital Surgery) · Philips Eye Institute (Minneapolis), HealthEast Midway Hospital, Abbott-Northwestern Hospital (Minneapolis) · 1690 University Avenue, Suite 200, St. Paul, MN 55104 · 612-646-2581

J. Daniel Nelson · Corneal Diseases & Transplantation (Dry Eyes, Anterior Segment—Cataract & Refractive, Optics & Refraction) · St. Paul-Ramsey Medical Center · St. Paul-Ramsey Medical Center, 640 Jackson Street, St. Paul, MN 55101 · 612-221-8745

Stillwater

Stephen S. Lane · Anterior Segment—Cataract & Refractive (Cornea External Disease) · VA Medical Center (Minneapolis) · Associated Eye Physicians, 232 North Main Street, Stillwater, MN 55082 · 612-439-8500

ORTHOPAEDIC SURGERY

Alexandria

Terence J. Kennedy · General Orthopaedic Surgery (Total Joint Replacement) · Douglas County Hospital · Alexandria Orthopaedic Associates, 1500 Irving Street, Alexandria, MN 56308 · 612-762-1144

Bemidji

Thomas E. Miller · General Orthopaedic Surgery · Lake Region Bone & Joint Surgeons, 3807 Greenleaf Avenue, NW, Bemidji, MN 56601-5817 · 218-751-9746

Duluth

Mark J. Carlson · General Orthopaedic Surgery · Orthopaedic Associates, 1000 East First Street, Suite 404, Duluth, MN 55804 · 218-722-5513

Bradley C. Edgerton · General Orthopaedic Surgery · Duluth Clinic, Department of Orthopaedics, 400 East Third Street, Duluth, MN 55805 · 218-725-4520

Edina

Allen L. Van Beek · Peripheral Nerve Surgery · North Memorial Health Care (Robbinsdale), Fairview-Southdale Hospital, Abbott-Northwestern Hospital (Minneapolis), Children's Health Care-Minneapolis (Minneapolis) · Plastic Surgery Specialists, 7373 France Avenue, South, Suite 510, Edina, MN 55435 · 612-588-0593; 612-830-1028

Minneapolis

David A. Fischer · Sports Medicine/Arthroscopy (Knee Surgery) · Fairview Riverside Medical Center, Abbott-Northwestern Hospital · Minneapolis Sports Medicine Center, 701 Twenty-Fifth Avenue, South, Suite 400, Minneapolis, MN 55454 · 612-339-7734

Ramon B. Gustilo · Reconstructive Surgery, Trauma (Total Joint Replacement, Fractures, Infections) · Hennepin County Medical Center, Abbott-Northwestern Hospital · Minneapolis Orthopaedic & Arthritis Institute, 825 South Eighth Street, Suite 550, Minneapolis, MN 55415 · 612-333-4521

Lyle O. Johnson · Pediatric Orthopaedic Surgery · Shriners Hospital for Crippled Children, 2025 East River Road, Minneapolis, MN 55414 · 612-335-5352

Richard F. Kyle · Trauma (Total Joint Replacement, Hip Surgery, Shoulder Surgery, Knee Surgery) · Hennepin County Medical Center · Hennepin County Medical Center, Department of Orthopaedic Surgery, 701 Park Avenue, South, Minneapolis, MN 55415 · 612-347-2812

Roby Calvin Thompson, Jr. · Trauma (Reconstructive Hip Surgery, General Surgical Oncology, Musculoskeletal Tumors) · University of Minnesota Hospital & Clinic · University of Minnesota Hospital & Clinic, 420 Delaware Street, SE, Box 492, Minneapolis, MN 55455 · 612-625-5648

Rochester

Miguel E. Cabanela · General Orthopaedic Surgery · Mayo Clinic, Department of Orthopaedic Surgery, 200 First Street, SW, Rochester, MN 55905 · 507-284-2226

Robert H. Cofield · Reconstructive Surgery (Shoulder) · Mayo Clinic · Mayo Clinic, Department of Orthopaedic Surgery, 200 First Street, SW, Rochester, MN 55905 · 507-284-2995

Bernard F. Morrey · Reconstructive Surgery (Hip, Knee, Elbow) · Mayo Clinic Mayo Clinic, 200 First Street, SW, Rochester, MN 55905 · 507-284-3659

Hamlet A. Peterson · Pediatric Orthopaedic Surgery · St. Mary's Hospital of Rochester, Mayo Clinic · Mayo Clinic, 200 First Street, SW, Rochester, MN 55905 · 507-284-2947

Douglas Jack Pritchard · Trauma · Rochester Methodist Hospital · Mayo Clinic, 200 First Street, SW, Rochester, MN 55905 · 507-284-2511

Franklin H. Sim · Trauma · Mayo Clinic · Mayo Clinic, 200 First Street, SW, Rochester, MN 55905 · 507-284-3661

Michael J. Stuart · Sports Medicine/Arthroscopy · Mayo Clinic, Department of Orthopaedic Surgery, 200 First Street, SW, Rochester, MN 55905 · 507-284-3462

Michael B. Wood · Peripheral Nerve Surgery · Mayo Clinic · Mayo Clinic, 200 First Street, SW, Rochester, MN 55905 · 507-284-2511

St. Cloud

Michael G. Orr · General Orthopaedic Surgery · St. Cloud Orthopaedics, 1555 Northway Drive, St. Cloud, MN 56303 · 612-259-4100

St. Paul

Peter J. Daly · General Orthopaedic Surgery (Total Joint Reconstruction, Sports Medicine/Arthroscopy, Shoulder Surgery, Reconstructive Surgery) · United Hospital, HealthEast Midway Hospital, HealthEast St. Joseph's Hospital, HealthEast Bethesda Lutheran Hospital & Rehabilitation Center, St. Paul-Ramsey Medical Center, Regina Medical Center (Hastings) · Landmark Orthopedics, 17 West Exchange Street, St. Paul, MN 55100 · 612-227-0200

James Gage · Pediatric Orthopaedic Surgery (Gait Analysis, Gait Pathology in Cerebral Palsy) · Gillette Children's Hospital · Gillette Children's Hospital, 200 East University Avenue, St. Paul, MN 55101 · 612-229-3840

Steven E. Koop · Pediatric Orthopaedic Surgery · Gillette Children's Hospital, 200 East University Avenue, St. Paul, MN 55101 · 612-221-8600

Lowell D. Lutter · Foot & Ankle Surgery · HealthEast Midway Hospital, Gillette Children's Hospital, United Hospital, Children's Healthcare—St. Paul · 1690 University Avenue, Suite 10, St. Paul, MN 55104 · 612-232-4770

Wayzata

David C. Templeman · Trauma (Pelvic, Acetabular Fractures, Articular Fractures, Nonunions & Malunions) · Hennepin County Medical Center (Minneapolis) · Wayzata Orthopaedics, 250 Central Avenue, North, Suite 303, Wayzata, MN 55391 · 612-476-0042

OTOLARYNGOLOGY

Duluth

David M. Choquette · General Otolaryngology · St. Luke's Hospital, St. Mary's Medical Center, Miller Dwan Medical Center, University Medical Center-Mesabi (Hibbing), Ely Bloomenson Community Hospital (Ely), Community Memorial Hospital (Cloquet) · Northland Ear, Nose, and Throat Associates, Northland Medical Center, Suite 403, 1000 East First Street, Duluth, MN 55805 · 218-727-8581

Todd J. Freeman · General Otolaryngology · Northland Ear, Nose, and Throat Associates, Northland Medical Center, Suite 403, 1000 East First Street, Duluth, MN 55805 · 218-727-8581

William Portilla · General Otolaryngology · Duluth Clinic, Department of Otolaryngology, 400 East Third Street, Duluth, MN 55805 · 218-722-8364

Minneapolis

George L. Adams · Head & Neck Surgery · University of Minnesota Hospital & Clinic · University of Minnesota Hospital & Clinic, 420 Delaware Street, SE, Box 396, Minneapolis, MN 55455 · 612-625-7400

Carl A. Brown · (Sinus & Nasal Surgery, Facial Plastic Surgery, Pediatric Airway, General Otolaryngology, Pediatric Otolaryngology) · Abbott-Northwestern Hospital, Children's Health Care—Minneapolis, Fairview Riverside Medical Center · Minneapolis Ear, Nose & Throat Clinic, 2211 Park Avenue, South, Minneapolis, MN 55404 · 612-871-1144

Samuel C. Levine · Otology · University of Minnesota Hospital & Clinic, VA Medical Center, Abbott-Northwestern Hospital, Hennepin County Medical Center · University of Minnesota Hospital & Clinic, 516 Delaware Street, SE, Box 396, Minneapolis, MN 55455 · 612-625-3200

Robert H. Maisel · Head & Neck Surgery (Partial Surgery for Voice Box Cancer, Laryngology) · Hennepin County Medical Center, University of Minnesota Hospital & Clinic · Hennepin County Medical Center, Department of Otolaryngology, 701 Park Avenue, South, Minneapolis, MN 55414 · 612-347-2424

Michael M. Paparella · Otology/Neurotology (Meniere's Disease, Otitis Media) · Fairview Riverside Medical Center · Minnesota Ear, Head & Neck Clinic, 701 Twenty-Fifth Avenue, South, Suite 200, Minneapolis, MN 55454-1449 · 612-339-2836

Rochester

George W. Facer · General Otolaryngology · Mayo Clinic, 200 First Street, SW, Rochester, MN 55905 · 507-282-2511

Stephen G. Harner · Otology/Neurotology (Acoustic Neuromas) · St. Mary's Hospital of Rochester, Mayo Clinic · Mayo Clinic, Department of Otolaryngology, 200 First Street, SW, Rochester, MN 55905 · 507-284-8532

Eugene B. Kern · Sinus & Nasal Surgery (Otorhinolaryngology, Cosmetic, Nasal Breathing Problems) · Mayo Clinic · Mayo Clinic, 200 First Street, SW, Rochester, MN 55905 · 507-284-1729

H. Bryan Neel III · Head & Neck Surgery, Laryngology · Mayo Clinic · Mayo Clinic, 200 First Street, SW, Rochester, MN 55905 · 507-284-2369

St. Paul

Stephen Liston · General Otolaryngology (Head & Neck Surgery) · Head & Neck Physicians & Surgeons Clinic, 310 North Smith Avenue, Suite 120, St. Paul, MN 55118 · 612-227-0821

Barbara N. Malone · Pediatric Otolaryngology · Children's Healthcare—St. Paul, Midwest Eye & Ear Institute, HealthEast St. Joseph's Hospital, United Hospital 393 North Dunlap Street, Suite 600, St. Paul, MN 55104 · 612-645-0691

Leighton Siegel · General Otolaryngology (Ear, Head, & Neck) · Head & Neck Physicians & Surgeons Clinic, 310 North Smith Avenue, Suite 120, St. Paul, MN 55118 · 612-227-0821

Robert W. Smith · (Pediatric Otolaryngology, Otology) · HealthEast Bethesda Lutheran Hospital & Rehabilitation Center, HealthEast Midway Hospital, HealthEast St. Joseph's Hospital, United Hospital, Gillette Children's Hospital · Central Medical Building, Suite 600, 393 North Dunlap Street, St. Paul, MN 55104 · 612-645-0691

PATHOLOGY

Duluth

Patrick C. J. Ward · General Pathology · University of Minnesota School of Medicine, Department of Pathology, 10 University Drive, Duluth, MN 55812 · 218-726-7911

Geoffrey A. Witrak · General Pathology · St. Mary's Medical Center, Department of Pathology, 407 East Third Street, Duluth, MN 55805 · 218-726-4090

Edina

Dale Craig Snover · Liver Pathology (Gastrointestinal Pathology, Transplantation Pathology) · Fairview-Southdale Hospital, Department of Pathology, 6401 France Avenue, South, Edina, MN 55435 · 612-924-5152

Minneapolis

Richard D. Brunning · Hematopathology · University of Minnesota Hospital & Clinic · University of Minnesota Hospital & Clinic, Mayo Building, Room D-223, 420 Delaware Street, SE, Box 609, Minneapolis, MN 55455 · 612-626-5704

Robert J. Gorlin · General Pathology (Rare Birth Defects, Syndromes of the Head & Neck, Hereditary Hearing Loss & Its Syndromes) · University of Minnesota Hospital & Clinic, Department of Oral Pathology, 420 Delaware Street, SE, Box 80, Minneapolis, MN 55455 · 612-624-6131

Charles A. Horwitz · General Pathology · Abbott-Northwestern Hospital, Department of Pathology, 800 East 28th Street, Minneapolis, MN 55407 · 612-863-4670

J. Carlos Manivel · General Pathology · University of Minnesota Hospital & Clinic, Department of Pathology, Mayo Building, 420 Delaware Street, SE, Box 76, Minneapolis, MN 55455 · 612-626-5848

Rochester

George M. Farrow · Surgical Pathology · Mayo Clinic · Mayo Clinic, 200 First Street, SW, Rochester, MN 55905 · 507-284-1954

Curtis A. Hanson · Hematopathology · Mayo Clinic · Mayo Clinic, 200 First Street, SW, Rochester, MN 55905 · 507-284-3045

Paul J. Kurtin · Hematopathology · Mayo Clinic, Department of Pathology, 200 First Street, SW, Rochester, MN 55905 · 507-280-9274

Jurgen Ludwig · Liver Pathology · Mayo Clinic · Mayo Clinic, 200 First Street, SW, Rochester, MN 55905 · 507-284-3867

Bernd W. Scheithauer · Neuropathology (Tumor) · Mayo Clinic · Mayo Clinic, 200 First Street, SW, Rochester, MN 55905 · 507-284-8350

John G. Strickler, Jr. · General Pathology · Mayo Clinic, Department of Pathology, 200 First Street, SW, Rochester, MN 55905 · 507-284-2511

K. Krishnan Unni · General Pathology · Mayo Clinic, Department of Pathology, 200 First Street, SW, Rochester, MN 55905 · 507-284-1193

Lester E. Wold · Surgical Pathology · Mayo Clinic · Mayo Clinic, Hilton Building, Suite 530, 200 First Street, SW, Rochester, MN 55905 · 507-284-8135

PEDIATRICS

Duluth

Rahul Aggarwal · Pediatric Critical Care · Duluth Clinic, Department of Pediatrics, 400 East Third Street, Duluth, MN 55805 · 218-722-8364

Roderick W. Krueger · Neonatal-Perinatal Medicine · Duluth Clinic, Department of Neonatology, 400 East Third Street, Duluth, MN 55805 · 218-722-8364

Minneapolis

Henry H. Balfour, Jr. · Pediatric Infectious Disease (Herpes Virus Infections) · University of Minnesota Hospital & Clinic · University of Minnesota Hospital & Clinic, 15-144 Phillips-Wangensteen Building, Harvard Street and East River Parkway, Box 437, Minneapolis, MN 55455-0392 · 612-626-5670

John L. Bass · Pediatric Cardiology · University of Minnesota Hospital & Clinic, Division of Pediatric Cardiology, 420 Delaware Street, SE, Box 94, Minneapolis, MN 55455 · 612-626-2755

Susan A. Berry · Metabolic Diseases (Genetics) · University of Minnesota Hospital & Clinic, Department of Pediatrics, 420 Delaware Street, SE, Minneapolis, MN 55455 · 612-624-7144

Blanche Chavers · Pediatric Nephrology · University of Minnesota Hospital & Clinic · University-Variety Hospital for Children, 420 Delaware Street, SE, Box 491, Minneapolis, MN 55455 · 612-626-2802

John A. Cich · Pediatric Hematology-Oncology · Children's Health Care—Minneapolis · Children's Health Care Minneapolis, Department of Hematology-Oncology, 2545 Chicago Avenue, South, Suite 402, Minneapolis, MN 55404 · 612-813-5940

Ann C. Dunnigan · Pediatric Cardiology (Electrophysiology) · University of Minnesota Hospital & Clinic · University of Minnesota Hospital & Clinic, 420 Delaware Street, SE, Box 94, Minneapolis, MN 55455 · 612-626-2755

Donnell D. Etzwiler · Pediatric Endocrinology (Diabetes) · International Diabetes Center, Park Nicollet Medical Center, Methodist Hospital · International Diabetes Center, 3800 Park Nicollet Boulevard, Minneapolis, MN 55416-2699 · 612-993-3393

Alfred J. Fish · Pediatric Nephrology · University of Minnesota Hospital & Clinic University of Minnesota Medical School, Division of Pediatric Nephrology, 420 Delaware Street, SE, Box 491, Minneapolis, MN 55455 · 612-626-2974

G. Scott Giebink · Pediatric Infectious Disease (Ear Infections, Immunizations) University of Minnesota Hospital & Clinic · University of Minnesota Hospital & Clinic, 420 Delaware Street, SE, Box 296, Minneapolis, MN 55455 · 612-624-6159

Margaret K. Hostetter · Pediatric Infectious Disease (International Adopted Children, General & Infectious Disease) · University of Minnesota Hospital & Clinic University of Minnesota Hospital & Clinic, Department of Pediatrics, 420 Delaware Street, SE, Box 296, Minneapolis, MN 55455 · 612-624-1112

Clifford E. Kashtan · Pediatric Nephrology (Kidney Transplantation, Hereditary Kidney Disease) · University of Minnesota Hospital & Clinic · University of Minnesota Medical School, Department of Pediatrics, 515 Delaware Street, SE, Box 491, Minneapolis, MN 55455 · 612-624-9193

John H. Kersey · Pediatric Hematology-Oncology (Bone Marrow Transplantation) University of Minnesota Hospital & Clinic · University of Minnesota Hospital & Clinic, 420 Delaware Street, SE, Box 86, Minneapolis, MN 55455 · 612-625-4659

Young Ki Kim · Pediatric Nephrology · University of Minnesota Hospital & Clinic, 420 Delaware Street, SE, Box 491, Minneapolis, MN 55455 · 612-624-5496

Michael Mauer · Pediatric Nephrology (Diabetic Kidney Disease) · University of Minnesota Hospital & Clinic · University of Minnesota Hospital & Clinic, 420 Delaware Street, SE, Box 491, Minneapolis, MN 55455 · 612-626-2780

Roy C. Maynard · Neonatal-Perinatal Medicine (Pediatric Pulmonology) · Children's Health Care—Minneapolis · 2545 Chicago Avenue, South, Suite 617, Minneapolis, MN 55404 · 612-863-3226

Alfred F. Michael, Jr. · Pediatric Nephrology (Glomerular Diseases) · University of Minnesota Hospital & Clinic · University of Minnesota Hospital & Clinic, Department of Pediatrics, 420 Delaware Street, SE, Box 391, Minneapolis, MN 55455 · 612-624-3113

James H. Moller · Pediatric Cardiology · Fairview Riverside Medical Center, Hennepin County Medical Center · University of Minnesota Medical School, 420 Delaware Street, SE, Box 288, Minneapolis, MN 55455 · 612-626-2790

Antoinette Moran · Pediatric Endocrinology · University of Minnesota Hospital & Clinic, Department of Pediatrics, 420 Delaware Street, SE, Box 404 Mayo, Minneapolis, MN 55455 · 612-624-4446

Joseph P. Neglia · Pediatric Hematology-Oncology · University of Minnesota Hospital & Clinic · University of Minnesota Hospital & Clinic, 420 Delaware Street, SE, Box 484, Minneapolis, MN 55455 · 612-626-2778

Mark E. Nesbit · Pediatric Hematology-Oncology (Pediatric Leukemia) · University of Minnesota Hospital & Clinic · University of Minnesota Hospital & Clinic, 420 Delaware Street, SE, Box 484, Minneapolis, MN 55455 · 612-626-2778

Thomas E. Nevins · Pediatric Nephrology (Dialysis, Kidney Transplantation) · University of Minnesota Hospital & Clinic · University of Minnesota Hospital & Clinic, 515 Delaware Street, SE, Box 491, Minneapolis, MN 55455 · 612-626-2922

Nathaniel R. Payne · Neonatal-Perinatal Medicine (Pediatric Infectious Disease) Abbott-Northwestern Hospital, Children's Health Care—Minneapolis · Minneapolis Children's Hospital, Department of Neonatology, 2525 Chicago Avenue, South, Minneapolis, MN 55404-4597 · 612-813-6295

Paul G. Quie · Pediatric Infectious Disease (White Blood Cell Disorders, Pediatric Immunology, Lyme Disease, Chronic Fatigue Syndrome, Pediatric Rheumatology) · University of Minnesota Hospital & Clinic · University of Minnesota Hospital & Clinic, 420 Delaware Street, SE, Box 296, Minneapolis, MN 55455 · 612-624-5146

Norma K. C. Ramsay · Pediatric Hematology-Oncology (Bone Marrow Transplantation) · University of Minnesota Hospital & Clinic · University of Minnesota Hospital & Clinic, 420 Delaware Street, SE, Box 366, Minneapolis, MN 55455 · 612-626-2778

Warren E. Regelmann · Pediatric Pulmonology · University of Minnesota, Cystic Fibrosis Center, Mayo Building, 420 Delaware Street, SE, Box 742, Minneapolis, MN 55455 · 612-624-0962

Albert P. Rocchini · Pediatric Cardiology (General, Interventional Catheterization) · Children's Health Care—Minneapolis, University of Minnesota Hospital & Clinic · University of Minnesota Hospital & Clinic, 420 Delaware Street, SE, Box 94, Minneapolis, MN 55455 · 612-626-2755

Sarah Jane Schwarzenberg · Pediatric Gastroenterology (Pediatric Hepatology, Pediatric Nutrition, Gastrointestinal Disease in Chronically Ill Children) · University of Minnesota Hospital & Clinic · University of Minnesota Hospital & Clinic, Department of Pediatric Gastroenterology, 420 Delaware Street, SE, Box 185, Minneapolis, MN 55455 · 612-624-4669

Harvey L. Sharp · Pediatric Gastroenterology · University of Minnesota Hospital & Clinic · University of Minnesota Hospital & Clinic, Department of Pediatric Gastroenterology, 420 Delaware Street, SE, Box 185, Minneapolis, MN 55455 · 612-624-1133

Alan R. Sinaiko · Pediatric Nephrology (Hypertension) · University of Minnesota Hospital & Clinic · University of Minnesota Hospital & Clinic, 420 Delaware Street, SE, Box 357, Minneapolis, MN 55455 · 612-626-2922

Martha L. Spencer · Pediatric Endocrinology · Park Nicollet Medical Center, 5000 West 39th Street, Minneapolis, MN 55416-3042 · 612-927-3530

Mendel Tuchman · Metabolic Diseases (Genetics) · University of Minnesota Hospital & Clinic, Department of Pediatrics, 516 Delaware Street, SE, Box 13-115 PWB, Minneapolis, MN 55455 · 612-624-5923

Warren Warwick · Pediatric Pulmonology (Cystic Fibrosis) · University of Minnesota Hospital & Clinic, 420 Delaware Street, SE, Box 742, Minneapolis, MN 55455-0392 · 612-624-7175

Sally A. Weisdorf · Pediatric Gastroenterology · University of Minnesota Hospital & Clinic, Department of Pediatric Gastroenterology, 420 Delaware Street, SE, Box 185, Minneapolis, MN 55455 · 612-624-3141

Chester B. Whitley · Metabolic Diseases (Genetics, Genetic Diseases, Gene Therapy) · University of Minnesota Hospital & Clinic · University of Minnesota Hospital & Clinic, Institute of Human Genetics and Department of Pediatrics, 420 Delaware Street, SE, Box 446 UMHC, Minneapolis, MN 55455 · 612-625-7422

William G. Woods · Pediatric Hematology-Oncology (Bone Marrow Transplantation, Childhood Cancer Screening, Pediatric Leukemia) · University of Minnesota Hospital & Clinic · University of Minnesota Hospital & Clinic, 420 Delaware Street, SE, Box 454, Minneapolis, MN 55455 · 612-626-2778

Gregory B. Wright · Pediatric Cardiology · Children's Health Care—Minneapolis Children's Heart Clinic, 2545 Chicago Avenue, South, Suite 106, Minneapolis, MN 55404 · 612-871-4660

Rochester

David J. Driscoll · Pediatric Cardiology (General) · Mayo Clinic · Mayo Clinic, 200 First Street, SW, Rochester, MN 55905 · 507-284-3372

Robert Feldt · Pediatric Cardiology · Mayo Clinic, Department of Pediatrics, 200 First Street, SW, Rochester, MN 55905 · 507-284-2511

Deborah Kay Freese · Pediatric Gastroenterology (Liver Disease, Pediatric Liver Transplant) · Mayo Clinic, Department of Pediatric & Adolescent Medicine, 200 First Street, SW, Rochester, MN 55905 · 507-284-3300

Joseph S. Gilchrist · Pediatric Hematology-Oncology · Mayo Clinic, Department of Pediatrics, 200 First Street, SW, Rochester, MN 55905 · 507-284-2511

Douglas D. Mair · Pediatric Cardiology (General) · Mayo Clinic · Mayo Clinic, 200 First Street, SW, Rochester, MN 55905 · 507-284-3351

Amy L. Manolis · Adolescent & Young Adult Medicine · Mayo Clinic, Department of Community, Pediatric and Adolescent Medicine, 200 First Street, SW, Rochester, MN 55905 · 507-284-5247

Coburn J. Porter · Pediatric Cardiology (Electrophysiology) · Mayo Clinic, Department of Pediatric Cardiology, 200 First Street, SW, Rochester, MN 55905 · 507-284-2911

Patricia S. Simmons · Pediatric & Adolescent Gynecology · Mayo Clinic · Mayo Clinic, Community Pediatric & Adolescent Medicine, 200 First Street, SW, Rochester, MN 55905 · 507-284-4466

John W. Yunginger · (Pediatric Allergy & Immunology) · Mayo Clinic · Mayo Clinic, 200 First Street, SW, Rochester, MN 55905 · 507-284-2922

Donald Zimmerman · Pediatric Endocrinology (General) · Mayo Clinic · Mayo Clinic, 200 First Street, SW, Rochester, MN 55905 · 507-284-3442

St. Paul

J. Michael Coleman · Neonatal-Perinatal Medicine · Children's Health Care—St. Paul Hospital, 345 North Smith Avenue, Suite 2100, St. Paul, MN 55102 · 612-220-6260

Catherine W. Gatto · Neonatal-Perinatal Medicine · Children's Healthcare—St. Paul, St. Paul-Ramsey Hospital · Children's Health Care—St. Paul Hospital, 345 North Smith Avenue, Suite 2100, St. Paul, MN 55102 · 612-220-6260

Erik A. Hagen · Neonatal-Perinatal Medicine · Children's Health Care—St. Paul Hospital, Department of Neonatology, 345 North Smith Avenue, Room 2100, St. Paul, MN 55102 · 612-220-6260

Paul T. Kubic · Pediatric Pulmonology · Children's Health Care—St. Paul Hospital, Pediatric Breathing Specialists, 345 North Smith Avenue, Suite 1100, St. Paul, MN 55102 · 612-220-6744

Carolyn J. Levitt · Abused Children · Children's Healthcare—St. Paul · Midwest Children's Resource Center, 360 Sherman Street, Suite 200, St. Paul, MN 55102 612-220-6750

Mark C. Mammel · Neonatal-Perinatal Medicine · St. Paul Children's Hospital, Department of Neonatal Medicine, 345 North Smith Avenue, St. Paul, MN 55102 612-220-6260

Christopher L. Moertel · Pediatric Hematology-Oncology (Hemophilia) · Children's Healthcare—St. Paul, United Hospital · 345 North Smith Avenue, St. Paul, MN 55102-2392 · 612-220-6732

John R. Priest · Pediatric Hematology-Oncology · 345 North Smith Avenue, St. Paul, MN 55102 · 612-220-6732

PEDIATRICS (GENERAL)

Brooklyn Center

Andrew A. Rzepka · Park Nicollet Medical Center, 6000 Earle Brown Drive, Brooklyn Center, MN 55430 · 612-993-4804

Duluth

Michael A. Bronson · Duluth Clinic, Department of Pediatrics, 400 East Third Street, Duluth, MN 55805 · 218-722-8364

Lori L. DeFrance · Duluth Clinic, Department of Pediatrics, 400 East Third Street, Duluth, MN 55805 · 218-722-8364

Jerome Kwako · Duluth Clinic, Department of Pediatrics, 400 East Third Street, Duluth, MN 55805 · 218-722-8364

Anne C. Stephen · Duluth Clinic, Department of Pediatrics, 400 East Third Street, Duluth, MN 55805 · 218-722-8364

Timothy D. Zager · Duluth Clinic, Department of Pediatrics, 400 East Third Street, Duluth, MN 55805 · 218-722-8364

Eagan

Theresa Ann Baker · Eagan Nicollet Medical Center, Department of Pediatrics, 1885 Plaza Drive, Eagan, MN 55122 · 612-683-4000

Edina

James R. Moore · (Chronic Conditions & Disabilities) · Southdale Pediatrics, 7250 France Avenue, South, Edina, MN 55435 · 612-831-4454

Fergus Falls

Lawrence F. Eisinger · Fergus Falls Medical Group, 615 South Mill Street, Fergus Falls, MN 56537-2738 · 218-739-2221

Allen E. Magnuson · Lake Region Hospital · Fergus Falls Medical Group, 615 South Mill Street, Fergus Falls, MN 56537 · 218-739-2228

Minneapolis

Robert W. Blum · (Adolescent Medicine) · University of Minnesota Hospital & Clinic · University of Minnesota Hospital & Clinic, Department of Pediatrics, 420 Delaware Street, SE, Box 721, Minneapolis, MN 55455 · 612-626-2796

Mace Goldfarb · Pediatric Associates, 3145 Hennepin Street, Minneapolis, MN 55408-2620 · 612-827-4055

Robert S. Karasov · Park Nicollet Clinic, 3800 Park Nicollet Boulevard, Minneapolis, MN 55416 · 612-927-3123

Anne M. Kelly · (Chronic Conditions & Disabilities, Difficult Diagnoses) · University of Minnesota Hospital & Clinic · University of Minnesota Hospital & Clinic, Department of Pediatrics, 420 Delaware Street, SE, Minneapolis, MN 55455 · 612-626-2820

Minnetonka

Renner S. Anderson · Park Nicollet Medical Center, 15111 Twelve Oaks Center Drive, Minnetonka, MN 55305 · 612-993-4570

Red Wing

Robert N. Schulenberg · (Attention Deficit Hyperactivity Disorder) · St. John's Regional Health Center · Interstate Medical Center, Highway 61 West, Red Wing, MN 55066 · 612-388-3503

Rochester

William J. Barbaresi · (Developmental Pediatrics) · Mayo Clinic, Department of Pediatrics, 200 First Street, SW, Rochester, MN 55905 · 507-284-2511

Daniel D. Broughton · Mayo Clinic, Department of Pediatric & Adolescent Medicine, 200 First Street, SW, Rochester, MN 55905 · 507-284-2511

Jay Lynn Hoecker · Mayo Clinic, Department of Pediatric & Adolescent Medicine, 200 First Street, SW, Rochester, MN 55905 · 507-284-5247

Richard D. Olsen · (Developmental Pediatrics) · Mayo Clinic, Department of Community Pediatrics, 200 First Street, SW, Rochester, MN 55905 · 507-284-2511

Thomas L. Peyla · (Adolescent Medicine) · Olmsted Medical Center · Olmsted Medical Center, Department of Pediatrics, 210 Ninth Street, Rochester, MN 55904 · 507-288-3443

St. Paul

James P. McCord · Children's Healthcare—St. Paul · St. Paul Children's Hospital, Pediatric Disease Consultants, 345 North Smith Avenue, St. Paul, MN 55102-2392 · 612-220-6700

Sandra K. Sackett · 2940 North Snelling Avenue, St. Paul, MN 55113 · 612-633-5603

White Bear Lake

Barbara A. Staub · (Chronic Conditions & Disabilities, General Pediatrics) · Children's Health Care—St. Paul (St. Paul) · Health Partners, 1430 Highway 96, White Bear Lake, MN 55110 · 612-426-1980

Willmar

Michael J. Hodapp · Affiliated Community Medical Center, 101 Willmar Avenue, SW, Willmar, MN 56201-3591 · 612-231-5000

Timothy V. Swanson · Affiliated Community Medical Center, 101 Willmar Avenue, SW, Willmar, MN 56201-3591 · 612-231-5000

Woodbury

Michael K. Nation · Children's Health Care—St. Paul (St. Paul) · Central Pediatrics, 7803 Afton Road, Woodbury, MN 55125 · 612-738-0470

PHYSICAL MEDICINE & REHABILITATION

Duluth

Matthew J. Eckman · General Physical Medicine & Rehabilitation (Rehabilitation of Strokes, Head Injuries, Spinal Cord Injuries, Back & Neck Pain) · Miller Dwan Medical Center, St. Mary's Medical Center, St. Luke's Hospital · Polinsky Medical Rehabilitation Center, 530 East Second Street, Duluth, MN 55805 · 218-722-8364 x4223

Kevin P. Murphy · General Physical Medicine & Rehabilitation · Duluth Clinic, Department of Physical Medicine, 400 East Third Street, Duluth, MN 55805 · 218-722-8364

Rochester

Robert W. DePompolo · General Physical Medicine & Rehabilitation · Mayo Clinic, Division of Physical Medicine & Rehabilitation, 200 First Street, SW, Rochester, MN 55905 · 507-284-0966

Margaret R. Lie · General Physical Medicine & Rehabilitation (Cancer Rehabilitation) · Mayo Clinic, 200 First Street, SW, Rochester, MN 55905 · 507-284-2511

St. Paul

Linda E. Krach · General Physical Medicine & Rehabilitation (Pediatric Rehabilitation) · Gillette Children's Hospital, 200 East University Avenue, St. Paul, MN 55101 · 612-291-2848

PLASTIC SURGERY

Duluth

Andrew Baertsch · General Plastic Surgery (Surgery of the Hand, Facial Aesthetic Surgery) · St. Luke's Hospital, Miller Dwan Medical Center, St. Mary's Medical Center · Northland Plastic Surgery, 925 East Superior Street, Suite 102, Duluth, MN 55805 · 218-724-7363

Edina

Michael C. Fasching · Head & Neck Surgery · 6545 France Avenue, South, Suite 240, Edina, MN 55435 · 612-920-2600

Allen L. Van Beek · Peripheral Nerve Surgery · North Memorial Health Care (Robbinsdale), Fairview-Southdale Hospital, Abbott-Northwestern Hospital (Minneapolis), Children's Health Care-Minneapolis (Minneapolis) · Plastic Surgery Specialists, 7373 France Avenue, South, Suite 510, Edina, MN 55435 · 612-588-0593; 612-830-1028

Rochester

Phillip G. Arnold · Reconstructive Surgery (Chest Wall Reconstruction, Reconstructive Surgery & the Aging Face) · Mayo Clinic · Mayo Clinic, Department of Plastic Surgery, 200 First Street, SW, Rochester, MN 55905 · 507-284-3214

PSYCHIATRY

Duluth

Ronald D. Franks · General Psychiatry (Mood & Anxiety Disorders, Psychopharmacology) · Miller Dwan Medical Center, St. Luke's Hospital, St. Mary's Medical Center · University of Minnesota School of Medicine, Office of the Dean, 10 University Drive, Suite 117, Duluth, MN 55812-2487 · 218-726-7571

Clyde R. Olson · General Psychiatry · Duluth Clinic, Department of Psychiatry, 400 East Third Street, Duluth, MN 55805 · 218-722-8364

Peder H. Svingen · Child & Adolescent Psychiatry · Duluth Clinic, Department of Psychiatry, 400 East Third Street, Duluth, MN 55805 · 218-722-8364

Edina

Deane C. Manolis · General Psychiatry · Minneapolis Psychiatric Clinic, 4010 West 65th Street, Suite 218, Edina, MN 55435 · 612-920-7203

Minneapolis

Gail A. Bernstein · Psychopharmacology, Child & Adolescent Psychiatry · University of Minnesota Hospital & Clinic, Department of Child & Adolescent Psychiatry, 420 Delaware Street, SE, Minneapolis, MN 55455 · 612-626-6577

Carrie M. Borchardt · Child & Adolescent Psychiatry · University of Minnesota Hospital & Clinic, Department of Child & Adolescent Psychiatry, 420 Delaware Street, SE, Minneapolis, MN 55455 · 612-626-6577

Paula J. Clayton · Mood & Anxiety Disorders, Psychopharmacology · University of Minnesota Hospital & Clinic · University of Minnesota Hospital & Clinic, 420 Delaware Street, SE, Box 77, Minneapolis, MN 55455 · 612-626-3853

Eduardo A. Colon · General Psychiatry (Consultation-Liaison Psychiatry, Mood & Anxiety Disorders, Neuropsychiatry) · Hennepin County Medical Center, Department of Psychiatry, 701 Park Avenue, South, Minneapolis, MN 55415 · 612-347-3604

Maurice William Dysken · Geriatric Psychiatry (Clinical Psychopharmacology) · VA Medical Center · Minneapolis Veterans Affairs Medical Center, One Veterans Drive, Minneapolis, MN 55417 · 612-725-2051

Elke D. Eckert · Eating Disorders (General Psychiatry, Psychopharmacology) · University of Minnesota Hospital & Clinic · University of Minnesota Hospital & Clinic, Department of Psychiatry, 420 Delaware Street, SE, Minneapolis, MN 55455 · 612-626-6871

Suck Won Kim · Mood & Anxiety Disorders · University of Minnesota Hospital & Clinic · University of Minnesota, Department of Psychiatry, 420 Delaware Street, SE, Box 392, Minneapolis, MN 55455 · 612-625-3210

Dean K. Knudson · (Geriatric Psychiatry, General Adult Psychiatry, Psychopharmacology) · Abbott-Northwestern Hospital · Minneapolis Psychiatric Institute, Wasie Center, Fourth Floor, 800 East 28th Street, Minneapolis, MN 55407-3799 612-863-5327

Mark Leffert · Psychoanalysis · 821 Marquette Avenue, Minneapolis, MN 55402 612-332-0817

Gabe J. Maletta · Geriatric Psychiatry (Psychopharmacology) · VA Medical Center Minneapolis Veterans Affairs Medical Center, Geriatrics and Extended Care, One Veterans Drive, Mail Code 11M, Minneapolis, MN 55417 · 612-725-2052

James E. Mitchell · Eating Disorders · University of Minnesota Hospital & Clinic University of Minnesota Hospital & Clinic, Department of Psychiatry, 420 Delaware Street, SE, Minneapolis, MN 55455 · 612-626-3633

Michael C. Moore · Child & Adolescent Psychiatry, Psychoanalysis · Foshay Tower, Suite 610, 821 Marquette Avenue, Minneapolis, MN 55402 · 612-339-0738

David Paulson · General Psychiatry · 914 South Eighth Street, Suite D-110, Minneapolis, MN 55404 · 612-347-2218

Michael K. Popkin · Mood & Anxiety Disorders · Hennepin County Medical Center · Hennepin County Medical Center, Department of Psychiatry, 701 Park Avenue, South, Mail Code 844, Minneapolis, MN 55415-1829 · 612-347-5764

Carlos H. Schenk · General Psychiatry · Hennepin County Medical Center, Child & Adolescent Psychiatry Unit, 701 Park Avenue, South, Minneapolis, MN 55415 612-347-2749

Sheila M. Specker · Addiction Psychiatry · University of Minnesota Hospital & Clinic · University of Minnesota Hospital & Clinic, Department of Psychiatry, 420 Delaware Street, SE, Minneapolis, MN 55455 · 612-626-3698

Joseph J. Westermeyer · Addiction Psychiatry (Cultural Psychiatry) · VA Medical Center, University of Minnesota Hospital & Clinic · Minneapolis Veterans Affairs Medical Center, Department of Psychiatry, One Veterans Drive, Mail Code 116A, Minneapolis, MN 55417 · 612-725-2037

Mark L. Willenbring · Addiction Psychiatry (Bioethics) · VA Medical Center · Minneapolis Veterans Affairs Medical Center, Department of Psychiatry, One Veterans Drive, Minneapolis, MN 55417 · 612-725-2228

Rochester

Gordon L. Moore · General Psychiatry · Mayo Clinic · Mayo Clinic, 200 First Street, SW, Rochester, MN 55905 · 507-284-2933

Robert M. Morse · Addiction Psychiatry · Mayo Clinic · Mayo Clinic, 200 First Street, SW, Rochester, MN 55905 · 507-284-2933

St. Paul

Willem Dieperink · Psychoanalysis · Lowry Medical Arts Building, Suite 1002, 350 St. Peter's Street, St. Paul, MN 55102 · 612-222-6096

Daniel R. Hanson · General Psychiatry (Mood Disorders, Schizophrenia) · St. Paul-Ramsey Medical Center · Ramsey Clinic, 640 Jackson Street, St. Paul, MN 55101-2595 · 612-221-2734

James M. Jaranson · General Psychiatry (Cultural Psychiatry, Refugee Trauma) St. Paul-Ramsey Medical Center · St. Paul-Ramsey Medical Center, Department of Psychiatry, 640 Jackson Street, St. Paul, MN 55101 · 612-221-2735

PULMONARY & CRITICAL CARE MEDICINE

Duluth

Paul J. Windberg · General Pulmonary & Critical Care Medicine · Duluth Clinic, Department of Pulmonary Medicine, 400 East Third Street, Duluth, MN 55805 218-722-8364

Norman G. Yunis · General Pulmonary & Critical Care Medicine · Duluth Clinic, Department of Pulmonary Medicine, 400 East Third Street, Duluth, MN 55805 218-722-8364

Paul E. Zimmerman · General Pulmonary & Critical Care Medicine · Duluth Clinic, Department of Pulmonary Medicine, 400 East Third Street, Duluth, MN 55805 · 218-722-8364

Minneapolis

Wilfred A. Corson · General Pulmonary & Critical Care Medicine · Minnesota Lung Center, 920 East 28th Street, Suite 700, Minneapolis, MN 55407 · 612-863-3750

Scott F. Davies · General Pulmonary & Critical Care Medicine (Fungal Infections of the Lung) · Hennepin County Medical Center · Hennepin County Medical Center, Department of Pulmonary Medicine, 701 Park Avenue, South, Minneapolis, MN 55415 · 612-347-2625

Paul R. Hamann · General Pulmonary & Critical Care Medicine · Minnesota Lung Center, 920 East 28th Street, Suite 700, Minneapolis, MN 55407 · 612-863-3750

Keith R. Harmon · General Pulmonary & Critical Care Medicine · Park Nicollet Medical Center, 3800 Park Nicollet Boulevard, Minneapolis, MN 55416 · 612-993-3242

Linda L. Hedemark · General Pulmonary & Critical Care Medicine (Tuberculosis, Lung Infections) · Hennepin County Medical Center · Hennepin County Tuberculosis Clinic, 525 Portland Avenue, South, Suite 210, Minneapolis, MN 55415 · 612-348-3031

Marshall Israel Hertz · General Pulmonary & Critical Care Medicine (Medical Care of Lung Transplant Patients, Bronchology) · University of Minnesota Hospital & Clinic · University of Minnesota Hospital & Clinic, 420 Delaware Street, SE, Box 398, Minneapolis, MN 55455 · 612-625-9922

Conrad Iber · General Pulmonary & Critical Care Medicine · Hennepin County Medical Center, Division of Pulmonary Medicine, 701 Park Avenue, South, Minneapolis, MN 55415 · 612-347-2625

Mitchell Kaye · General Pulmonary & Critical Care Medicine · 920 East 28th Street, Suite 700, Minneapolis, MN 55407 · 612-863-3750

James W. Leatherman · Asthma (Acutely Ill Asthmatics) · University of Minnesota Hospital & Clinic, Hennepin County Medical Center · Hennepin County Medical Center, Department of Pulmonary Medicine, 701 Park Avenue, South, Minneapolis, MN 55415 · 612-347-2625

Dennis E. Niewoehner · General Pulmonary & Critical Care Medicine · Minneapolis Veterans Affairs Medical Center, Department of Pulmonary Medicine, One Veterans Drive, Minneapolis, MN 55417 · 612-725-4400

Richard C. Woellner · General Pulmonary & Critical Care Medicine (Occupational & Environmental Lung Disease) · Methodist Hospital · Park Nicollet Medical Center, 3800 Park Nicollet Boulevard, Minneapolis, MN 55416 · 612-927-3242

Robbinsdale

Robert L. Colbert · General Pulmonary & Critical Care Medicine · Respiratory Consultants, 3366 Oakdale Avenue, North, Suite 509, Robbinsdale, MN 55422 · 612-520-2940

Rochester

W. Mark Brutinel · General Pulmonary & Critical Care Medicine · Mayo Clinic, Department of Pulmonary & Critical Care Medicine, 200 First Street, SW, Rochester, MN 55905 · 507-284-2494

Richard A. DeRemee · General Pulmonary & Critical Care Medicine · Mayo Clinic · Mayo Clinic, Department of Pulmonary & Critical Care Medicine, 200 First Street, SW, Rochester, MN 55905 · 507-284-2957

Charles W. Drage · General Pulmonary & Critical Care Medicine · Mayo Clinic, Department of Pulmonary & Critical Care Medicine, 200 First Street, SW, Rochester, MN 55905 · 507-284-2447

William F. Dunn · General Pulmonary & Critical Care Medicine · Mayo Clinic, Department of Pulmonary & Critical Care Medicine, 200 First Street, SW, Rochester, MN 55905 · 507-284-3811

Eric S. Edell · Bronchology · Mayo Clinic, Department of Pulmonary & Critical Care Medicine, 200 First Street, SW, Rochester, MN 55905 · 507-284-2511

Peter C. Gay · General Pulmonary & Critical Care Medicine · Mayo Clinic, Department of Pulmonary & Critical Care Medicine, 200 First Street, SW, Rochester, MN 55905 · 507-284-2511

Delmar J. Gillespie · General Pulmonary & Critical Care Medicine · Mayo Clinic, Department of Pulmonary & Critical Care Medicine, 200 First Street, SW, Rochester, MN 55905 · 507-284-2511

Douglas R. Gracey · General Pulmonary & Critical Care Medicine · Mayo Clinic, Department of Pulmonary & Critical Care Medicine, 200 First Street, SW, Rochester, MN 55905 · 507-284-2495

Rolf D. Hubmayr · General Pulmonary & Critical Care Medicine · Mayo Clinic, Division of Pulmonary & Critical Care Medicine, 200 First Street, SW, Rochester, MN 55905 · 507-255-5444

Andrew H. Limper · General Pulmonary & Critical Care Medicine · Mayo Clinic, Department of Pulmonary & Critical Care Medicine, 200 First Street, SW, Rochester, MN 55905 · 507-284-3478

John C. McDougall · General Pulmonary & Critical Care Medicine · Mayo Clinic Mayo Clinic, Department of Pulmonary & Critical Care Medicine, 200 First Street, SW, Rochester, MN 55905 · 507-284-2079

David E. Midthun · General Pulmonary & Critical Care Medicine · Mayo Clinic, Department of Pulmonary & Critical Care Medicine, 200 First Street, SW, Rochester, MN 55905 · 507-284-0561

Steven G. Peters · General Pulmonary & Critical Care Medicine · Mayo Clinic, Department of Pulmonary & Critical Care Medicine, 200 First Street, SW, Rochester, MN 55905 · 507-284-2511

Udaya B. S. Prakash · Bronchology, Lung Infections, General Pulmonary & Critical Care Medicine (Rare & Uncommon Lung Diseases, Laser Therapy in Lung Diseases, Diseases of Pleura, Lung Cancer, Pulmonary Hypertension, Emphysema) · Mayo Clinic · Mayo Clinic, 200 First Street, SW, Rochester, MN 55905 · 507-284-4162

Edward C. Rosenow III · General Pulmonary & Critical Care Medicine (Pulmonary Medicine) · Mayo Clinic · Mayo Clinic, Department of Pulmonary & Critical Care Medicine, 200 First Street, SW, Rochester, MN 55905 · 507-284-2964

Jay H. Ryu · General Pulmonary & Critical Care Medicine · Mayo Clinic, Department of Pulmonary & Critical Care Medicine, 200 First Street, SW, Rochester, MN 55905 · 507-284-2511

Paul D. Scanlon · General Pulmonary & Critical Care Medicine · Mayo Clinic, Department of Pulmonary & Critical Care Medicine, 200 First Street, SW, Rochester, MN 55905 · 507-284-2511

John P. Scott · General Pulmonary & Critical Care Medicine · Mayo Clinic, Department of Pulmonary & Critical Care Medicine, 200 First Street, SW, Rochester, MN 55905 · 507-266-8900

John W. Shepard, Jr. · General Pulmonary & Critical Care Medicine (Sleep Disorders) · Mayo Clinic, Sleep Disorders Center, 200 First Street, SW, Rochester, MN 55905 · 507-266-8900

Ulrich Specks · General Pulmonary & Critical Care Medicine · Mayo Clinic, Department of Pulmonary & Critical Care Medicine, 200 First Street, SW, Rochester, MN 55905 · 507-284-2511

Bruce A. Staats · General Pulmonary & Critical Care Medicine (Sleep Disorders) · Mayo Clinic, Department of Pulmonary & Critical Care Medicine, 200 First Street, SW, Rochester, MN 55905 · 507-284-2511

James P. Utz · General Pulmonary & Critical Care Medicine · Mayo Clinic, Department of Pulmonary & Critical Care Medicine, 200 First Street, SW, Rochester, MN 55905 · 507-284-5398

David E. Williams · General Pulmonary & Critical Care Medicine · Mayo Clinic, Department of Pulmonary & Critical Care Medicine, 200 First Street, SW, Rochester, MN 55905 · 507-284-3764

St. Cloud

Terence R. Pladson · General Pulmonary & Critical Care Medicine · St. Cloud Hospital · Centracare Clinic, 1200 Sixth Avenue, North, St. Cloud, MN 56303 · 612-252-5131

St. Paul

Thomas B. Dunkel · General Pulmonary & Critical Care Medicine · 17 West Exchange Street, Suite 710, St. Paul, MN 55100 · 612-232-4300

James R. Flink · General Pulmonary & Critical Care Medicine (Asthma, Occupational Lung Disease) · United Hospital · Pulmonary & Critical Care Associates, 255 North Smith Avenue, Suite 201, St. Paul, MN 55102 · 612-224-5895

Lee M. Kamman · General Pulmonary & Critical Care Medicine · St. Paul Lung Center, 255 North Smith Avenue, Suite 201, St. Paul, MN 55102 · 612-224-5895

John J. Marini · General Pulmonary & Critical Care Medicine (Acute Respiratory Failure, Mechanical Ventilation, Adult Respiratory Distress Syndrome, General Internal Medicine) · St. Paul-Ramsey Medical Center · St. Paul-Ramsey Medical Center, Department of Pulmonary & Critical Care Medicine, 640 Jackson Street, St. Paul, MN 55101 · 612-221-3135

RADIATION ONCOLOGY

Duluth

Roger T. Collins · General Radiation Oncology · Miller Dwan Medical Center, Department of Radiation Oncology, 502 East Second Street, Duluth, MN 55805 218-720-1313

David McNaney · General Radiation Oncology (Breast Cancer, Lung Cancer, Prostate Cancer, Genito-Urinary Cancer, Gynecologic Cancer) · Miller Dwan Medical Center, Department of Radiation Oncology, 502 East Second Street, Duluth, MN 55805 · 218-720-1313

Rodolfo E. Urias · General Radiation Oncology · Miller Dwan Medical Center, Department of Radiation Oncology, 502 East Second Street, Duluth, MN 55805 218-720-1313

Minneapolis

Kathryn Ellen Dusenberry · General Radiation Oncology · University of Minnesota Hospital & Clinic · University of Minnesota Hospital & Clinic, Department of Radiation Oncology, Harvard Street at East River Parkway, Minneapolis, MN 55455 · 612-626-3000

Tae H. Kim · Pediatric Radiation Oncology (General Radiation Oncology) · Abbott-Northwestern Hospital · Abbott-Northwestern Hospital, Department of Radiation Oncology, 800 East 28th Street, Minneapolis, MN 55407 · 612-863-4060

Chung K. Lee · General Radiation Oncology (Hodgkin's Disease, Non-Hodgkin's Lymphomas, Hyperthermia, Breast Cancer, Head & Neck Cancer) · University of Minnesota Hospital & Clinic · University of Minnesota Hospital & Clinic, Department of Radiation Oncology, Harvard Street at East River Road, Room 1-208, Box 494, Minneapolis, MN 55455-0110 · 612-626-6700

Seymour H. Levitt · Breast Cancer, Lymphomas (Hodgkin's Disease) · University of Minnesota Hospital & Clinic · University of Minnesota Hospital & Clinic, Harvard Street at East River Road, Box 436, Minneapolis, MN 55455 · 612-626-3000

Rochester

John D. Earle · General Radiation Oncology, Lymphomas · Mayo Clinic · Mayo Clinic, 200 First Street, SW, Rochester, MN 55905 · 507-284-2511

Robert L. Foote · Head & Neck Cancer · Mayo Clinic · Mayo Clinic, 200 First Street, SW, Rochester, MN 55905 · 507-284-9500

Leonard L. Gunderson · Gastroenterologic Cancer (Intraoperative Irradiation [IORT], Soft Tissue Sarcomas) · Mayo Clinic · Mayo Clinic, 200 First Street, SW, Rochester, MN 55905 · 507-284-2949

Paula J. Schomberg · General Radiation Oncology · Mayo Clinic · Mayo Clinic, Department of Radiation Oncology, 200 First Street, SW, Rochester, MN 55905 · 507-284-2511

St. Cloud

Jon A. Maier · General Radiation Oncology · St. Cloud Hospital, 1406 Sixth Avenue, North, St. Cloud, MN 56303 · 612-255-5693

St. Paul

Roger A. Potish · Gynecologic Cancer · University of Minnesota Hospital & Clinic (Minneapolis), United Hospital · United Hospital, 345 Sherman Street, St. Paul, MN 55102 · 612-220-5525

RADIOLOGY

Duluth

William D. Witrak · General Radiology · Duluth Clinic, Department of Radiology, 400 East Third Street, Duluth, MN 55805 · 218-722-8364

Minneapolis

David W. Hunter · General Radiology (Vascular & Interventional Radiology) · University of Minnesota Hospital & Clinic · University of Minnesota Hospital & Clinic, Department of Radiology, 420 Delaware Street, SE, Minneapolis, MN 55455 · 612-626-2826

James W. Walsh · General Radiology (Computed Tomography Imaging, Magnetic Resonance Imaging) · University of Minnesota Hospital & Clinic, Department of Radiology, 420 Delaware Street, SE, Minneapolis, MN 55455 · 612-625-7434

Rochester

Lawrence Randolph Brown · Chest · Mayo Clinic, Department of Radiology, 200 First Street, SW, Rochester, MN 55905 · 507-284-2511

Glenn S. Forbes · Neuroradiology · Mayo Clinic · Mayo Clinic, Department of Radiology, 200 First Street, SW, Rochester, MN 55905 · 507-284-2511

Steven J. Swenson · Chest · Mayo Clinic · Mayo Clinic, Department of Radiology, 200 First Street, SW, Rochester, MN 55905 · 507-284-2511

St. Paul

Joseph Tashjian · General Radiology (Chest Radiology) · St. Paul-Ramsey Medical Center, 640 Jackson Street, St. Paul, MN 55101 · 612-221-3797

RHEUMATOLOGY

Duluth

Stephen L. Hadley · General Rheumatology · Duluth Clinic, Department of Rheumatology, 400 East Third Street, Duluth, MN 55805 · 218-722-8364

Robert D. Leff · General Rheumatology · Duluth Clinic, Department of Rheumatology, 400 East Third Street, Duluth, MN 55805 · 218-722-8364

Edina

Jeffrey C. Felt · General Rheumatology · 7250 France Avenue, South, Suite 215, Edina, MN 55435-4312 · 612-893-1959

Minneapolis

Erskine M. Caperton · General Rheumatology · Abbott-Northwestern Hospital, Fairview Riverside Medical Center · Arthritis Associates of Minnesota, 63 South Ninth Street, Suite 711, Minneapolis, MN 55402 · 612-332-4396

Ronald P. Messner · General Rheumatology (Lupus, Vasculitis) · University of Minnesota Hospital & Clinic · University of Minnesota Hospital & Clinic, Department of Medicine, Section of Rheumatology, 515 Delaware Street, SE, Minneapolis, MN 55455 · 612-625-1155

Rochester

Doyt LaDean Conn · General Rheumatology · Mayo Clinic · Mayo Clinic, 200 First Street, SW, Rochester, MN 55905 · 507-284-2002

Gene G. Hunder · Vasculitis (Polymyalgia Rheumatica, Giant Cell [Temporal] Arteritis) · Mayo Clinic · Mayo Clinic, Division of Rheumatology, 200 First Street, SW, Rochester, MN 55905 · 507-284-2060

SURGERY

Duluth

Richard O. Adams · General Surgery · Duluth Clinic, Department of Surgery, 400 East Third Street, Duluth, MN 55805 · 218-722-8364

Charles K. Bertel · General Surgery · Duluth Clinic, Department of Surgery, 400 East Third Street, Duluth, MN 55805 · 218-722-8364

Thomas M. Nelson · General Surgery · Northland Gastroenterology & Surgery, 915 East First Street, Third Floor, Duluth, MN 55805 · 218-725-6050

Thomas H. Wiig · General Surgery · Duluth Clinic, Department of Surgery, 400 East Third Street, Duluth, MN 55805 · 218-722-8364

Edina

David R. Joesting · General Vascular Surgery · Surgical Consultants, Fairview-Southdale Physicians Building, Suite 550, 6363 France Avenue, South, Edina, MN 55435 · 612-927-7004

Minneapolis

John P. Delaney · Endocrine Surgery (Breast Surgery, Gastroenterologic Surgery, General Surgery) · University of Minnesota Hospital & Clinic · University of Minnesota Hospital & Clinic, 516 Delaware Street, SE, Box 195, Minneapolis, MN 55455 · 612-626-3000

David L. Dunn · Transplantation (General Surgery) · University of Minnesota Hospital & Clinic · University of Minnesota, Department of Surgery, 420 Delaware Street, SE, Box 242, Minneapolis, MN 55455 · 612-626-1999

William G. Gamble · Breast Surgery · 3800 Park Nicollet Boulevard, Minneapolis, MN 55416-2527 · 612-927-3180

Arthur J. Matas · Transplantation · University of Minnesota Hospital & Clinic · University of Minnesota Hospital & Clinic, 516 Delaware Street, Suite 58, Box 328, Minneapolis, MN 55455-0301 · 612-625-6460

David E. R. Sutherland · Transplantation (Kidney & Pancreas Transplantation, Diabetes, Pancreas Surgery) · University of Minnesota Hospital & Clinic · University of Minnesota Hospital & Clinic, 420 Delaware Street, SE, Box 280, Minneapolis, MN 55455 · 612-625-7600

Rochester

Thomas C. Bower · General Vascular Surgery · Mayo Clinic, Department of Surgery, 200 First Street, SW, Rochester, MN 55905 · 507-284-2644

Kenneth J. Cherry · General Vascular Surgery (Aortic Surgery, Graft Infection) · Mayo Clinic, St. Mary's Hospital of Rochester, Rochester Methodist Hospital · Mayo Clinic, Division of Vascular Surgery, 200 First Street, SW, Rochester, MN 55905 · 507-284-4494

Roger R. Dozois · Gastroenterologic Surgery (Inflammatory Bowel Disease) · Mayo Clinic · Mayo Clinic, Division of Colon & Rectal Surgery, 200 First Street, SW, Rochester, MN 55905 · 507-284-2218

Peter Gloviczki · General Vascular Surgery (Venous Disease, Vascular Malformations & Lymphoedema, Aortic Surgery, Limb Salvage Procedures) · Mayo Clinic · Mayo Clinic, Division of Vascular Surgery, 200 First Street, SW, West 6B, Rochester, MN 55905 · 507-284-2644

Clive S. Grant · Endocrine Surgery · Mayo Clinic · Mayo Clinic, 200 First Street, SW, Rochester, MN 55905 · 507-284-2166

John W. Hallett, Jr. · General Vascular Surgery (Infrainguinal Bypass Surgery, Aneurysms) · Mayo Clinic · Mayo Clinic, Division of Vascular Surgery, 200 First Street, SW, Rochester, MN 55905 · 507-284-4751

Ruud A. F. Krom · Transplantation (Liver Transplantation) · Mayo Clinic · Mayo Clinic, EI-3G Liver Transplant, 200 First Street, SW, Rochester, MN 55905 · 507-266-1580

David M. Nagorney · Gastroenterologic Surgery (Hepatic Surgery) · Mayo Clinic, Rochester Methodist Hospital, St. Mary's Hospital of Rochester · Mayo Clinic, 200 First Street, SW, West Sixth, Rochester, MN 55905 · 507-284-2644

Peter C. Pairolero · General Vascular Surgery · Mayo Clinic, Department of Surgery, 200 First Street, SW, Rochester, MN 55905 · 507-282-2511; 507-284-2808

John H. Pemberton · Gastroenterologic Surgery (Inflammatory Bowel Disease) · Mayo Clinic · Mayo Clinic, Department of Surgery, 200 First Street, SW, Rochester, MN 55905 · 507-284-2359

Michael G. Sarr · Gastroenterologic Surgery (Pancreatic Surgery, Bariatric Surgery, Gastrointestinal Motility Disorders) · Mayo Clinic · Mayo Clinic, 201 First Street, SW, Rochester, MN 55905 · 507-284-2644

Sylvester Sterioff · Transplantation (Kidney, Liver & Pancreas Transplantation) Rochester Methodist Hospital, St. Mary's Hospital of Rochester · Mayo Clinic, 200 First Street, SW, Rochester, MN 55905 · 507-284-8392

Jon van Heerden · Endocrine Surgery (Endocrine-Thyroid Tumors, Pancreatic Islet-Cell Tumors, Hyperparathyroidism) · Mayo Clinic · Mayo Clinic, 200 First Street, SW, Rochester, MN 55905 · 507-284-3364

St. Paul

David C. Anderson · General Surgery · Minnesota Surgical Associates, 280 North Smith Avenue, Suite 450, St. Paul, MN 55102-2424 · 612-224-1347

Robert L. Telander · Pediatric Surgery (Newborn Surgical Problems, Inflammatory Bowel Disease, Childhood Cancer, Pediatric Non-Cardiac Thoracic Surgery, Pediatric Colon & Rectal Surgery) · Children's Healthcare—St. Paul, Children's Health Care—Minneapolis · Pediatric Surgical Associates, 280 North Smith Avenue, Suite 810, St. Paul, MN 55401 · 612-228-0401

SURGICAL ONCOLOGY

Minneapolis

David A. Rothenberger · Colon & Rectal Cancer · University of Minnesota Hospital & Clinic · University of Minnesota Hospital & Clinic, 420 Delaware Street, SE, Box 450, Minneapolis, MN 55455 · 612-625-3288; 612-291-1151

Rochester

John H. Donohue · General Surgical Oncology · Mayo Clinic, 200 First Street, SW, Rochester, MN 55905 · 507-284-2683

Roger R. Dozois · Colon & Rectal Cancer · Mayo Clinic · Mayo Clinic, Division of Colon & Rectal Surgery, 200 First Street, SW, Rochester, MN 55905 · 507-284-2218

David M. Nagorney · Gastrointestinal Cancer (Liver Cancer) · Mayo Clinic, Rochester Methodist Hospital, St. Mary's Hospital of Rochester · Mayo Clinic, 200 First Street, SW, West Sixth, Rochester, MN 55905 · 507-284-2644

THORACIC SURGERY

Duluth

Per H. Wickstrom · General Thoracic Surgery · Duluth Clinic, Department of Cardiothoracic Surgery, 400 East Third Street, Duluth, MN 55805 · 218-722-8364

Minneapolis

R. Morton Bolman III · Adult Cardiothoracic Surgery, Transplantation (Heart Transplantation, Lung Transplantation, Heart & Lung Transplantation) · University of Minnesota Hospital & Clinic · University of Minnesota Hospital & Clinic, Division of Cardiovascular and Thoracic Surgery, 410 East River Road, Box 207 UMHC, Minneapolis, MN 55455 · 612-625-3902

Frazier Eales · General Thoracic Surgery · Minnesota Thoracic, 920 East 28th Street, Suite 440, Minneapolis, MN 55407 · 612-863-3999

Robert W. Emery · General Thoracic Surgery (Adult Cardiothoracic Surgery, Transplantation, Thoracic Oncological Surgery) · Abbott-Northwestern Hospital, United Hospital (St. Paul), Fairview-Southdale Hospital, Fairview Riverside Hospital, St. Joseph's Medical Center (Brainerd), St. Cloud Hospital (St. Cloud) · Minneapolis Cardiology, 920 East 28th Street, Suite 420, Minneapolis, MN 55407 612-863-3950

Hovald K. Helseth, Jr. · Pediatric Cardiac Surgery (Adult Cardiothoracic Surgery) Children's Health Care—Minneapolis · Children's Heart Clinic, 2545 Chicago Avenue, South, Suite 106, Minneapolis, MN 55404 · 612-871-4660

Sara J. Shumway · Adult Cardiothoracic Surgery (Heart & Lung Transplantation) University of Minnesota Hospital & Clinic · University of Minnesota Hospital & Clinic, 420 Delaware Street, SE, Box 207, Minneapolis, MN 55455 · 612-626-0976

Rochester

Mark S. Allen · General Thoracic Surgery · Mayo Clinic, Department of Thoracic Surgery, 200 First Street, SW, Rochester, MN 55905 · 507-284-2644

Gordon K. Danielson · Adult Cardiothoracic Surgery, Pediatric Cardiac Surgery St. Mary's Hospital of Rochester · Mayo Clinic, 200 First Street, SW, Rochester, MN 55905 · 507-255-7062

Claude Deschamps · General Thoracic Surgery · Mayo Clinic · Mayo Clinic, Department of Thoracic Surgery, 200 First Street, SW, Rochester, MN 55905 · 507-284-2644

Thomas A. Orszulak · General Thoracic Surgery · Mayo Clinic, Department of Cardiac Surgery, 200 First Street, SW, Rochester, MN 55905 · 507-255-7067

Peter C. Pairolero · Thoracic Oncological Surgery, General Thoracic Surgery (Esophageal Cancer) · Mayo Clinic · Mayo Clinic, 200 First Street, SW, Rochester, MN 55905 · 507-282-2511; 507-284-2808

Francisco J. Puga · Pediatric Cardiac Surgery · St. Mary's Hospital of Rochester Mayo Clinic, 200 First Street, SW, Rochester, MN 55905 · 507-284-2644

Hartzell V. Schaff · Adult Cardiothoracic Surgery (Coronary Bypass Surgery, Cardiac Surgery) · Mayo Clinic, St. Mary's Hospital of Rochester, Rochester Methodist Hospital · Mayo Clinic, 200 First Stree*, SW, Rochester, MN 55905 · 507-255-7068

Victor F. Trastek · Thoracic Oncological Surgery, General Thoracic Surgery (Esophageal Cancer, Lung Cancer, Esophageal Reflux Disease, Barret's Disease) Mayo Clinic · Mayo Clinic, 200 First Street, SW, Rochester, MN 55905 · 507-284-2942

UROLOGY

Duluth

Curt H. Hutchens · General Urology · Northland Urology Associates, 1000 East First Street, Duluth, MN 55805 · 218-727-8414

Minneapolis

John C. Hulbert · Endourology (Ureteroscopy, Percutaneous Renal Surgery, Laparoscopic Urologic Surgery) · University of Minnesota Hospital & Clinic · University of Minnesota Hospital & Clinic, 420 Delaware Street, SE, Box 394, Minneapolis, MN 55455 · 612-625-3209

Jon L. Pryor · General Urology (Impotence) · University of Minnesota Hospital & Clinic, Department of Urology, 420 Delaware Street, SE, Box 394, Minneapolis, MN 55455 · 612-625-0662

Pratap K. Reddy · Endourology, Urologic Oncology (Reconstructive Surgery) · University of Minnesota Hospital & Clinic · University of Minnesota Hospital & Clinic, Department of Urologic Surgery, 420 Delaware Street, SE, Box 394, Minneapolis, MN 55455 · 612-625-2486; 612-625-9933

Rochester

David M. Barrett · Neuro-Urology & Voiding Dysfunction, Impotence, Urologic Oncology (Genito-Urinary Cancer) · Mayo Clinic · Mayo Clinic, 200 First Street, SW, Rochester, MN 55905 · 507-284-2248

Michael L. Blute · Urologic Oncology (Genito-Urinary Cancer) · Mayo Clinic · Mayo Clinic, 200 First Street, SW, Rochester, MN 55905 · 507-284-3982

Douglas A. Husmann · Pediatric Urology · Mayo Clinic, Department of Urology, 200 First Street, SW, Rochester, MN 55905 · 507-284-2959

Stephen A. Kramer · Pediatric Urology · Mayo Clinic, St. Mary's Hospital of Rochester · Mayo Clinic, 200 First Street, SW, Rochester, MN 55905 · 507-284-3249

Michael M. Lieber · Urologic Oncology · Mayo Clinic · Mayo Clinic, 200 First Street, SW, Rochester, MN 55905 · 507-284-4427

David E. Patterson · Endourology · St. Mary's Hospital of Rochester, Mayo Clinic Mayo Clinic, Department of Urology, 200 First Street, SW, Rochester, MN 55905 507-284-4015

Joseph W. Segura · Endourology (Stone Disease, Ureteroscopy, Percutaneous Stone Removal) · Mayo Clinic · Mayo Clinic, 200 First Street, SW, Rochester, MN 55905 · 507-284-2297

Horst Zincke · Urologic Oncology · Mayo Clinic · Mayo Clinic, Department of Urology, 200 First Street, SW, Rochester, MN 55905 · 507-284-3981

MISSOURI

ALLERGY & IMMUNOLOGY

Cape Girardeau

Jean Chapman · General Allergy & Immunology · Southeast Missouri Hospital, St. Francis Medical Center · 23 Doctors' Park, Cape Girardeau, MO 63703 · 573-335-1218

Chesterfield

John A. Wood · General Allergy & Immunology (Pulmonary Diseases) · 224 South Woodsmill Road, Suite 500 South, Chesterfield, MO 63017 · 314-878-6260

Columbia

Peter Konig · General Allergy & Immunology (Asthma, Pediatric Pulmonology) · University Hospital & Children's Hospital · University Hospital & Children's Hospital, Department of Child Health, One Hospital Drive, Columbia, MO 65212 · 573-882-6993

Joplin

David L. Straub · General Allergy & Immunology · St. John's Regional Medical Center, Freeman Hospital · 2700 McClelland Boulevard, Suite 105, Joplin, MO 64804 · 417-782-1343

Kansas City

Jay M. Portnoy · General Allergy & Immunology (Immunodeficiency) · Children's Mercy Hospital · Children's Mercy Hospital, Department of Allergy & Immunology, 2401 Gillham Road, Kansas City, MO 64108-9898 · 816-234-3097

St. Louis

Harvey R. Colten · General Allergy & Immunology (Pulmonology) · St. Louis Children's Hospital · St. Louis Children's Hospital, Department of Pediatrics, One Children's Place, Room 830ST, St. Louis, MO 63110 · 314-454-2129

Alan P. Knutsen · General Allergy & Immunology (Pediatric only, Immunodeficiency, AIDS) · Cardinal Glennon Children's Hospital, 1465 South Grand Boulevard, St. Louis, MO 63104 · 314-268-4014

Phillip E. Korenblat · General Allergy & Immunology (Asthma) · Barnes West County Hospital (Creve Coeur), Barnes-Jewish Hospital · Associated Specialists in Medicine, 1040 North Mason Road, Suite 115, St. Louis, MO 63141 · 314-542-0606

Raymond G. Slavin · General Allergy & Immunology (Sinusitis, Asthma) · St. Louis University Hospital · St. Louis University Doctors Office Building, 3660 Vista Avenue, St. Louis, MO 63110 · 314-577-8456

Thomas F. Smith · General Allergy & Immunology (Pediatric Pulmonology, Asthma, Sinusitis, Clinical & Lab Immunology) · St. Louis Children's Hospital · St. Louis Children's Hospital, Division of Allergy & Pulmonology, One Children's Place, Room 2N78, St. Louis, MO 63110 · 314-454-2694

Robert C. Strunk · General Allergy & Immunology (Pediatric Allergy & Immunology, Asthma, Allergy) · St. Louis Children's Hospital · Washington University School of Medicine, Children's Annex, Sixth Floor, Room 603, 400 South Kingshighway Boulevard, St. Louis, MO 63110 · 314-454-2284

ANESTHESIOLOGY

Columbia

Bruce J. Gordon · General Anesthesiology (Obstetric Anesthesia, Pain) · Boone Hospital Center · Columbia Anesthesia Associates, 1506 East Broadway, Suite 302, Columbia, MO 65201 · 573-449-1207

E. Scott McCord · General Anesthesiology · University of Missouri Medical Center, Sameday Surgery Center, Columbia, MO 65212 · 573-882-2568

Angela R. Stewart · General Anesthesiology · Boone Hospital Center · Columbia Anesthesia Associates, 1506 East Broadway, Suite 302, Columbia, MO 65201 · 573-449-1207

Joplin

Kalai Huff · General Anesthesiology (Cardiothoracic Anesthesiology, Healthcare Management, Obstetric Anesthesia) · St. John's Regional Medical Center · Anesthesia Professionals, 1703 West 30th Street, Suite A, Joplin, MO 64804 · 417-624-7844

Ira Joe Pryor · General Anesthesiology · Southwest Anesthesiology, 3333 McIntosh Circle, Suite Six, P.O. Box 3930, Joplin, MO 64803 · 417-781-6661

Kansas City

Susan S. Porter · Neuroanesthesia · Saint Luke's Hospital of Kansas City, Department of Anesthesia, 4400 Wornall Road, Kansas City, MO 64111 · 816-932-2033

Springfield

Jack M. Bagby · General Anesthesiology · Professional Anesthesia, 1900 South National Avenue, Suite 1800, Springfield, MO 65804 · 417-887-6323

St. Louis

Demetrius G. Lappas · Adult Cardiovascular · Barnes-Jewish Hospital · Washington University School of Medicine, 660 South Euclid Avenue, Campus Box 8054, St. Louis, MO 63110 · 314-362-6584

CARDIOVASCULAR DISEASE

Cape Girardeau

James B. Chapman · General Cardiovascular Disease · Cardiovascular Associates, 25 Doctors Park, Cape Girardeau, MO 63703 · 573-334-6008

Gordon L. Haycraft · General Cardiovascular Disease (Interventional Cardiology, Lipid Abnormalities) · St. Francis Medical Center, Southeast Missouri Hospital · Cape Girardeau Physician Associates, 14 Doctors Park, Cape Girardeau, MO 63703-4993 · 573-334-9641

Columbia

Gregory C. Flaker · General Cardiovascular Disease (Cardiac Electrophysiology, Cardiac Arrhythmias, Cardiac Catheterization, Pacemakers) · University Hospital & Children's Hospital · University Hospital & Children's Hospital, One Hospital Drive, Columbia, MO 65212 · 573-882-2296

Jerry D. Kennett · General Cardiovascular Disease (Cardiac Catheterization) · Boone Hospital Center, University Hospital & Children's Hospital, Columbia Regional Hospital · 401 Keene Street, Columbia, MO 65201 · 573-876-1630

Lenard L. Politte · General Cardiovascular Disease · Boone Hospital Center · The Cardiology Clinic, 401 Keene Street, Columbia, MO 65201 · 573-874-3300

H. K. Reddy · General Cardiovascular Disease (Interventional Cardiology, Percutaneous Catheter-Based Interventions, Congestive Heart Failure & Cardiac Transplantation, Exercise Stress Testing) · University Hospital & Children's Hospital, Division of Cardiology, One Hospital Drive, Columbia, MO 65212 · 573-882-8450

Richard R. Webel · General Cardiovascular Disease (Interventional Cardiology) · University Hospital & Children's Hospital, Division of Cardiology, One Hospital Drive, Columbia, MO 65212 · 573-882-2296

Karl T. Weber · Heart Failure (Clinical Exercise Testing, General Cardiovascular Disease) · University Hospital & Children's Hospital · University of Missouri, Columbia, School of Medicine, Medical Science Center, Room MA432, Columbia, MO 65212 · 573-882-8581

Joplin

Francis H. Corcoran · General Cardiovascular Disease (Invasive Cariology, Angioplasty) · St. John's Regional Medical Center · Heart Care Associates, 2817 McClelland Boulevard, Suite 224, Joplin, MO 64803-2788 · 417-781-5387

Thomas B. Moore · General Cardiovascular Disease (Adult Cardiology, Cardiac Rehabilitation) · St. John's Regional Medical Center · Heart Care Associates, 2817 McClelland Boulevard, Suite 224, P.O. Box 2788, Joplin, MO 64805-2788 · 417-781-5387

Robert J. Stuppy · General Cardiovascular Disease (Primary and Secondary Prevention of Cardiovascular Disease) · St. John's Regional Medical Center · Heart Care Associates, 2817 McClelland Boulevard, Suite 224, P.O. Box 2788, Joplin, MO 64803-2788 · 417-781-5387

Kansas City

Timothy M. Bateman · General Cardiovascular Disease (Nuclear Cardiology) · Mid-America Heart Institute · Cardiovascular Consultants, 4330 Wornall Road, Suite 2000, Kansas City, MO 64111 · 816-931-1883

William N. Brodine · General Cardiovascular Disease · Kansas City Cardiology, 6420 Prospect Avenue, Suite T-509, Kansas City, MO 64132 · 816-523-4525

Robert D. Conn · General Cardiovascular Disease · Saint Luke's Hospital of Kansas City · Cardiovascular Consultants, 4330 Wornall Road, Suite 2000, Kansas City, MO 64111 · 816-931-1883

James R. Eynon · General Cardiovascular Disease · Kansas City Cardiology, 6420 Prospect Avenue, Suite T-509, Kansas City, MO 64132 · 816-523-4525

Randall E. Genton · General Cardiovascular Disease · Mid-America Cardiology Associates, 4321 Washington Avenue, Suite 4000, Kansas City, MO 64111 · 816-531-5510

M. Eugene Kendall · General Cardiovascular Disease · Kansas City Cardiology, 6420 Prospect Avenue, Suite T-509, Kansas City, MO 64132 · 816-523-4525

Lynn H. Kindred · General Cardiovascular Disease · Mid-America Cardiology Associates, 4321 Washington Avenue, Suite 4000, Kansas City, MO 64111 · 816-531-5510

Ben D. McCallister · General Cardiovascular Disease · Saint Luke's Hospital of Kansas City, Mid-America Heart Institute · Cardiovascular Consultants, 4330 Wornall Road, Suite 2000, Kansas City, MO 64111 · 816-931-1883

David R. McConahay · General Cardiovascular Disease · Cardiovascular Consultants, 4330 Wornall Road, Suite 2000, Kansas City, MO 64111 · 816-931-1884

Barry D. Rutherford · General Cardiovascular Disease (Angioplasty, Acute Myocardiac Infarction, Cardiac Rehabilitation, Clinical Exercise Testing) · Saint Luke's Hospital of Kansas City, Mid-America Heart Institute · Cardiovascular Consultants, 4330 Wornall Road, Suite 2000, Kansas City, MO 64111-3210 · 816-931-1883

James L. Vacek · General Cardiovascular Disease · Mid-America Cardiology Associates, 4321 Washington Avenue, Suite 4000, Kansas City, MO 64111 · 816-531-5510

Springfield

Paul C. Freiman · General Cardiovascular Disease · Springfield Clinic, 3231 South National Avenue, Springfield, MO 65807 · 417-883-7422

Myron W. Mizell · Cardiac Catheterization (Interventional Cardiology) · Cardiology Group, 1965 South Fremont Street, Suite 2950, Springfield, MO 65804 · 417-882-1984

St. Louis

Preben Bjerregaard · General Cardiovascular Disease (Cardiac Electrophysiology, Cardiac Arrhythmias) · St. Louis University Hospital · St. Louis University Health Science Center, Division of Cardiology, 3635 Vista Avenue at Grand Boulevard, St. Louis, MO 63110-0250 · 314-577-8894

Alan C. Braverman · General Cardiovascular Disease (Marfan Syndrome, Aortic Diseases) · Barnes-Jewish Hospital · Barnes-Jewish Hospital, East Pavilion Building, Suite 16419, One Barnes Hospital Plaza, St. Louis, MO 63110 · 314-362-1291

Michael E. Cain · General Cardiovascular Disease (Cardiac Electrophysiology, Cardiac Arrhythmias, Clinical Cardiac Electrophysiology & Pacing) · Barnes-Jewish Hospital · Washington University School of Medicine, Division of Cardiology, 660 South Euclid Avenue, Campus Box 8086, St. Louis, MO 63110-1010 · 314-362-1508

Bernard R. Chaitman · Clinical Exercise Testing, General Cardiovascular Disease (Nuclear Cardiology) · St. Louis University Hospital · St. Louis University School of Medicine, Health Sciences Center, 13th Floor, 3635 Vista Avenue at Grand Boulevard, P.O. Box 15250, St. Louis, MO 63110-0250 · 314-577-8890

Edward M. Geltman · Cardiac Positron Emission Tomography (PET), Heart Failure (Congestive Heart Failure, Transplantation Medicine) · Barnes-Jewish Hospital · Washington University School of Medicine, 660 South Euclid Avenue, Campus Box 8086, St. Louis, MO 63110 · 314-362-5317

Morton J. Kern · Cardiac Catheterization · St. Louis University Hospital · St. Louis University Health Sciences Center, 3635 Vista Avenue at Grand Boulevard, P.O. Box 15250, St. Louis, MO 63110-0250 · 314-577-8860

Arthur J. Labovitz · Echocardiography · St. Louis University Hospital, Health Science Center, 3535 Vista Avenue at Grand Boulevard, St. Louis, MO 63110 · 314-577-8898

Bruce D. Lindsey · Echocardiography · Washington University School of Medicine, Division of Cardiology, 660 South Euclid Avenue, Campus Box 8086, St Louis, MO 63110 · 314-362-1045

Philip A. Ludbrook · Cardiac Catheterization (Adult Congenital Heart Disease) Barnes-Jewish Hospital · Washington University Medical Center, Cardiac Unit, 660 South Euclid Avenue, Campus Box 8086, St. Louis, MO 63110 · 314-362-3794

D. Douglas Miller · Nuclear Cardiology (Cardiac Disease in Women, Clinical Exercise Testing, General Cardiovascular Disease) · St. Louis University Hospital St. Louis University Health Sciences Center, 3635 Vista Avenue at Grand Boulevard, St. Louis, MO 63110-0250 · 314-577-8897

Leslie W. Miller · Transplantation Medicine (Post-Heart Transplantation Care, Heart Failure) · St. Louis University Hospital · St. Louis University Health Sciences Center, Division of Cardiology, 3635 Vista Avenue at Grand Boulevard, P.O. Box 15250, St. Louis, MO 63110-0250 · 314-577-8896

CLINICAL PHARMACOLOGY

St. Louis

Paula M. Fracasso · Barnes-Jewish Hospital · Washington University School of Medicine, 660 South Euclid Avenue, Campus Box 8056, St. Louis, MO 63110 · 314-362-7229

COLON & RECTAL SURGERY

Columbia

Walter Russell Peters, Jr. · General Colon & Rectal Surgery (Colon & Rectal Cancer, Gastroenterologic Surgery) · Boone Hospital Center, Columbia Regional Hospital · Columbia Surgical Associates, 3401 Berrywood Drive, Suite 104, Columbia, MO 65201-6598 · 573-443-8773

Kansas City

John W. Heryer · General Colon & Rectal Surgery · Colo-Rectal Surgery Associates, 4320 Wornall Road, Kansas City, MO 64111-3210 · 816-531-5648

St. Louis

Elisa H. Birnbaum · General Colon & Rectal Surgery · Barnes-Jewish Hospital · Barnes-Jewish Hospital, Department of Colon & Rectal Surgery, 216 South Kingshighway Boulevard, St. Louis, MO 63110 · 314-454-7177

James W. Fleshman · General Colon & Rectal Surgery · Barnes-Jewish Hospital Barnes-Jewish Hospital, Department of Colon & Rectal Surgery, 216 South Kingshighway Boulevard, St. Louis, MO 63110 · 314-454-7177

Ira Joe Kodner · General Colon & Rectal Surgery, Colon & Rectal Cancer (Inflammatory Bowel Disease [Crohn's & Ulcerative Colitis], Construction & Management of Intestinal Stomas [Colostomy & Ileostomy]) · Barnes-Jewish Hospital · Barnes-Jewish Hospital, 216 South Kingshighway Boulevard, St. Louis, MO 63110 · 314-454-7177

Anthony M. Vernava III · General Colon & Rectal Surgery (Colon & Rectal Cancer) · St. Louis University Hospital, St. Mary's Health Center · St. Louis University Health Sciences Center, Department of General Surgery, FDT Building, 3635 Vista Avenue at Grand Boulevard, P.O. Box 15250, St. Louis, MO 63110-0250 · 314-577-8562

DERMATOLOGY

Cape Girardeau

Henry S. Brown · Clinical Dermatology · 1326 Copper Road, Cape Girardeau, MO 63701 · 573-334-8500

Columbia

Philip C. Anderson · Clinical Dermatology · University Hospital & Children's Hospital, One Hospital Drive, Columbia, MO 65212 · 573-882-3141

David P. Clark · Clinical Dermatology · University Hospital & Children's Hospital, Department of Dermatology, One Hospital Drive, Room M173, Columbia, MO 65212 · 573-882-6144

James A. Roller · Clinical Dermatology · Boone Hospital Center, Columbia Regional Hospital · 3401 Berrywood Drive, Suite 202, Columbia, MO 65201 · 573-875-1527

Joplin

Mark S. Matlock · Clinical Dermatology · General Dermatology and Skin Cancer Surgery, 2817 McClelland Boulevard, Suite 125, Joplin, MO 64804 · 417-624-0440

Jess S. Simmons, Jr. · Clinical Dermatology (Acne, Skin Cancer Surgery) · Boulevard Professional Park, Suite 107, 2700 McClelland Boulevard, Joplin, MO 64804 417-623-5599

Springfield

Troy E. Major · Clinical Dermatology · 1000 East Primrose Street, Springfield, MO 65807 · 417-881-7220

St. Louis

Lynn A. Cornelius · Clinical Dermatology (Wound Healing, Vascular Biology) · Barnes-Jewish Hospital · Barnes-Jewish Hospital, Division of Dermatology, 216 South Kingshighway Boulevard, St. Louis, MO 63110 · 314-454-8290

Arthur Z. Eisen · Cutaneous Immunology · Barnes-Jewish Hospital · Washington University School of Medicine, Division of Dermatology, 660 South Euclid Avenue, Campus Box 8123, St. Louis, MO 63110 · 314-362-8180; 314-362-2643

Karen E. Forsman · Clinical Dermatology · Washington University School of Medicine, Barnes West Dermatology, 1040 North Mason Road, Suite 120, St. Louis, MO 63141 · 314-434-1991

Susan B. Mallory · Pediatric Dermatology (Genetic Skin Diseases, Vascular Lesions of the Skin) · St. Louis Children's Hospital, Barnes-Jewish Hospital · St. Louis Children's Hospital, One Children's Place, Room A281, St. Louis, MO 63110 · 314-454-2714

Neal S. Penneys · Clinical Dermatology (Dermatopathology) · St. Louis University Hospital · St. Louis University, Department of Dermatology, 1402 South Grand Boulevard, St. Louis, MO 63104 · 314-268-5215

Lester T. Reese · Clinical Dermatology · Barnes-Jewish Hospital, Missouri Baptist Medical Center · 522 North New Ballas Road, St. Louis, MO 63141 · 314-567-5873

Elaine Siegfried · Pediatric Dermatology · St. Louis University Hospital, Barnes-Jewish Hospital, Bethesda General Hospital, Cardinal Glennon Children's Hospital, St. John's Mercy Medical Center · St. Louis University, Department of Dermatology, 1402 South Grand Boulevard, St. Louis, MO 63104 · 314-577-6064

Robert E. Ziegler · Clinical Dermatology (Acne, Skin Cancer) · Barnes-Jewish Hospital, St. Anthony's Medical Center, St. Mary's Health Center, St. Joseph Hospital of Kirkwood (Kirkwood) · 7937 Big Bend Boulevard, St. Louis, MO 63119 · 314-962-4511

ENDOCRINOLOGY & METABOLISM

Cape Girardeau

Daniel S. Duick · Thyroid (Diabetes, General Endocrinology & Metabolism) · St. Francis Medical Center, Southeast Missouri Hospital · Endocrinology Associates, 1435 Mt. Auburn Road, Cape Girardeau, MO 63701 · 573-335-0006

Columbia

George T. Griffing · General Endocrinology & Metabolism (Diabetes, Thyroid) University Hospital & Children's Hospital · University Hospital & Children's Hospital, University of Missouri School of Medicine, Division of Endocrinology, Diabetes & Metabolism, One Hospital Drive, Columbia, MO 65212 · 573-882-2273

Springfield

Ralph J. Duda, Jr. · General Endocrinology & Metabolism (Osteoporosis, Diabetes Mellitus) · St. John's Regional Health Center · Springfield Clinic, 3231 South National Avenue, Springfield, MO 65807 · 417-888-5660; 417-883-7422

Larry E. Koppers · General Endocrinology & Metabolism (Diabetes Mellitus, Pituitary Tumors, Thyroid Disease) · Cox Medical Centers-North, Cox Medical Centers-South · Center for Internal Medicine, 1443 North Robberson Avenue, Suite 600, Springfield, MO 65802 · 417-269-4450

Edward J. Kryshak · General Endocrinology & Metabolism (Diabetes) · St. John's Regional Health Center · Springfield Clinic, 3231 South National Avenue, Springfield, MO 65807-7396 · 417-888-5660

Gregory A. Ledger · General Endocrinology & Metabolism (Metabolic Bone Disease, Diabetes) · St. John's Regional Health Center · Springfield Clinic, 3231 South National Avenue, Springfield, MO 65807-7396 · 417-888-5660

St. Louis

Louis V. Avioli · Paget's Disease (Osteoporosis, Menopause) · Barnes-Jewish Hospital · Washington University Medical Center, Steinberg Building, Seventh Floor, 216 South Kingshighway Boulevard, St. Louis, MO 63110 · 314-454-8410

William Clutter · Thyroid · Washington University School of Medicine, Department of Endocrinology & Metabolism, 4570 Children's Place, St. Louis, MO 63110 · 314-362-7601

Philip E. Cryer · Diabetes (General Endocrinology & Metabolism) · Barnes-Jewish Hospital · Washington University School of Medicine, 660 South Euclid Avenue, Campus Box 8127, St. Louis, MO 63110 · 314-362-7617

Anne C. Goldberg · (Lipids) · Barnes-Jewish Hospital · Washington University School of Medicine, Department of Internal Medicine, 660 South Euclid Avenue, Campus Box 8046, St. Louis, MO 63110-1093 · 314-362-3500

Julio V. Santiago · Diabetes (Adult & Pediatric) · St. Louis Children's Hospital, Barnes-Jewish Hospital · St. Louis Children's Hospital, Department of Pediatric Metabolism, One Children's Place, Campus Box 8116, St. Louis, MO 63110 · 314-454-6051

Gustav Schonfeld · General Endocrinology & Metabolism (Lipids, Diabetes) · Barnes-Jewish Hospital · Washington University School of Medicine, 660 South Euclid Avenue, Campus Box 8046, St. Louis, MO 63110-1093 · 314-362-3500

Clay Semenkovich · Diabetes (Lipids, General Endocrinology & Metabolism) · Barnes-Jewish Hospital · Washington University School of Medicine, 660 South Euclid Avenue, Campus Box 8046, St. Louis, MO 63110 · 314-362-3500

Donald A. Skor · Diabetes (Lipids) · Barnes-Jewish Hospital · Barnes-Jewish Hospital, One Barnes Hospital Plaza, Suite 17416, St. Louis, MO 63110-1013 · 314-362-5100

FAMILY MEDICINE

Cape Girardeau

S. Kent Griffith · Regional Primary Care, 69 Doctors Park, Cape Girardeau, MO 63703 · 573-334-4766

Columbia

Jeffery L. Belden · (Occupational Medicine, Geriatric Medicine, General Family Medicine) · Boone Hospital Center · Family Health Care, 1506 East Broadway, Suite 220, Columbia, MO 65201-5895 · 573-449-0808

Robert L. Blake, Jr. · University Hospital & Children's Hospital, Department of Family and Community Medicine, One Hospital Drive, Columbia, MO 65212 · 573-882-4433

Jack M. Coldwill · University Hospital & Children's Hospital, Department of Family and Community Medicine, One Hospital Drive, Columbia, MO 65212 · 573-882-1758

Anne B. Fitzsimmons · University Hospital & Children's Hospital · University Hospital & Children's Hospital, Department of Family and Community Medicine, One Hospital Drive, Columbia, MO 65212 · 573-882-1584

Elizabeth A. Garrett · University Hospital & Children's Hospital · University Hospital & Children's Hospital, Department of Family and Community Medicine, Medical School Building, Room M231, One Hospital Drive, Columbia, MO 65212 · 573-882-0974

Michael L. Le Fevre · (Obstetrics) · University Hospital & Children's Hospital · University Hospital & Children's Hospital, Department of Family Medicine, Health Sciences Center, Room MA303, Columbia, MO 65212 · 573-882-6191

Georgia B. Nolph · (Geriatric Medicine, Women's Health, General Family Medicine) · University Hospital & Children's Hospital · Green Meadows Building A, 3217 South Providence Road, Columbia, MO 65203 · 573-882-6191; 573-882-2163

Erika N. Ringdahl · University Hospital & Children's Hospital, Division of Family Medicine, One Hospital Drive, Columbia, MO 65212 · 573-882-4991

Harold A. Williamson · University Hospital & Children's Hospital · University Hospital & Children's Hospital, Department of Family Medicine, Health Sciences Center, Room MA303, Columbia, MO 65212 · 573-882-4991

Steven C. Zweig · Green Meadows Family Medicine Clinic, 3217 South Providence Road, Columbia, MO 65203 · 573-882-6191

Florissant

William E. Hines · (Smoking Cessation Programs, Health Education, General Family Medicine) · Christian Hospital Northeast-Northwest (St. Louis), Deaconess Medical Center-Central Campus (St. Louis) · Hines Family Care Center, Hines Medical Building, Suite C, 13300 New Halls Ferry Road, Florissant, MO 63033 · 314-830-1900

Fulton

Allen J. Daugird · 110 North Hospital Drive, Fulton, MO 65251 · 573-642-5911

Joplin

William D. Kessler, Jr. · Building B, Suite 204, 2700 McClelland Boulevard, Joplin, MO 64804 · 417-782-6767

Timothy O'Keefe · Building B, Suite 204, 2700 McClelland Boulevard, Joplin, MO 64804 · 417-782-6767

Springfield

James Blaine · (Control of Drunk Driving, Child Advocacy, Tobacco Control Concerning Children) · Springfield Clinic, 3231 South National Avenue, Springfield, MO 65807-7396 · 417-883-7422

Richard T. Honderick · Springfield Clinic, 3231 South National Avenue, Springfield, MO 65807 · 417-885-0834

Mark A. Newport · Springfield Clinic, 3231 South National Avenue, Springfield, MO 65807 · 417-883-7422

W. Timothy Wilson · Springfield Family Medicine, 1965 South Fremont Street, Suite 1900, Springfield, MO 65804 · 417-883-0023

St. Louis

Thomas A. Johnson, Jr. · (Clinical Preventive Medicine, General Family Medicine) · St. John's Mercy Medical Center · St. John's Family Medicine, 615 South New Ballas Road, St. Louis, MO 63141 · 314-569-6010

Trenton

David L. Ryan · 903 Custer Street, Trenton, MO 64683 · 816-359-4317

GASTROENTEROLOGY

Cape Girardeau

Dean A. Edwards · General Gastroenterology · St. Francis Medical Center, Southeast Missouri Hospital · Gastroenterology Associates of Southeast Missouri, 21 Doctors Park, Cape Girardeau, MO 63703 · 573-334-8870

Columbia

Donald C. Gerhardt · General Gastroenterology (Esophageal Motility) · Boone Hospital Center, Columbia Regional Hospital · Boone Clinic, Department of Gastroenterology, 401 Keene Street, Columbia, MO 65201 · 573-874-3300

Paul D. King · Hepatology · University Hospital & Children's Hospital, One Hospital Drive, Columbia, MO 65212 · 573-882-1013

John B. Marshall · General Gastroenterology (Endoscopy, Esophageal Disease) · University Hospital & Children's Hospital, Harry S. Truman Memorial Veterans Hospital · University Hospital & Children's Hospital, Division of Gastroenterology, Medical Science Building, Room MA421, One Hospital Drive, Columbia, MO 65212 · 573-882-1013

Joplin

Phil W. Harrison · General Gastroenterology · 1001 McIntosh Road, Joplin, MO 64804 · 417-623-5250

Kansas City

Mark J. Allen · General Gastroenterology · Saint Luke's Hospital of Kansas City Mid-America Gastrointestinal Consultants, 4321 Washington Avenue, Suite 5600, Kansas City, MO 64111-5905 · 816-561-2000

John H. Helzberg · General Gastroenterology (Endoscopy, Hepatology) · Mid-America Gastrointestinal Consultants, 4321 Washington Avenue, Suite 5600, Kansas City, MO 64111-5905 · 816-561-2000

Mark S. McPhee · General Gastroenterology · Saint Luke's Hospital of Kansas City · Mid-America Gastrointestinal Consultants, 4321 Washington Avenue, Suite 5600, Kansas City, MO 64111-5905 · 816-561-2000

Springfield

Robert E. Kipfer · General Gastroenterology · Cox Medical Centers-South · Ferrell-Duncan Clinic, 1001 East Primrose Street, P.O. Box 9007, Springfield, MO 65808-9007 · 417-885-7250

St. Louis

Giuseppe Aliperti · Endoscopy (Pancreatic Disease, General Gastroenterology) · Barnes-Jewish Hospital · Barnes-Jewish Hospital, Division of Gastroenterology, One Barnes Hospital Plaza, St. Louis, MO 63110 · 314-362-5678

David H. Alpers · General Gastroenterology (Nutrition, Functional Bowel Disease, Inflammatory Bowel Disease, Peptic Disorders) · Barnes-Jewish Hospital · Washington University School of Medicine, Division of Gastroenterology, 660 South Euclid Avenue, Campus Box 8124, St. Louis, MO 63110 · 314-362-8940

Bruce R. Bacon · Hepatology (Hepatitis, Hepatic Iron Metabolism) · St. Louis University Hospital · St. Louis University, Health Sciences Center, 3635 Vista Avenue at Grand Boulevard, St. Louis, MO 63110 · 314-577-8764

Ray E. Clouse · General Gastroenterology, Esophageal Disease · Barnes-Jewish Hospital · Washington University School of Medicine, Division of Gastroenterology, One Barnes Hospital Plaza, St. Louis, MO 63110 · 314-362-5035

Adrian M. DiBisceglie · (Hepatology) · St. Louis University Hospital · St. Louis University Health Sciences Center, Internal Medicine Administration, 1402 South Grand Boulevard, St. Louis, MO 63104 · 314-577-8762

Marion Peters · Hepatology · Barnes-Jewish Hospital · Washington University School of Medicine, 660 South Euclid Avenue, Campus Box 8124, St. Louis, MO 63110 · 314-747-1124

Burton A. Shotz · Endoscopy · 10287 Clayton Road, St. Louis, MO 63124 · 314-997-0554

Gary R. Zuckerman · Endoscopy · Barnes-Jewish Hospital · Barnes-Jewish Hospital, Gastroenterology Division, One Barnes Hospital Plaza, St. Louis, MO 63110 314-362-5674

GERIATRIC MEDICINE

Columbia

Thomas Edes · Harry S. Truman Memorial Veterans Hospital, Department of Medicine, 800 Hospital Drive, Columbia, MO 65201 · 573-443-2511

David R. Mehr · (Infections in Nursing Home Residents, Geriatric Assessment, Family Medicine) · University Hospital & Children's Hospital · University Hospital & Children's Hospital, Department of Family and Community Medicine, One Hospital Drive, Columbia, MO 65212 · 573-882-6676

Kansas City

Peter S. Holt · 4320 Wornall Road, Suite 208, Kansas City, MO 64114 · 816-531-0552

St. Louis

David W. Bentley · (Infectious Disease, Nursing Home-Acquired Infections) · VA Medical Center, St. Louis University Hospital · VA Medical Center, Jefferson Barracks Division, GRECC, Suite 11G/JB, One Jefferson Barracks Drive, St. Louis, MO 63125 · 314-894-6510

Fran E. Kaiser · (Erectile Dysfunction [Impotence], Menopause, Women's Health, General Geriatrics, Diabetes) · St. Louis University Hospital · St. Louis University Hospital, Division of Geriatric Medicine, 1402 South Grand Boulevard, Room M238, St. Louis, MO 63104 · 314-577-8462

Douglas K. Miller · St. Louis University Health Sciences Center, Department of Internal Medicine, Division of Geriatric Medicine, 1402 South Grand Boulevard, Room M238, St. Louis, MO 63104 · 314-577-6055

John E. Morley · (Diabetes, General Geriatric Medicine) · St. Louis University Hospital · St. Louis University Hospital, Department of Geriatrics, 1402 South Grand Boulevard, Room M238, St. Louis, MO 63114 · 314-577-8462

HAND SURGERY

Cape Girardeau

Ricky Lents · General Hand Surgery · Orthopaedic Associates, 48 Doctors Park, Cape Girardeau, MO 63703 · 573-335-8257

Columbia

Gregory H. Croll · General Hand Surgery · University Hospital & Children's Hospital, Division of Plastic Surgery, One Hospital Drive, Columbia, MO 65212 573-882-2275

James F. Eckenrode · General Hand Surgery · Boone Hospital Center, Columbia Regional Hospital · Columbia Orthopaedic Group, 400 Keene Street, P.O. Box 0, Columbia, MO 65205 · 573-443-2402

Barry J. Gainor · General Hand Surgery (Peripheral Nerve Surgery, Reconstructive Surgery) · University Hospital & Children's Hospital · University Hospital & Children's Hospital, Orthopaedic Surgery Office M562, One Hospital Drive, Columbia, MO 65212 · 573-882-3105

C. Linwood Puckett · General Hand Surgery · University Hospital & Children's Hospital · University Hospital & Children's Hospital, Division of Plastic Surgery, One Hospital Drive, Room M349, Columbia, MO 65212 · 573-882-2275

Joplin

John M. Veitch · General Hand Surgery (General Orthopaedic Surgery) · St. John's Regional Medical Center, Mount Carmel Medical Center (Pittsburg, KS) · Midwest Orthopaedic Surgery, 3126 Jackson Street, Suite 201, P.O. Box 2507, Joplin, MO 64803 · 417-781-2807

St. Louis

Paul R. Manske · Reconstructive Surgery (General Hand Surgery, Tendons, Congenital, Nerve Surgery [Nerve Compression], Wrist Problems) · Barnes-Jewish Hospital, St. Louis Children's Hospital · Barnes-Jewish Hospital, Department of Orthopaedics, One Barnes Hospital Plaza, Suite 11300, St. Louis, MO 63110 · 314-747-2510

INFECTIOUS DISEASE

Chesterfield

Leon R. Robison · General Infectious Disease (HIV/AIDS, Osteomyelitis) · St. Luke's Hospital · St. Luke's Hospital, Department of Internal Medicine, North Medical Building, Suite 750, 222 South Woodsmill Road, Chesterfield, MO 63017-3405 · 314-275-8600

Columbia

Gordon D. Christensen · General Infectious Disease · University Hospital & Children's Hospital, Division of Infectious Diseases, One Hospital Drive, Columbia, MO 65212 · 573-882-3107

E. Dale Everett · General Infectious Disease · University Hospital & Children's Hospital, Division of Infectious Diseases, One Hospital Drive, Columbia, MO 65212 · 573-882-3107

William Salzer · General Infectious Disease (AIDS, Infection in the Immuno-compromised) · University & Children's Hospitals & Clinics, Ellis Fischel Cancer Center of University of Missouri, Harry S. Truman Memorial Veterans Hospital · University Hospital & Children's Hospital, Department of Infectious Disease, One Hospital Drive, Columbia, MO 65212 · 573-882-3107

Joplin

Eden M. Esguerra · General Infectious Disease (Adults, Hospital-Acquired Infections, Bone & Joint Infections) · St. John's Regional Medical Center, Freeman Hospital · 2817 McClelland Boulevard, Suite 121, Joplin, MO 64804 · 417-781-8688

Kansas City

Michael R. Driks · General Infectious Disease · Baptist Medical Center · Baptist Medical Center, Infectious Disease Clinic, 6601 Rockhill Road, Kansas City, MO 64131 · 816-276-7820

David S. McKinsey · General Infectious Disease (Antifungal Therapy, Endocarditis, AIDS) · Research Medical Center · Infectious Disease Associates of Kansas City, 2361 East Meyer Boulevard, Kansas City, MO 64132 · 816-276-4038

David L. Smith · General Infectious Disease (HIV, Pneumonia) · Research Medical Center · Research Medical Center, 2316 East Meyer Boulevard, Kansas City, MO 64132 · 816-276-3979

Springfield

Wolfe B. Gerecht · General Infectious Disease · Cox Medical Centers-South, St. John's Regional Health Center · Ferrell-Duncan Clinic, 1001 East Primrose Street, P.O. Box 9007, Springfield, MO 65808-9007 · 417-885-7300

Alastair Haddow · General Infectious Disease · Internal Medicine Group, 1900 South National Avenue, Suite 2200, Springfield, MO 65804 · 417-887-4000

St. Louis

J. William Campbell · General Infectious Disease (AIDS, Bone Infections) · Barnes-Jewish Hospital · Grant Medical Clinic, 114 North Taylor Avenue, St. Louis, MO 63108-2199 · 314-534-8600

Gerald Medoff · AIDS, Fungal Infections · Barnes-Jewish Hospital · Washington University Medical Center, Infectious Diseases Division, 660 South Euclid Avenue, Campus Box 8051, St. Louis, MO 63110 · 314-362-4413

William G. Powderly · AIDS (Fungal Infections) · Barnes-Jewish Hospital · Washington University School of Medicine, 4511 Forest Park Parkway, Suite 304, St. Louis, MO 63108 · 314-454-0058

Gregory A. Storch · AIDS (Virology) · St. Louis Children's Hospital, Barnes-Jewish Hospital · St. Louis Children's Hospital, One Children's Place, Room 2N68, St. Louis, MO 63110-1013 · 314-454-6079

INTERNAL MEDICINE (GENERAL)

Clayton

Paul G. Schneider · St. Mary's Health Center (St. Louis), Missouri Baptist Medical Center (St. Louis) · Mid-County Internal Medicine, Bellevue West Medical Building, Suite 350, 1031 Bellevue Avenue, Clayton, MO 63117 · 314-781-8662

Columbia

Richard Burns · (Geriatric Medicine, Hypertension) · University Hospital & Children's Hospital · University of Missouri, Columbia School of Medicine, Department of Internal Medicine, 3113 South Providence Road, Columbia, MO 65203 · 573-882-4464

Donald M. Delwood · (Emergency Medicine, Critical Care Medicine) · Boone Hospital Center, Columbia Regional Hospital · 500 Keene Street, Suite 305, Columbia, MO 65201 · 573-874-3300

R. Dennis Marienfeld · Harry S. Truman Memorial Veterans Hospital · Harry S. Truman Memorial Veterans Hospital, Ambulatory Care, 800 Hospital Drive, Columbia, MO 65201-5297 · 573-882-4141

Lyndell D. Scoles · Boone Hospital Center · Boone Clinic, 401 Keene Street, Columbia, MO 65201 · 573-874-3300

R. Wade Shondelmeyer · Boone Hospital Center · Boone Clinic, 401 Keene Street, Columbia, MO 65201 · 573-874-3300

Jan Swaney · (Geriatric Medicine, General Internal Medicine) · University Hospital & Children's Hospital · Internal Medicine Green Meadows, 3213 South Providence Road, Columbia, MO 65203 · 573-882-4464

Paul K. Tichenor · University of Missouri, Columbia, School of Medicine, Department of Internal Medicine, 3113 South Providence Road, Columbia, MO 65203 · 573-882-4464

Joplin

Dennis W. Smith · (Preventive Medicine, Echocardiography, Exercise Physiology, General Internal Medicine) · St. John's Regional Medical Center, Freeman Hospital · 2817 McClelland Boulevard, Suite 155, Joplin, MO 64804 · 417-623-5610

Kansas City

James I. Mertz · 4320 Wornall Road, Suite 208, Kansas City, MO 64111 · 816-531-0552

Carnie Nulton · Kansas City Internal Medicine, 6420 Prospect Avenue, Suite T-101, Kansas City, MO 64132 · 816-363-4100

J. Chris Perryman · Saint Luke's Hospital of Kansas City · St. Luke's Internal Medicine Clinic, 4321 Washington Road, Suite 3000, Kansas City, MO 64111 · 816-932-3100

Overland County

Robert Karsh · Overland Medical Center, 2428 Woodson Road, Overland County, MO 63114 · 314-427-2424

Springfield

Richard D. Cunningham · 1900 South National Avenue, Suite 3200, Springfield, MO 65804 · 417-888-7701

Norman P. Knowlton III · Springfield Clinic, 1965 South Fremont Street, Suite 3500, Springfield, MO 65804-2243 · 417-888-7730

Steven M. Leitch · St. John's Regional Health Center · Springfield Clinic, Department of Internal Medicine, 3231 South National Avenue, Springfield, MO 65807 · 417-888-5668

Dominick M. Meldi · Springfield Clinic, Department of Internal Medicine, 3231 South National Avenue, Springfield, MO 65807 · 417-882-9785

Theresa A. Olsen · Springfield Clinic, Department of Internal Medicine, 3231 South National Avenue, Springfield, MO 65807 · 417-883-7422

James T. Rogers · Internal Medicine Associates, 1900 South National Avenue, Suite 3400, Springfield, MO 65804-2240 · 417-887-7002

Melvin O. Walker, Jr. · (Panic Disorders) · St. John's Regional Health Center · Internal Medicine Group, 1900 South National Avenue, Suite 2200, Springfield, MO 65804 · 417-887-4000

St. Louis

Benjamin Borowsky · (Endocrinology & Metabolism, Diabetes, Thyroid) · Barnes-Jewish Hospital · Central Medical Group, 4932 Forest Park Boulevard, St. Louis, MO 63108 · 314-367-2757

J. William Campbell · Grant Medical Clinic, 114 North Taylor Avenue, St. Louis, MO 63108 · 314-534-8600

John S. Daniels · (Diabetes) · Barnes-Jewish Hospital, Department of Medicine, One Barnes Hospital Plaza, Suite 17416, St. Louis, MO 63110 · 314-362-5100

Lewis C. Fischbein · (Rheumatology, General Internal Medicine) · Barnes-Jewish Hospital · University Medical Consultants, East Pavilion Building, Suite 16422, One Barnes Hospital Plaza, St. Louis, MO 63110 · 314-367-9595

John M. Grant · Grant Medical Clinic, 114 North Taylor Avenue, St. Louis, MO 63108-2102 · 314-534-8600

Neville Grant · (Endocrinology & Metabolism) · Barnes-Jewish Hospital, St. Luke's Hospital (Chesterfield) · Grant Medical Clinic, 114 North Taylor Avenue, St. Louis, MO 63108-2102 · 314-534-8600

Robert M. Heaney · (Preventive Medicine, Cancer Screening, Osteoporosis) · St. Louis University Hospital · St. Louis University Hospital, Division of General Internal Medicine, 1402 South Grand Boulevard, St. Louis, MO 63104 · 314-577-6143

Micki Klearman · (Rheumatology) · Barnes-Jewish Hospital · University Medical Consultants, East Pavilion Building, Suite 16422, One Barnes Hospital Plaza, St. Louis, MO 63110 · 314-367-9595

Deborah L. Parks · (General Internal Medicine, General Rheumatology, Rheumatoid Arthritis, Lupus, Auto-Immune Disease, Women's Health) · Barnes-Jewish Hospital · Maryland Medical Group, 4652 Maryland Avenue, St. Louis, MO 63108-1913 · 314-367-3113

Marybeth Pereira · (General Internal Medicine, Rheumatology) · Barnes-Jewish Hospital · University Medical Consultants, East Pavilion Building, Suite 16422, One Barnes Hospital Plaza, St. Louis, MO 63131-1436 · 314-367-9595

Robert J. Saltman · (Endocrinology, Diabetes, General Internal Medicine) · Barnes-Jewish Hospital, Barnes West County Hospital (Creve Coeur) · Barnes West Medical Consultants, 1040 North Mason Road, Suite 123, St. Louis, MO 63141-6361 · 314-576-6633

Robert J. Schneider · Associated Internists, 675 Old Ballas Road, Suite 103, St. Louis, MO 63141-7011 · 314-567-1902

Bernard L. Shore · (General Internal Medicine, Pulmonary Diseases) · Barnes-Jewish Hospital · Maryland Medical Group, 4652 Maryland Avenue, St. Louis, MO 63108 · 314-367-3113

Donald A. Skor · (Diabetes, Lipids) · Barnes-Jewish Hospital · Barnes-Jewish Hospital, One Barnes Hospital Plaza, Suite 17416, St. Louis, MO 63110-1013 · 314-362-5100

H. Douglas Walden · (General Internal Medicine, Consultative Medicine) · St. Louis University Hospital, St. Mary's Health Center · St. Louis University Doctors Office Building, 3660 Vista Avenue, St. Louis, MO 63110 · 314-577-6100

MEDICAL ONCOLOGY & HEMATOLOGY

Cape Girardeau

Stanley D. Sides · General Medical Oncology & Hematology (Disorders of Bleeding, Thrombosis) · St. Francis Medical Center, Southeast Missouri Hospital · Cape Girardeau Physician Associates, 14 Doctors Park, Cape Girardeau, MO 63703-4993 · 573-334-9641

Benjamin H. Yuen · General Medical Oncology & Hematology (General Internal Medicine) · Southeast Missouri Hospital, St. Francis Medical Center · Cape Girardeau Physician Associates, 14 Doctors Park, Cape Girardeau, MO 63703-4993 573-334-9641

Columbia

Donald Doll · General Medical Oncology & Hematology (AIDS, Myelodys Plastic Syndromes) · University Hospital & Children's Hospital, Harry S. Truman Memorial Veterans Hospital · University Hospital & Children's Hospital, Department of Medical Oncology & Hematology, One Hospital Drive, Columbia, MO 65212 573-882-6964

Joseph J. Muscato · General Medical Oncology & Hematology (Breast Cancer, Neuro-Oncology) · Boone Hospital Center, Columbia Regional Hospital · Hematology-Oncology Associates, 105 Keene Street, Columbia, MO 65201 · 573-874-7800

Michael C. Perry · Breast Cancer (Lung Cancer, Cancer Chemotherapy, General Medical Oncology & Hematology, Pain Management) · Ellis Fischel Cancer Center of University of Missouri · University of Missouri-Ellis Fischel Cancer Center, 115 Business Loop 70 West, Room 116.71, Columbia, MO 65203 · 573-882-4979

Joplin

Mark J. Skelley · General Medical Oncology & Hematology · Oncology and Hematology Center, 2727 McClelland Boulevard, P.O. Box 2786, Joplin, MO 64803 · 417-782-7722

Kansas City

Verda Hunter · Gynecologic Cancer (Surgery and Chemotherapy Treatment, Disorders of the Vulva, Reconstructive Pelvic Surgery, General Obstetrics & Gynecology) · Research Medical Center, Baptist Medical Center, Saint Joseph Health Center, Menorah Medical Center · Oncology Hematology Associates, Plaza Medical Building, Suite 103, 1000 East 50th Street, Kansas City, MO 64110 816-276-8968

Richard J. Mundis · General Medical Oncology & Hematology · 1010 Carondelet Drive, Suite 401, Kansas City, MO 64114 · 816-941-2992

Jesse A. Roberts · General Medical Oncology & Hematology · Saint Luke's Hospital of Kansas City, North Kansas City Hospital (North Kansas City), Liberty Hospital (Liberty) · Heartland Hematology-Oncology Associates, 2001 Northeast Parvin Road, Kansas City, MO 64116 · 816-455-8136

Frank T. Slovick · General Medical Oncology & Hematology · Heartland Hematology-Oncology Associates, 2001 Northeast Parvin Road, Kansas City, MO 64116 816-454-1659

St. Charles

Daniel W. Luedke · General Medical Oncology & Hematology · Missouri Cancer Care, 330 First Capital Drive, St. Charles, MO 63301 · 314-947-4007

St. Louis

Matthew A. Arquette · General Medical Oncology & Hematology · Barnard Cancer Center, 4960 Children's Place, Campus Box 8056, St. Louis, MO 63110 · 314-362-4843

Nancy L. Bartlett · Lymphomas · Barnard Cancer Center, 4960 Children's Place, Campus Box 8056, St. Louis, MO 63110 · 314-362-4843

Morey Blinder · General Medical Oncology & Hematology (Disorders of Bleeding, Thrombosis, Blood Banking/Transfusion Medicine) · Barnes-Jewish Hospital Barnard Cancer Center, 660 South Euclid Avenue, St. Louis, MO 63110 · 314-362-8857

Michael Bolger · General Medical Oncology & Hematology (Breast Cancer, Leukemia, Disorders of Bleeding, Thrombosis) · Missouri Baptist Medical Center, St. Luke's Hospital (Chesterfield) · The Cancer Center, 3015 North Ballas Road, St. Louis, MO 63131 · 314-569-5151

Goronwy O. Broun, Jr. · Gynecologic Cancer · St. Louis University Hospital · St. Louis University Health Sciences Center, FDT Building, Eighth Floor, 3635 Vista Avenue at Grand Boulevard, St. Louis, MO 63110 · 314-577-8854

George J. Broze, Jr. · Disorders of Bleeding, Thrombosis · Barnes-Jewish Hospital · Barnes-Jewish Hospital, Division of Hematology, 216 South Kingshighway Boulevard, St. Louis, MO 63110 · 314-362-8811

Paula M. Fracasso · General Medical Oncology & Hematology (Breast Cancer, Gynecologic Cancer) · Barnes-Jewish Hospital · Washington University School of Medicine, 660 South Euclid Avenue, Campus Box 8056, St. Louis, MO 63110 · 314-362-7229

Daniel C. Ihde · Lung Cancer (Neuro-Oncology, Endocrine Cancer) · Barnes-Jewish Hospital · Wohl Hospital, 4960 Children's Place, Room 103, St. Louis, MO 63110 · 314-362-4819

Alan P. Lyss · Breast Cancer (Lung Cancer, Colorectal Cancer, Gastrointestinal Cancer) · Missouri Baptist Medical Center, Barnes-Jewish Hospital, St. Luke's Hospital (Chesterfield) · Missouri Baptist Cancer Center, 3015 North New Ballas Road, St. Louis, MO 63131-2374 · 314-569-5151

Joanne E. Mortimer · Breast Cancer (Medical Oncology only) · Barnard Cancer Center · Barnard Cancer Center, 660 South Euclid Avenue, Campus Box 8056, St. Louis, MO 63110 · 314-362-7597

Joel Picus · Genito-Urinary Cancer (Gastrointestinal Cancer, General Medical Oncology & Hematology) · Barnes-Jewish Hospital, St. Louis Children's Hospital Washington University School of Medicine, Barnard Cancer Center, 660 South Euclid Avenue, Campus Box 8056, St. Louis, MO 63110 · 314-362-7229

NEPHROLOGY

Cape Girardeau

Frank W. Braxton · General Nephrology (Dialysis [Acute & Chronic], Kidney Disease) · Southeast Missouri Hospital, St. Francis Medical Center · 1349 Mount Auburn Road, Cape Girardeau, MO 63701 · 573-334-9564

Chesterfield

Thomas Pohlman · General Nephrology · St. Luke's Hospital, Department of Nephrology, 222 South Woodsmill Road, Room 750 North, Chesterfield, MO 63017 · 314-275-8600

Columbia

John H. Bauer · Hypertension (Diabetic Renal Disease, Hypertensive Renal Disease) · University Hospital & Children's Hospital, Harry S. Truman Memorial Veterans Hospital · University Hospital & Children's Hospital, Department of Medicine, Health Science Center, Room N425, One Hospital Drive, Columbia, MO 65212 · 573-882-4894

Ramesh Khanna · General Nephrology, Dialysis, Kidney Disease (Diabetes) · University & Children's Hospitals & Clinics, Ellis Fischel Cancer Center of University of Missouri · University Hospital & Children's Hospital, Health Sciences Center, Room MA436, One Hospital Drive, Columbia, MO 65212 · 573-882-7991

Karl D. Nolph · Dialysis, Kidney Disease (Peritoneal Dialysis, Diabetic Kidney Disease) · University Hospital & Children's Hospital · University Hospital & Children's Hospital, Health Sciences Center, Room MA436, One Hospital Drive, Columbia, MO 65212 · 573-882-7991

Zbylut J. Twardowski · Dialysis, Kidney Disease (Kidney Transplantation) · University Hospital & Children's Hospital · University Hospital & Children's Hospital, Health Sciences Center, Room MA436, One Hospital Drive, Columbia, MO 65212 · 573-882-7991

John C. Van Stone · Dialysis · University Hospital & Children's Hospital · Medical Specialist Clinic, Dialysis Clinic, 3300 Lamone Industrial Boulevard, Columbia, MO 65201 · 573-882-8788

Joplin

R. Robert Hatlelid · General Nephrology (Dialysis, Kidney Transplantation) · St. John's Regional Medical Center · Joplin Nephrology Associates, 1800 West 30th Street, Joplin, MO 64804-1520 · 417-782-5000

Kansas City

James I. Mertz · General Nephrology · 4320 Wornall Road, Suite 208, Kansas City, MO 64111 · 816-531-0552

St. Louis

Daniel C. Brennan · Kidney Transplantation · Barnes-Jewish Hospital, Queeny Tower, Suite 6107, One Barnes Hospital Plaza, St. Louis, MO 63110 · 314-362-8351

James A. Delmez · Kidney Disease · Chromalloy American Kidney Center, One Barnes Hospital Plaza, Box 8129, St. Louis, MO 63110 · 314-362-7205

Stephen L. Gluck · General Nephrology (Acid-Base Disorders, Renal Tubular Acidosis) · Barnes-Jewish Hospital · Washington University School of Medicine, Renal Division, 660 South Euclid Avenue, Campus Box 8126, St. Louis, MO 63110 · 314-362-8232

Keith A. Hruska · General Nephrology · Barnes-Jewish Hospital, Renal Division, 216 South Kingshighway Boulevard, St. Louis, MO 63110 · 314-454-7970

Saulo Klahr · General Nephrology · Barnes-Jewish Hospital · Washington University School of Medicine, Jewish Hospital of St. Louis, 216 South Kingshighway Boulevard, St. Louis, MO 63110 · 314-454-7107

Kevin J. Martin · General Nephrology (Hypertension, Bone Disease) · St. Louis University Hospital · St. Louis University Hospital, Department of Nephrology, 3635 Vista Avenue at Grand Boulevard, Ninth Floor, St. Louis, MO 63110 · 314-577-8765

Aubrey R. Morrison · Kidney Disease (General Nephrology) · Barnes-Jewish Hospital · Washington University School of Medicine, Renal Division, 660 South Euclid Avenue, Campus Box 8103, St. Louis, MO 63110 · 314-362-2597

Eduardo Slatopolsky · Kidney Disease · Chromalloy American Kidney Center, One Barnes Hospital Plaza, Box 8129, St. Louis, MO 63110 · 314-362-7205

NEUROLOGICAL SURGERY

Cape Girardeau

David G. Yingling · General Neurological Surgery · Cape Neurosurgical Associates, 3129 Blattner Drive, Cape Girardeau, MO 63703 · 573-339-0900

Columbia

Edward V. Colapinto · Tumor Surgery (Stereotactic Radiosurgery) · University & Children's Hospitals & Clinics, Ellis Fischel Cancer Center of University of Missouri · University of Missouri School of Medicine, Division of Neurosurgery, One Hospital Drive, Room N521, Columbia, MO 65212 · 573-882-4908

David F. Jimenez · Pediatric Neurological Surgery · University Hospital & Children's Hospital, Division of Neurosurgery, One Hospital Drive, Columbia, MO 65212 · 573-882-4908

John J. Oró · General Neurological Surgery (Skull-Base Surgery, Spinal Surgery, Vascular Neurological Surgery) · University Hospital & Children's Hospital, Harry S. Truman Memorial Veterans Hospital · University of Missouri, Columbia, School of Medicine, Health Science Center, Room N521, One Hospital Drive, Columbia, MO 65212 · 573-882-4908

Joplin

Hish S. Majzoub · General Neurological Surgery · Joplin Neurosurgical Associates, 2902 B McClelland Boulevard, Suite Seven, Joplin, MO 64804 · 417-781-4733

Kansas City

Robert A. Morantz · Tumor Surgery (Brain Tumors, Gamma Knife Radiosurgery, General Neurological Surgery) · Research Medical Center, Baptist Medical Center, Saint Joseph Health Center · Midwest Neurosurgery, 6420 Prospect Avenue, Suite T-411, Kansas City, MO 64132 · 816-363-2500

St. Louis

Ralph G. Dacey, Jr. · General Neurological Surgery, Tumor Surgery, Vascular Neurological Surgery · Barnes-Jewish Hospital · Barnes-Jewish Hospital, 660 South Euclid Avenue, Campus Box 8057, St. Louis, MO 63110 · 314-362-3571

Robert L. Grubb, Jr. · General Neurological Surgery (Vascular Neurological Surgery, Skull-Base Surgery) · Barnes-Jewish Hospital, St. Louis Children's Hospital Washington University School of Medicine, 660 South Euclid Avenue, Campus Box 8057, St. Louis, MO 63110 · 314-362-3567

T. S. Park · Pediatric Neurological Surgery (Epilepsy Surgery, Cerebral Palsy) · St. Louis Children's Hospital · St. Louis Children's Hospital, Department of Neurosurgery, One Children's Place, St. Louis, MO 63110 · 314-454-2811

NEUROLOGY

Cape Girardeau

Abdul B. Chaudhari · General Neurology · Neurology Clinic, 66 Doctors Park, Cape Girardeau, MO 63703 · 573-334-7175

David Lee · General Neurology · Neurological Associates, 3004 Gordhamville Road, Cape Girardeau, MO 63701 · 573-651-3188

Columbia

Steven H. Horowitz · Electromyography, Neuromuscular Disease · University Hospital & Children's Hospital, Department of Neurology, One Hospital Drive, Box M-741, Columbia, MO 65212 · 573-882-3134

Joplin

Christopher R. Andrew · General Neurology (Electromyography) · Freeman Hospital · 1020 McIntosh Circle, Suite 201, Joplin, MO 64804 · 417-623-3330

Springfield

Michael H. Luzecky · General Neurology · St. John's Regional Health Center · Springfield Clinic/Neurological Associates of the Ozarks, 1965 South Fremont Street, Suite 2800, Springfield, MO 65804 · 417-881-5590

Rodney D. Quinn · General Neurology (Clinical Neurophysiology) · Cox Medical Centers-North, Cox Medical Centers-South · Ferrell-Duncan Clinic, 1001 East Primrose Street, P.O. Box 9007, Springfield, MO 65808-9007 · 417-885-7360

George F. Wong III · General Neurology (Movement Disorders, Epilepsy) · Ferrell-Duncan Clinic, 1001 East Primrose Street, P.O. Box 9007, Springfield, MO 65808-9007 · 417-885-7360

St. Louis

David B. Clifford · Infectious & Demyelinating Diseases (AIDS, Epilepsy, Neuropharmacology, General Neurology) · Washington University School of Medicine, Department of Neurology, 660 South Euclid Avenue, Campus Box 8111, St. Louis, MO 63110 · 314-362-3296

Anne H. Cross · Infectious & Demyelinating Diseases · Barnes-Jewish Hospital Washington University School of Medicine, Department of Neurology, 660 South Euclid Avenue, Campus Box 8111, St. Louis, MO 63110 · 314-362-3293

J. Michael Hatlelid · General Neurology (Epilepsy, Movement Disorders) · St. Mary's Health Center, Barnes-Jewish Hospital, St. Luke's Hospital (Chesterfield), Deaconess Medical Center-Central Campus · Neurology Associates, 1034 South Brentwood Boulevard, Suite 854, St. Louis, MO 63117 · 314-725-2010

William R. Logan · General Neurology · St. John's Mercy Medical Center · St. John's Mercy Medical Center, 621 South New Ballas Road, Suite 5003, St. Louis, MO 63141 · 314-569-6507

Joel S. Perlmutter · Movement Disorders · Barnes-Jewish Hospital · Washington University School of Medicine, Department of Neurology, 4525 Scott Avenue, Campus Box 8225, St. Louis, MO 63110 · 314-362-6908

Alan Pestronk · Neuromuscular Disease · Barnes-Jewish Hospital, St. Louis Children's Hospital · Washington University School of Medicine, 660 South Euclid Avenue, Campus Box 8111, St. Louis, MO 63110 · 314-362-6981

William J. Powers · Strokes (Cerebral Vascular Disease) · Barnes-Jewish Hospital Washington University School of Medicine, East Building, 4525 Scott Avenue, St. Louis, MO 63110 · 314-362-7116

John B. Selhorst · Neuro-Ophthalmology (General Adult Neurology) · St. Louis University Hospital · St. Louis University School of Medicine, 3660 Vista Avenue at Grand Boulevard, St. Louis, MO 63110-0250 · 314-577-8026

John L. Trotter · Infectious & Demyelinating Diseases (Demyelinating Diseases only, Multiple Sclerosis) · Barnes-Jewish Hospital, St. Louis Children's Hospital Washington University School of Medicine, 660 South Euclid Avenue, Campus Box 8111, St. Louis, MO 63110 · 314-362-3293

NEUROLOGY, CHILD

Springfield

Eugene Tenorio · General Child Neurology (Epilepsy, Attention Deficit Disorder) · Cox Medical Centers-South, St. John's Regional Health Center · Pediatric Neurology of the Ozarks, 1000 East Primrose Street, Suite 440, Springfield, MO 65807 · 417-269-1010

St. Louis

Denis I. Altman · General Child Neurology · St. Louis Child Neurology Services, Tower B, Suite 5009, 621 South New Ballas Road, St. Louis, MO 63141 · 314-569-6515

Blaise F. D. Bourgeois · Epilepsy · St. Louis Children's Hospital · St. Louis Children's Hospital, Department of Pediatric Neurology, One Children's Place, St. Louis, MO 63110 · 314-454-6120

Philip R. Dodge · General Child Neurology · St. Louis Children's Hospital · St. Louis Children's Hospital, Department of Pediatric Neurology, One Children's Place, Room 12E25, St. Louis, MO 63110 · 314-454-2699

W. Edwin Dodson · Epilepsy (Anti-Epileptic Drug Therapy, General Child Neurology) · Barnes-Jewish Hospital, St. Louis Children's Hospital · St. Louis Children's Hospital, Department of Neurology, One Children's Place, Room 12E25, St. Louis, MO 63110 · 314-454-6120

Suresh Kotagal · General Child Neurology (Pediatric Sleep Disorders) · Cardinal Glennon Children's Hospital, St. Louis University Hospital · Cardinal Glennon Children's Hospital, Department of Neurology, 1465 South Grand Boulevard, St. Louis, MO 63104 · 314-577-5338

John F. Mantovani · General Child Neurology (Child Development) · St. John's Mercy Medical Center, St. Louis Children's Hospital, Cardinal Glennon Children's Hospital · St. Louis Child Neurology Services, Tower B, Suite 5009, 621 South New Ballas Road, St. Louis, MO 63141 · 314-569-6515

Michael J. Noetzel · General Child Neurology (Cerebral Palsy, Pediatric Neurorehabilitation) · St. Louis Children's Hospital, Barnes-Jewish Hospital · St. Louis Children's Hospital, Department of Pediatric Neurology, One Children's Place, Room 12E25, St. Louis, MO 63110 · 314-454-6120

Arthur L. Prensky · General Child Neurology (Metabolic Diseases, Headache) · St. Louis Children's Hospital · St. Louis Children's Hospital, One Children's Place, Room 12E25, St. Louis, MO 63110 · 314-454-6085

NUCLEAR MEDICINE

Springfield

Edward W. Gotti · General Nuclear Medicine (Bone Density) · St. John's Regional Health Center, Department of Nuclear Medicine, 1235 East Cherokee Street, Springfield, MO 65804 · 417-885-2865

St. Louis

Farrokh Dehdashti · General Nuclear Medicine (Oncology, Breast, Prostate) · Barnes-Jewish Hospital, St. Louis Children's Hospital · Mallinckrodt Institute of Radiology at Washington University, Division of Nuclear Medicine, 510 South Kingshighway Boulevard, St. Louis, MO 63110-1076 · 314-362-7418

Keith Fischer · General Nuclear Medicine · Washington University School of Medicine, Department of Nuclear Medicine, 216 South Kingshighway Boulevard, St. Louis, MO 63110 · 314-454-7235

James W. Fletcher · General Nuclear Medicine (Health Care Policy & Research, Cost-Effectiveness & Diagnostic Imaging) · St. Louis University Hospital · St. Louis University School of Medicine, Department of Nuclear Medicine, 3635 Vista Avenue at Grand Boulevard, St. Louis, MO 63110 · 314-577-8047

Robert J. Gropler · General Nuclear Medicine (Nuclear Cardiology, Magnetic Resonance Imaging, General Cardiovascular Disease) · Barnes-Jewish Hospital, St. Louis Children's Hospital · Mallinckrodt Institute of Radiology at Washington University, Division of Nuclear Medicine, 510 South Kingshighway Boulevard, St. Louis, MO 63110-1076 · 314-362-7418

Val Lowe · General Nuclear Medicine (Positron Emission Tomography, Oncology) · St. Louis University Hospital, Department of Nuclear Medicine, 3635 Vista Avenue at Grand Boulevard, St. Louis, MO 63110 · 314-577-8048

Thomas R. Miller · General Nuclear Medicine · Barnes-Jewish Hospital · Mallinckrodt Institute of Radiology at Washington University, 510 South Kingshighway Boulevard, St. Louis, MO 63110 · 314-362-2807

Henry D. Royal · Radiation Accidents & Radiation Injury, General Nuclear Medicine · Mallinckrodt Institute of Radiology, Barnes-Jewish Hospital, St. Louis Children's Hospital · Mallinckrodt Institute of Radiology at Washington University, 510 South Kingshighway Boulevard, St. Louis, MO 63110-1076 · 314-362-2809

Barry A. Siegel · General Nuclear Medicine (Clinical Positron Emission Tomography [PET], Nuclear Radiology) · Barnes-Jewish Hospital, St. Louis Children's Hospital · Mallinckrodt Institute of Radiology at Washington University, 510 South Kingshighway Boulevard, St. Louis, MO 63110 · 314-362-2809

OBSTETRICS & GYNECOLOGY

Cape Girardeau

Scott G. Pringle · General Obstetrics & Gynecology · Cape OBGYN Associates, 55 Doctors Park, Cape Girardeau, MO 63703 · 573-334-5249

Jacob P. Pyeatte, Jr. · General Obstetrics & Gynecology · Cape OBGYN Associates, 55 Doctors Park, Cape Girardeau, MO 63703 · 573-334-5249

Chesterfield

Joseph E. Belew · General Obstetrics & Gynecology (Infertility) · St. Luke's Hospital, Missouri Baptist Medical Center (St. Louis), Barnes-Jewish Hospital (St. Louis) · Obstetrical Associates of St. Louis, 224 South Woodsmill Road, Suite 750, Chesterfield, MO 63017-3470 · 314-576-9797

William E. Houck · General Obstetrics & Gynecology · Barnes-Jewish Hospital (St. Louis), St. Luke's Hospital, Missouri Baptist Medical Center (St. Louis) · Obstetrical Associates of St. Louis, 224 South Woodsmill Road, Suite 750, Chesterfield, MO 63017 · 314-576-9797

Jorge A. Pineda · Reproductive Endocrinology (Assisted Reproductive Techniques Procedures, Endoscopy, Endometriosis, Uterine Anomalies) · St. Luke's Hospital · St. Luke's Hospital Advanced Reproductive Specialists, 226 South Woodsmill Road, Suite 64 West, Chesterfield, MO 63017 · 314-542-9422

Kevin Shaberg · General Obstetrics & Gynecology · 224 South Woodsmill Road, Suite 720 South, Chesterfield, MO 63017 · 314-576-6166

Columbia

John Cassels · General Obstetrics & Gynecology · GYN Fertility Clinic, 3211 South Providence Road, Columbia, MO 65203 · 573-882-7199

William T. Griffin · General Obstetrics & Gynecology (Reproductive Surgery) · University Hospital & Children's Hospital · Green Meadows Fertility Center, 3211 South Providence Road, Suite 301, Columbia, MO 65203 · 573-882-6600

Donald C. Patterson · Gynecologic Cancer (Gynecologic Surgery, Urogynecology) · Boone Hospital Center, Columbia Regional Hospital, University Hospital & Children's Hospital · 500 Keene Street, Suite 206, Columbia, MO 65201 · 573-442-2221

William D. Trumbower · General Obstetrics & Gynecology · Boone Hospital Center · Women's Health Associates, 601 East Broadway Street, Suite 100, Columbia, MO 66201 · 573-443-6401

Susan E. Winkelmann · General Obstetrics & Gynecology · University Hospital & Children's Hospital, Department of Obstetrics & Gynecology, One Hospital Drive, Columbia, MO 65212 · 573-882-7938

Joplin

T. Keith Grebe · General Obstetrics & Gynecology · Freeman Hospital · OB-GYN Associates of Joplin, 1221 McIntosh Circle, Joplin, MO 64804 · 417-624-1711

Howard H. Roberts · General Obstetrics & Gynecology (Gynecology only) · Building A, 3101 McClelland Boulevard, Joplin, MO 64804 · 417-624-1714

Herbert J. Schmidt · General Obstetrics & Gynecology (Gynecologic Cancer) · Building A, 3101 McClelland Boulevard, Joplin, MO 64804 · 417-624-1714

Kansas City

James A. Thorp · Maternal & Fetal Medicine · Saint Luke's Hospital of Kansas City · Saint Luke's Perinatal Center, Outpatient Center Two, 4400 Wornall Road, Kansas City, MO 64111 · 816-932-3585

John D. Yeast · Maternal & Fetal Medicine (General Obstetrics & Gynecology) Saint Luke's Hospital of Kansas City · Saint Luke's Hospital of Kansas City, Outpatient Center Two, 4400 Wornall Road, Kansas City, MO 64111 · 816-932-3585

James P. Youngblood · General Obstetrics & Gynecology · Truman Medical Center, Department of Obstetrics & Gynecology, 2301 Holmes Street, Kansas City, MO 64108 · 816-556-3454

Richmond Heights

Randall W. Tobler · General Obstetrics & Gynecology · Richmond Medical Center, 6744 Clayton Road, Suite 325, Richmond Heights, MO 63117 · 314-647-4334

Springfield

Leonard Bell · General Obstetrics & Gynecology · Women's Clinic, 1900 South National Avenue, Suite 1916, Springfield, MO 65804 · 417-887-5500

Alfred J. Bonebrake · General Obstetrics & Gynecology (Gynecology only) · Women's Clinic, 1900 South National Avenue, Suite 1960, Springfield, MO 65804

Kathleen L. Graves · General Obstetrics & Gynecology · Medical Plaza, 3850 South National Street, Suite 400, Springfield, MO 63017 · 417-269-6850

John W. Williams · General Obstetrics & Gynecology · Springfield OBGYN, 100 East Primrose Street, Suite 200, Springfield, MO 65807 · 417-887-0966

St. Louis

Scott W. Biest · General Obstetrics & Gynecology · Barnes-Jewish Hospital, Missouri Baptist Medical Center, St. Luke's Hospital (Chesterfield) · Consultants in Women's Health Care, 522 North New Ballas Road, Suite 350, St. Louis, MO 63141 · 314-432-8181

Bruce Bryan · General Obstetrics & Gynecology · Barnes-Jewish Hospital, St. Luke's Hospital (Chesterfield), Missouri Baptist Medical Center · OBGYN Associates, 1034 Brentwood Boulevard, St. Louis, MO 63110 · 314-725-9300

James P. Crane · Genetics (Ultrasound, General Obstetrics & Gynecology, Maternal & Fetal Medicine) · Barnes-Jewish Hospital · Washington School of Medicine, Department of Obstetrics & Gynecology, 660 South Euclid Avenue, St. Louis, MO 63110 · 314-362-6249

Cathleen Rae Faris · General Obstetrics & Gynecology · St. Mary's Health Center, Barnes-Jewish Hospital · West End Women's Health, 4949 West Pine Drive, Suite 2H, St. Louis, MO 63108 · 314-361-6339

Diana L. Gray · Genetics (Prenatal Diagnosis, Ob/Gyn Ultrasound) · Barnes-Jewish Hospital · Barnes-Jewish Hospital, 216 South Kingshighway Boulevard, St. Louis, MO 63110 · 314-454-8135

Mark J. Jostes · General Obstetrics & Gynecology · Barnes-Jewish Hospital, Missouri Baptist Medical Center, St. Luke's Hospital (Chesterfield) · 3009 North Ballas Road, Suite 366-C, St. Louis, MO 63131 · 314-569-2424

Ming-Shian Kao · (Gynecologic Surgery, Gynecologic Cancer) · St. Mary's Health Center, St. Louis University Hospital, Deaconess Medical Center-Central Campus · St. Louis University Health Sciences Center, Department of Obstetrics & Gynecology, 1031 Bellevue Avenue, Suite 400, St. Louis, MO 63117 · 314-781-7455

Rebecca P. McAllister · General Obstetrics & Gynecology (Female Urinary Incontinence, Pelvic Prolapse Menopause) · Barnes-Jewish Hospital · Barnes-Jewish Hospital, Department of Obstetrics & Gynecology, One Barnes Hospital Plaza, Suite 16306, St. Louis, MO 63110 · 314-362-4211

Diane F. Merritt · General Obstetrics & Gynecology (Gynecology only, Pediatric & Adolescent Gynecology, Menopause) · Barnes-Jewish Hospital, St. Louis Children's Hospital · Barnes-Jewish Hospital, Department of Reproductive Endocrinology, 4911 Barnes Hospital Plaza, St. Louis, MO 63110 · 314-362-8048

David G. Mutch · Gynecologic Cancer · Barnes-Jewish Hospital · Barnes-Jewish Hospital, Department of Gynecological Oncology, 4911 Barnes Hospital Plaza, St. Louis, MO 63110 · 314-362-7135

D. Michael Nelson · Maternal & Fetal Medicine · Barnes-Jewish Hospital · Washington University School of Medicine, Department of Obstetrics & Gynecology, 4911 Barnes Hospital Plaza, St. Louis, MO 63110 · 314-747-0739

Randall R. Odem · Reproductive Endocrinology (Reproductive Surgery, Assisted Reproductive Technologies) · Barnes-Jewish Hospital · Washington University School of Medicine, Department of Reproductive Endocrinology, 4911 Barnes Hospital Plaza, St. Louis, MO 63110 · 314-362-7144

Michael J. Paul · Maternal & Fetal Medicine · Missouri Baptist Medical Center, Barnes-Jewish Hospital · Center for Women's Wellness, 3015 North Ballas Road, Third Floor West, St. Louis, MO 63131 · 314-995-8955

Janet S. Rader · Gynecologic Cancer (High-Risk Gynecological Cancer Families, Cervical Cancer Screening) · Barnes-Jewish Hospital, Missouri Baptist Medical Center, St. Louis Children's Hospital · St. Louis Maternity Hospital, Department of Gynecological Oncology, 4911 Barnes Hospital Plaza, St. Louis, MO 63110 · 314-362-7135

Valerie Ratts · Reproductive Endocrinology (Pediatric & Adolescent Gynecology) Barnes-Jewish Hospital, St. Louis Children's Hospital · Washington University School of Medicine, Department of Reproductive Endocrinology, 4911 Barnes Hospital Plaza, St. Louis, MO 63110 · 314-362-7144

Jerome D. Sachar · General Obstetrics & Gynecology · Consultants in Women's Health Care, 522 North New Ballas Road, Suite 350, St. Louis, MO 63141 · 314-432-8181

James R. Schreiber · Reproductive Endocrinology (General Obstetrics & Gynecology, Reproductive Surgery) · Barnes-Jewish Hospital, St. Louis Regional Medical Center · Barnes-Jewish Hospital, Department of Obstetrics & Gynecology, 4911 Barnes Hospital Plaza, St. Louis, MO 63110 · 314-362-7139

Ronald C. Strickler · Reproductive Endocrinology · Barnes-Jewish Hospital · Barnes-Jewish Hospital, 216 South Kingshighway Boulevard, St. Louis, MO 63110 · 314-454-8920

David L. Weinstein · General Obstetrics & Gynecology (Endometriosis, Vaginal Birth after Cesarean Section) · Barnes-Jewish Hospital, Missouri Baptist Medical Center, St. Luke's Hospital (Chesterfield) · Consultants in Women's Health Care, 522 North New Ballas Road, Suite 350, St. Louis, MO 63141 · 314-432-8181

Daniel B. Williams · Reproductive Endocrinology (Reproductive Surgery) · Barnes-Jewish Hospital · Washington University School of Medicine, Department of Reproductive Endocrinology, 4911 Barnes Hospital Plaza, St. Louis, MO 63110-1094 · 314-362-7144

OPHTHALMOLOGY

Cape Girardeau

Charles H. Cozean, Jr. · General Ophthalmology (Anterior Segment—Cataract & Refractive, Glaucoma, Research & Development) · St. Francis Medical Center · 56 Doctors' Park, Cape Girardeau, MO 63703 · 573-344-4401

Richard Keis · General Ophthalmology · Keis Ophthalmology Associates, 1429 Mount Auburn Road, Cape Girardeau, MO 63701 · 573-335-9175

Chesterfield

Jack Hartstein · General Ophthalmology (Anterior Segment—Cataract & Refractive, Contact Lenses) · St. Luke's Hospital, Barnes-Jewish Hospital (St. Louis), Missouri Baptist Medical Center (St. Louis), St. John's Mercy Medical Center (St. Louis), Deaconess Medical Center (St. Louis), St. Mary's Health Center (St. Louis) · 224 South Woodsmill Road, Suite 700, Chesterfield, MO 63017 · 314-361-2525

Columbia

John W. Cowden · Corneal Diseases & Transplantation (Anterior Segment—Cataract & Refractive) · University Hospital & Children's Hospital, Harry S. Truman Memorial Veterans Hospital · Mason Institute of Ophthalmology, One Hospital Drive, Columbia, MO 65212 · 573-882-1029

Lenworth N. Johnson · Neuro-Ophthalmology (General Ophthalmology) · University Hospital & Children's Hospital · University Hospital & Children's Hospital, Mason Institute of Ophthalmology, One Hospital Drive, Columbia, MO 65212 · 573-884-6180

Joplin

John Yuhas · General Ophthalmology · Regional Eye Center, 1531 West 32nd Street, Joplin, MO 64804 · 417-781-3631

Kansas City

Gerhard W. Cibis · Pediatric Ophthalmology (Electrophysiology, Ophthalmic Genetics) · Children's Mercy Hospital, Saint Luke's Hospital of Kansas City, Research Medical Center, University of Kansas Medical Center (Kansas City, KS) Country Club Plaza, Suite 421, 4620 J. C. Nichols Parkway, Kansas City, MO 64112-1681 · 816-561-0306

Daniel S. Durrie · Corneal Diseases & Transplantation, Anterior Segment—Cataract & Refractive · Saint Luke's Hospital of Kansas City, Children's Mercy Hospital · Hunkeler Eye Centers, 4321 Washington Avenue, Suite 6000, Kansas City, MO 64111 · 816-931-4733

John D. Hunkeler · Anterior Segment—Cataract & Refractive · Saint Luke's Hospital of Kansas City · Hunkeler Eye Centers, 4321 Washington Avenue, Suite 6000, Kansas City, MO 64111 · 816-931-4733

Charles M. Lederer, Jr. · General Ophthalmology (Glaucoma, Anterior Segment—Cataract & Refractive) · Saint Joseph Health Center, Baptist Medical Center, Truman Medical Center, Western Missouri Medical Center · Glaucoma Care of the Midwest, 6650 Troost Way, Suite 310, Kansas City, MO 64131 · 816-333-3525

Michael C. Stiles · Glaucoma · Saint Luke's Hospital of Kansas City, University of Kansas Medical Center (Kansas City, KS) · Hunkeler Eye Centers, 4321 Washington Avenue, Suite 6000, Kansas City, MO 64111-5900 · 816-931-4733

Springfield

Paul N. Arnold · Anterior Segment—Cataract & Refractive (Corneal Diseases & Transplantation, Glaucoma) · Arnold Cataract and Eye Surgery Center, Cox Medical Centers-North, Cox Medical Centers-South, St. John's Regional Health Center, Columbia Hospital of the Ozarks-South · Arnold Cataract and Eye Surgery Center, 1265 East Primrose Street, Springfield, MO 65804 · 417-886-3937

St. Joseph

James A. Murphy · General Ophthalmology (Anterior Segment—Cataract & Refractive, Glaucoma) · Heartland Health System · 2921 North Belt Highway, Suite M9, St. Joseph, MO 64506 · 816-233-2020

St. Louis

George M. Bohigian · General Ophthalmology (Anterior Segment—Cataract & Refractive, Corneal Diseases & Transplantation) · Barnes-Jewish Hospital, St. Luke's Hospital (Chesterfield), Outpatient Surgery Center of St. Louis · 450 North New Ballas Road, St. Louis, MO 63141 · 314-569-1155

Isaac Boniuk · Vitreo-Retinal Surgery (Retinal Diseases) · Barnes-Jewish Hospital, St. Luke's Hospital (Chesterfield) · Barnes Retina Institute, East Pavilion Building, Suite 17413, One Barnes Hospital Plaza, St. Louis, MO 63110 · 314-367-1181

Sophia Chung · Neuro-Ophthalmology · St. Louis University Hospital, Barnes-Jewish Hospital, Bethesda General Hospital · Anheuser-Busch Eye Institute, St. Louis University Medical Center, 1755 South Grand Avenue, St. Louis, MO 63104 · 314-577-6037

Philip L. Custer · Oculoplastic & Orbital Surgery · Barnes-Jewish Hospital, St. Louis Children's Hospital · Barnes-Jewish Hospital, One Barnes Hospital Plaza, Suite 17305, St. Louis, MO 63110 · 314-361-2698

Lawrence A. Gans · General Ophthalmology (Corneal Diseases & Transplantation, Anterior Segment—Cataract & Refractive, Glaucoma) · Barnes-Jewish Hospital, Christian Hospital Northeast-Northwest, St. Luke's Hospital (Chesterfield), DePaul Health Center (Bridgeton), Carlinville Area Hospital (Carlinville, IL), St. Francis Hospital (Litchfield, IL) · Eye Health Care Associates, 215 Dunn Road, St. Louis, MO 63031 · 314-921-2020

Gilbert Grand · Medical Retinal Diseases (Vitreo-Retinal Surgery) · Barnes-Jewish Hospital, St. Luke's Hospital (Chesterfield), Missouri Baptist Medical Center · Barnes Retina Institute, East Pavilion Building, Suite 17413, One Barnes Hospital Plaza, St. Louis, MO 63110 · 314-367-1181

William M. Hart, Jr. · Neuro-Ophthalmology · Barnes-Jewish Hospital · Washington University School of Medicine, 660 South Euclid Avenue, Campus Box 8096, St. Louis, MO 63110 · 314-362-7163

John B. Holds · Oculoplastic & Orbital Surgery (Ocular Oncology) · St. John's Mercy Medical Center, St. Louis University Hospital · Anheuser-Busch Eye Institute, 621 South New Ballas Road, Suite 5018B, St Louis, MO 63141-8200 · 314-567-3567

Henry J. Kaplan · Uveitis (Macular Disease) · Barnes-Jewish Hospital, St. Louis Children's Hospital · Washington University School of Medicine, Department of Ophthalmology & Visual Sciences, 660 South Euclid Avenue, Campus Box 8096, St. Louis, MO 63110 · 314-362-3937

Michael A. Kass · Glaucoma · Barnes-Jewish Hospital, Washington University Eye Center · Washington University School of Medicine, Department of Ophthalmology & Visual Sciences, 660 South Euclid Avenue, Campus Box 8096, St. Louis, MO 63110 · 314-362-3937

Allan E. Kolker · Glaucoma · Barnes-Jewish Hospital, Washington University Eye Center · Washington University School of Medicine, Department of Ophthalmology & Visual Sciences, 660 South Euclid Avenue, Campus Box 8096, St. Louis, MO 63110 · 314-362-3937

Thomas K. Krummenacher · Vitreo-Retinal Surgery (Diabetic Retinopathy, Macular Degeneration, Retinal Detachment, Uveitis) · St. Luke's Hospital (Chesterfield), St. John's Mercy Medical Center, St. Mary's Health Center, Deaconess Medical Center, Missouri Baptist Medical Center, Christian Hospital Northeast-Northwest · Retina & Vitreous Consultants, 1034 South Brentwood Boulevard, Suite 1625, St. Louis, MO 63117-1208 · 314-727-6711

Anthony J. Lubniewski · Corneal Diseases & Transplantation (External Disease, Intraocular Lens Implants) · Barnes-Jewish Hospital · Washington University School of Medicine, Department of Ophthalmology & Visual Sciences, 660 South Euclid Avenue, Box 8096, St. Louis, MO 63110-1093 · 314-362-3937

Gregg T. Lueder · (Pediatric Ophthalmology, Adult Strabismus, Retinoblastoma) St. Louis Children's Hospital, Barnes-Jewish Hospital · St. Louis Children's Hospital, One Children's Place, Room 2S89, St. Louis, MO 63110 · 314-454-6026

Travis A. Meredith · Vitreo-Retinal Surgery, Medical Retinal Diseases (Vitreo-Retinal Diseases) · Anheuser-Busch Eye Institute, St. Luke's Hospital (Chesterfield), Barnes-Jewish Hospital, Missouri Baptist Medical Center · Retina Consultants, Barnes Retina Institute, East Pavilion Building, Suite 17413, One Barnes Hospital Plaza, St. Louis, MO 63110 · 314-367-1181

R. Joseph Olk · Medical Retinal Diseases, Vitreo-Retinal Surgery · Barnes-Jewish Hospital · The Retina Center, Barnes West County Hospital, 1040 North Mason Road, Suite 219, St. Louis, MO 63110-1093 · 314-275-2020

Jay S. Pepose · Corneal Diseases & Transplantation (Refractive Surgery) · Barnes-Jewish Hospital · Washington University School of Medicine, Department of Ophthalmology & Visual Sciences, 660 South Euclid Avenue, Campus Box 8096, St. Louis, MO 63110 · 314-362-3937

John J. Purcell, Jr. · General Ophthalmology (Anterior Segment—Cataract & Refractive, Corneal Diseases & Transplantation) · St. Mary's Health Center · Eye Microsurgery of St. Louis, 6400 Clayton Road, Suite 416, St. Louis, MO 63117-1850 · 314-647-2277

David J. Schanzlin · Corneal Diseases & Transplantation, Anterior Segment—Cataract & Refractive (Cornea & External Disease) · Anheuser-Busch Eye Institute · Anheuser-Busch Eye Institute, 1755 South Grand Boulevard, St. Louis, MO 63104 · 314-577-8265

Matthew A. Thomas · Medical Retinal Diseases (Vitreo-Retinal Surgery) · Barnes-Jewish Hospital, St. Luke's Hospital (Chesterfield), Missouri Baptist Medical Center · Barnes Retina Institute, East Pavilion Building, Suite 17413, One Barnes Hospital Plaza, St. Louis, MO 63110 · 314-367-1181

Lawrence Tychsen · Pediatric Ophthalmology (Pediatric & Adult Strabismus) · St. Louis Children's Hospital, Barnes-Jewish Hospital · St. Louis Children's Hospital, One Children's Place, Room 2S89, St. Louis, MO 63110 · 314-454-6026; 800-KIDS-218

Mitchel L. Wolf · Medical Retinal Diseases (Electrodiagnostic Testing, General Ophthalmology) · Barnes-Jewish Hospital · Barnes-Jewish Hospital, Department of Ophthalmology, 4932 Forest Park, Suite 6B, St. Louis, MO 63108 · 314-454-7885

ORTHOPAEDIC SURGERY

Cape Girardeau

Ricky Lents · General Orthopaedic Surgery · Orthopaedic Associates, 48 Doctors Park, Cape Girardeau, MO 63703 · 573-335-8257

Michael C. Trueblood · General Orthopaedic Surgery · Orthopaedic Associates, 48 Doctors Park, Cape Girardeau, MO 63703 · 573-335-8257

Columbia

Mark A. Adams · Sports Medicine/Arthroscopy (Knee Surgery) · Columbia Regional Hospital, University Hospital & Children's Hospital, Boone Hospital Center · Columbia Orthopaedic Group, 400 Keene Street, P.O. Box 0, Columbia, MO 65205 · 573-443-2402

Jeffrey O. Anglen · Trauma (Reconstructive Surgery) · University Hospital & Children's Hospital · University Hospital & Children's Hospital, Department of Orthopaedic Surgery, One Hospital Drive, Room M562, Columbia, MO 65212 · 573-882-3104

Thomas R. Highland · Spinal Surgery · Boone Hospital Center, Columbia Regional Hospital · Columbia Orthopaedic Group, 400 Keene Street, P.O. Box 0, Columbia, MO 65205 · 573-443-2402

Patrick Smith · (Sports Medicine/Arthroscopy, Knee Surgery, Shoulder Surgery) Columbia Regional Hospital, Boone Hospital Center, University Hospital & Children's Hospital · Columbia Orthopaedic Group, 400 Keene Street, P.O. Box 0, Columbia, MO 65201 · 573-443-2402

Joplin

David Black · General Orthopaedic Surgery (Reconstructive Surgery, Sports Medicine/Arthroscopy) · St. John's Regional Medical Center, Mount Carmel Medical Center (Pittsburg, KS) · Midwest Orthopaedic Surgery, St. John's Orthopaedic Center, 3126 Jackson Street, P.O. Box 2507, Joplin, MO 64803 · 417-781-2807

Springfield

Fred G. McQueary · General Orthopaedic Surgery · Orthopaedic Clinic, 2115 South Fremont Street, Suite 1000, Springfield, MO 65804 · 417-882-6040

Richard A. Seagrave · General Orthopaedic Surgery · Springfield Clinic, 3231 South National Avenue, Springfield, MO 65807 · 417-883-7422

St. Louis

Keith H. Bridwell · Spinal Surgery (Complex Spinal Surgery [Pediatric & Adult], Spinal Deformities & Disorders [Pediatric & Adult]) · Barnes-Jewish Hospital, St. Louis Children's Hospital, Shriners Hospital for Crippled Children · Barnes-Jewish Hospital, Department of Orthopaedics, One Barnes Hospital Plaza, Suite 11300 West Pavilion, St. Louis, MO 63110 · 314-362-4080

Clayton R. Perry · Trauma · Barnes-Jewish Hospital · Barnes-Jewish Hospital, Department of Orthopaedic Surgery, One Barnes Hospital Plaza, Suite 11300, St. Louis, MO 63110 · 314-362-4080

Perry L. Schoenecker · Pediatric Orthopaedic Surgery · Shriners Hospital for Crippled Children, St. Louis Children's Hospital, Barnes-Jewish Hospital · Shriners Hospital for Crippled Children, 2001 South Lindbergh Boulevard, St. Louis, MO 63131-3597 · 314-432-3600

Charles J. Sutherland · Reconstructive Surgery (Knee Surgery, Hip Surgery) · Barnes-Jewish Hospital, One Barnes Hospital Plaza, Suite 11300, St. Louis, MO 63110 · 314-362-4080

Leo A. Whiteside · Reconstructive Surgery (Knee Surgery, Hip Surgery) · Biomechanical Research Laboratory, Barnes West County Hospital (Creve Coeur) · Missouri Bone & Joint Center, 10 Barnes West Drive, Suite 100, St. Louis, MO 63141 · 314-205-2223

OTOLARYNGOLOGY

Cape Girardeau

Walter A. Schroeder · General Otolaryngology (Facial Plastic Surgery, Head & Neck Surgery) · St. Francis Medical Center, Southeast Missouri Hospital · 3203 Blattner Drive, Cape Girardeau, MO 63703 · 573-334-5007

Columbia

Paul R. Cook · General Otolaryngology (Otolaryngic Allergy, Rhinology, Sinus & Nasal Surgery) · University Hospital & Children's Hospital, Audrain Medical Center (Mexico), Harry S. Truman Memorial Veterans Hospital · University of Missouri School of Medicine, Department of Otolaryngology, One Hospital Drive, Room MA314, Columbia, MO 65212 · 573-882-8175

David S. Parsons · Pediatric Otolaryngology (Sinus & Nasal Surgery, Laryngology, Bronchoesophagology) · University Hospital & Children's Hospital, Audrain Medical Center (Mexico) · University Hospital & Children's Hospital, Division of Otolaryngology, One Hospital Drive, Room MA314, Columbia, MO 65212 · 573-882-8173

Independence

Frederick W. Hahn, Jr. · General Otolaryngology · 4801 Cliff Avenue, Independence, MO 64055 · 816-478-3555

Joplin

Frank W. Shagets · Facial Plastic Surgery, Head & Neck Surgery (Sinus & Nasal Surgery) · St. John's Regional Medical Center, Freeman Hospital · 2700 McClelland Boulevard, Room 305, Joplin, MO 64804 · 417-623-5111

Kansas City

Charles M. Luetje II · Otology · Midwest Ear Institute, Trinity Lutheran Hospital, Saint Luke's Hospital of Kansas City · Otologic Center, 3100 Broadway, Suite 509, Kansas City, MO 64111 · 816-531-7373

R. Vanneman Spake · General Otolaryngology · Mid-America Ear, Nose & Throat Associates, 4320 Wornall Road, Suite 300, Kansas City, MO 64111 · 816-931-8440

Bradley S. Thedinger · Otology (Neurotology) · Trinity Lutheran Hospital, Saint Luke's Hospital of Kansas City, Children's Mercy Hospital · Otologic Center, 3100 Broadway, Suite 509, Kansas City, MO 64111 · 816-531-7373

Springfield

Floyd R. Barnhill · General Otolaryngology · Regional Ear, Nose & Throat Clinic, 1965 South Fremont Street, Suite 1950, Springfield, MO 65804 · 417-887-5750

St. Louis

James H. Boyd · Head & Neck Surgery (Skull-Base Surgery, Thyroid/Parathyroid Surgery) · St. Louis University Hospital, Cardinal Glennon Children's Hospital, St. John's Mercy Medical Center, St. Mary's Health Center · St. Louis University Hospital, Department of Otolaryngology, 3660 Vista Avenue, Suite 312, St. Louis, MO 63110 · 314-577-6110

Gregory H. Branham · Facial Plastic Surgery · St. Louis University Hospital, St. John's Mercy Medical Center, Cardinal Glennon Children's Hospital, St. Mary's Health Center · St. Louis University Hospital, Department of Otolaryngology, 3635 Vista Avenue at Grand Boulevard, St. Louis, MO 63110 · 314-577-8884

Thomas K. Donovan · General Otolaryngology · St. John's Mercy Medical Center, Tower Building B, Suite 7008, 621 South New Ballas Road, St. Louis, MO 63141 · 314-997-4430

John F. Eisenbeis · Laryngology (Voice Disorders, Sinus & Nasal Surgery, General Otolaryngology) · St. Louis University Hospital, St. John's Mercy Medical Center, Cardinal Glennon Children's Hospital, St. Mary's Health Center · St. Louis University Hospital, 3660 Vista Avenue, Suite 312, St. Louis, MO 63110 · 314-577-6110; 314-577-8884

John M. Fredrickson · Head & Neck Surgery (Free Flap Reconstruction, Implantable Middle Ear Hearing Aid) · Barnes-Jewish Hospital · Barnes-Jewish Hospital, McMillan Building, Room 9906, 517 South Euclid Avenue, St. Louis, MO 63110 · 314-362-7550

William H. Friedman · Sinus & Nasal Surgery · Park Central Institute, Deaconess Medical Center-Central Campus · Park Central Institute, 6125 Clayton Avenue, Suite 430, St. Louis, MO 63139-3269 · 314-768-3222

Joel A. Goebel · Otology (Dizziness & Balance Problems, Otology/Neurotology) · Barnes-Jewish Hospital · Barnes-Jewish Hospital, McMillan Building, 517 South Euclid Avenue, Campus Box 8115, St. Louis, MO 63110 · 314-362-7509

Bruce H. Haughey · Head & Neck Surgery (Facial Surgery, Microvascular Reconstructive Surgery, Sinus, Skull-Base & Nasal Disorders, Laryngology) · Barnes-Jewish Hospital, St. Louis Children's Hospital · Barnes-Jewish Hospital, McMillan Building, Room 990, 517 South Euclid Avenue, Campus Box 8115, St. Louis, MO 63110 · 314-362-0365

Jacques A. Herzog · Otology/Neurotology · St. Luke's Hospital (Chesterfield), Christian Hospital-Northeast, Barnes-Jewish Hospital · Center for Hearing and Balance Disorders, 11155 Dunn Road, Suite 209-E, St. Louis, MO 63136 · 314-741-3388

G. Robert Kletzker · Otology (Neurotology, Skull-Base Surgery) · Barnes-Jewish Hospital, St. John's Mercy Medical Center, Missouri Baptist Medical Center, St. Louis Children's Hospital · Midwest Otologic Group, Tower C, Suite 597, 621 South New Ballas Road, St. Louis, MO 63141 · 314-432-5151

Rodney P. Lusk · Pediatric Otolaryngology, Sinus & Nasal Surgery · St. Louis Children's Hospital · St. Louis Children's Hospital, One Children's Place, Room 3S35, St. Louis, MO 63110-1077 · 314-454-2333

Harlan R. Muntz · Pediatric Otolaryngology · St. Louis Children's Hospital · St. Louis Children's Hospital, One Children's Place, Room 3S35, St. Louis, MO 63110 · 314-454-6162

J. Gail Neely · Otology/Neurotology · Barnes-Jewish Hospital, St. Louis Children's Hospital · Washington University School of Medicine, 517 South Euclid Avenue, Campus Box 8115, St. Louis, MO 63110 · 314-362-7344

Donald G. Sessions · Head & Neck Surgery · Barnes-Jewish Hospital, 517 South Euclid Avenue, Campus Box 8115, St. Louis, MO 63110 · 314-362-7526

Peter G. Smith · Otology/Neurotology, Skull-Base Surgery · St. John's Mercy Medical Center, Barnes-Jewish Hospital, St. Louis Children's Hospital, Missouri Baptist Medical Center · Midwest Otologic Group, Tower C, Suite 597, 621 South New Ballas Road, St. Louis, MO 63141 · 314-432-5151

Gershon J. Spector · Head & Neck Surgery (Skull-Base Surgery, Otology/Neurotology) · Barnes-Jewish Hospital · Barnes-Jewish Hospital, 517 South Euclid Avenue, Campus Box 8115, St. Louis, MO 63110 · 314-362-7526

John A. Stith · Pediatric Otolaryngology · Cardinal Glennon Children's Hospital, Department of Pediatric Otolaryngology, 1465 South Grand Boulevard, St. Louis, MO 63104 · 314-577-5675

Stanley E. Thawley · Sinus & Nasal Surgery · Barnes-Jewish Hospital, St. Louis Children's Hospital · Barnes-Jewish Hospital, 517 South Euclid Avenue, Campus Box 8115, St. Louis, MO 63110 · 314-362-7524

J. Regan Thomas · Facial Plastic Surgery · St. Louis University Hospital, Missouri Baptist Medical Center, St. Luke's Hospital (Chesterfield) · Facial Plastic Surgery Center, 3009 North Ballas Road, Suite 269, St. Louis, MO 63131 · 314-997-4651

Mark A. Varvares · Head & Neck Surgery (Head & Neck Reconstructive Surgery, Airway Reconstruction, Facial Plastic Surgery, General Otolaryngology, Laryngology) · St. Louis University Hospital, St. John's Mercy Medical Center, St. Mary's Health Center · St. Louis University Hospital, Department of Otolaryngology, 3660 Vista Avenue, Suite 312, St. Louis, MO 63110 · 314-577-8884

PATHOLOGY

Columbia

Timothy S. Loy · (Surgical Pathology) · University Hospital & Children's Hospital, Department of Pathology, Room M214B, One Hospital Drive, Columbia, MO 65212-0002 · 573-882-1223

Joplin

Margaret E. McDonald · General Pathology · St. John's Regional Medical Hospital, 2727 McClelland Boulevard, Joplin, MO 64804 · 417-625-2928

St. Louis

Louis P. Dehner · Surgical Pathology, Dermatopathology (Pediatric Pathology) · Barnes-Jewish Hospital, St. Louis Children's Hospital · Barnes-Jewish Hospital, Division of Anatomic Pathology, One Barnes Hospital Plaza, St. Louis, MO 63110 314-362-0150

Deborah J. Gersell · (Surgical Pathology, Obstetrical & Gynecological Pathology) Washington University School of Medicine, Division of Surgical Pathology, Barnes Hospital Plaza, St. Louis, MO 63110 · 314-362-0115

Christine G. Janney · (Anatomic/Surgical Pathology, Gynecologic Pathology, Liver/Gastrointestinal Pathology, Bone/Soft Tissue Pathology) · St. Louis University Hospital, Department of Pathology, 3635 Vista Avenue at Grand Boulevard, St. Louis, MO 63110-0250 · 314-577-8782

Mark R. Wick · Surgical Pathology (Dermatopathology, Immunopathology) · Barnes-Jewish Hospital · Barnes-Jewish Hospital, Division of Surgical Pathology, One Barnes Hospital Plaza, St. Louis, MO 63110 · 314-362-0101

PEDIATRICS

Chesterfield

Michelle Kemp · (Pediatric Allergy & Immunology) · Allergy & Asthma Care, 1585 Woodlake Drive, Suite 201, Chesterfield, MO 63017 · 314-878-2788

Columbia

Guillo J. Barbero · Pediatric Gastroenterology (Motility Gastrointestinal Disturbances, Psychosomatic Disturbances in Gastrointestinal Pediatric Illness, General Pediatrics) · University Hospital & Children's Hospital, Department of Child Health, One Hospital Drive, Columbia, MO 65212 · 573-882-6119

Michael S. Cooperstock · Pediatric Infectious Disease · University Hospital & Children's Hospital · University Hospital & Children's Hospital, Department of Child Health, One Hospital Drive, Columbia, MO 65212 · 573-882-6161

David E. Goldstein · Pediatric Endocrinology (Diabetes) · University Hospital & Children's Hospital · University Hospital & Children's Hospital, Department of Child Health, One Hospital Drive, Columbia, MO 65212 · 573-882-6979

Ted Groshong · Pediatric Nephrology · University Hospital & Children's Hospital · University of Missouri School of Medicine, Medical Science Building, Room MA202, Office of Medical Education, Columbia, MO 65212 · 573-882-4141

Nasrollah Hakami · Pediatric Hematology-Oncology · University Hospital & Children's Hospital, Department of Child Health, One Hospital Drive, Columbia, MO 65212 · 573-882-3961

Richard Ephraim Hillman · Metabolic Diseases (Genetics) · University Hospital & Children's Hospital · University Hospital & Children's Hospital, Department of Child Health, One Hospital Drive, Room M749, Columbia, MO 65212-0002 · 573-882-6991

Elizabeth James · Neonatal-Perinatal Medicine · University Hospital & Children's Hospital · University Hospital & Children's Hospital, Department of Child Health, One Hospital Drive, Columbia, MO 65212 · 573-882-2272

Zuhdi A. Lababidi · Pediatric Cardiology (Interventional Cardiology) · University Hospital & Children's Hospital · Children's Hospital & Clinic, Department of Pediatric Cardiology, One Hospital Drive, Columbia, MO 65212 · 573-882-2501

Edward A. Wright · (Pediatric Rehabilitation) · University Hospital & Children's Hospital · University Hospital & Children's Hospital, Howard A. Rusk Rehabilitation Center, Room 501, One Hospital Drive, Columbia, MO 65212 · 573-882-3101

Kansas City

John V. Anderson · Neonatal-Perinatal Medicine · Saint Luke's Hospital of Kansas City, Perinatal Pediatrics, 4401 Wornall Road, Kansas City, MO 64111 · 816-932-2493

Susan E. Duthie · Pediatric Critical Care · Children's Mercy Hospital, Department of Critical Care and Anesthesiology, 2401 Gillham Road, Kansas City, MO 64108-9898 · 816-234-3041

Abbas Emami · Pediatric Hematology-Oncology · Children's Mercy Hospital, Department of Hematology-Oncology, 2401 Gillham Road, Kansas City, MO 64108 · 816-234-3265

Alan S. Gamis · Pediatric Hematology-Oncology (Pediatric Bone Marrow Transplantation) · Children's Mercy Hospital · Children's Mercy Hospital, Department of Hematology-Oncology, 2401 Gillham Road, Kansas City, MO 64108 · 816-234-3265

Robert T. Hall · Neonatal-Perinatal Medicine · Children's Mercy Hospital, Neonatal Office, 2401 Gillham Road, Kansas City, MO 64108 · 816-234-3591

Campbell P. Howard · Pediatric Endocrinology (Diabetes) · Children's Mercy Hospital · Children's Mercy Hospital, Department of Endocrinology, 2401 Gillham Road, Kansas City, MO 64108-9898 · 816-234-3072

Mary Anne Jackson · Pediatric Infectious Disease · Children's Mercy Hospital · Children's Mercy Hospital, Department of Infectious Disease, 2401 Gillham Road, Kansas City, MO 64108-9898 · 816-234-3795

Michael S. McCubbin · Pediatric Pulmonology · Children's Mercy Hospital, Department of Pulmonary Medicine, 2401 Gillham Road, Kansas City, MO 64108 816-234-3033

Lloyd C. Olson · Pediatric Infectious Disease · Children's Mercy Hospital · Children's Mercy Hospital, Department of Infectious Disease, 2401 Gillham Road, Kansas City, MO 64108-9898 · 816-234-3370

Charles C. Roberts · Pediatric Gastroenterology · Children's Mercy Hospital · Children's Mercy Hospital, Department of Gastroenterology, 2401 Gillham Road, Kansas City, MO 64108 · 816-234-3016

Bradley A. Warady · Pediatric Nephrology (Dialysis, Kidney Transplantation) · Children's Mercy Hospital · Children's Mercy Hospital, Section of Pediatric Nephrology, 2401 Gillham Road, Kansas City, MO 64108 · 816-234-3010

Gerald M. Woods · Pediatric Hematology-Oncology · Children's Mercy Hospital, Department of Hematology-Oncology, 2401 Gillham Road, Kansas City, MO 64108 · 816-234-3265

St. Louis

Thomas Aceto, Jr. · Pediatric Endocrinology (General, Growth Disorders) · Cardinal Glennon Children's Hospital · Cardinal Glennon Children's Hospital, 1465 South Grand Boulevard, St. Louis, MO 63104 · 314-577-5648

Richard Barry · Pediatric Critical Care (Emergency Medicine) · Cardinal Glennon Children's Hospital, 1465 South Grand Boulevard, St. Louis, MO 63104-1003 314-577-5668

Barbara R. Cole · Pediatric Nephrology (Hypertension, Polycystic Kidney Disease) · St. Louis Children's Hospital · St. Louis Children's Hospital, Department of Pediatrics, One Children's Place, Room 1060, St. Louis, MO 63110 · 314-454-6043

Harvey R. Colten · Pediatric Pulmonology · St. Louis Children's Hospital · St. Louis Children's Hospital, Department of Pediatrics, One Children's Place, Room 830ST, St. Louis, MO 63110 · 314-454-2129

S. Bruce Dowton · (Genetics, Metabolic Diseases) · Washington University School of Medicine, Department of Pediatrics, One Children's Place, St. Louis, MO 63110 · 314-454-6093

Robert J. Fallon · Pediatric Hematology-Oncology · Cardinal Glennon Children's Hospital, Department of Pediatric Hematology-Oncology/Stem Cell Transplant, 1465 South Grand Boulevard, St. Louis, MO 63104 · 314-577-5638

Robert E. Kane III · Pediatric Gastroenterology (Pediatric Hepatology, Pediatric Liver Transplantation) · Cardinal Glennon Children's Hospital, St. Louis University Hospital, Saint Charles (St. Charles) · Cardinal Glennon Children's Hospital, Department of Gastroenterology, 1465 South Grand Boulevard, St. Louis, MO 63104-1095 · 314-577-5647

James P. Keating · Pediatric Gastroenterology (Diagnosis) · St. Louis Children's Hospital · St. Louis Children's Hospital, One Children's Place, Room 3S36, St. Louis, MO 63110 · 314-454-6006

William J. Keenan · Neonatal-Perinatal Medicine · Cardinal Glennon Children's Hospital, Department of Neonatal Medicine, 1465 South Grand Boulevard, St. Louis, MO 63104-1003 · 314-577-5642

James S. Kemp · Pediatric Pulmonology (Sudden Infant Death Syndrome) · St. Louis Children's Hospital · St. Louis Children's Hospital, Allergy and Pulmonary Medicine, Department of Pediatrics, One Children's Place, St. Louis, MO 63110 314-454-2694

Robert M. Kennedy · (Pediatric Emergency Medicine, Pain Management) · St. Louis Children's Hospital · St. Louis Children's Hospital, Department of Emergency Medicine, One Children's Place, St. Louis, MO 63110-0177 · 314-454-2341

Robert E. Lynch · Pediatric Critical Care (Pediatric Nephrology) · Cardinal Glennon Children's Hospital, St. John's Mercy Medical Center · Cardinal Glennon Children's Hospital, 1465 South Grand Boulevard, Room 2905, St. Louis, MO 63104 · 314-577-5600

George B. Mallory · Pediatric Pulmonology (Pediatric Lung Transplantation) · St. Louis Children's Hospital, Barnes-Jewish Hospital · St. Louis Children's Hospital, Allergy and Pulmonary Medicine, Department of Pediatrics, One Children's Place, St. Louis, MO 63110 · 314-454-2694

James A. Monteleone · Abused Children · Cardinal Glennon Children's Hospital Cardinal Glennon Children's Hospital, 1465 South Grand Boulevard, St. Louis, MO 63104 · 314-268-6406

Terry L. Moore · Pediatric Rheumatology (General Rheumatology, Immunology) Cardinal Glennon Children's Hospital, St. Louis University Hospital · St. Louis University Health Sciences Center, Division of Rheumatology, Doisy Hall, Room R211A, 1402 South Grand Boulevard, St. Louis, MO 63104 · 314-577-8467

Blakeslee E. Noyes · Pediatric Pulmonology (Asthma, Cystic Fibrosis, Lung Transplantation) · Cardinal Glennon Children's Hospital · Cardinal Glennon Children's Hospital, 1465 South Grand Boulevard, St. Louis, MO 63104 · 314-268-6439

Chris L. Ohlemeyer · Adolescent & Young Adult Medicine (Adolescent Gynecology) · Cardinal Glennon Children's Hospital · Cardinal Glennon Children's Hospital, 1465 South Grand Boulevard, St. Louis, MO 63104-1095 · 314-268-6406

J. Julio Perez Fontan · Pediatric Critical Care · St. Louis Children's Hospital · St. Louis Children's Hospital, One Children's Place, St. Louis, MO 63110 · 314-454-2527

Robert J. Rothbaum · Pediatric Gastroenterology (Nutrition, Inflammatory Bowel Disease, Cystic Fibrosis) · St. Louis Children's Hospital · St. Louis Children's Hospital, Division of Pediatric Gastroenterology and Nutrition, One Children's Place, Room A264, St. Louis, MO 63110 · 314-454-6173

Bruce K. Rubin · Pediatric Pulmonology (Cystic Fibrosis, Asthma) · Cardinal Glennon Children's Hospital, St. John's Mercy Medical Center · Cardinal Glennon Children's Hospital, Department of Pediatric Pulmonary Medicine, 1465 South Grand Boulevard, St. Louis, MO 63104 · 314-268-6439

Julio V. Santiago · Pediatric Endocrinology (Diabetes) · St. Louis Children's Hospital, Barnes-Jewish Hospital · St. Louis Children's Hospital, Department of Pediatric Metabolism, One Children's Place, Campus Box 8116, St. Louis, MO 63110 · 314-454-6046

Anthony J. Scalzo · Pediatric Critical Care (Emergency Medicine, Medical Toxicology) · Cardinal Glennon Children's Hospital, 1465 South Grand Boulevard, St. Louis, MO 63104-1003 · 314-577-5668

Alan Leigh Schwartz · Pediatric Hematology-Oncology (Pediatric Cancer) · St. Louis Children's Hospital · St. Louis Children's Hospital, One Children's Place, Room 3S36, St. Louis, MO 63110 · 314-454-6128

Penelope Greta Shackelford · Pediatric Infectious Disease · St. Louis Children's Hospital · St. Louis Children's Hospital, One Children's Place, Room 1102, St. Louis, MO 63110 · 314-454-6050

Gregory A. Storch · Pediatric Infectious Disease (Pediatric AIDS, Virology, Diagnosis of Viral Infections, Polymerase Chain Reaction) · St. Louis Children's Hospital, Barnes-Jewish Hospital · St. Louis Children's Hospital, One Children's Place, Room 2N68, St. Louis, MO 63110-1013 · 314-454-6079

Arnold W. Strauss · Pediatric Cardiology (General Pediatrics, Molecular Genetics) · St. Louis Children's Hospital · Washington University School of Medicine, St. Louis Children's Hospital, Department of Pediatrics, Division of Cardiology, One Children's Place, Room 1S40, St. Louis, MO 63110 · 314-454-6095

Sherida Tollefsen · Pediatric Endocrinology (Growth Hormone, Diabetes) · St. Louis Children's Hospital · St. Louis Children's Hospital, One Children's Place, St. Louis, MO 63110 · 314-454-6051

Teresa J. Vietti · Pediatric Hematology-Oncology (Pediatric Cancer Chemotherapy) · St. Louis Children's Hospital, Shriners Hospital for Crippled Children, Barnes-Jewish Hospital · St. Louis Children's Hospital, Department of Hematology & Oncology, One Children's Place, Room 9S, St. Louis, MO 63110 · 314-454-6228

Donna A. Wall · Pediatric Hematology-Oncology (Stem Cell Transplantation, Cord Blood Transplantation) · Cardinal Glennon Children's Hospital · Cardinal Glennon Children's Hospital, Department of Pediatric Hematology-Oncology, 1465 South Grand Boulevard, St. Louis, MO 63104-1095 · 314-577-5638

John B. Watkins · Pediatric Gastroenterology (Liver Disease, Nutrition) · St. Louis Children's Hospital · St. Louis Children's Hospital, One Children's Place, Room 2S36, St. Louis, MO 63110 · 314-454-6299

Neil H. White · Pediatric Endocrinology (Diabetes) · St. Louis Children's Hospital · St. Louis Children's Hospital, Department of Pediatrics, Endocrinology and Metabolism Division, One Children's Place, St. Louis, MO 63110 · 314-454-6051

Ellen G. Wood · Pediatric Nephrology · Cardinal Glennon Children's Hospital, 1465 South Grand Boulevard, St. Louis, MO 63104 · 314-577-5662

PEDIATRICS (GENERAL)

Cape Girardeau

Jerry H. Allen · 800 East Fifth Street, Cape Girardeau, MO 63090 · 573-239-7892

Gary S. Olson · (Attention Deficit Disorder, Attention Deficit Hyperactivity Disorder, General Pediatrics) · Southeast Missouri Hospital, St. Francis Medical Center · Cape Girardeau Physician Associates, 14 Doctors Park, Cape Girardeau, MO 63701 · 573-334-9641

Connie D. Simmons · (Sports Medicine, General Pediatrics) · Southeast Missouri Hospital, St. Francis Medical Center · Cape Girardeau Physician Associates, 24 South Mount Auburn, Cape Girardeau, MO 63703 · 573-334-9641

Chesterfield

Gordon R. Bloomberg · (Pediatric Allergy, Pediatric Asthma) · St. Louis Children's Hospital (St. Louis), St. Luke's Hospital, St. John's Mercy Medical Center (St. Louis) · 226 South Woodsmill Road, Suite 36W, Chesterfield, MO 63017 · 314-453-9666

Thomas C. McKinney · (Infectious Diseases) · St. Louis Children's Hospital (St. Louis), St. Luke's Hospital, St. John's Mercy Medical Center (St. Louis) · St. Louis Pediatrics Associates, 226 South Woodsmill Road, Suite 32 West, Chesterfield, MO 63017 · 314-576-1616

Juanita Polito-Colvin · St. Louis Pediatrics Associates, 226 South Woodsmill Road, Suite 32 West, Chesterfield, MO 63017 · 314-576-1616

George Sato · St. Louis Children's Hospital (St. Louis), St. John's Mercy Medical Center (St. Louis), St. Luke's Hospital · St. Louis Pediatrics Associates, 226 South Woodsmill Road, Suite 32, Chesterfield, MO 63017 · 314-576-1616

Richard W. Sato · St. Louis Pediatrics Associates, 226 South Woodsmill Road, Suite 32 West, Chesterfield, MO 63017 · 314-576-1616

Columbia

Charles Carnahan · Boone Hospital Center · Boone Clinic, 401 Keene Street, Columbia, MO 65201 · 573-874-3300

Robert J. Harris · (Asthma, General Infectious Disease, Attention Deficit Disorder) · Boone Hospital Center, University Hospital & Children's Hospital, Columbia Regional Hospital · Boone Clinic, 401 Keene Street, Columbia, MO 65201 573-874-3300

Joseph W. Mayo · Boone Hospital Center · 201 West Broadway Street, Suite G, Columbia, MO 65203 · 573-443-0937

Creve Coeur

Elliot F. Gellman · (General Pediatrics, Pediatric Hematology-Oncology, Psychological/ Social Development) · St. Louis Children's Hospital (St. Louis), St. John's Mercy Medical Center (St. Louis) · Pediatric & Adolescent Medical Consultants, 456 North New Ballas Road, Suite 220, Creve Coeur, MO 63141 · 314-567-7337

W. Gary Sherman · St. Louis Children's Hospital (St. Louis), St. John's Mercy Medical Center (St. Louis) · Pediatric & Adolescent Medical Consultants, 456 North New Ballas Road, Suite 220, Creve Coeur, MO 63141 · 314-567-7337

Joplin

Dian L. Doody · Freeman Hospital · 1030 McIntosh Circle, Suite One, Joplin, MO 64804 · 417-782-2002

Kansas City

Kurt Metzl · (Attention Deficit Disorder, Behavior Problems) · Saint Joseph Health Center, Baptist Medical Center, Children's Mercy Hospital · 930 Carondelet Drive, Suite 302, Kansas City, MO 64114 · 816-942-5437

Charles V. Moylan · Saint Luke's Hospital of Kansas City · Pediatric Associates, 4400 Broadway Street, Suite 206, Kansas City, MO 64111 · 816-561-8100

Jeffrey A. Waters · Saint Luke's Hospital of Kansas City, Children's Mercy Hospital · Pediatric Associates, 4400 Broadway Street, Suite 206, Kansas City, MO 64111 · 816-561-8100

Sikeston

Joseph C. Blanton · (Adolescent Medicine, Neonatal-Perinatal Medicine, Attention Deficit Disorders) · Missouri Delta Medical Center · Ferguson Medical Group, 1012 North Main Street, Sikeston, MO 63801 · 573-471-0330

Springfield

Frederic L. Hamburg · Pediatric Associates, 1000 East Primrose Street, Suite 560, Springfield, MO 65807 · 417-882-1600

Christopher H. Snyder, Jr. · Pediatric Associates, 1000 East Primrose Street, Suite 503, Springfield, MO 65807 · 417-882-1600

Don D. Sponenberg · (Attention Deficit Disorder, Asthma, General Pediatrics) · St. John's Regional Health Center · Springfield Clinic, 3231 South National Avenue, Springfield, MO 65807 · 417-885-0810

St. Louis

Charles H. Dougherty · St. Louis Children's Hospital · Health Key Medical Group, 13131 Tesson Ferry Road, St. Louis, MO 63128 · 314-842-5239

David E. Hartenbach · St. Louis Children's Hospital, St. John's Mercy Medical Center, St. Luke's Hospital (Chesterfield), Missouri Baptist Medical Center, St. Mary's Health Center · Health Key Pediatrics, 77 West Port Plaza, Suite 168, St. Louis, MO 63146 · 314-878-3221

Nancy E. Holmes · Central Pediatrics, 8512 Delmar Street, Suite 217, St. Louis, MO 63124 · 314-997-7004

Richard L. Lazaroff · Health Key Pediatrics, 77 West Port Plaza, Suite 168, St. Louis, MO 63146 · 314-878-3221

Allison C. Nash · 3737 North Kingshighway Boulevard, St. Louis, MO 63115 · 314-261-5250

Jay E. Noffsinger · (Sports Medicine, Lead Poisoning in Children) · Cardinal Glennon Children's Hospital · Cardinal Glennon Children's Hospital, Department of Pediatrics, 1465 South Grand Boulevard, St. Louis, MO 63104 · 314-577-5643

Steven I. Plax · St. Louis Children's Hospital · The Children's Clinic, 8025 Dale Street, St. Louis, MO 63117 · 314-644-2566

Paul S. Simons · (Developmental & Behavioral Pediatrics) · St. Louis Children's Hospital · Health Key Pediatrics, 4488 Forest Park Parkway, St. Louis, MO 63108 314-535-7855

Patricia B. Wolff · (Endocrinology, General Pediatrics, Diabetes, Thyroid) · St. Louis Children's Hospital, St. John's Mercy Medical Center · Health Key Pediatrics, 4488 Forest Park Parkway, St. Louis, MO 63108 · 314-535-7855

PHYSICAL MEDICINE & REHABILITATION

Columbia

Robert R. Conway · General Physical Medicine & Rehabilitation (Work-Related Injuries, Electrodiagnostic Medicine) · University Hospital & Children's Hospital University Hospital & Children's Hospital, Howard A. Rusk Rehabilitation Center, Room 501, One Hospital Drive, Columbia, MO 65212 · 573-882-3101; 314-882-8142

Edward A. Wright · General Physical Medicine & Rehabilitation (Pediatric Rehabilitation) · University Hospital & Children's Hospital · University Hospital & Children's Hospital, Howard A. Rusk Rehabilitation Center, Room 501, One Hospital Drive, Columbia, MO 65212 · 573-882-3101

Joplin

Laurie L. Behm · General Physical Medicine & Rehabilitation · 2817 McClelland Boulevard, Joplin, MO 64804 · 417-782-7750

Springfield

Russell R. Bond, Jr. · General Physical Medicine & Rehabilitation (Traumatic Brain Injury Rehabilitation, Sports Medicine) · Cox Medical Centers-North, Cox Medical Centers-South · Southwest Physical Medicine and Rehabilitation, Cox Medical Center South, 3801 South National Avenue, 800 West, Springfield, MO 65807 · 417-269-6868

PLASTIC SURGERY

Columbia

Constance M. Barone · General Plastic Surgery (Craniofacial Surgery, Pediatric Plastic Surgery, Maxillofacial Surgery, Facial Aesthetic Surgery) · University Hospital & Children's Hospital · University Hospital & Children's Hospital, Division of Plastic Surgery, One Hospital Drive, Columbia, MO 65212 · 573-882-2275

Gregory H. Croll · General Plastic Surgery · University Hospital & Children's Hospital, Division of Plastic Surgery, One Hospital Drive, Columbia, MO 65212 573-882-2275

C. Linwood Puckett · Reconstructive Surgery, Facial Aesthetic Surgery (Hand Surgery, General Plastic Surgery) · University Hospital & Children's Hospital · University Hospital & Children's Hospital, Division of Plastic Surgery, One Hospital Drive, Room M349, Columbia, MO 65212 · 573-882-2275

Springfield

Rodney K. Geter · Reconstructive Surgery (Body Contouring, Surgery of the Hand) · St. John's Regional Health Center · Springfield Clinic, Plastic and Reconstructive Surgery, 3231 South National Avenue, Springfield, MO 65807 · 417-885-0878

St. Louis

Susan E. Mackinnon · Peripheral Nerve Surgery (Thoracic Outlet Disorders, Brachial Plexus Surgery, Facial Palsy, Nerve Reconstruction, Painful Nerve Surgery, Nerve Transplantation) · Barnes-Jewish Hospital, St. Louis Children's Hospital · Barnes-Jewish Hospital, East Pavilion Building, Suite 17424, One Barnes Hospital Plaza, St. Louis, MO 63110 · 314-362-4587

Jeffrey L. Marsh · Pediatric Plastic Surgery, Craniofacial Surgery, Reconstructive Surgery (Cleft Lip & Palate Surgery, Facial Aesthetic Surgery) · St. Louis Children's Hospital · St. Louis Children's Hospital, Department of Pediatric Plastic Surgery, One Children's Place, St. Louis, MO 63110 · 314-454-6020

Paul M. Weeks · Reconstructive Surgery (Surgery of the Hand, Peripheral Nerve Surgery) · Barnes-Jewish Hospital, St. Louis Children's Hospital · Barnes-Jewish Hospital, Department of Plastic Surgery, One Barnes Hospital Plaza, Suite 17424, St. Louis, MO 63110 · 314-362-4593

V. Leroy Young · General Plastic Surgery · Cosmetic Surgery Associates, 1040 North Mason Road, Suite 206, St. Louis, MO 63141-6366 · 314-878-0520

PSYCHIATRY

Ballwin

Haruo Kusama · Child & Adolescent Psychiatry · 13611 Barrett Office Drive, Suite 203, Ballwin, MO 63021 · 314-822-8660

Chesterfield

Kimberli E. McCallum · Child & Adolescent Psychiatry, Eating Disorders (Psychoanalysis) · St. Luke's Hospital · Child, Adolescent & Family Center, 425 South Woodsmill Road, Suite 160, Chesterfield, MO 63017 · 314-579-0609

Clayton

Stuart J. Ozar · General Psychiatry, Psychoanalysis · 141 North Meramec Street, Suite 205, Clayton, MO 63105 · 314-725-2828

Columbia

M. Marga Dick · General Psychiatry (Mood & Anxiety Disorders, Psychoanalysis) 209D East Green Meadows Road, Columbia, MO 65203 · 573-449-5800

Suzanne M. King · Geriatric Psychiatry · Mid-Missouri Mental Health Center · University of Missouri, Columbia School of Medicine, Department of Psychiatry and Neurology, One Hospital Drive, Columbia, MO 65201 · 573-882-3176

Joplin

William J. Klontz · General Psychiatry · 2817 McClelland Boulevard, Suite 124, Joplin, MO 64804 · 417-782-9120

Springfield

Philip J. LeFevre · Geriatric Psychiatry (General Psychiatry, Electroconvulsive Therapy, Mood & Anxiety Disorders, Psychopharmacology, Schizophrenia) · St. John's Regional Health Center · 1965 South Fremont, Suite 3000, Springfield, MO 65804 · 417-883-5141

St. Louis

John T. Biggs · General Psychiatry · 1034 South Brentwood Boulevard, Suite 800, St. Louis, MO 63117 · 314-863-2244

Karen R. Boesch · Geriatric Psychiatry · 1035 Bellevue Street, Suite 412, St. Louis, MO 63117 · 314-647-4488

Wilson M. Compton III · Addiction Psychiatry (Substance Abuse) · Washington University School of Medicine, Department of Psychiatry, 4940 Children's Place, St. Louis, MO 63110 · 314-362-2413

John G. Csernansky · Psychopharmacology · Malcolm Bliss Mental Health Center · Malcolm Bliss Mental Health Center, 5400 Arsenal Street, St. Louis, MO 63139 · 314-644-7800

Paul A. Dewald · Psychoanalysis (Psychotherapy) · St. Louis Psychoanalytic Institute, St. Louis University Hospital · St. Louis Psychoanalytic Institute, 4524 Forest Park Boulevard, St. Louis, MO 63108 · 314-367-5817

Wayne C. Drevetz · General Psychiatry (Brain Imaging, Mood & Anxiety Disorders, Neuropsychiatry, Psychopharmacology) · Barnes-Jewish Hospital · Washington University School of Medicine, Department of Psychiatry, 4940 Children's Place, St. Louis, MO 63110-1093 · 314-362-2459

M. Robin Eastwood · Geriatric Psychiatry · St. Louis University Hospital · University of St. Louis School of Medicine, Department of Psychiatry, 1221 South Grand Boulevard, St. Louis, MO 63104 · 314-577-8724

Cynthia A. Florin · Psychoanalysis (General Psychiatry, Psychopharmacology) · Barnes-Jewish Hospital · Washington University School of Medicine, Department of Psychiatry, 24 South Kingshighway Boulevard, St. Louis, MO 63108 · 314-362-2436

Barbara Geller · Child & Adolescent Psychiatry (Mood & Anxiety Disorders, Psychopharmacology) · Barnes-Jewish Hospital, St. Louis Children's Hospital · Washington University School of Medicine, Department of Psychiatry, 4940 Children's Place, St. Louis, MO 63110 · 314-362-7365

George T. Grossberg · Geriatric Psychiatry (Alzheimer's Disease, Mood & Anxiety Disorders) · St. Louis University Hospital · St. Louis University Hospital, Division of Geriatric Psychiatry, 1221 South Grand Boulevard, St. Louis, MO 63104 · 314-577-8726

Samuel B. Guze · General Psychiatry (Affective Disorders, Alcoholism Disorders, Diagnostic Evaluation, Somatization Disorders, Psychopharmacology, Schizophrenia) · Barnes-Jewish Hospital · Washington University School of Medicine, 4940 Children's Place, St. Louis, MO 63110 · 314-362-7772

Duane Q. Hagen · General Psychiatry (Occupational Psychiatry, Mood & Anxiety Disorders, Psychopharmacology, Suicidology) · St. John's Mercy Medical Center St. John's Mercy Medical Center, Tower Building B, Suite 2008, 621 South New Ballas Road, St. Louis, MO 63141 · 314-569-6295

Donald P. Hay · Geriatric Psychiatry (Affective Disorders, Agitation in Dementia Patients, Electroconvulsive Therapy, Psychopharmacology) · St. Louis University Hospital · St. Louis University School of Medicine, 1221 South Grand Boulevard, St. Louis, MO 63104 · 314-577-8727

Richard W. Hudgens · General Psychiatry · Barnes-Jewish Hospital, Department of Psychiatry, 4940 Children's Place, St. Louis, MO 63110-1093 · 314-362-2622

Keith E. Isenberg · General Psychiatry (Geriatric Psychiatry, Psychopharmacology, Schizophrenia) · Barnes-Jewish Hospital · Washington University School of Medicine, Department of Psychiatry, 4940 Children's Place, Campus Box 8134, St. Louis, MO 63110 · 314-362-1819

Michael R. Jarvis · General Psychiatry (Geriatric Psychiatry, Psychopharmacology) · Barnes-Jewish Hospital · University of Missouri School of Medicine, Department of Psychiatry, 4940 Children's Place, St. Louis, MO 63110 · 314-362-3072

William A. Kelly · Psychoanalysis · St. Louis Psychoanalytic Institute · St. Louis Psychoanalytic Institute, 4524 Forest Park Boulevard, St. Louis, MO 63108 · 314-367-6299

Joan Luby · Child & Adolescent Psychiatry (Infant & Preschool Psychiatry) · St. Louis Children's Hospital, Barnes-Jewish Hospital · Washington University School of Medicine, Division of Child Psychiatry, 4940 Children's Place, St. Louis, MO 63110 · 314-454-2303

Richard E. Mattison · Child & Adolescent Psychiatry · Barnes-Jewish Hospital, St. Louis Children's Hospital · Washington University School of Medicine, Department of Psychiatry, 4940 Children's Place, St. Louis, MO 63110 · 314-454-2303

C. Leon McGahee · Geriatric Psychiatry · Wohl Institute, 1221 South Grand Boulevard, St. Louis, MO 63104 · 314-577-8728

Robert W. Meyers · Psychoanalysis · St. Louis University Hospital · St. Louis Psychoanalytic Institute, 4524 Forest Park Boulevard, Room 103, St. Louis, MO 63108 · 314-367-8424

Jule P. Miller · Psychoanalysis · St. Louis Psychoanalytic Institute, 4524 Forest Park Boulevard, St. Louis, MO 63108 · 314-367-2660

K. Lynne Moritz · Psychoanalysis (Mood & Anxiety Disorders, Child Analysis) · St. Louis University Hospital · St. Louis Psychoanalytic Institute, 4524 Forest Park Boulevard, St. Louis, MO 63108 · 314-367-7979

John W. Newcomer · Schizophrenia (Geriatric Psychiatry, Psychopharmacology) Barnes-Jewish Hospital, Department of Psychiatry, One Barnes Hospital Plaza, St. Louis, MO 63110-1002 · 314-362-5939

Carol S. North · General Psychiatry (Schizophrenia, Dissociative Disorders, Post-Traumatic Stress Disorders) · Barnes-Jewish Hospital · Washington University School of Medicine, Department of Psychiatry, 4940 Children's Place, St. Louis, MO 63110 · 314-362-2586

Eric J. Nuetzel · Psychoanalysis · St. Louis Psychoanalytic Institute, 4524 Forest Park Boulevard, St. Louis, MO 63108 · 314-367-2726

Stephen L. Post · Psychoanalysis · St. Louis Psychoanalytic Institute, 4524 Forest Park Boulevard, St. Louis, MO 63108 · 314-361-8333

Mary Ramsey · (Psychoanalysis, Mood & Anxiety Disorders) · 777 South New Ballas Road, Suite 330W, St. Louis, MO 63141 · 314-432-3404

Theodore Reich · Mood & Anxiety Disorders (Genetics) · Washington University School of Medicine, Department of Psychiatry, Barnes Hospital Plaza, St. Louis, MO 63110 · 314-362-2149

Thomas F. Richardson · General Psychiatry · Barnes-Jewish Hospital · Pavilion Associates, One Barnes Hospital Plaza, St. Louis, MO 63110 · 314-362-3901

Eugene H. Rubin · Geriatric Psychiatry · Barnes-Jewish Hospital · Washington University School of Medicine, Department of Psychiatry, 4940 Children's Place, Campus Box 8134, St. Louis, MO 63110 · 314-362-2462

Marcel T. Saghir · General Psychiatry · 1034 South Brentwood Boulevard, Suite 1200, St. Louis, MO 63117 · 314-862-4448

Moisy Shopper · Psychoanalysis (Adult, Adolescent & Child Psychoanalysis, Forensic Psychiatry) · Cardinal Glennon Children's Hospital · St. Louis Psychoanalytic Institute, 4524 Forest Park Boulevard, St. Louis, MO 63108-2168 · 314-361-4646

Nathan M. Simon · Psychoanalysis · St. Louis University Hospital, Barnes-Jewish Hospital · St. Louis Psychoanalytic Institute, 4524 Forest Park Boulevard, St. Louis, MO 63108 · 314-367-6299

James B. Smith · General Psychiatry · 4660 Maryland Avenue, Suite 210, St. Louis, MO 63108 · 314-367-3050

Betty Sonnenwirth · Psychoanalysis · 141 North Meramec Street, Suite 108, St. Louis, MO 63105 · 314-727-8400

Richard D. Todd · Child & Adolescent Psychiatry (Mood & Anxiety Disorders, Psychopharmacology) · Barnes-Jewish Hospital, St. Louis Children's Hospital · Washington University School of Medicine, Department of Psychiatry, 4940 Children's Place, Campus Box 8134, St. Louis, MO 63110 · 314-362-8650

Eugene E. Trunnell · Psychoanalysis (Brief Psychotherapy, Dreams, Dissociative Disorders, General Psychiatry, Mood & Anxiety Disorders, Psychopharmacology) St. Louis University Hospital · St. Louis Psychoanalytic Institute, 4524 Forest Park Boulevard, St. Louis, MO 63108 · 314-361-4844

Harold D. Wolff · General Psychiatry (Geriatric Psychiatry) · Barnes-Jewish Hospital · 605 Old Ballas Road, Suite 100, St. Louis, MO 63141-7070 · 314-569-2525

Sean H. Yutzy · Forensic Psychiatry (General Psychiatry) · Barnes-Jewish Hospital · Washington University School of Medicine, Department of Psychiatry, 4940 Children's Place, St. Louis, MO 63110-1093 · 314-362-2440

Charles F. Zorumski · General Psychiatry (Neuropsychiatry, Psychopharmacology) · Barnes-Jewish Hospital · Washington University School of Medicine, Department of Psychiatry, 4940 Children's Place, St. Louis, MO 63110 · 314-362-8650

PULMONARY & CRITICAL CARE MEDICINE

Cape Girardeau

Khalid I. Khan · General Pulmonary & Critical Care Medicine · Pulmonary Clinic, 62 Doctors Park, Cape Girardeau, MO 63703 · 573-335-5359

Columbia

R. Phillip Dellinger · General Pulmonary & Critical Care Medicine (Asthma) · University Hospital & Children's Hospital, Harry S. Truman Memorial Veterans Hospital · University of Missouri, Columbia, Department of Internal Medicine, Pulmonary & Critical Care Division, One Hospital Drive, Columbia, MO 65212 · 573-882-2991

Joplin

Rick L. Scacewater · General Pulmonary & Critical Care Medicine · 1531 West 32nd Street, Suite 201, Joplin, MO 64804 · 417-782-8350

Kansas City

James S. Bower · General Pulmonary & Critical Care Medicine · Kansas City Pulmonary Clinic, 6420 Prospect Avenue, Suite 303, Kansas City, MO 64132 · 816-333-1919

Charles J. Brook · General Pulmonary & Critical Care Medicine (Sleep Disorders Medicine) · Kansas City Pulmonary Clinic, 6420 Prospect Avenue, Suite 303, Kansas City, MO 64132 · 816-333-1919

Garth F. Harrison · General Pulmonary & Critical Care Medicine (Sleep Disorders Medicine) · Research Medical Center · Kansas City Pulmonary Clinic, 6420 Prospect Avenue, Suite 303, Kansas City, MO 64132 · 816-333-1919

Vincent Lem · General Pulmonary & Critical Care Medicine · Saint Luke's Hospital of Kansas City · Midwest Pulmonary Consultants, 4321 Washington Street, Suite 5100, Kansas City, MO 64111 · 816-756-2255

Daniel L. Schlozman · General Pulmonary & Critical Care Medicine · Kansas City Pulmonary Clinic, 6420 Prospect Avenue, Suite 303, Kansas City, MO 64132 816-333-1919

St. Louis

Thomas Morgan Hyers · General Pulmonary & Critical Care Medicine (Adult Respiratory Distress Syndrome, Pulmonary Thromboembolism) · St. Louis University Hospital · St. Louis University Health Sciences Center, 3635 Vista Avenue at Grand Boulevard, P.O. Box 15250, St. Louis, MO 63110-0250 · 314-577-8856

Cesar Keller · General Pulmonary & Critical Care Medicine (Lung Transplantation) · St. Louis University Hospital · St. Louis University Health Sciences Center, Division of Pulmonology, FDT Building, Seventh Floor, 3635 Vista Avenue at Grand Boulevard, St. Louis, MO 63104 · 314-577-8856

Marin H. Kollef · General Pulmonary & Critical Care Medicine (Critical Care) · Barnes-Jewish Hospital · Washington University School of Medicine, Division of Pulmonary & Critical Care Medicine, 660 South Euclid Avenue, Campus Box 8052, St. Louis, MO 63110 · 314-362-3776

Stephen S. Lefrak · General Pulmonary & Critical Care Medicine (Critical Care) Barnes-Jewish Hospital · Barnes-Jewish Hospital, 216 South Kingshighway Boulevard, St. Louis, MO 63110 · 314-454-7116

Jill A. Musika Ohar · General Pulmonary & Critical Care Medicine (Occupational Lung Disease, Asthma, Pulmonary Vascular Diseases) · St. Louis University Hospital · St. Louis University Health Sciences Center, 3635 Vista Avenue at Grand Boulevard, P.O. Box 15250, St. Louis, MO 63110-0250 · 314-577-8856

Daniel P. Schuster · General Pulmonary & Critical Care Medicine (Critical Care) Barnes-Jewish Hospital · Washington University School of Medicine, Department of Internal Medicine, Division of Pulmonary & Critical Care Medicine, 660 South Euclid Avenue, St. Louis, MO 63110 · 314-362-3776

Robert M. Senior · General Pulmonary & Critical Care Medicine (Chronic Obstructive Pulmonary Disease, Asthma, Bronchology) · Barnes-Jewish Hospital · Barnes-Jewish Hospital, 216 South Kingshighway Boulevard, St. Louis, MO 63110 · 314-454-7524; 314-454-7113

Deborah Shure · General Pulmonary & Critical Care Medicine (Lung Cancer, Pulmonary Hypertension) · Barnes-Jewish Hospital · Barnes-Jewish Hospital, 216 South Kingshighway Boulevard, St. Louis, MO 63110 · 314-454-7117

Elbert P. Trulock III · (Lung Transplantation, Emphysema, Pulmonary Fibrosis, Pulmonary Hypertension) · Barnes-Jewish Hospital · Washington University School of Medicine, Division of Pulmonary & Critical Care Medicine, 660 South Euclid Avenue, Campus Box 8052, St. Louis, MO 63110-1093 · 314-362-6905

RADIATION ONCOLOGY

Bridgeton

Venkata Devineni · General Radiation Oncology · DePaul Health Center, 12303 DePaul Drive, Bridgeton, MO 63044 · 314-344-6090

Columbia

Steven J. Westgate · General Radiation Oncology · Ellis Fischel Cancer Center, Division of Radiation Oncology, 115 Business Loop 70 West, Columbia, MO 65203 · 573-882-8644

Jefferson City

Mark Bryer · General Radiation Oncology (Gastroenterologic Cancer) · Ellis Fischel Cancer Center of University of Missouri (Columbia) · Mid-Missouri Medical Foundation, 3400 West Truman Boulevard, Jefferson City, MO 65109 · 573-893-5252

Kansas City

Scott C. Cozad · General Radiation Oncology · North Kansas City Hospital (North Kansas City) · Parvin Road Radiation Oncology Center, 2001 Northeast Parvin Road, Kansas City, MO 64116 · 816-452-2751

Arthur Elman · General Radiation Oncology · Saint Luke's Hospital of Kansas City, Department of Radiation Oncology, 4400 Wornall Road, Box 30064, Kansas City, MO 64111 · 816-932-2575

R. Bruce Hoskins · General Radiation Oncology · Radiation Oncology Associates, 1004 Carondelet Way, Suite 100, Kansas City, MO 64114 · 816-942-5800

Vickie Massey · General Radiation Oncology (Brachytherapy) · Trinity Lutheran Hospital, Department of Radiation Oncology, 3030 Baltimore Road, Kansas City, MO 64108 · 816-751-2930

Steven S. Nigh · General Radiation Oncology · Therapeutic Radiologists, 6400 Prospect Avenue, Suite 240, Kansas City, MO 64132 · 816-363-2677

Jay S. Robinow · General Radiation Oncology · Therapeutic Radiologists, 6400 Prospect Avenue, Suite 240, Kansas City, MO 64132 · 816-363-2677

Springfield

J. Drew Rogers · General Radiation Oncology · Radiation Oncology of the Ozarks, 1423 North Jefferson Avenue, Springfield, MO 65802 · 417-882-9960

St. Charles

John M. Bedwinek · Breast Cancer · St. Joseph Health Center · St. Joseph Health Center, Department of Radiation Oncology, 330 First Capitol Drive, Suite 100, St. Charles, MO 63301 · 314-947-5055

St. Louis

Bahman Emami · Head & Neck Cancer (Lung Cancer, 3-D Conformal Radiotherapy) · Mallinckrodt Institute of Radiology, Barnes-Jewish Hospital · Mallinckrodt Institute of Radiology at Washington University, 510 South Kingshighway Boulevard, St. Louis, MO 63110 · 314-362-8525

Perry W. Grigsby · Gynecologic Cancer · Barnes-Jewish Hospital · Mallinckrodt Institute of Radiology at Washington University, 510 South Kingshighway Boulevard, St. Louis, MO 63110 · 314-362-8502

James E. Marks · Head & Neck Cancer (Brain Tumors) · Missouri Baptist Medical Center · Missouri Baptist Medical Center, Radiation Oncology, 3015 North New Ballas Road, St. Louis, MO 63131 · 314-569-5157

Jeff M. Michalski · Pediatric Radiation Oncology, Genito-Urinary Cancer (Sarcomas) · Barnes-Jewish Hospital, St. Louis Children's Hospital · Washington University School of Medicine, Department of Radiation Oncology, 4939 Children's Place, Suite 5500, St. Louis, MO 63110 · 314-362-8566

Robert J. Myerson · (Hyperthermia, Gastroenterologic Cancer) · Barnes-Jewish Hospital · Barnes-Jewish Hospital, 216 South Kingshighway Boulevard, P.O. Box 14109, St. Louis, MO 63110 · 314-454-7236

Carlos A. Perez · Lung Cancer, Gynecologic Cancer, Genito-Urinary Cancer, Breast Cancer · Radiation Oncology Center, Mallinckrodt Institute of Radiology · Mallinckrodt Institute of Radiology at Washington University, Radiation Oncology Center, 510 South Kingshighway Boulevard, St. Louis, MO 63110 · 314-362-8542

Joseph R. Simpson · Brain Cancer (Brain Tumors, Ear, Nose, Throat Cancers, Stereotactic Brain Irradiation) · Barnes-Jewish Hospital, Missouri Baptist Medical Center · Barnes-Jewish Hospital, 4939 Children's Place, Suite 5500, Campus Box 8224, St. Louis, MO 63110 · 314-362-8516

Marie E. Taylor · Breast Cancer · Barnes-Jewish Hospital · Mallinckrodt Institute of Radiology at Washington University, 510 South Kingshighway Boulevard, St. Louis, MO 63110 · 314-362-8567

Todd H. Wasserman · Lymphomas (Hodgkin's Disease, Non-Hodgkin's Lymphomas, General Radiation Oncology) · Barnes-Jewish Hospital · Washington University School of Medicine, 4939 Children's Place, Suite 5500, St. Louis, MO 63110-1001 · 314-362-8501

RADIOLOGY

Springfield

Douglas Hacker · Magnetic Resonance Imaging, Neuroradiology · Springfield Radiological Group, 1675 Seminole Street, Suite J, Springfield, MO 65804 · 417-881-5033

James M. Sauer · Magnetic Resonance Imaging, Neuroradiology (Head & Neck Radiology) · St. John's Regional Health Center · St. John's Hospital, Springfield Clinic, 1235 East Cherokee Street, Springfield, MO 65804 · 417-881-5033

St. Louis

D. Claire Anderson · Chest · Barnes-Jewish Hospital, Washington University School of Medicine · Mallinckrodt Institute of Radiology at Washington University, 510 South Kingshighway Boulevard, St. Louis, MO 63110 · 314-362-2927

DeWitte T. Cross III · Neuroradiology (Interventional Neuroradiology) · Barnes-Jewish Hospital · Mallinckrodt Institute of Radiology at Washington University, 510 South Kingshighway Boulevard, St. Louis, MO 63110 · 314-362-5950

Jay P. Heiken · (Abdominal Imaging, Body Computed Tomography, Magnetic Resonance Imaging) · Barnes-Jewish Hospital · Mallinckrodt Institute of Radiology at Washington University, 510 South Kingshighway Boulevard, St. Louis, MO 63110 · 314-362-1053

William H. McAlister · Pediatric Radiology · St. Louis Children's Hospital, Department of Radiology, One Children's Place, St. Louis, MO 63110 · 314-454-6229

William D. Middleton · General Radiology (Ultrasonography) · Barnes-Jewish Hospital · Mallinckrodt Institute of Radiology at Washington University, 510 South Kingshighway Boulevard, St. Louis, MO 63110 · 314-362-1053

Barbara S. Monsees · General Radiology (Mammography) · Mallinckrodt Institute of Radiology at Washington University, 510 South Kingshighway Boulevard, St. Louis, MO 63110 · 314-362-2912; 314-362-5880

Daniel Picus · (Vascular & Interventional Radiology, Cardiovascular Disease, General Radiology) · Barnes-Jewish Hospital, St. Louis Children's Hospital · Mallinckrodt Institute of Radiology at Washington University, 510 South Kingshighway Boulevard, St. Louis, MO 63110-1016 · 314-362-2900

Stuart S. Sagel · Chest (Cardiovascular Disease, Computed Body Tomography) · Barnes-Jewish Hospital · Mallinckrodt Institute of Radiology at Washington University, 510 South Kingshighway Boulevard, St. Louis, MO 63110 · 314-362-2927

Marilyn J. Siegel · Pediatric Radiology · St. Louis Children's Hospital · Mallinckrodt Institute of Radiology at Washington University, 510 South Kingshighway Boulevard, St. Louis, MO 63110-1076 · 314-454-6229

William R. Totty · General Radiology (Bone Radiology, Magnetic Resonance Imaging) · Barnes-Jewish Hospital · Mallinckrodt Institute of Radiology at Washington University, 510 South Kingshighway Boulevard, St. Louis, MO 63110 · 314-362-2911

RHEUMATOLOGY

Cape Girardeau

Philip W. Taylor · General Rheumatology · Cape Girardeau Physician Associates, 14 Doctors Park, Cape Girardeau, MO 63701 · 573-334-9641

Columbia

Donald R. Kay · General Rheumatology · Boone Hospital Center · Boone Clinic, Department of Rheumatology, 401 Keene Street, Columbia, MO 65201 · 573-874-3300

Geetha Reddy · General Rheumatology (Systemic Lupus Erythematosus, Rheumatoid Arthritis, Antiphospholipid Antibody Syndrome) · University Hospital & Children's Hospital · University Hospital & Children's Hospital, Department of Rheumatology, One Hospital Drive, Columbia, MO 65212 · 573-882-8095

Gordon C. Sharp · General Rheumatology (Lupus, Scleroderma/Mixed Connective Tissue Disease) · University Hospital & Children's Hospital · University Hospital & Children's Hospital, Health Sciences Center, Room MA427, One Hospital Drive, Columbia, MO 65212 · 573-882-8730

Sara E. Walker · General Rheumatology (Clinical Immunology, Systemic Lupus Erythematosus) · Harry S. Truman Memorial Veterans Hospital, University Hospital & Children's Hospital · Harry S. Truman Memorial Veterans Hospital, 800 Hospital Drive, Columbia, MO 65201 · 573-443-2511 x6656

Joplin

Michael E. Joseph · General Rheumatology · 2700 McClelland Boulevard, Building A, Suite 104, Joplin, MO 64804 · 417-624-0050

Kansas City

John K. Layle · General Rheumatology · Medical Plaza II, Suite 40, 4330 Wornall Road, Kansas City, MO 64111 · 816-531-0930

Anne M. Regier · General Rheumatology · 665 Troost Street, Suite 103, Kansas City, MO 64131 · 816-361-1910

Springfield

Stephen Armstrong · General Rheumatology · Ferrell-Duncan Clinic, 1001 East Primrose Street, Springfield, MO 65807 · 417-885-7120

Joseph L. Mayus · General Rheumatology · Ferrell-Duncan Clinic, 1001 East Primrose Street, Springfield, MO 65807 · 417-885-7120

St. Louis

John P. Atkinson · General Rheumatology (Systemic Lupus Erythematosus, Complement, Autoimmunity, Clinical & Lab Immunology, Immunodeficiency, Edematous Conditions) · Barnes-Jewish Hospital · Washington University School of Medicine, 4570 Children's Place, St. Louis, MO 63110 · 314-362-7601

Andrew R. Baldassare · General Rheumatology · DePaul Health Center (Bridgeton), St. John's Mercy Medical Center, Saint Charles (St. Charles) · Arthritis Consultants, 522 North New Ballas Road, Suite 240, St. Louis, MO 63141 · 314-567-5100

SURGERY

Cape Girardeau

John P. Christy · General Surgery (General Surgical Oncology, General Thoracic Surgery) · Doctor's Regional Medical Center (Poplar Bluff) · Kneibert Clinic, 686 Lester Street, Cape Girardeau, MO 63901 · 573-686-2411

Robert S. Hunt · General Surgery (Breast Surgery, Endocrine Surgery) · Southeast Missouri Hospital, St. Francis Medical Center · Cape Girardeau Surgical Clinic, 10 Doctors Park, Cape Girardeau, MO 63703 · 573-334-3074

Jerry L. Kinder · General Surgery · Cape Girardeau Surgical Clinic, 10 Doctors Park, Cape Girardeau, MO 63703 · 573-334-3074

Ronald Richmond · General Surgery (Surgical Critical Care) · Southeast Missouri Hospital, St. Francis Medical Center · Cape Girardeau Surgical Clinic, 10 Doctors Park, Cape Girardeau, MO 63701 · 573-334-3074

Columbia

Vincent P. Gurucharri · General Surgery (Laparoscopy, General Thoracic Surgery, Gastroenterologic Surgery, Head & Neck Surgery, General Surgical Oncology) · Boone Hospital Center, Columbia Regional Hospital · Columbia Surgical Associates, 3401 Berrywood Drive, Suite 104, Columbia, MO 65201 · 573-443-8773

Mary Alice Helikson · Pediatric Surgery (Surgical Critical Care, Trauma) · University Hospital & Children's Hospital · University Hospital & Children's Hospital, Department of Surgery, One Hospital Drive, Suite N307, Columbia, MO 65212 · 573-882-4156

Paul W. Humphrey · General Surgery (General Vascular Surgery, Laparoscopic Surgery, Breast Surgery, Endocrine Surgery, Gastroenterologic Surgery) · Boone Hospital Center, Columbia Regional Hospital · Columbia Surgical Associates, 3401 Berrywood Drive, Suite 104, Columbia, MO 65201-6598 · 573-443-8773

Debra Koivunen · Endocrine Surgery (Breast Surgery, General Surgery) · University Hospital & Children's Hospital, Harry S. Truman Memorial Veterans Hospital · University Hospital & Children's Hospital, Division of General Surgery, One Hospital Drive, Columbia, MO 65212 · 573-882-6127

Michael H. Metzler · General Surgery (Trauma, Surgical Critical Care) · University Hospital & Children's Hospital · University Hospital & Children's Hospital, Department of Surgery, One Hospital Drive, Columbia, MO 65212 · 573-882-8157

Brent W. Miedema · General Surgery (Gastroenterologic Surgery, Gastrointestinal Cancer, Gastrointestinal Motility) · University Hospital & Children's Hospital, Harry S. Truman Memorial Veterans Hospital · University Hospital & Children's Hospital, Division of General Surgery, One Hospital Drive, Columbia, MO 65212 · 573-882-3276

W. Kirt Nichols · General Vascular Surgery (General Surgery) · University Hospital & Children's Hospital · University Hospital & Children's Hospital, Division of Vascular/General Surgery, One Hospital Drive, Columbia, MO 65212 · 573-882-7136

Donald Silver · General Vascular Surgery (Thrombosis, Arterial & Venous Thromboembolism, Ischemia Reperfusion Injury) · University Hospital & Children's Hospital · University of Missouri, Columbia, School of Medicine, Department of Surgery, One Hospital Drive, Columbia, MO 65212 · 573-882-8178

Boyd Terry · General Surgery (Bariatric Surgery) · University Hospital & Children's Hospital, Department of Surgery, Division of General Surgery, One Hospital Drive, Columbia, MO 65212 · 573-882-7156

Curt M. Vogel · General Vascular Surgery · University Hospital & Children's Hospital, Boone Hospital Center, Columbia Regional Hospital · Columbia Surgical Associates, 3401 Berrywood Drive, Suite 104, Columbia, MO 65201-6598 · 573-443-8773

Hannibal

Michael J. Bukstein · General Surgery (General Vascular Surgery, General Surgical Oncology, General Thoracic Surgery) · Hannibal Regional Hospital, Blessing Hospital (Quincy, IL) · Hannibal Clinic, 711 Grand Avenue, Hannibal, MO 63401-0311 · 573-221-5250

Joplin

W. C. Dandridge, Jr. · (Breast Surgery, Trauma) · St. John's Regional Medical Center, McCune-Brooks Hospital (Carthage), Freeman Hospital · Joplin Surgical Associates, 3126 Jackson Street, Suite 102, P.O. Box 3058, Joplin, MO 64803 · 417-781-4404; 417-358-1454

Sikeston

Fred H. Thornton · General Surgery (General Surgical Oncology, Thoracic Oncological Surgery) · Missouri Delta Medical Center · 1012 North Main Street, Sikeston, MO 63801 · 573-471-0330

Springfield

Michael E. Ashley · General Surgery · Springfield Clinic, 3231 South National Avenue, Springfield, MO 65807 · 417-888-5671

St. Louis

Brent T. Allen · General Vascular Surgery (General Surgery) · Barnes-Jewish Hospital · Barnes-Jewish Hospital, Queeny Tower, Suite 5103, One Barnes Hospital Plaza, St. Louis, MO 63110 · 314-362-7408

Todd K. Howard · Transplantation (Liver Transplantation, Kidney Transplantation, Hepatic Resections, General Surgery, Surgical Critical Care) · Barnes-Jewish Hospital, St. Louis Children's Hospital · Barnes-Jewish Hospital, Queeny Tower, Suite 6107, One Barnes Hospital Plaza, St. Louis, MO 63110 · 314-362-5701

Joseph J. Hurley · General Vascular Surgery · St. John's Mercy Medical Center St. John's Mercy Medical Center, Department of Surgery, 621 South New Ballas Road, Suite 6005, St. Louis, MO 63141 · 314-569-4200

Donald L. Kaminski · General Surgery (Gastroenterologic Surgery, Liver & Pancreatic Surgery) · St. Louis University Hospital · St. Louis University Hospital, Department of Surgery, 3635 Vista Avenue at Grand Boulevard, P.O. Box 15250, St. Louis, MO 63110-0250 · 314-577-8353; 314-577-6131

Jerome F. Levy · Breast Surgery (Laparoscopic Procedures, Reconstructive Breast Surgery) · Barnes-Jewish Hospital · Barnes-Jewish Hospital, St. Louis Surgery, One Barnes Hospital Plaza, St. Louis, MO 63110 · 314-367-9400

Jeffrey A. Norton · Endocrine Surgery (Cancer) · Barnes-Jewish Hospital · Barnes-Jewish Hospital, Department of Surgery, One Barnes Hospital Plaza, Campus Box 8109, St. Louis, MO 63110 · 314-362-7320

Gregorio A. Sicard · General Vascular Surgery (Aortic Surgery, Carotid Artery Surgery) · Barnes-Jewish Hospital · Barnes-Jewish Hospital, One Barnes Hospital Plaza, Suite 5103, St. Louis, MO 63110 · 314-362-7841

Nathaniel J. Soper · Gastroenterologic Surgery (Laparoscopic Surgery, General Surgery) · Barnes-Jewish Hospital · Barnes-Jewish Hospital, One Barnes Hospital Plaza, Suite 6108, St. Louis, MO 63110 · 314-362-6900

Steven Strasberg · Gastroenterologic Surgery (Hepatobiliary-Pancreatic Surgery) Barnes-Jewish Hospital, St. Louis Children's Hospital · Barnes-Jewish Hospital, Department of Surgery, Queeny Tower, Suite 6108, One Barnes Hospital Plaza, St. Louis, MO 63110 · 314-362-7147

Jessie L. Ternberg · Pediatric Surgery (Oncology, Shoer Bowel Problems) · St. Louis Children's Hospital · St. Louis Children's Hospital, Department of Pediatric Surgery, One Children's Place, Room 5W12, St. Louis, MO 63110 · 314-454-6022

Samuel A. Wells · Endocrine Surgery (Surgical Oncology) · Barnes-Jewish Hospital · Washington University School of Medicine, 660 South Euclid Avenue, Campus Box 8109, St. Louis, MO 63110 · 314-362-8020

SURGICAL ONCOLOGY

Cape Girardeau

Robert S. Hunt · General Surgical Oncology · Southeast Missouri Hospital, St. Francis Medical Center · Cape Girardeau Surgical Clinic, 10 Doctors Park, Cape Girardeau, MO 63703 · 573-334-3074

Columbia

David M. Ota · Colon & Rectal Cancer, Breast Cancer (Laparoscopic Colon Surgery) · Ellis Fischel Cancer Center of University of Missouri · Ellis Fischel Cancer Center, 115 Business Loop 70 West, Columbia, MO 65203 · 573-882-8454

Kansas City

Paul G. Koontz, Jr. · General Surgical Oncology (Breast Surgery, Endocrine Surgery) · Saint Luke's Hospital of Kansas City · 4320 Wornall Road, Suite 308, Kansas City, MO 64111 · 816-753-7460

Howard Rosenthal · (Orthopaedic Oncology, Musculoskeletal Oncology, Adult and Pediatric Bone and Soft Tissue Tumors, Metabolic Bone Diseases) · Trinity Lutheran Hospital, North Kansas City Hospital (North Kansas City), Menorah Medical Center (Overland Park, KS), Children's Mercy Hospital · Drisko, Fee & Parkins Limb Preservation Institute, 2929 Baltimore Road, Suite 500, Kansas City, MO 64108 · 816-531-0370

Darryl Wallace · General Surgical Oncology (Gynecologic Cancer) · Saint Luke's Hospital of Kansas City · Oncology Center, 4323 Wornall Road, Kansas City, MO 64111 · 816-932-3300

St. Louis

Michael Brunt · General Surgical Oncology · Barnes-Jewish Hospital, Department of Surgery, 216 South Kingshighway Boulevard, St. Louis, MO 63110 · 314-454-7194

Gerard M. Doherty · General Surgical Oncology (Endocrine Surgery, Breast Surgery) · Barnes-Jewish Hospital · Barnes-Jewish Hospital, Department of Surgery, Queeny Tower, Suite 5108, One Barnes Hospital Plaza, St. Louis, MO 63110 · 314-362-8370

Ira Joe Kodner · Colon & Rectal Cancer · Barnes-Jewish Hospital · Barnes-Jewish Hospital, 216 South Kingshighway Boulevard, St. Louis, MO 63110 · 314-454-7177

Jeffrey F. Moley · General Surgical Oncology, Breast Cancer (Endocrine Surgery) Barnes-Jewish Hospital, VA Medical Center · Barnes-Jewish Hospital, Queeny Tower, Suite 5108, One Barnes Hospital Plaza, St. Louis, MO 63110 · 314-362-5210

David G. Mutch · General Surgical Oncology (Gynecologic Cancer) · Barnes-Jewish Hospital · Barnes-Jewish Hospital, Department of Gynecological Oncology, 4911 Barnes Hospital Plaza, St. Louis, MO 63110 · 314-362-7135

Jeffrey A. Norton · General Surgical Oncology · Barnes-Jewish Hospital, Department of Surgery, One Barnes Hospital Plaza, Campus Box 8109, St. Louis, MO 63110 · 314-362-7320

Gordon W. Philpott · Breast Cancer · Barnes-Jewish Hospital · Barnes-Jewish Hospital, Department of Surgery, 216 South Kingshighway Boulevard, St. Louis, MO 63110 · 314-454-7170

Diane M. Radford · Breast Cancer · Washington University School of Medicine, 660 South Euclid Avenue, Campus Box 8109, St. Louis, MO 63110 · 314-362-7931

Anthony M. Vernava III · Colon & Rectal Cancer · St. Louis University Hospital, St. Mary's Health Center · St. Louis University Health Sciences Center, Department of General Surgery, FDT Building, 3635 Vista Avenue at Grand Boulevard, P.O. Box 15250, St. Louis, MO 63110-0250 · 314-577-8562

Eric D. Whitman · General Surgical Oncology (Melanoma, Immunotherapy, Cancer Biotherapy) · Barnes-Jewish Hospital, St. Louis Children's Hospital · Barnes-Jewish Hospital, Queeny Tower, Suite 5108, One Barnes Hospital Drive, St. Louis, MO 63110 · 314-362-5270

THORACIC SURGERY

Columbia

Jack J. Curtis · General Thoracic Surgery (Adult Cardiothoracic Surgery, Transplantation) · University Hospital & Children's Hospital · University Hospital & Children's Hospital, Department of Cardiothoracic Surgery, One Hospital Drive, Columbia, MO 65212 · 573-882-6954

Todd L. Demmy · Adult Cardiothoracic Surgery (Thoracic Oncological Surgery, Transplantation) · University & Children's Hospitals & Clinics, Ellis Fischel Cancer Center of University of Missouri · University Hospital & Children's Hospital, Department of Cardiothoracic Surgery, One Hospital Drive, Columbia, MO 65212 573-882-6954

Kansas City

Jeffrey M. Piehler · General Thoracic Surgery · Saint Luke's Hospital of Kansas City · Mid-America Thoracic & Cardiovascular Surgeons, Medical Plaza Building II, Suite 50, 4320 Wornall Road, Kansas City, MO 64111 · 816-931-7743

St. Louis

Joel D. Cooper · General Thoracic Surgery, Transplantation (Lung Transplantation, Thoracic Oncological Surgery) · Barnes-Jewish Hospital · Barnes-Jewish Hospital, Queeny Tower, Suite 3108, One Barnes Hospital Plaza, St. Louis, MO 63110 · 314-362-6021

James L. Cox · Adult Cardiothoracic Surgery (Electrophysiology) · Barnes-Jewish Hospital · Barnes-Jewish Hospital, Queeny Tower, Suite 3108, One Barnes Hospital Plaza, St. Louis, MO 63110 · 314-362-6185

T. Bruce Ferguson, Jr. · Adult Cardiothoracic Surgery (Surgical Electrophysiology, Pacemakers & Defibrillator Therapy) · Barnes-Jewish Hospital · Barnes-Jewish Hospital, Queeny Tower, Suite 3108, One Barnes Hospital Plaza, St. Louis, MO 63110 · 314-362-6183

William Gay · Adult Cardiothoracic Surgery · Barnes-Jewish Hospital · Barnes-Jewish Hospital, Division of Cardiothoracic Surgery, Queeny Tower, Suite 3108, One Barnes Hospital Plaza, St. Louis, MO 63110 · 314-747-1315

Charles B. Huddleston · Pediatric Cardiac Surgery · St. Louis Children's Hospital, Department of Cardiology, One Barnes Hospital Plaza, Suite 3108, St. Louis, MO 63110 · 314-454-6165

Nicholas T. Kouchoukos · Adult Cardiothoracic Surgery (Aortic & Great Vessel Surgery) · Barnes-Jewish Hospital, St. Louis Children's Hospital, · Barnes-Jewish Hospital, 216 South Kingshighway Boulevard, St. Louis, MO 63110 · 314-454-7175

Keith S. Naunheim · General Thoracic Surgery (Thoracic Oncological Surgery, Thoracoscopy) · St. Louis University Hospital, St. Mary's Health Center · St. Louis University Health Sciences Center, Department of Surgery, 3635 Vista Avenue at Grand Boulevard, P.O. Box 15250, St. Louis, MO 63110-0250 · 314-577-8360

Michael K. Pasque · Adult Cardiothoracic Surgery (Cardiac Transplantation, General Thoracic Surgery) · Barnes-Jewish Hospital · Barnes-Jewish Hospital, Queeny Tower, Suite 3103, One Barnes Hospital Plaza, St. Louis, MO 63110 · 314-362-6237

G. Alexander Patterson · General Thoracic Surgery, Transplantation (Lung Transplantation, Lung Surgery) · Barnes-Jewish Hospital · Barnes-Jewish Hospital, Queeny Tower, Suite 3108, One Barnes Hospital Plaza, St. Louis, MO 63110 314-362-6025

William F. Sasser · General Thoracic Surgery (Thoracic Outlet Disorders, Thoracic Oncological Surgery, Pacemakers, Endoscopy, Esophageal Disease) · St. John's Mercy Medical Center, Christian Hospital Northeast, Missouri Baptist Medical Center, DePaul Hospital (Bridgeton) · 621 South New Ballas Road, Suite 542A, St. Louis, MO 63141 · 314-567-1841

UROLOGY

Cape Girardeau

John P. Hall · General Urology · Urological Associates, Three Doctors Park, Cape Girardeau, MO 63703 · 573-334-7748

Columbia

Gilbert Ross, Jr. · General Urology (Transplantation) · University Hospital & Children's Hospital · University Hospital & Children's Hospital, Division of Urology, One Hospital Drive, Room N510, Mail Code DC080.0, Columbia, MO 65212 · 573-882-1151

Dana J. Weaver-Osterholtz · General Urology · University Hospital & Children's Hospital · University Hospital & Children's Hospital, Department of Urology, One Hospital Drive, Columbia, MO 65212 · 573-882-1151

Joplin

G. Scott Brehm · General Urology · Joplin Urology, 2817 McClelland Boulevard, Suite 123, Joplin, MO 64804 · 417-623-3703

Springfield

Harry L. Ellis · General Urology · Urology Surgical Associates, 1965 South Fremont Street, Suite 3100, Springfield, MO 65804 · 417-882-0300

St. Louis

Gerald L. Andriole · Urologic Oncology · Barnes-Jewish Hospital · Barnes-Jewish Hospital, Division of Urology, 4690 Children's Place, St. Louis, MO 63110 · 314-362-8200

Arnold D. Bullock · General Urology (Prostate Cancer, Impotence, Urologic Oncology) · Barnes-Jewish Hospital · Barnes-Jewish Hospital, 216 South Kingshighway Boulevard, Suite 3304, Campus Box 8242, St. Louis, MO 63110 · 314-454-7178

William J. Catalona · Urologic Oncology (Prostate Cancer) · Barnes-Jewish Hospital · Washington University School of Medicine, Division of Urologic Surgery, 4960 Children's Place, St. Louis, MO 63110 · 314-362-8206

Ralph V. Clayman · Endourology (Stone Disease, Ureteroscopy, Percutaneous Stone Removal, Laparoscopy [Kidney Removal & Renal Reconstruction]) · Barnes-Jewish Hospital · Washington University School of Medicine, Department of Urologic Surgery, 4960 Children's Place, St. Louis, MO 63110 · 314-362-8208

M'liss A. Hudson · Urologic Oncology (Bladder Cancer, General Urology) · Barnes-Jewish Hospital · Barnes-Jewish Hospital, 4960 Children's Plaza, Campus Box 8242, St. Louis, MO 63110 · 314-362-8200

Carl G. Klutke · Neuro-Urology & Voiding Dysfunction · Barnes-Jewish Hospital Barnes-Jewish Hospital, 4960 Children's Plaza, Campus Box 8242, St. Louis, MO 63110 · 314-362-8200

Elspeth M. McDougall · General Urology · Washington University School of Medicine, 4960 Children's Place, 10130 Wohl Clinic, St. Louis, MO 63110 · 314-362-9271

MONTANA

ALLERGY & IMMUNOLOGY

Billings

Kathleen Cecilia Davis · General Allergy & Immunology (Asthma, Urticaria/ Angioedema, Immunodeficiency) · Deaconess Medical Center Health System, Saint Vincent Hospital & Health Center · Deaconess Medical Center Health System, 2800 Tenth Avenue, North, P.O. Box 37000, Billings, MT 59107 · 406-256-2500

David Redfern · General Allergy & Immunology · Billings Clinic, 2825 Eighth Avenue, North, P.O. Box 35100, Billings, MT 59107 · 406-238-2500

Macij Tomaszewski · General Allergy & Immunology · 1020 North 27th Street, Suite 315, Billings, MT 59101 · 406-252-3222

Helena

Richard S. Buswell · (Asthma, Rhinitis, Urticaria) · St. Peter's Community Hospital · South Hills Medical Center, 2600 Winne, Helena, MT 59601 · 406-442-0507

Missoula

Donald Nevin Gillespie · (Seasonal Pollen Allergies, Regional Allergens, Pediatric Asthma) · St. Patrick Hospital, Community Medical Center · 610 West Spruce Street, Missoula, MT 59802 · 406-728-6472

ANESTHESIOLOGY

Billings

David T. Danes · General Anesthesiology · 1145 North 29th Street, Suite 7B, Billings, MT 59103 · 406-657-4165

David Khoe · General Anesthesiology · Anesthesiology Services, 2520 Seventeenth Street, West, Suite B4, Billings, MT 59102 · 406-259-1686

Brian McGuire · General Anesthesiology · Deaconess Medical Center Health System, Department of Surgery, 2800 Tenth Avenue, North, P.O. Box 37000, Billings, MT 59107 · 406-657-4165

Thomas A. Robinson · General Anesthesiology · 2520 Seventeenth Street, West, Suite B4, Billings, MT 59102 · 406-259-1686

Marvin Warren · General Anesthesiology · Anesthesiology Services, 2520 Seventeenth Street, West, Suite B4, Billings, MT 59102 · 406-259-1686

Great Falls

Eric J. Anderson · General Anesthesiology · 1006 First Avenue, South, P.O. Box 2827, Great Falls, MT 59403 · 406-727-6311

Brian G. Bertha · General Anesthesiology · 1006 First Avenue, South, P.O. Box 2827, Great Falls, MT 59403 · 406-727-6311

Mark P. Peterson · General Anesthesiology · 1006 First Avenue, South, P.O. Box 2827, Great Falls, MT 59403 · 406-727-6311

Missoula

John W. Bradford · General Anesthesiology · 2620 Glen Drive, Missoula, MT 59801 · 406-721-7751

Teresa A. Garland · General Anesthesiology · 3700 Russell Street, Suite C-118, Missoula, MT 59801 · 406-721-6029

Steven C. Kemple · General Anesthesiology · 327 East Broadway, Missoula, MT 59802 · 406-721-2604

CARDIOVASCULAR DISEASE

Billings

John R. Burg · General Cardiovascular Disease · Billings Clinic, 2825 Eighth Avenue, North, P.O. Box 35100, Billings, MT 59101 · 406-238-2000

Herman David Sorensen · General Cardiovascular Disease · Billings Clinic, Welch Heart Center, 1020 North 27th Street, Billings, MT 59101 · 406-238-2500

Great Falls

Daniel R. Walker · General Cardiovascular Disease · 2718 Fifteenth Avenue, South, Great Falls, MT 59405 · 406-727-8780

L. M. Willson, Jr. · (Cardiac Catheterization, Echocardiography, Heart Failure) · Columbus Hospital, Montana Deaconess Medical Center · 400 Fifteenth Avenue, South, Suite 208, Great Falls, MT 59405 · 406-727-9979

Helena

Richard D. Paustian · General Cardiovascular Disease · 32 Medical Park Drive, Helena, MT 59601 · 406-449-7943

Missoula

Joseph C. Cleveland · (Adult Cardiothoracic Surgery, Coronary Artery Bypass, Valvular Heart Surgery) · St. Patrick Hospital · 554 West Broadway, Missoula, MT 59802 · 406-728-4558

Alan Gabster · General Cardiovascular Disease · 601 West Spruce Street, Suite J, Missoula, MT 59802 · 406-543-4649

James H. Oury · (Aortic and Mitral Valve Repair, Pulmonary Autograft Procedure for Aortic Valve Replacement in Athletes, Coronary Artery Bypass) · St. Patrick Hospital · 554 West Broadway, Missoula, MT 59802 · 406-728-4558

George Henry Reed · General Cardiovascular Disease · St. Patrick Hospital · 601 West Spruce Street, Missoula, MT 59802 · 406-721-3005

W. Stan Wilson · General Cardiovascular Disease · 601 West Spruce Street, Missoula, MT 59802 · 406-721-4080

COLON & RECTAL SURGERY

Billings

Paul F. Grmoljez · General Colon & Rectal Surgery · Billings Clinic, 2825 Eighth Avenue, North, P.O. Box 35100, Billings, MT 59101 · 406-238-2325

Terry A. Housinger · General Colon & Rectal Surgery · Deaconess Medical Center Health System, Saint Vincent Hospital & Health Center · Billings Clinic, 2825 Eighth Avenue, North, P.O. Box 35100, Billings, MT 59107 · 406-238-2500

Robert N. Hurd · General Colon & Rectal Surgery (General Surgery, Trauma, Breast Surgery) · Deaconess Medical Center Health System · Billings Clinic, 2825 Eighth Avenue, North, P.O. Box 35100, Billings, MT 59107-5100 · 406-238-2500

DERMATOLOGY

Billings

Albert C. Reynaud · Clinical Dermatology · Deaconess Medical Center Health System, 2800 Tenth Avenue, North, P.O. Box 37000, Billings, MT 59107-5100 · 406-238-2500

William Smoot · Clinical Dermatology · Yellowstone Dermatology, 1020 North 27th Street, Suite 410, Billings, MT 59101 · 406-248-3113

Great Falls

David Baldridge · (Mohs Micrographic Surgery, Skin Cancer Surgery & Reconstruction) · Montana Deaconess Medical Center, Columbus Hospital · College Park Center, 2300 Twelfth Avenue, South, Great Falls, MT 59405 · 406-727-1131

Kathryn Kay Hansen · Clinical Dermatology (Surgical Dermatology, Pediatric Dermatology) · Great Falls Clinic, 1400 Twenty-Ninth Street, South, P.O. Box 5012, Great Falls, MT 59403 · 406-454-2171

Helena

Stephen D. Behlmer · Clinical Dermatology (Dermatologic Surgery, Reconstructive Surgery) · St. Peter's Community Hospital · Associated Dermatology, 50 South Last Chance Gulch, Helena, MT 59601 · 406-442-3534

Missoula

Lance R. Hinther · Clinical Dermatology · 2825 Fort Missoula Road, Missoula, MT 59801 · 406-549-7556

EATING DISORDERS

Billings

D. Frank Johnson · Obesity · Health Care Clinic, 1600 Poly Drive, Suite 305, Billings, MT 59102 · 406-248-4580

ENDOCRINOLOGY & METABOLISM

Billings

Diane Christina Roland · General Endocrinology & Metabolism · Deaconess Medical Center Health System, 2800 Tenth Avenue, North, P.O. Box 37000, Billings, MT 59107 · 406-256-2500

Great Falls

Philip A. Krezowski · General Endocrinology & Metabolism · Great Falls Clinic, 1400 Twenty-Ninth Street, South, P.O. Box 5012, Great Falls, MT 59403 · 406-454-2171

Missoula

Nancy R. Eyler · General Endocrinology & Metabolism (Diabetes, Thyroid) · Community Medical Center, St. Patrick Hospital · 2831 Fort Missoula Road, Missoula, MT 59801 · 406-549-4529

FAMILY MEDICINE

Billings

Leonard W. Etchart · Billings West Internal Medicine, 1650 Avenue D, Billings, MT 59102 · 406-248-1138

Helena

William Mark Batey · Family Practice Center, 405 Saddle Drive, Helena, MT 59601 · 406-442-0120

Earl E. Book · St. Peter's Community Hospital · Livery Square, Suite 208, 33 Neill Avenue, Helena, MT 59601 · 406-443-5354

Robert M. Shepard · Family Health Clinic of Helena, 820 North Montana Avenue, Helena, MT 59601 · 406-442-3300

Michael Steven Strekall · Family Practice Center, 405 Saddle Drive, Helena, MT 59601 · 406-442-0120

Missoula

Eric J. Kress · Family Practice, 631 West Alder, Missoula, MT 59802 · 406-721-1850

Robert D. Marks · 2831 Fort Missoula Road, Suite 302, Missoula, MT 59801 · 406-542-1232

Judith McDonald · Family Practice, 631 West Alder, Missoula, MT 59802 · 406-721-1850

GASTROENTEROLOGY

Billings

Mark J. Dell'Aglio · General Gastroenterology · Billings Clinic, 2825 Eighth Avenue, North, P.O. Box 35100, Billings, MT 59101 · 406-238-2500

John Clifford Finke · General Gastroenterology · Billings Clinic, 2825 Eighth Avenue, North, P.O. Box 35100, Billings, MT 59101 · 406-238-2500

Mark Clifford Rumans · General Gastroenterology · Deaconess Medical Center Health System, 2800 Tenth Avenue, North, P.O. Box 37000, Billings, MT 59107 · 406-256-2500

Great Falls

John T. Molloy · General Gastroenterology · Big Sky Health Care, 400 Thirteenth Avenue, South, Suite 203, Great Falls, MT 59405 · 406-727-4584

Helena

Kenneth V. Eden · General Gastroenterology · Internal Medicine Associates, 121 North Last Chance Gulch, Helena, MT 59601 · 406-442-1994

Missoula

James A. Cain · General Gastroenterology · 601 West Spruce Street, Suite F, Missoula, MT 59802 · 406-728-4160

Kimberly John Curtis · General Gastroenterology · 601 West Spruce Street, Suite F, Missoula, MT 59802 · 406-728-4160

Richard Glynn Murney, Jr. · General Gastroenterology · Western Montana Clinic, 515 West Front Street, Missoula, MT 59807 · 406-721-5600

GERIATRIC MEDICINE

Billings

Patricia Coon · (General Geriatric Medicine, Geriatric Assessment, Alzheimer's Disease, Dementing Illnesses) · Deaconess Medical Center Health System, Saint Vincent Hospital & Health Center · Billings Clinic, 2825 Eighth Avenue, North, P.O. Box 35100, Billings, MT 59107 · 406-238-2500

Helena

V. Lee Harrison · Internal Medicine Associates, 121 North Last Chance Gulch, Helena, MT 59601 · 406-442-1994

Missoula

Jenny Davis Murney · Western Montana Clinic, 515 West Front Street, P.O. Box 7609, Missoula, MT 59807 · 406-721-5600

Ann M. Murphy · Western Montana Clinic, 515 West Front Street, P.O. Box 7609, Missoula, MT 59807 · 406-721-5600

HAND SURGERY

Billings

Thomas R. Johnson · General Hand Surgery · Orthopaedic Surgeons, 1232 North 30th Street, Billings, MT 59101 · 406-245-3149

Great Falls

Charles D. Jennings · General Hand Surgery (General Orthopaedic Surgery) · Great Falls Orthopaedic Associates, Doctors Plaza, Suite 16, 2800 Eleventh Avenue, South, Great Falls, MT 59405 · 406-761-1410

Missoula

Thomas R. Rickard · (Microsurgery, Pediatric Hand Surgery, Arthritis) · Community Medical Center, St. Patrick Hospital · Northern Rockies Orthopaedic Specialists, 2831 Fort Missoula Road, Suite 232, Missoula, MT 59801 · 406-728-6101

INFECTIOUS DISEASE

Billings

David Calhoun · General Infectious Disease · Deaconess Medical Center Health System, 2800 Tenth Avenue, North, P.O. Box 37000, Billings, MT 59107 · 406-256-2500

Frederick W. Kahn · General Infectious Disease (Respiratory Infections, Critical Care Medicine) · Saint Vincent Hospital & Health Center · Respiratory Center, 1145 North 29th Street, Suite 300, Billings, MT 59101 · 406-238-6800

Ronald H. Smith · General Infectious Disease · Community Medical Center (Missoula) · Billings Clinic, 2825 Eighth Avenue, North, P.O. Box 35100, Billings, MT 59107-5100 · 406-238-2500

Butte

John Pullman · General Infectious Disease · Mercury Street Medical Group, 300 West Mercury Street, Butte, MT 59701 · 406-782-1261

Great Falls

Raymond A. Geyer · General Infectious Disease (AIDS, Hospital-Acquired Infections, Fungal Infections) · Montana Deaconess Medical Center, Columbus Hospital · Great Falls Clinic, 1400 Twenty-Ninth Street, South, P.O. Box 5012, Great Falls, MT 59403 · 406-454-2171

Missoula

George F. Risi · General Infectious Disease · Missoula Medical Oncology and Infectious Disease, 615 West Alder, Missoula, MT 59802 · 406-728-2539

Les Whitney · General Infectious Disease · Western Montana Clinic, 515 West Front Street, P.O. Box 7609, Missoula, MT 59807 · 406-721-5600

INTERNAL MEDICINE (GENERAL)

Billings

Steven Jay Gerstner · Deaconess Medical Center Health System, 2800 Tenth Avenue, North, P.O. Box 37000, Billings, MT 59107 · 406-256-2500

Lucinda Mae Husby · Deaconess Medical Center Health System, 2800 Tenth Avenue, North, P.O. Box 37000, Billings, MT 59107 · 406-256-2500

Charles R. McClave II · 1145 North 29th Street, Suite 200, Billings, MT 59101 406-245-1140

Neal Barry Sorensen · 1230 North 30th Street, Billings, MT 59101 · 406-238-6900

Charles Allen Wittnam · (General Internal Medicine, Thyroid Disease) · Deaconess Medical Center Health System, Saint Vincent Hospital & Health Center · 1020 North 27th Street, Suite 301A, Billings, MT 59101 · 406-245-4441

Great Falls

Bobby L. Maynard · Great Falls Clinic, 1400 Twenty-Ninth Street, South, P.O. Box 5012, Great Falls, MT 59403 · 406-454-2171

John T. Molloy · Big Sky Health Care, 400 Thirteenth Avenue, South, Suite 203, Great Falls, MT 59405 · 406-727-4584

Helena

Michael D. Hixon · 65 Medical Park Drive, Helena, MT 59601 · 406-442-1231

Missoula

Rebecca S. Anderson · 2831 Fort Missoula Road, Suite 131, Missoula, MT 59801 406-721-0636

H. Eric Hughson · (Occupational Medicine) · St. Patrick Hospital · Western Montana Clinic, 515 West Front Street, P.O. Box 7609, Missoula, MT 59807 · 406-721-5600 x336

Mary C. Langenderfer · Western Montana Clinic, 515 West Front Street, Missoula, MT 59802 · 406-721-5600

Stanley Seagraves · St. Patrick Hospital, Community Medical Center · Western Montana Clinic, 515 West Front Street, P.O. Box 7609, Missoula, MT 59807 · 406-721-5600

Beth E. Thompson · Blue Mountain Clinic, 1916 Brooks Street, P.O. Box 136, Missoula, MT 59801 · 406-721-1646

Wesley W. Wilson · (Diabetes, Hematology) · St. Patrick Hospital · Western Montana Clinic, Department of Internal Medicine, 515 West Front Street, P.O. Box 7609, Missoula, MT 59802 · 406-721-5600

MEDICAL ONCOLOGY & HEMATOLOGY

Billings

Neel Hammond · General Medical Oncology & Hematology (Solid Tumors, Breast Cancer, Lung Cancer, Colon Cancer, Cancer Control & Prevention) · Saint Vincent Hospital & Health Center · Internal Medicine Associates, 1230 North 30th Street, Billings, MT 59101 · 406-238-6900

Roger Gene Santala · General Medical Oncology & Hematology · Deaconess Medical Center Health System, Saint Vincent Hospital & Health Center · Deaconess Medical Center Health System, 2825 Eighth Avenue, North, P.O. Box 37000, Billings, MT 59107 · 406-238-2714

Donald I. Twito · General Medical Oncology & Hematology · Billings Clinic, 2825 Eighth Avenue, North, P.O. Box 35100, Billings, MT 59107 · 406-238-2544

Brock P. Whittenberger · General Medical Oncology & Hematology · Billings Clinic, 2825 Eighth Avenue, North, P.O. Box 35100, Billings, MT 59101 · 406-238-2500

Great Falls

Karl Anton Guter · General Medical Oncology & Hematology · Columbus Hospital, Montana Deaconess Medical Center · Great Falls Clinic, 1400 Twenty-Ninth Street, South, P.O. Box 5012, Great Falls, MT 59403 · 406-454-2171

Grant W. Harrer · General Medical Oncology & Hematology · Big Sky Health Care, 400 Thirteenth Avenue, South, Suite 203, Great Falls, MT 59405 · 406-727-4584

Missoula

Eric F. Berglund · General Medical Oncology & Hematology · Western Montana Clinic, 515 West Front Street, P.O. Box 7609, Missoula, MT 59807 · 406-721-5600

Stephen F. Speckart · General Medical Oncology & Hematology · Missoula Medical Oncology and Infectious Disease, 615 West Alder, Missoula, MT 59802 406-728-2539

John M. Trauscht · General Medical Oncology & Hematology (General Internal Medicine, General Geriatric Medicine) · St. Patrick Hospital, Community Medical Center · Western Montana Clinic, 515 West Front Street, Missoula, MT 59802 · 406-721-5600

NEPHROLOGY

Billings

Donald L. Hicks · General Nephrology · Billings Clinic, 2825 Eighth Avenue, North, P.O. Box 35100, Billings, MT 59107-5100 · 406-238-2500

James D. Knostman · General Nephrology · Billings Clinic, 2825 Eighth Avenue, North, P.O. Box 35100, Billings, MT 59107-5100 · 406-238-2500

Great Falls

Thomas Walter Rosenbaum · General Nephrology · Great Falls Clinic, 1400 Twenty-Ninth Street, South, P.O. Box 5012, Great Falls, MT 59403 · 406-454-2171

Missoula

Margaret Eddy · General Nephrology (Glomerular Diseases, Hypertension) · St. Patrick Hospital, Community Medical Center · Western Montana Clinic, 515 West Front Street, Missoula, MT 59802 · 406-721-5600

John Henry Reiter · General Nephrology · Western Montana Clinic, 515 West Front Street, Missoula, MT 59802 · 406-721-5600

NEUROLOGICAL SURGERY

Billings

Eugen J. Dolan · General Neurological Surgery (Trauma) · Deaconess Medical Center Health System, Saint Vincent Hospital & Health Center · Billings

Clinic, 2825 Eighth Avenue, North, P.O. Box 35100, Billings, MT 59101 · 406-238-2500

Lashman W. Soriya · General Neurological Surgery (Microsurgery for Brain and Spinal Disorders, Pituitary Tumor Surgery, Radiofrequency Thermocoagulation for Tic Doloreaux) · Deaconess Medical Center Health System · Billings Clinic, 2825 Eighth Avenue, North, P.O. Box 35100, Billings, MT 59107-5100 · 406-238-2500

Great Falls

Howard Lee Finney III · General Neurological Surgery · 400 Fifteenth Avenue, South, Suite 103, Great Falls, MT 59405 · 406-727-4105

Dale M. Schaefer · General Neurological Surgery (Spinal Surgery, Tumor Surgery, Vascular Neurological Surgery) · Montana Deaconess Medical Center, Columbus Hospital · 1300 Twenty-Eighth Street, South, Suite Seven, Great Falls, MT 59405 · 406-454-0375

Missoula

Richard C. Dewey · General Neurological Surgery (Pediatric Neurosurgery, Spinal Surgery) · St. Patrick Hospital, Community Medical Center · Neurological Associates, 601 West Spruce Street, Suite E, Missoula, MT 59802 · 406-728-6520

Henry H. Gary · General Neurological Surgery · Neurological Associates, 601 West Spruce Street, Suite E, Missoula, MT 59802 · 406-728-6520

NEUROLOGY

Billings

Patrick J. Cahill · General Neurology · Deaconess Medical Center Health System, 2800 Tenth Avenue, North, P.O. Box 37000, Billings, MT 59107 · 406-256-2500

Roger S. Williams · General Neurology (Stroke, Multiple Sclerosis) · Deaconess Medical Center Health System · Deaconess Medical Center Health System, 2825 Eighth Avenue, North, Billings, MT 59101 · 406-238-2399

Great Falls

Dennis W. Dietrich · (Demyelinating Diseases, Degenerative Diseases, Electromyography) · Columbus Hospital, Montana Deaconess Medical Center · Columbus Professional Building, 400 Thirteenth Avenue, South, Suite 101, Great Falls, MT 59405 · 406-727-3720

Helena

Charles B. Anderson · General Neurology · St. Peter's Community Hospital, Neurology Services, 2475 Broadway, Helena, MT 59601 · 406-444-2288

Missoula

Stephen F. Johnson · General Neurology · Western Montana Clinic, 515 West Front Street, P.O. Box 7609, Missoula, MT 59807 · 406-721-5600 x238

NEUROLOGY, CHILD

Billings

Gail L. Kennedy · General Child Neurology · Deaconess Medical Center Health System, Saint Vincent Hospital & Health Center · Deaconess Medical Center Health System, 2800 Tenth Avenue, North, P.O. Box 37000, Billings, MT 59107 406-256-2500

Helena

Donald J. Wight · General Child Neurology (Epilepsy) · St. Peter's Community Hospital, Children's Neurology Center, 2475 Broadway, Helena, MT 59601 · 406-444-2288

OBSTETRICS & GYNECOLOGY

Billings

Danielle Emery · General Obstetrics & Gynecology · Billings Clinic, 2825 Eighth Avenue, North, P.O. Box 35100, Billings, MT 59107 · 406-238-2500

Douglas T. Ezell · (Infertility, Ultrasound) · Saint Vincent Hospital & Health Center, Deaconess Medical Center Health System · Billings OBGYN Associates, College Park Professional Center, Suite 202, 2520 Seventeenth Street, West, Billings, MT 59102 · 406-248-3607

James R. Harris · General Obstetrics & Gynecology · Deaconess Medical Center Health System, 2800 Tenth Avenue, North, P.O. Box 37000, Billings, MT 59107 406-256-2500

Daniel M. Molloy · General Obstetrics & Gynecology · 1239 North Broadway, Suite Six, Billings, MT 59101 · 406-245-4100

Thomas C. Olson · General Obstetrics & Gynecology (Genital Relaxation/Prolapse, Hysteroscopy, Urinary Incontinence) · Deaconess Medical Center Health System, Saint Vincent Hospital & Health Center · Billings Clinic, 2825 Eighth Avenue, North, P.O. Box 35100, Billings, MT 59107-5100 · 406-238-2500

Mark E. Randak · General Obstetrics & Gynecology · Billings Clinic, 2825 Eighth Avenue, North, P.O. Box 35100, Billings, MT 59101 · 406-238-2500

Great Falls

Peter L. Burleigh · General Obstetrics & Gynecology · Great Falls Clinic, 1400 Twenty-Ninth Street, South, P.O. Box 5012, Great Falls, MT 59403 · 406-454-2171

Marci J. Eck · General Obstetrics & Gynecology · 400 Thirteenth Avenue, South, Suite 104, Great Falls, MT 59405 · 406-452-9989

Robert J. McClure · General Obstetrics & Gynecology (Reproductive Endocrinology, Reproductive Surgery) · Montana Deaconess Medical Center, Columbus Hospital · Great Falls Clinic, 1400 Twenty-Ninth Street, South, P.O. Box 5012, Great Falls, MT 59403 · 406-454-2171

Helena

Jack W. McMahon, Jr. · General Obstetrics & Gynecology · Helena OBGYN Associates, 45 Medical Park Drive, Suite A, Helena, MT 59601 · 406-442-1914

Missoula

Craig W. McCoy · (High-Risk Obstetrics, Operative Laparoscopy) · Community Medical Center · Missoula Ob-Gyn Associates, Missoula Community Physicians Center, 2825 Fort Missoula Road, Missoula, MT 59801 · 406-728-8190

Stephen Dale Smith · General Obstetrics & Gynecology · Community Medical Center · 2825 Fort Missoula Road, Suite 115, Missoula, MT 59801 · 406-728-4292

OPHTHALMOLOGY

Billings

James S. Good · General Ophthalmology · Billings Clinic, Department of Ophthalmology, 2528 Eighth Avenue, North, Billings, MT 59101 · 406-238-2500

J. Thomas Priddy · General Ophthalmology · Billings Clinic, 2825 Eighth Avenue, North, P.O. Box 35100, Billings, MT 59107 · 406-238-2500

Great Falls

E. Gary Petersen · General Ophthalmology · 1300 Twenty-Eighth Street, South, Suite 10, Great Falls, MT 59405 · 406-761-5231

Helena

Richard J. Hopkins · General Ophthalmology · 121 North Last Chance Gulch, Helena, MT 59601 · 406-443-4040

Missoula

Richard W. Beighle · General Ophthalmology (Anterior Segment—Cataract & Refractive, Glaucoma) · Community Medical Center, St. Patrick Hospital · Rocky Mountain Eye & Ear Center, 700 West Kent, Missoula, MT 59801 · 406-728-3502

Paul K. Overland · General Ophthalmology · 715 Kensington Road, Suite 22, Missoula, MT 59801 · 406-543-3551

James G. Randall · (Small Incision Cataract Surgery, Vitreo-Retinal Surgery, Retinal Detachment, Diabetic Retinopathy) · Rocky Mountain Eye Surgery Center · Rocky Mountain Eye & Ear Center, 700 West Kent, Missoula, MT 59801-6700 · 406-728-3502

John D. Salisbury · General Ophthalmology · Rocky Mountain Eye & Ear Center, 700 West Kent, Missoula, MT 59801 · 406-728-3502

ORTHOPAEDIC SURGERY

Billings

Wheeler T. Daniels · General Orthopaedic Surgery (Total Joint Replacement) · Saint Vincent Hospital & Health Center · Orthopaedic Associates, Yellowstone Medical Building, Suite 100, 1145 North 29th Street, Billings, MT 59101 · 406-238-6700

James Tyson Lovitt · General Orthopaedic Surgery · Orthopaedic Surgeons, 1232 North 30th Street, Billings, MT 59101 · 406-245-3149

Robert S. Schultz · General Orthopaedic Surgery (Sports Medicine/Arthroscopy, Trauma) · Deaconess Medical Center Health System, Saint Vincent Hospital & Health Center · Billings Clinic, Orthopaedic Department, 2825 Eighth Avenue, North, P.O. Box 35100, Billings, MT 59107-5200 · 406-256-2633

Peter V. Teal · General Orthopaedic Surgery · Orthopaedic Surgeons, 1232 North 30th Street, Billings, MT 59101 · 406-245-3149

Great Falls

Paul M. Melvin · General Orthopaedic Surgery · Great Falls Orthopaedic Associates, Doctors Plaza, Suite 16, 2800 Eleventh Avenue, South, Great Falls, MT 59405 · 406-761-1410

Helena

Kenneth V. Carpenter · General Orthopaedic Surgery · Helena Orthopaedic Clinic, One Medical Park Drive, Helena, MT 59601 · 406-442-4811

M. Brooke Hunter · General Orthopaedic Surgery · St. Peter's Community Hospital · Orthopaedic Clinic, One Medical Park Drive, Helena, MT 59601 · 406-442-4811

Missoula

Patrick R. Robins · General Orthopaedic Surgery · Missoula Orthopedic Associates, 700 West Kent Avenue, Missoula, MT 59801 · 406-721-4233

Robert John Seim · General Orthopaedic Surgery · 700 West Kent Avenue, Missoula, MT 59801 · 406-721-4436

Michael A. Sousa · General Orthopaedic Surgery · 601 West Spruce Street, Suite C, Missoula, MT 59802 · 406-728-1498

OTOLARYNGOLOGY

Billings

Steven A. Butler · General Otolaryngology · Ear, Nose and Throat Associates, 1145 North 29th Street, Suite 401, Billings, MT 59101 · 406-252-5616

Gordon E. Henneford · General Otolaryngology · Ear, Nose and Throat Associates, 1145 North 29th Street, Suite 401, Billings, MT 59101 · 406-252-5616

Great Falls

John A. Schvaneveldt · General Otolaryngology · Great Falls Clinic, 1400 Twenty-Ninth Street, South, P.O. Box 5012, Great Falls, MT 59403 · 406-771-3423

Missoula

Daniel E. Braby · General Otolaryngology · Rocky Mountain Eye & Ear Center, 700 West Kent, Missoula, MT 59801 · 406-728-3506

Thomas C. Hoshaw · Otology (General Otolaryngology) · St. Patrick Hospital, Community Medical Center · Rocky Mountain Eye & Ear Center, 700 West Kent, Missoula, MT 59801-6700 · 406-728-3506

PATHOLOGY

Billings

Gordon L. Cox · General Pathology · 2800 Tenth Avenue, North, P.O. Box 37000, Billings, MT 59107-7000 · 406-657-4071

Charles C. Schirmer · General Pathology · Deaconess Medical Center Health System, 2800 Tenth Avenue, North, P.O. Box 37000, Billings, MT 59107 · 406-657-4069

Dennis D. Schreffler · General Pathology · Deaconess Medical Center Health System, 2800 Tenth Avenue, North, P.O. Box 37000, Billings, MT 59107 · 406-657-4069

Mark C. Sheiko · General Pathology · 2800 Tenth Avenue, North, P.O. Box 37000, Billings, MT 59107-7000 · 406-657-4070

Great Falls

John R. Henneford · General Pathology · Columbus Hospital, Pathology Department, 500 Fifteenth Avenue, South, P.O. Box 5013, Great Falls, MT 59403 · 406-727-3333

Cheryl M. Reichert · (Surgical Pathology, Breast Pathology, Blood Banking) · Columbus Hospital, Pathology Laboratory, 500 Fifteenth Avenue, South, Great Falls, MT 59405 · 406-771-5021

PEDIATRICS (GENERAL)

Billings

Frederick E. Gunville · Deaconess Medical Center Health System, 2800 Tenth Avenue, North, P.O. Box 37000, Billings, MT 59107 · 406-256-2500

Paul H. Kelker · Billings Clinic, 2825 Eighth Avenue, North, Billings, MT 59107 406-238-2308

Great Falls

Jack L. Haling · Great Falls Clinic, 1400 Twenty-Ninth Street, South, Great Falls, MT 59405 · 406-727-9777

Jeffrey P. Hinz · Great Falls Clinic, 1400 Twenty-Ninth Street, South, P.O. Box 5012, Great Falls, MT 59403 · 406-454-2171

Mark A. Underwood · (General Pediatrics, Neonatology) · Montana Deaconess Medical Center, Columbus Hospital · Great Falls Clinic, 400 Thirteenth Avenue, South, Suite 106, Great Falls, MT 59405 · 406-727-9777

Helena

John A. Reynolds · Helena Pediatric Clinic, 1122 North Montana Avenue, Helena, MT 59601 · 406-449-5563

Jeffrey H. Strickler · 1122 North Montana Avenue, Helena, MT 59601 · 406-449-5563

Missoula

Daniel A. Harper · 2825 Fort Missoula Road, Missoula, MT 59801 · 406-721-0858

PHYSICAL MEDICINE & REHABILITATION

Great Falls

James D. Hinde · General Physical Medicine & Rehabilitation (Pain Management, Electrodiagnostic Medicine) · Montana Deaconess Medical Center, Columbus Hospital · Montana Plains Rehabilitation, 1300 Twenty-Eighth Street, South, Suite 9A, Great Falls, MT 59405-5926 · 406-455-5490

Bill J. Tacke · General Physical Medicine & Rehabilitation (Electrodiagnostic Medicine, Pain Management) · Montana Deaconess Medical Center · Montana Plains Rehabilitation, 1300 Twenty-Eighth Street, South, Suite 9A, Great Falls, MT 59405-5296 · 406-455-5490

Helena

Allen M. Weinert, Jr. · General Physical Medicine & Rehabilitation · St. Peter's Community Hospital, Neurosciences Department, 2475 Broadway, Helena, MT 59601 · 406-444-2288

Missoula

Dean E. Ross · General Physical Medicine & Rehabilitation · 2825 Fort Missoula Road, Missoula, MT 59801 · 406-721-8441

PLASTIC SURGERY

Billings

Anthony Joseph De Angelis · General Plastic Surgery · 1020 North 27th Street, Suite 310, Billings, MT 59101 · 406-252-5700

Walter J. Peet · General Plastic Surgery · 1020 North 27th Street, Suite 400, Billings, MT 59101 · 406-245-3238

Great Falls

Christopher W. Conner · General Plastic Surgery · Great Falls Clinic, 1400 Twenty-Ninth Street, South, P.O. Box 5012, Great Falls, MT 59403 · 406-454-2171

John E. O'Connor · General Plastic Surgery · Montana Plastic Surgeons, 2519 Thirteenth Avenue, South, Great Falls, MT 59405 · 406-727-6544

Missoula

Donald E. Murray · General Plastic Surgery · 614 West Spruce Street, Missoula, MT 59802 · 406-728-3811

PSYCHIATRY

Billings

John T. Blodgett · Child & Adolescent Psychiatry · Deaconess Behavioral Health Clinic, Transwestern Building III, Suite 502, 550 North 31st Street, Billings, MT 59107 · 406-255-8550

Duncan D. Burford, Sr. · General Psychiatry · 2520 Seventeenth Street, West, Suite 103, Billings, MT 59102 · 406-252-6082

David B. Carlson · General Psychiatry (Psychopharmacology) · Deaconess Behavioral Health Clinic, Transwestern Building III, Suite 502, 550 North 31st Street, Billings, MT 59107 · 406-255-8550

Joseph D. Rich · General Psychiatry (Child & Adolescent Psychiatry, Forensic Psychiatry, Psychopharmacology) · Deaconess Psychiatric Center · Deaconess Psychiatric Center, 2800 Tenth Avenue, North, P.O. Box 37000, Billings, MT 59107-7000 · 406-657-3900

Thomas W. Van Dyke · General Psychiatry · Mental Health Center, 1245 North 29th Street, Billings, MT 59101 · 406-252-5658

Fort Harrison

H. Russell Sampley · General Psychiatry (Neuropsychiatry) · VA Medical Center VA Medical Center, Department of Veteran Affairs, Fort Harrison, MT 59636 · 406-442-6410

Great Falls

James L. Day · General Psychiatry (Community Psychiatry, Rural Psychiatry) · Montana Deaconess Medical Center · Cascade Counseling, 1300 Twenty-Eighth Street, South, Suite One, P.O. Box 3089, Great Falls, MT 59403 · 406-761-2100

Donald E. Engstrom · General Psychiatry (Mood & Anxiety Disorders, Psychopharmacology, Schizophrenia) · Montana Deaconess Medical Center · Great Falls Clinic, 1400 Twenty-Ninth Street, South, P.O. Box 5012, Great Falls, MT 59403 406-771-3450

Jeanne Garcia · General Psychiatry (Mood & Anxiety Disorders, Electroconvulsive Therapy) · Montana Deaconess Medical Center · Psychiatric Associates, 2800 Eleventh Avenue, South, Suite 23, Great Falls, MT 59405 · 406-771-1967

Jack D. Hornby · General Psychiatry · Cascade Counseling, 1300 Twenty-Eighth Street, South, Suite One, P.O. Box 3089, Great Falls, MT 59403 · 406-761-2100

Helena

Nanci-Ames Curtis · General Psychiatry · Behavioral Health Services, 50 South Last Chance Gulch, Suite Five, Helena, MT 59601 · 406-444-2233

William A. Fulton · General Psychiatry · Shodair Hospital, 840 Helena Avenue, P.O. Box 5539, Helena, MT 59604-5539 · 406-444-7500

Nathan A. Munn · General Psychiatry · 50 South Last Chance Gulch, Helena, MT 59601 · 406-444-2233

C. John Tupper, Jr. · General Psychiatry · Shodair Hospital, 840 Helena Avenue, P.O. Box 5539, Helena, MT 59604-5539 · 406-444-7557

Kalispell

Alan S. Quint · General Psychiatry (Mood & Anxiety Disorders) · Pathways Treatment Center, Kalispell Regional Hospital · 17 Second Street, East, Suite 205, Kalispell, MT 59901 · 406-755-3148

Missoula

Scott E. Elrod · General Psychiatry · Providence Offices, Providence Center, Suite S304, 900 North Orange, Missoula, MT 59802 · 406-728-2000

Noel L. Hoell · General Psychiatry (Mood & Anxiety Disorders, Psychopharmacology) · St. Patrick Hospital · 554 West Broadway, Suite 500, Missoula, MT 59802 · 406-721-6050

Michael J. Silverglat · General Psychiatry (Neuropsychiatry, Geriatric Psychiatry) St. Patrick Hospital · 554 West Broadway, Suite 500, Missoula, MT 59802 · 406-721-6050

Warm Springs

Virginia Lee Hill · General Psychiatry (Forensic Psychiatry, Schizophrenia) · Montana State Hospital · Montana State Hospital, Warm Springs, MT 59756 · 406-693-7000

PULMONARY & CRITICAL CARE MEDICINE

Billings

Walter R. Fairfax · General Pulmonary & Critical Care Medicine · Billings Clinic, 2825 Eighth Avenue, North, P.O. Box 35100, Billings, MT 59107 · 406-238-2500

Robert K. Merchant · General Pulmonary & Critical Care Medicine · Billings Clinic, 2825 Eighth Avenue, North, Billings, MT 59101 · 406-238-2500

R. James Rollins · General Pulmonary & Critical Care Medicine · Billings Clinic, 2825 Eighth Avenue, North, P.O. Box 35100, Billings, MT 59107 · 406-238-2500

Nicholas J. Wolter · General Pulmonary & Critical Care Medicine · Billings Clinic, 2825 Eighth Avenue, North, P.O. Box 35100, Billings, MT 59107 · 406-238-2500

Great Falls

Richard Dyer Blevins · General Pulmonary & Critical Care Medicine (Asthma, Bronchology) · Montana Deaconess Medical Center, Columbus Hospital · Great Falls Clinic, 1400 Twenty-Ninth Street, South, P.O. Box 5012, Great Falls, MT 59403 · 406-454-2171

Missoula

William B. Bekemeyer · General Pulmonary & Critical Care Medicine · Western Montana Clinic, 515 West Front Street, Missoula, MT 59807 · 406-721-5600

Shull Lemire · General Pulmonary & Critical Care Medicine · St. Patrick Hospital, Community Medical Center · 2825 Fort Missoula Road, Suite 317, Missoula, MT 59801 · 406-721-8608

C. Paul Loehnen · General Pulmonary & Critical Care Medicine · 601 West Spruce Street, Suite F, Missoula, MT 59802 · 406-728-5324

RADIATION ONCOLOGY

Billings

Frank R. Lamm · General Radiation Oncology · Northern Rockies Regional Cancer Treatment Center, 1041 North 29th Street, P.O. Box 369, Billings, MT 59103 · 406-248-2212

John Terry · General Radiation Oncology · Deaconess Medical Center Health System, Saint Vincent Hospital & Health Center · Northern Rockies Regional Cancer Treatment Center, 1041 North 29th Street, P.O. Box 369, Billings, MT 59103-0369 · 406-248-2212

Great Falls

Robert D. Pfeffer · General Radiation Oncology · Columbus Hospital, Radiation Oncology Department, 500 Fifteenth Avenue, South, Great Falls, MT 59405 · 406-727-3333

Carl R. Shonk · General Radiation Oncology · Columbus Hospital, Radiation Oncology Department, 500 Fifteenth Avenue, South, Great Falls, MT 59405 · 406-727-3333

Missoula

Katherine L. Markette · General Radiation Oncology · St. Patrick Hospital, 325 Owen Street, Missoula, MT 59802 · 406-542-0341

RADIOLOGY

Billings

Douglas G. Bell · General Radiology (Diagnostic Radiology, Neuroradiology, Magnetic Resonance Imaging) · Deaconess Medical Center Health System · Deaconess Medical Center Health System, Radiology Department, 2800 Tenth Avenue, North, P.O. Box 37000, Billings, MT 59107 · 406-657-4190

Wiley R. Bland · General Radiology · Eastern Radiology, 1145 North 29th Street, Suite 500, Billings, MT 59101 · 406-259-5521

Dean A. Bruschwein · General Radiology · Deaconess Medical Center Health System, 1108 North 27th Street, Billings, MT 59107 · 406-657-4190

Lawrence L. Herbert · General Radiology (Diagnostic Radiology) · Deaconess Medical Center Health System · Deaconess Medical Center Health System, Radiology Department, 2800 Tenth Avenue, North, Billings, MT 59107 · 406-657-4190

Daniel Mitchell · General Radiology · P.O. Box 1524, Billings, MT 59103 · 406-252-2305

Jerry Dane Wolf · General Radiology · 1108 North 27th Street, P.O. Box 1524, Billings, MT 59103 · 406-252-2305

Great Falls

John C. Hackethorn · General Radiology · Columbus Hospital, 500 Fifteenth Avenue, South, Great Falls, MT 59405 · 406-771-5146

Helena

Dennis L. Palmer · General Radiology · St. Peter's Community Hospital, 2475 Broadway, Helena, MT 59601 · 406-444-2300

Missoula

Sarsfield P. Dougherty · General Radiology (Vascular & Interventional Radiology) · St. Patrick Hospital, Community Medical Center · Missoula Radiology, 3205 Russell Street, P.O. Box 2039, Missoula, MT 59806 · 406-721-4906

Thomas A. Layne · General Radiology · St. Patrick Hospital, Department of Radiology, 500 West Broadway, Missoula, MT 59802 · 406-543-7271

Albert R. Ward · General Radiology · Missoula Radiology, 3205 Russell Street, P.O. Box 2039, Missoula, MT 59806 · 406-721-4906

RHEUMATOLOGY

Billings

Susan C. English · General Rheumatology (Systemic Lupus, Osteoporosis) · Deaconess Medical Center Health System, Saint Vincent Hospital & Health Center · Billings Clinic, 2825 Eighth Avenue, North, P.O. Box 35100, Billings, MT 59107-5100 · 406-238-2500

Phillip E. Griffin, Jr. · General Rheumatology · Billings Clinic, 2825 Eighth Avenue, North, P.O. Box 35100, Billings, MT 59101 · 406-238-2404

Great Falls

Elton J. Adams · General Rheumatology · Big Sky Health Care, 400 Thirteenth Avenue, South, Suite 203, Great Falls, MT 59405 · 406-727-4584

Missoula

Margaret R. Schlesinger · General Rheumatology · Western Montana Clinic, 515 West Front Street, P.O. Box 7609, Missoula, MT 59807 · 406-721-5600 x245

SURGERY

Billings

Dennistoun Brown · Pediatric Surgery · Deaconess Medical Center Health System, 2800 Tenth Avenue, North, P.O. Box 37000, Billings, MT 59107 · 406-256-2500

John H. Cook · General Surgery · Surgical Associates, 1230 North 30th Street, Suite A, Billings, MT 59101 · 406-252-8494

John R. Gregory · General Surgery · Billings Clinic, 2825 Eighth Avenue, North, P.O. Box 35100, Billings, MT 59107-5100 · 406-238-2500

Paul F. Grmoljez · General Surgery · Billings Clinic, 2825 Eighth Avenue, North, P.O. Box 35100, Billings, MT 59101 · 406-238-2325

Terry A. Housinger · General Surgery · Billings Clinic, 2825 Eighth Avenue, North, P.O. Box 35100, Billings, MT 59107 · 406-238-2500

John D. Middleton · General Surgery (General Vascular Surgery, General Thoracic Surgery) · Saint Vincent Hospital & Health Center, Deaconess Medical Center Health System · Surgical Associates, 1230 North 30th Street, Suite A, Billings, MT 59101-0176 · 406-252-8494

Bozeman

Charles F. Rinker · General Surgery (Trauma) · Bozeman Deaconess Hospital · Surgical Associates of Bozeman, 925 Highland Boulevard, Suite 2200, Bozeman, MT 59715 · 406-587-0704

Great Falls

William R. McGregor · General Surgery (General Surgical Oncology, General Colon & Rectal Surgery) · Columbus Hospital, Montana Deaconess Medical Center · Prospect Heights Medical Center, 401 Fifteenth Avenue, South, Suite 206, Great Falls, MT 59405 · 406-761-6611

James E. Mungus · General Vascular Surgery (General Surgery) · Montana Deaconess Medical Center, Columbus Hospital · Great Falls Clinic, 1400 Twenty-Ninth Street, South, P.O. Box 5012, Great Falls, MT 59403 · 406-771-3000

Michael B. Orcutt · General Surgery · Great Falls Clinic, 1400 Twenty-Nine Street, South, P.O. Box 5012, Great Falls, MT 59403 · 406-454-2171

Helena

Dale G. Johnson · General Surgery · Medical Park Surgical Clinic, 400 Saddle Drive, Helena, MT 59601 · 406-442-0099

Missoula

Lori A. Grimsley · General Surgery · 900 North Orange Street, Suite 107, Missoula, MT 59802 · 406-542-7525

David M. Hayes · General Surgery (Head & Neck Surgery) · Rocky Mountain Eye & Ear Center, 700 West Kent, Missoula, MT 59801 · 406-728-3506

J. Bradley Pickardt · General Surgery (Breast Surgery, Gastroenterologic Surgery, General Vascular Surgery, Trauma, General Surgical Oncology, General Thoracic Surgery) · Western Montana Clinic, 515 West Front Street, P.O. Box 7609, Missoula, MT 59807 · 406-721-5600

Charles J. Swannack · General Surgery · Western Montana Clinic, 515 West Front Street, P.O. Box 7609, Missoula, MT 59807 · 406-721-5600

THORACIC SURGERY

Billings

Hewes D. Agnew · General Thoracic Surgery · Billings Clinic, 2825 Eighth Avenue, North, P.O. Box 35100, Billings, MT 59101 · 406-238-2321

Timothy A. Dernbach · General Thoracic Surgery (General Vascular Surgery, Adult Cardiothoracic Surgery) · Saint Vincent Hospital & Health Center · 1145 North 29th Street, Suite 305, Billings, MT 59101 · 406-238-6820

J. Scott Millikan · General Thoracic Surgery (General Vascular Surgery, Adult Cardiothoracic Surgery) · Deaconess Medical Center Health System · Billings Clinic, 2825 Eighth Avenue, North, P.O. Box 35100, Billings, MT 59107-5100 · 406-238-2500

Robert J. Wilmouth · Adult Cardiothoracic Surgery (General Thoracic Surgery, General Vascular Surgery, Thoracic Oncological Surgery) · Deaconess Medical Center Health System, Saint Vincent Hospital & Health Center · Billings Clinic, 2825 Eighth Avenue, North, P.O. Box 35100, Billings, MT 59107 · 406-238-2500

Helena

Dale G. Johnson · General Thoracic Surgery · Medical Park Surgical Clinic, 400 Saddle Drive, Helena, MT 59601 · 406-442-0099

UROLOGY

Billings

Robert E. Cadoff · General Urology · 1145 North 29th Street, Suite 503, Billings, MT 59101 · 406-256-7102

Lawrence W. Klee · General Urology (Pediatric Urology, Urologic Oncology) · Billings Clinic, 2825 Eighth Avenue, North, P.O. Box 35100, Billings, MT 59107-5100 · 406-238-2449

Richard B. Melzer · General Urology · Billings Clinic, 2825 Eighth Avenue, North, P.O. Box 35100, Billings, MT 59101 · 406-238-2500

C. Dale Vermillion · General Urology (Pediatric Urology) · Billings Clinic, 2825 Eighth Avenue, North, P.O. Box 35100, Billings, MT 59107-5100 · 406-238-2500

Great Falls

James C. Bull · General Urology · 400 Fifteenth Avenue, South, Great Falls, MT 59405 · 406-452-9546

W. Peter Horst · General Urology · Great Falls Clinic, 1400 Twenty-Ninth Street, South, P.O. Box 5012, Great Falls, MT 59403 · 406-454-2171

Helena

Ronald Mow · General Urology · St. Peter's Community Hospital · 65 Medical Park Drive, Helena, MT 59601 · 406-442-2113

Vern G. Tolstedt · General Urology · 65 Medical Park Drive, Helena, MT 59601 406-442-3550

Missoula

David E. Guth · General Urology (Impotence, Pediatric Urology) · St. Patrick Hospital, Missoula Community Hospital, Marcus Daly Memorial Hospital (Hamilton) · Urology Associates, 601 West Spruce Street, Missoula, MT 59802 · 406-728-3366

Roger S. Munro · General Urology (Neuro-Urology & Voiding Dysfunction, Urologic Oncology, Endourology, Impotence) · St. Patrick Hospital, Community Medical Center · Missoula Medical Plaza, Suite 206, 900 North Orange Street, Missoula, MT 59802 · 406-543-1967

Byron C. Olson · General Urology · Urology Associates, 601 West Spruce Street, Missoula, MT 59802 · 406-728-3366

NEBRASKA

ALLERGY & IMMUNOLOGY

Lincoln

Melvin Hoffman · General Allergy & Immunology · Allergy, Asthma & Immunology Associates, Gateway Professional Building, Suite 208, 600 North Cotner Boulevard, Lincoln, NE 68505 · 402-464-5969

Frederic Kiechel III · General Allergy & Immunology (Asthma, Chronic Infection) · Bryan Memorial Hospital, St. Elizabeth Community Health Center, Lincoln General Hospital · Allergy, Asthma & Immunology Associates, Gateway Professional Building, Suite 208, 600 North Cotner Boulevard, Lincoln, NE 68505 402-464-5969

Omaha

Russell J. Hopp · General Allergy & Immunology (Pediatric Allergy & Immunology, Immunodeficiency) · St. Joseph Hospital, Children's Hospital · Creighton University, Department of Pediatrics, 601 North 30th Street, Suite 6820, Omaha, NE 68131 · 402-280-4580

Roger Kobayashi · General Allergy & Immunology, Immunodeficiency (AIDS) · Children's Hospital, Archbishop Bergan Mercy Medical Center, UCLA Medical Center (Los Angeles, CA) · Allergy, Asthma, and Immunology Associates, 2808 South 80th Avenue, Omaha, NE 68124 · 402-391-1800

Kevin R. Murphy · General Allergy & Immunology · Midwest Allergy & Asthma Clinic, 8552 Cass Street, Omaha, NE 68114 · 402-397-7400

Thomas C. Nilsson · General Allergy & Immunology · Midwest Allergy & Asthma Clinic, 8552 Cass Street, Omaha, NE 68114 · 402-397-7400

Robert G. Townley · General Allergy & Immunology (Asthma, Internal Medicine, Bronchial Hyperresponsiveness) · St. Joseph Hospital, VA Medical Center · Creighton University School of Medicine, 2500 California Plaza, Omaha, NE 68178 · 402-280-4180

Mark C. Wilson · General Allergy & Immunology (Pediatric Allergy & Immunology) · Children's Hospital, Department of Pediatric Pulmonology, 8301 Dodge Street, Omaha, NE 68114 · 402-390-5624

Papillion

Thomas B. Casale · General Allergy & Immunology (Asthma) · Asthma & Allergy Center, 410 East Gold Coast Road, Suite 326, Papillion, NE 68128 · 402-592-2055

CARDIOVASCULAR DISEASE

Lincoln

Christopher C. Caudill · General Cardiovascular Disease (Interventional Cardiology, Preventative Cardiology, Heart Failure, Transplantation Medicine) · Bryan Memorial Hospital, Lincoln General Hospital, St. Elizabeth Community Health Center · Cardiology Consultants, 1500 South 48th Street, Suite 800, Lincoln, NE 68506 · 402-489-6554

Joseph R. Gard · General Cardiovascular Disease · Nebraska Heart Institute, 1500 South 48th Street, Suite 800, Lincoln, NE 68506-5248 · 402-489-6554

Charles S. Wilson · General Cardiovascular Disease (Cardiac Catheterization, Echocardiography, Clinical Exercise Testing, Pacemakers) · Bryan Memorial Hospital · Nebraska Heart Institute, 1500 South 48th Street, Suite 800, Lincoln, NE 68506 · 402-489-6554

Omaha

Thomas R. Brandt · General Cardiovascular Disease · Omaha Cardiovascular Center, 8901 West Dodge Road, Omaha, NE 68114 · 402-393-6588

Maria-Teresa Olivari · Transplantation Medicine, Heart Failure (Post-Heart Transplantation Care, Congestive Heart Failure, Cardiac Rehabilitation, Clinical Exercise Testing) · University of Nebraska Medical Center · University of Nebraska Medical Center, Department of Internal Medicine, Cardiology Division,

600 South 42nd Street, Room UH 6162, Box 982265, Omaha, NE 68198-2265 · 402-559-5151

CLINICAL PHARMACOLOGY

Lincoln

Leslie A. Spry · Wedgewood Medical Center, 1919 South 40th Street, Suite 104, Lincoln, NE 68502-5755 · 402-488-6750

COLON & RECTAL SURGERY

Omaha

Garnet J. Blatchford · General Colon & Rectal Surgery · Archbishop Bergan Mercy Medical Center, Immanuel Medical Center, Nebraska Methodist Hospital, St. Joseph Hospital, Midlands Community Hospital (Papillion), University of Nebraska Medical Center, Bishop Clarkson Memorial Hospital, Children's Hospital · 711 Professional Tower, 105 South 17th Street, Omaha, NE 68102-1401 · 402-344-7666

Mark A. Christensen · General Colon & Rectal Surgery (Colon & Rectal Cancer, Inflammatory Bowel Disease) · Immanuel Medical Center, Archbishop Bergan Mercy Medical Center, Nebraska Methodist Hospital, St. Joseph Hospital, Midlands Community Hospital (Papillion), Bishop Clarkson Memorial Hospital · 711 Professional Tower, 105 South 17th Street, Omaha, NE 68102 · 402-344-7666

Alan G. Thorson · General Colon & Rectal Surgery, Colon & Rectal Cancer · Nebraska Methodist Hospital, St. Joseph Hospital, Immanuel Medical Center, Archbishop Bergan Mercy Medical Center, Bishop Clarkson Memorial Hospital, University of Nebraska Medical Center, Midlands Community Hospital (Papillion), Children's Hospital · 711 Professional Tower, 105 South 17th Street, Omaha, NE 68102 · 402-344-7666

DERMATOLOGY

Lincoln

Rodney Steven W. Basler · Clinical Dermatology · South Lincoln Dermatology Group, 2625 Stockwell Street, Lincoln, NE 68502-5755 · 402-421-3335

David A. Bigler · Clinical Dermatology (Dermatologic Oncology) · Gateway Dermatologic Surgeons, 600 North Cotner Boulevard, Suite 311, Lincoln, NE 68505 402-467-4361

Ann E. B. Lott · Clinical Dermatology · Gateway Dermatologic Surgeons, 600 North Cotner Boulevard, Suite 311, Lincoln, NE 68505 · 402-467-4361

Robyn Gembol Ryan · Clinical Dermatology (Skin Cancer Surgery & Reconstruction, Laser Surgery) · St. Elizabeth Community Health Center · Sutton Ryan Dermatology, 1710 South 70th Street, Lincoln, NE 68506-1601 · 402-483-7700

Margaret Kontras Sutton · Clinical Dermatology (Aging Skin, Skin Cancer Surgery & Reconstruction) · St. Elizabeth Community Health Center · Sutton Ryan Dermatology, 1710 South 70th Street, P.O. Box 6068, Lincoln, NE 68506-0068 · 402-483-7700

Stuart P. Westburg · Clinical Dermatology (Acne, Geriatric Dermatology) · Lincoln General Hospital, Bryan Memorial Hospital, St. Elizabeth Community Health Center · Lincoln Dermatology Clinic, 2756 O Street, Lincoln, NE 68510-1341 · 402-474-4497

Omaha

Suzanne W. Braddock · Clinical Dermatology · Braddock Dermatology, Westgate Professional Center, 2808 South 80th Avenue, Omaha, NE 68124-3253 · 402-390-0333

ENDOCRINOLOGY & METABOLISM

Lincoln

Monte M. Scott · General Endocrinology & Metabolism · Wedgewood Medical Center, 120 Wedgewood Drive, Lincoln, NE 68510 · 402-489-8821

Omaha

Timothy O. Wahl · General Endocrinology & Metabolism (Diabetes, Thyroid) · Bishop Clarkson Memorial Hospital, Nebraska Methodist Hospital · Internal Medicine Associates, Doctor's Building, North Tower, Room 650, 4242 Farnam Street, Omaha, NE 68131-2850 · 402-552-2600

FAMILY MEDICINE

Bellevue

Daniel E. Halm · University Medical Associates, 3604 Summit Plaza, Bellevue, NE 68124-2138 · 402-595-2275

Elkhorn

William P. Fitzgibbons · Skyline Medical Center, 20845 West Dodge Road, Elkhorn, NE 68022 · 402-289-4031

Lincoln

Jon Joy Hinrichs · Holmes Lake Family Health Center, 6900 Van Dorn Road, Suite 24, Lincoln, NE 68506-2882 · 402-489-3200

Dale E. Michels · (Geriatric Medicine) · Bryan Memorial Hospital, St. Elizabeth Community Health Center · Lincoln Family Medical Group, 7441 O Street, Suite 400, Lincoln, NE 68510-2468 · 402-488-7400

Omaha

Timothy Raymond Malloy · (Geriatric Medicine) · University of Nebraska Medical Center, Department of Family Medicine, 600 South 42nd Street, Omaha, NE 68198-9350 · 402-559-7200

Morris B. Mellion · (Sports Medicine) · Nebraska Methodist Hospital, Children's Hospital, University of Nebraska Medical Center · Sports Medicine Center, 2255 South 132nd Street, Omaha, NE 68144-2501 · 402-333-0303

Michael A. Sitorius · (Adolescent Medicine, Sports Medicine, Obesity) · University of Nebraska Medical Center, Department of Family Medicine, 600 South 42nd Street, Omaha, NE 68198-3075 · 402-559-5279

GASTROENTEROLOGY

Lincoln

David R. Dyke · General Gastroenterology · Bryan Memorial Hospital, Lincoln General Hospital, St. Elizabeth Community Health Center · Gastroenterology Specialties, 1500 South 48th Street, Suite 712, Lincoln, NE 68506-5243 · 402-489-8444

Omaha

Michael F. Sorrell · Hepatology · University of Nebraska Medical Center · University of Nebraska Medical Center, 600 South 42nd Street, Omaha, NE 68198-2000 · 402-559-7912

GERIATRIC MEDICINE

Omaha

Catherine M. Eberle · (Geriatric Rehabilitation) · University of Nebraska Medical Center · University of Nebraska Medical Center, Department of Geriatrics, 600 South 42nd Street, Box 985620, Omaha, NE 68198-5620 · 402-559-4427

Thomas V. Jones · University of Nebraska Medical Center, 600 South 42nd Street, Omaha, NE 68198-5620 · 402-559-7512

Brenda Keller · University of Nebraska Medical Center, 600 South 42nd Street, Omaha, NE 68198-5620 · 402-559-4427

Jane F. Potter · University of Nebraska Medical Center · University of Nebraska Medical Center, 600 South 42nd Street, Box 985620, Omaha, NE 68198-5620 · 402-559-4427

Susan G. Scholer · Omaha Internal Medicine Physicians, 808 South 52nd Street, Omaha, NE 68106-1802 · 402-551-8900

Monica R. Vandivort · (Optimizing Functional Status, Quality of Life Issues) · University of Nebraska Medical Center, VA Medical Center · University of Nebraska Medical Center, 600 South 42nd Street, Omaha, NE 68198 · 402-559-4427

HAND SURGERY

Lincoln

William F. Garvin · General Hand Surgery · Bryan Memorial Hospital, Lincoln General Hospital, St. Elizabeth Community Health Center · Nebraska Orthopaedic Associates, 6940 Van Dorn Road, Lincoln, NE 68506 · 402-488-3322

Omaha

Robert M. Cochran · General Hand Surgery · Orthopaedic Surgeons, 8300 Dodge Street, Suite 320, Omaha, NE 68114 · 402-393-2525

INFECTIOUS DISEASE

Lincoln

Richard A. Morin · General Infectious Disease · 1919 South 40th Street, Suite 214, Lincoln, NE 68506-5247 · 402-489-1110

Omaha

Edward A. Dominguez · General Infectious Disease (Herpes Virus Infections, Transplantation Infections) · University of Nebraska Medical Center · University of Nebraska Medical Center, Department of Infectious Disease, 600 South 42nd Street, Omaha, NE 68198-5400 · 402-559-8650

Laurel C. Preheim · General Infectious Disease · St. Joseph Hospital, University of Nebraska Medical Center · VA Medical Center, 4101 Woolworth Avenue, Omaha, NE 68105-1873 · 402-449-0650

INTERNAL MEDICINE (GENERAL)

Lincoln

Arthur S. Annin · Antelope Creek Physicians, 2200 South 40th Street, Suite 104, Lincoln, NE 68506 · 402-489-5577

Jeffery A. Grubbe · Wedgewood Medical Center, 120 Wedgewood Drive, Lincoln, NE 68510 · 402-489-8821

Robert L. Haag · East Lincoln Internal Medicine, 1101 South 70th Street, Suite 100, Lincoln, NE 68510 · 402-483-2926

Timothy J. Stivrins · East Lincoln Internal Medicine, 1101 South 70th Street, Suite 100, Lincoln, NE 68510 · 402-483-2926

Omaha

Steven T. Bailey · Internal Medicine Midwest, 525 North 132nd Street, Suite 225, Omaha, NE 68154-4043 · 402-496-2800

T. J. Holmes · Omaha Internal Medicine Physicians, 808 South 52nd Street, Omaha, NE 68106-1802 · 402-551-8900

David V. O'Dell · (General Internal Medicine, General Family Practice) · University of Nebraska Medical Center, VA Medical Center · University of Nebraska Medical Center, Department of Internal Medicine, 600 South 42nd Street, Omaha, NE 68198-3331 · 402-559-7299

Richard K. Osterholm · (Cerebral Vascular Disease, Thrombotic Disorders) · Bishop Clarkson Memorial Hospital, University of Nebraska Medical Center · Internal Medicine Associates, Doctor's Building, North Tower, Room 650, 4242 Farnam Street, Omaha, NE 68131 · 402-552-2600

Susan G. Scholer · Omaha Internal Medicine Physicians, 808 South 52nd Street, Omaha, NE 68106-1802 · 402-551-8900

Edward J. Taylor · Internal Medicine Associates, Doctor's Building, North Tower, Room 650, 4242 Farnam Street, Omaha, NE 68131 · 402-552-2600

MEDICAL ONCOLOGY & HEMATOLOGY

Lincoln

Daniel F. Moravec, Jr. · General Medical Oncology & Hematology · Wedgewood Medical Center, 120 Wedgewood Drive, Lincoln, NE 68510-2482 · 402-489-8821

Omaha

James O. Armitage · Bone Marrow Transplantation, Lymphomas · University of Nebraska Medical Center, Department of Internal Medicine, 600 South 42nd Street, Omaha, NE 68198-3332 · 402-559-7290

Philip J. Bierman · Lymphomas (Bone Marrow Transplantation) · University of Nebraska Medical Center · University of Nebraska Medical Center, Department of Internal Medicine, 600 South 42nd Street, Box 983330, Omaha, NE 68198-3330 · 402-559-5520

Michael R. Bishop · Leukemia (Bone Marrow Transplantation) · University of Nebraska Medical Center, Department of Internal Medicine, 600 South 42nd Street, Omaha, NE 68198 · 402-559-6000

John F. Foley · Breast Cancer (Lung Cancer) · University of Nebraska Medical Center · University of Nebraska Medical Center, 600 South 42nd Street, Box 983330, Omaha, NE 68198-3330 · 402-559-6313

William D. Haire · Disorders of Bleeding, Thrombosis (Thrombotic Disorders) · University of Nebraska Medical Center · University of Nebraska College of Medicine, 600 South 42nd Street, Box 983330, Omaha, NE 68198-3330 · 402-559-7599

Anne Kessinger · Breast Cancer (Bone Marrow Transplantation, General Medical Oncology & Hematology, Gynecologic Cancer) · University of Nebraska Medical Center · University of Nebraska Medical Center, Department of Oncology/Hematology, 600 South 42nd Street, Box 983330, Omaha, NE 68198-3330 · 402-559-5170

Elizabeth C. Reed · Breast Cancer · University of Nebraska Medical Center, Department of Internal Medicine, 600 South 42nd Street, Omaha, NE 68105-3330 · 402-559-5600

Margaret Tempero · Gastrointestinal Cancer · University of Nebraska Medical Center · University of Nebraska Medical Center, Department of Internal Medicine, 600 South 42nd Street, Box 986805, Omaha, NE 68198-6805 · 402-559-7081

Julie M. Vose · Lymphomas · University of Nebraska Medical Center, Department of Internal Medicine, 600 South 42nd Street, Box 983330, Omaha, NE 68198-3330 · 402-559-5166

NEPHROLOGY

Lincoln

Scott P. Liggett · General Nephrology (Cardiac Transplantation) · Bryan Memorial Hospital · Consultative Nephrology, First Tier Building, Suite 407, 100 North 56th Street, Lincoln, NE 68504 · 402-466-8259

Leslie A. Spry · General Nephrology · Wedgewood Medical Center, 1919 South 40th Street, Suite 104, Lincoln, NE 68506 · 402-488-6750

Omaha

Michael D. Hammeke · General Nephrology (Dialysis, Kidney Disease) · University of Nebraska Medical Center · University of Nebraska Medical Center, 600 South 42nd Street, Box 983040, Omaha, NE 68198-3040 · 402-559-9293

NEUROLOGICAL SURGERY

Lincoln

Benjamin R. Gelber · General Neurological Surgery · 1500 South 48th Street, Suite 511, Lincoln, NE 68502-3763 · 402-488-3002

Eric W. Pierson · General Neurological Surgery · 1500 South 48th Street, Suite 511, Lincoln, NE 68502-3763 · 402-475-4948

NEUROLOGY

Lincoln

Lewiston W. Birkmann · General Neurology · Neurology Associates, 1530 South 70th Street, Suite 201, Lincoln, NE 68506 · 402-483-7226

David L. Smith · General Neurology (Parkinson's Disease) · Bryan Memorial Hospital, Lincoln General Hospital, St. Elizabeth Community Health Center · Neurology Associates, 1530 South 70th Street, Suite 201, Lincoln, NE 68506 · 402-483-7226

Omaha

Rifaat M. Bashir · General Neurology (Neuro-Oncology) · University of Nebraska Medical Center · University of Nebraska Medical Center, Department of Internal Medicine, 600 South 42nd Street, Box 982045, Omaha, NE 68198-2045 · 402-559-4496

Richard H. Legge · Neuro-Ophthalmology (Pediatric Ophthalmology) · Archbishop Bergan Mercy Medical Center, Bishop Clarkson Memorial Hospital, Boys Town National Research Hospital, Douglas County Hospital, Immanuel Medical Center, Children's Hospital, Methodist Richard Young Hospital, Nebraska Methodist Hospital, St. Joseph Hospital, University of Nebraska Medical Center, VA Medical Center · 7810 Davenport Street, Omaha, NE 68114 · 402-397-1815

NEUROLOGY, CHILD

Omaha

Richard D. Torkelson · (Pediatric and Adult Epilepsy) · University of Nebraska Medical Center, Children's Hospital · University of Nebraska Medical Center, Division of Neurology, 600 South 42nd Street, Box 982045, Omaha, NE 68198-2045 · 402-559-4193

NUCLEAR MEDICINE

Omaha

Glenn V. Dalrymple · General Nuclear Medicine · University of Nebraska Medical Center · University of Nebraska Medical Center, 600 South 42nd Street, Omaha, NE 68198-1045 · 402-559-5280

OBSTETRICS & GYNECOLOGY

Lincoln

Stephen G. Swanson · General Obstetrics & Gynecology (Urogynecology, Pelvic Prolapse, Reproductive Endocrinology, Laparoscopic Surgery) · Bryan Memorial Hospital, St. Elizabeth Community Health Center, Lincoln General Hospital · Women's Clinic of Lincoln, 220 Lyncrest Drive, Lincoln, NE 68510 · 402-434-3382

Omaha

Murray J. Casey · Gynecologic Oncology · Creighton University Women's Health Center, St. Joseph Hospital · Creighton University, Women's Health Center, 601 North 30th Street, Suite 4700, Omaha, NE 68131 · 402-280-4440

OPHTHALMOLOGY

Lincoln

Gregory E. Sutton · General Ophthalmology · Eye Surgical Associates, 1710 South 70th Street, Lincoln, NE 68506 · 402-489-8838

Larry W. Wood · General Ophthalmology · Eye Surgical Associates, 1710 South 70th Street, Lincoln, NE 68506 · 402-489-8838

Omaha

Carl B. Camras · Glaucoma · University of Nebraska Medical Center · University of Nebraska Medical Center, 600 South 42nd Street, Box 985540, Omaha, NE 68198-5540 · 402-559-4276

Michael A. Halsted · Anterior Segment—Cataract & Refractive (Corneal Disease) Eye Physicians of Omaha, 4353 Dodge Street, Omaha, NE 68131 · 402-552-2020

Peter J. Whitted · General Ophthalmology (Anterior Segment—Cataract & Refractive, Corneal Diseases & Transplantation) · Bishop Clarkson Memorial Hospital, Nebraska Methodist Hospital, Immanuel Medical Center, Children's Hospital, Archbishop Bergan Mercy Medical Center · Eye Physicians of Omaha, 4353 Dodge Street, Omaha, NE 68131-2709 · 402-552-2020

ORTHOPAEDIC SURGERY

Lincoln

Patrick E. Clare · Sports Medicine/Arthroscopy · Nebraska Orthopaedic Associates, 6940 Van Dorn Road, Lincoln, NE 68506 · 402-488-3322

William F. Garvin · General Orthopaedic Surgery (General Hand Surgery, Foot & Ankle Surgery) · Bryan Memorial Hospital, Lincoln General Hospital, St. Elizabeth Community Health Center · Nebraska Orthopaedic Associates, 6940 Van Dorn Road, Lincoln, NE 68506 · 402-488-3322

David P. Heiser · General Orthopaedic Surgery · Nebraska Orthopaedic Associates, 6940 Van Dorn Road, Lincoln, NE 68506 · 402-488-3322

Omaha

Robert M. Cochran · General Orthopaedic Surgery · Orthopaedic Surgeons, 8300 Dodge Street, Suite 320, Omaha, NE 68114 · 402-393-2525

Timothy C. Fitzgibbons · Foot & Ankle Surgery · Alegent Health Memorial Hospital (Schuyler), Archbishop Bergan Mercy Medical Center · 7710 Mercy Road, Suite 224, Omaha, NE 68124 · 402-399-8550

Kevin L. Garvin · (Hip Surgery, Knee Surgery, Reconstructive Surgery) · University of Nebraska Medical Center · University of Nebraska Medical Center, Department of Orthopaedic Surgery, 600 South 42nd Street, Box 981080, Omaha, NE 68198-1080 · 402-559-4375

James R. Neff · Tumor Surgery (Musculoskeletal Oncologic Surgery, Musculoskeletal Pathology, Adult Reconstructive Surgery, Trauma) · University of Nebraska Medical Center · University of Nebraska Medical Center, 600 South 42nd Street, Omaha, NE 68198-1080 · 402-559-8000

OTOLARYNGOLOGY

Lincoln

Michael F. Rapp · General Otolaryngology · St. Elizabeth Community Health Center, Bryan Memorial Hospital, Lincoln General Hospital, Tri-County Area Hospital (Lexington) · Associated Ear, Nose & Throat Surgeons, 1530 South 70th Street, Lincoln, NE 68506 · 402-489-2266

F. Edward Stivers · General Otolaryngology · Ear, Nose and Throat Specialists, 5440 South Street, Suite 1100, Lincoln, NE 68506-2116 · 402-488-5600

Omaha

Patrick E. Brookhouser · Pediatric Otolaryngology (Otology) · Boys Town National Research Hospital · Boys Town National Research Hospital, 555 North 30th Street, Omaha, NE 68131-2136 · 402-498-6540

Britt A. Thedinger · Otology/Neurotology (Cochlear Implants, Medical & Surgical Treatment of Adult & Pediatric Hearing Impairment Diseases of the Ear, Balance Disorders, Facial Nerve Dysfunction, Balance Retraining, Pediatric Otolaryngology) · Bishop Clarkson Memorial Hospital, Archbishop Bergan Mercy Medical Center, Nebraska Methodist Hospital, Children's Memorial Hospital, Immanuel Medical Center, Memorial Hospital of Dodge County (Fremont) · Ear Specialists of Omaha, 4242 Farnam Street, Suite 142, Omaha, NE 68131 · 402-552-3277; 800-228-3277

Anthony J. Yonkers · Head & Neck Surgery (Cleft Lip, Cleft Palate, Facial Plastic & Reconstructive Surgery) · University of Nebraska Medical Center · University of Nebraska Medical Center, 600 South 42nd Street, Omaha, NE 68198-1225 · 402-559-8007

PATHOLOGY

Lincoln

Robert F. Shapiro · General Pathology (Microbiology, Cytology, Medical Management) · Pathology Medical Services, 1919 South 40th Street, Suite 333, Lincoln, NE 68506 · 402-473-5586

Larry D. Toalson · General Pathology · Pathology Medical Service, 1919 South 40th Street, Suite 333, P.O. Box 6960, Lincoln, NE 68506-6960 · 402-483-5053

Omaha

Samuel M. Cohen · General Pathology (Surgical Pathology) · University of Nebraska Medical Center, 600 South 42nd Street, Box 983135, Omaha, NE 68198-3135 · 402-559-6388

Sonny L. Johansson · General Pathology (Surgical Pathology) · University of Nebraska Medical Center, Department of Pathology and Microbiology, 600 South 42nd Street, Box 983135, Omaha, NE 68198-3135 · 402-559-7681

Dennis D. Weisenburger · Hematopathology · University of Nebraska Medical Center, Department of Pathology and Microbiology, 600 South 42nd Street, Omaha, NE 68198-3135 · 402-559-4186

PEDIATRICS

Omaha

Dean L. Antonson · Pediatric Gastroenterology (Eating Disorders, Organ Transplantation) · University of Nebraska Medical Center, Department of Pediatric Gastroenterology and Nutrition, 600 South 42nd Street, Omaha, NE 68198-5160 402-559-7294

Bruce A. Buehler · (Pediatric Genetics, Pediatric Metabolic Diseases) · University of Nebraska Medical Center, Children's Hospital, St. Joseph Hospital, Boys Town National Research Hospital · University of Nebraska Medical Center, Department of Pediatrics/MRI, 600 South 42nd Street, Omaha, NE 68198-5450 · 402-559-6400

John P. Cheatham · Pediatric Cardiology · Children's Hospital, Department of Pediatric Cardiology, 8301 Dodge Street, Omaha, NE 68114 · 402-559-5341

Peter F. Coccia · Pediatric Hematology-Oncology (Bone Marrow Transplantation, Pediatric Leukemia) · University of Nebraska Medical Center · University of Nebraska Medical Center, 600 South 42nd Street, Box 982168, Omaha, NE 68198-2168 · 402-559-7257

John L. Colombo · Pediatric Pulmonology (Cystic Fibrosis, Acute and Chronic Lung Injury in Children) · University of Nebraska Medical Center, Children's Hospital, St. Joseph Hospital · University of Nebraska Medical Center, 600 East 42nd Street, Omaha, NE 68198-5190 · 402-559-6275

David A. Danford · Pediatric Cardiology · University of Nebraska Medical Center, Department of Pediatric Cardiology, 600 South 42nd Street, Omaha, NE 68198-2166 · 402-390-5692

Carl H. Gumbiner · Pediatric Cardiology (Pediatric Critical Care) · Children's Hospital, Department of Pediatric Cardiology, 8301 Dodge Street, Omaha, NE 68114 · 402-390-5612

Mark T. Houser · Pediatric Nephrology · University of Nebraska Medical Center, Department of Pediatrics, 600 South 42nd Street, Box 982169, Omaha, NE 68198-2169 · 402-559-7344

John Dale Kugler · Pediatric Cardiology (Pediatric Arrhythmias and Electrophysiology, Ablation of Arrhythmias) · University of Nebraska Medical Center, Children's Hospital · University of Nebraska Medical Center, 600 South 42nd Street, Box 982166, Omaha, NE 68198-2166 · 402-390-3647

Jon A. Vanderhoof · Pediatric Gastroenterology (Nutrition, Pediatric Liver Transplant, Short Bowel Syndrome) · St. Joseph Hospital, Children's Hospital, University of Nebraska Medical Center · Pediatric Gastroenterology and Nutrition, 8300 Dodge Street, Suite 330, Omaha, NE 68114 · 402-390-3033

Mark C. Wilson · Pediatric Pulmonology · Children's Hospital, Department of Pediatric Pulmonology, 8301 Dodge Street, Omaha, NE 68114-4114 · 402-390-5624

PEDIATRICS (GENERAL)

Lincoln

Thomas D. Calvert · Lincoln Pediatric Group, 4701 Normal Boulevard, Lincoln, NE 68506 · 402-489-3834

Jeffrey J. David · Lincoln Pediatric Group, 4701 Normal Boulevard, Lincoln, NE 68506 · 402-489-3834

Douglas D. Ebers · St. Elizabeth Community Health Center, Lincoln General Hospital, Bryan Memorial Hospital · Lincoln Pediatric Group, 4701 Normal Boulevard, Lincoln, NE 68506 · 402-489-3834

Charles G. Erickson · (Behavioral Pediatrics) · St. Elizabeth Community Health Center · Lincoln Pediatric Group, 4701 Normal Boulevard, Lincoln, NE 68506-5592 · 402-489-3834

Michael A. Schmidt · (Genetics) · Pediatric & Medical Genetics, 600 North Cotner Boulevard, Suite 119, Lincoln, NE 68505 · 402-464-5551

Omaha

Mark J. Domet · Gold Circle Pediatrics, 13930 Gold Circle, Omaha, NE 68144 · 402-333-0422

Joseph Straley · Children's Hospital, Nebraska Methodist Hospital, Archbishop Bergan Mercy Medical Center, Immanuel Medical Center, Bishop Clarkson Memorial Hospital · Kids' Doctors, 8701 West Dodge Road, Suite 404, Omaha, NE 68114 · 402-390-5437

John Norman Walburn · University of Nebraska Medical Center · University of Nebraska Medical Center, General Pediatric Clinic, 600 South 42nd Street, Omaha, NE 68198-9400 · 402-559-5978

Robert D. Woodford · Pediatric Associates, 9202 West Dodge Road, Suite 101, Omaha, NE 68114 · 402-397-7337

PLASTIC SURGERY

Omaha

Richard John Bruneteau · General Plastic Surgery (Facial Aesthetic Surgery, Craniofacial Surgery, Pediatric Plastic Surgery) · Children's Hospital, Nebraska Methodist Hospital, Boys Town National Research Hospital, Archbishop Bergan Mercy Medical Center, Immanuel Medical Center · Aesthetic Surgical Images, 8900 West Dodge Road, Omaha, NE 68114 · 402-390-0100

R. Coleen Stice · General Plastic Surgery (General Hand Surgery, Aging Skin, Skin Cancer Surgery & Reconstruction, Wound Healing) · Metropolitan Plastic & Reconstructive Surgery, 6510 Sorensen Parkway, Suite 102, Omaha, NE 68152-2138 · 402-572-3310

PSYCHIATRY

Norfolk

George W. Bartholow · General Psychiatry · Norfolk Regional Center, 1700 North Victory Road, P.O. Box 1209, Norfolk, NE 68702 · 402-370-3311

Omaha

Subhash C. Bhatia · General Psychiatry (Geriatric Psychiatry, Addiction Psychiatry) · VA Medical Center, St. Joseph Center for Mental Health · Creighton University, Department of Psychiatry, 602 South 45nd Street, Omaha, NE 68198-5575 · 402-559-9235

William J. Burke · Geriatric Psychiatry · University of Nebraska Medical Center, Department of Psychiatry, 600 South 42nd Street, Omaha, NE 68198 · 402-559-5012

Chung-Chou Chu · Mood & Anxiety Disorders (Schizophrenia, Psychopharmacology) · St. Joseph Center for Mental Health · University of Nebraska Medical Center, Outpatient Psychiatry, 600 South 42nd Street, Box 985575, Omaha, NE 68198-5575 · 402-559-5055

Mark H. Fleisher · Mental Retardation/Mental Health (Diagnosis & Treatment of Mental Disorders in Individuals with Developmental Disabilities and/or Mental Retardation) · University of Nebraska Medical Center · University of Nebraska Medical Center, Department of Psychiatry, 600 South 42nd Street, Box 985575, Omaha, NE 68198-5575 · 402-559-5055

David G. Folks · Geriatric Psychiatry (General Psychiatry) · University of Nebraska Medical Center, St. Joseph Center for Mental Health, VA Medical Center University of Nebraska Medical Center, Department of Psychiatry, 600 South 42nd Street, Box 985575, Omaha, NE 68198-5575 · 402-559-5100

Carl H. Greiner · (Psychotherapy, Mood & Anxiety Disorders) · St. Joseph Center for Mental Health · University of Nebraska Medical Center, Department of Psychiatry, 602 South 42nd Street, Omaha, NE 68198 · 402-559-5004

Blaine Shaffer · General Psychiatry (Cultural Psychiatry) · St. Joseph Center for Mental Health · Creighton-Nebraska Psychiatric Clinic, 11920 Burt Street, Suite 170, Omaha, NE 68154 · 402-595-2213

PULMONARY & CRITICAL CARE MEDICINE

Lincoln

Bob J. Bleicher · General Pulmonary & Critical Care Medicine · Pulmonary Specialties, 1500 South 48th Street, Suite 605, Lincoln, NE 68506 · 402-483-1919

M. Jack Mathews · General Pulmonary & Critical Care Medicine · Wedgewood Medical Center, 120 Wedgewood Drive, Suite A, Lincoln, NE 68510-2482 · 402-489-8821

Omaha

Walter J. O'Donohue, Jr. · General Pulmonary & Critical Care Medicine (Asthma, Lung Infections) · St. Joseph Hospital · St. Joseph Hospital at Creighton University Medical Center, 601 North 30th Street, Suite 5850, Omaha, NE 68131-2197 · 402-280-4184

Stephen I. Rennard · General Pulmonary & Critical Care Medicine · University of Nebraska Medical Center · University of Nebraska Medical Center, 600 South 42nd Street, Omaha, NE 68198-5300 · 402-559-7313

Joseph H. Sisson · General Pulmonary & Critical Care Medicine · University of Nebraska Medical Center · University of Nebraska Medical Center, Pulmonary & Critical Care Medicine Section, 600 South 42nd Street, Omaha, NE 68198-5300 · 402-559-4087

Stephen B. Smith · General Pulmonary & Critical Care Medicine · Internal Medicine Associates, Doctor's Building, North Tower, Room 650, 4242 Farnam Street, Omaha, NE 68131 · 402-552-2600

RADIOLOGY

Omaha

Jud W. Gurney · Chest · University of Nebraska Medical Center · University of Nebraska Medical Center, Department of Radiology, 600 South 42nd Street, Box 981045, Omaha, NE 68198-1045 · 402-559-4000

Thomas J. Imray · General Radiology (Genito-Urinary Radiology, Chest Radiology, Cardiovascular Disease) · University of Nebraska Medical Center, VA Medical Center · University of Nebraska Medical Center, Department of Radiology, 600 South 42nd Street, Omaha, NE 68198-1045 · 402-559-6396

Timothy C. McCowan · (Vascular & Interventional Radiology, Cardiovascular Disease) · University of Nebraska Medical Center, Department of Radiology, 600 South 42nd Street, Box 981045, Omaha, NE 68198-1045 · 402-559-4477

RHEUMATOLOGY

Lincoln

Arthur Lawrence Weaver · General Rheumatology (Rheumatoid Arthritis, Osteoarthritis) · Bryan Memorial Hospital · Arthritis Center of Nebraska, 2121 South 56th Street, Lincoln, NE 68506 · 402-489-0333

Omaha

Lynell W. Klassen · General Rheumatology (Immunology) · University of Nebraska Medical Center, 600 South 42nd Street, Omaha, NE 68198 · 402-559-4000

James R. O'Dell · General Rheumatology (Rheumatoid Arthritis) · University of Nebraska Medical Center, VA Medical Center · University of Nebraska Medical Center, Department of Rheumatology, 600 South 42nd Street, Box 983025, Omaha, NE 68198-3025 · 402-559-7288

William R. Palmer · General Rheumatology · Bishop Clarkson Memorial Hospital, Nebraska Methodist Hospital, Archbishop Bergan Mercy Medical Center · Internal Medicine Associates, Doctor's Building, North Tower, Room 650, 4242 Farnam Street, Omaha, NE 68131 · 402-552-2600

SURGERY

Lincoln

David Harold Bingham · General Vascular Surgery · Surgical Associates of Lincoln, 2221 South 17th Street, Suite 106, Lincoln, NE 68502-3763 · 402-476-7561

Michael R. Norris · General Surgery · Surgical Associates of Lincoln, 2221 South 17th Street, Suite 106, Lincoln, NE 68502-3763 · 402-476-7561

John L. Reed · General Surgery · Prairie Surgical Associates, 1919 South 40th Street, Suite 107, Lincoln, NE 68506 · 402-486-3400

Lloyd E. Tenney · General Surgery · Surgical Associates of Lincoln, 2221 South 17th Street, Suite 106, Lincoln, NE 68502-3763 · 402-476-7561

Omaha

Robert J. Fitzgibbons, Jr. · General Surgery (Laparoscopy, Gastroenterologic Surgery) · St. Joseph Hospital, Archbishop Bergan Mercy Medical Center · Creighton University, Department of Surgery, 601 North 30th Street, Suite 3740, Omaha, NE 68131-2197 · 402-280-4503

Ronald A. Hinder · Gastroenterologic Surgery (Laparoscopy, Endoscopy, Esophageal Disease) · St. Joseph Hospital, Archbishop Bergan Mercy Medical Center · St. Joseph Hospital at Creighton University Medical Center, Department of Surgery, 601 North 30th Street, Suite 3740, Omaha, NE 68131-2197 · 402-280-4090

Layton F. Rikkers · Gastroenterologic Surgery (General Surgery, Hepatic Surgery, Biliary Surgery, Liver Cancer) · University of Nebraska Medical Center · University of Nebraska Medical Center, 600 South 42nd Street, Omaha, NE 68198-3280 · 402-559-8272

Byers W. Shaw, Jr. · Transplantation (Liver Transplantation) · University of Nebraska Medical Center · University of Nebraska Medical Center, 600 South 42nd Street, Omaha, NE 68198-3280 · 402-559-4076

John W. Smith · General Vascular Surgery · Nebraska Methodist Hospital · Methodist Hospital, Department of Surgery, 8300 Dodge Street, Omaha, NE 68114 · 402-393-6624

Robert J. Stratta · Transplantation (Pancreas Transplantation, Kidney Transplantation, Transplantation Infections, General Surgery, Surgical Critical Care) · University of Nebraska Medical Center, Bishop Clarkson Memorial Hospital · University of Nebraska Medical Center, Department of Surgery, 600 South 42nd Street, Box 983280, Omaha, NE 68198-3280 · 402-559-4076

SURGICAL ONCOLOGY

Omaha

Philip D. Schneider · General Surgical Oncology · University of Nebraska Medical Center, Department of Surgery, 600 South 42nd Street, Box 983280, Omaha, NE 68198-3280 · 402-559-4017

Alan G. Thorson · Colon & Rectal Cancer · Nebraska Methodist Hospital, St. Joseph Hospital, Immanuel Medical Center, Archbishop Bergan Mercy Medical Center, Bishop Clarkson Memorial Hospital, University of Nebraska Medical Center, Midlands Community Hospital (Papillion), Children's Hospital · 711 Professional Tower, 105 South 17th Street, Omaha, NE 68102 · 402-344-7666

THORACIC SURGERY

Lincoln

Deepak M. Gangahar · General Thoracic Surgery (Adult Cardiothoracic Surgery, Heart & Lung Transplant, Peripheral Vascular Surgery) · Nebraska Heart Institute, 1500 South 48th Street, Suite 800, Lincoln, NE 68506-5248 · 402-489-6553

Omaha

Kim F. Duncan · Pediatric Cardiac Surgery · University of Nebraska Medical Center, Department of Surgery, Section of Cardiothoracic Surgery, 600 South 42nd Street, Omaha, NE 68198-2315 · 402-559-4424

Timothy A. Galbraith · (Adult Cardiothoracic Surgery, Cardiac Transplantation, Mechanical Circulatory Assistance) · University of Nebraska Medical Center · University of Nebraska Medical Center, Department of Surgery, Section of Cardiothoracic Surgery, 600 South 42nd Street, Omaha, NE 68198-2315 · 402-559-4424

Rudy Paul Lackner · General Thoracic Surgery (Thoracic Oncological Surgery, Transplantation) · University of Nebraska Medical Center, VA Medical Center · University of Nebraska Medical Center, Department of Surgery, Section of Thoracic Surgery, 600 South 42nd Street, Box 982315, Omaha, NE 68198-2315 · 402-559-4424

UROLOGY

Lincoln

Alan H. Domina · General Urology (Impotence, Incontinence, Endourology, Neuro-Urology & Voiding Dysfunction, Urologic Oncology) · Lincoln General Hospital, Bryan Memorial Hospital, St. Elizabeth Community Health Center · 4740 A Street, Suite 206, Lincoln, NE 68510 · 402-489-8888

Sushil S. Lacy · General Urology · 4740 A Street, Suite 206, Lincoln, NE 68510 402-489-8888

Omaha

Rodney J. Taylor · General Urology · University of Nebraska Medical Center, Department of Urologic Surgery, 600 South 42nd Street, Omaha, NE 68198-2360 402-559-4292

NEW MEXICO

ALLERGY & IMMUNOLOGY

Albuquerque

Bruce H. Feldman · General Allergy & Immunology · 8010 Mountain Road, NE, Albuquerque, NM 87110 · 505-265-6782

Shirley Murphy · General Allergy & Immunology (Cystic Fibrosis, Allergy, Asthma) · University Hospital, Children's Hospital of New Mexico · University of New Mexico Medical Center, Ambulatory Care Center, Third Floor, 2211 Lomas Boulevard, NE, Albuquerque, NM 87131 · 505-272-5551

Los Alamos

Richard W. Honsinger · General Allergy & Immunology (General Internal Medicine) · Los Alamos Medical Center, St. Vincent Hospital (Santa Fe), University Hospital (Albuquerque) · Allergy & Asthma Associates, Los Alamos Medical Center, 3917 West Road, Los Alamos, NM 87544 · 505-662-4351

ANESTHESIOLOGY

Albuquerque

C. Hilary Compton · General Anesthesiology · Lovelace Medical Center, Department of Anesthesiology, 5400 Gibson Boulevard, SE, Albuquerque, NM 87108 · 505-262-7197

Elliot S. Marcus · General Anesthesiology (Pediatric Anesthesiology, Adult Cardiovascular Anesthesia, Neuroanesthesia) · University of New Mexico Health

Sciences Center, Department of Anesthesiology, 2211 Lomas Boulevard, NE, Albuquerque, NM 87131-5216 · 505-272-2610

Santa Fe

Ervin Hinds · Pain · Calle Medico, Suite Four, Santa Fe, NM 87505 · 505-983-3275

CARDIOVASCULAR DISEASE

Albuquerque

Michael H. Crawford · Echocardiography · University Hospital · University of New Mexico Medical Center, Department of Cardiology, 2211 Lomas Boulevard, NE, Albuquerque, NM 87131-5271 · 505-272-6020

Roswell

Jerome Dominick · General Cardiovascular Disease · 1600 Southeast Main Street, Roswell, NM 88201 · 505-623-1370

Santa Fe

H. William Adkison · General Cardiovascular Disease · Santa Fe Cardiology Associates, 1651 Galisteo Street, Suite Four, Santa Fe, NM 87505 · 505-984-8012

R. Brad Stamm · General Cardiovascular Disease (Nuclear Cardiology) · St. Vincent Hospital · New Mexico Heart Institute, Santa Fe Division, 1651 Galisteo Street, Suite Four, Santa Fe, NM 87505 · 505-984-8012

COLON & RECTAL SURGERY

Albuquerque

Don M. Morris · General Colon & Rectal Surgery (Colon & Rectal Cancer, Inherited Gastrointestinal Malignancies) · University Hospital, University of New Mexico Cancer Center · University of New Mexico Medical Center, Department of Surgery, 2211 Lomas Boulevard, NE, Albuquerque, NM 87131-5341 · 505-272-4161

Santa Fe

Raphael I. Shapiro · General Colon & Rectal Surgery · St. Vincent Hospital, USPHS-IHS Santa Fe Hospital · Santa Fe Surgical Associates, 435 St. Michaels Drive, Suite B-202, Santa Fe, NM 87505 · 505-988-3975

DERMATOLOGY

Albuquerque

William G. Chapman · Clinical Dermatology (Mohs Surgery for Skin Cancer, Laser Surgery) · Dermatology Consultants, 8316 Kaseman Court, NE, Albuquerque, NM 87110 · 505-292-5850

Roswell

John Henry · Clinical Dermatology · 207 North Union Street, Roswell, NM 88201 505-624-2330

Santa Fe

Karen Van de Velde · Clinical Dermatology · 435 St. Michaels Drive, Suite B204, Santa Fe, NM 87505 · 505-986-5025

ENDOCRINOLOGY & METABOLISM

Albuquerque

R. Philip Eaton · General Endocrinology & Metabolism · University of New Mexico Health Sciences Center, Department of Internal Medicine, Division of Endocrinology, Ambulatory Care Center, Fifth Floor, 2211 Lomas Boulevard, NE, Albuquerque, NM 87131-5271 · 505-272-4656

Patricia Kapsner · General Endocrinology & Metabolism · University of New Mexico Medical Center, Department of Medicine, 2211 Lomas Boulevard, NE, Albuquerque, NM 87131 · 505-272-2147

David S. Schade · Diabetes · University Hospital · University of New Mexico Medical Center, Department of Medicine and Endocrinology, 2211 Lomas Boulevard, NE, Albuquerque, NM 87131 · 505-272-4657

B. Sylvia Vela · General Endocrinology & Metabolism · VA Medical Center, 2100 Ridgecrest Drive, SE, Mail Code 111, Albuquerque, NM 87108 · 505-265-1711

Santa Fe

Robert M. Bernstein · General Endocrinology & Metabolism (Diabetes) · 1533 South St. Francis Drive, Suite B, Santa Fe, NM 87505 · 505-982-2860

FAMILY MEDICINE

Albuquerque

Arthur Kaufman · (General Family Practice, General Internal Medicine, Adolescent Medicine) · University Hospital · University of New Mexico Health Services and Science Center, Department of Family and Community Medicine, 2400 Tucker Avenue, NE, Albuquerque, NM 87131 · 505-277-2165

Christopher McGrew · University of New Mexico Health Sciences Center School of Medicine, Department of Orthopaedics, Ambulatory Care Center, Second Floor West, 2211 Lomas Boulevard, NE, Albuquerque, NM 87131-5296 · 505-272-4107

Martha C. McGrew · University of New Mexico Medical Center, Department of Family Practice, 2211 Lomas Boulevard, NE, Albuquerque, NM 87131 · 505-277-2165

Caryn McHarney-Brown · University of New Mexico Health Sciences Center, Department of Family & Community Medicine, 2400 Tucker Avenue, NE, Third Floor, Albuquerque, NM 87131-5241 · 505-277-2165

Carol L. Merovka · 8020 Constitution Place, Suite 203, Albuquerque, NM 87110 · 505-298-1344

Robin J. Tuchler · First Family Health Care, 5550 Wyoming Boulevard, Albuquerque, NM 87109 · 505-821-5010

Berthold E. Umland · (General Family Practice, Mind-Body Issues, Gender Dysphoria) · University Hospital · University of New Mexico Health Services and Science Center, The Family Practice Center, 2400 Tucker Avenue, NE, Box 5241, Albuquerque, NM 87131 · 505-277-2165

Christopher Urbina · (Public Health, Border Health) · University of New Mexico Health Services and Science Center, Department of Family and Community Medicine, 2400 Tucker Avenue, NE, Albuquerque, NM 87131-5241 · 505-277-2165

Roswell

Charles Fenzi · 808 North Union Street, Roswell, NM 88201 · 505-622-1411

Santa Fe

Fen Sartorius · Rodeo Family Medicine, 4001 Rodeo Road, Santa Fe, NM 87505 · 505-471-8994

Steven L. Wright · (Addiction Medicine) · Rodeo Family Medicine, 4001 Rodeo Road, Santa Fe, NM 87505 · 505-471-8994

GASTROENTEROLOGY

Albuquerque

Sanjeev Arora · General Gastroenterology (Therapeutic Endoscopy) · University of New Mexico Health Sciences Center, Department of Internal Medicine, Division of Gastroenterology, Ambulatory Care Center, Fifth Floor, 2211 Lomas Boulevard, NE, Albuquerque, NM 87106 · 505-272-4755

Howard K. Gogel · Endoscopy · Southwest Gastroenterology, 201 Cedar Street, SE, Suite 702, Albuquerque, NM 87106 · 505-243-8018

Santa Fe

Cornelius P. Dooley · General Gastroenterology · Northern New Mexico Gastroenterology Associates, 1651 Galisteo Road, Suite 12, Santa Fe, NM 87505 · 505-983-5631

David Hoverson · General Gastroenterology · 1651 Galisteo Road, Suite 12, Santa Fe, NM 87505 · 505-983-5631

Alfred W. Pinkerton · General Gastroenterology · 1650 Hospital Drive, Suite 200, Santa Fe, NM 87505 · 505-982-4276

GERIATRIC MEDICINE

Albuquerque

Robert D. Lindeman · (General Geriatric Medicine, Geriatric Nephrology) · University Hospital · University of New Mexico Health Sciences Center, Department of Medicine, Division of Gerontology, Ambulatory Care Center, Fifth Floor, 2211 Lomas Boulevard, NE, Albuquerque, NM 87131 · 505-272-6082

Richard J. Roche · Presbyterian Hospital, St. Joseph Medical Center, St. Joseph Northeast Heights Hospital · Internal and Family Medicine Associates, 6100 Pan American Freeway, NE, Suite 200, Albuquerque, NM 87109 · 505-823-1010

HAND SURGERY

Albuquerque

Moheb S. Moneim · Peripheral Nerve Surgery (Microsurgery) · University of New Mexico Medical Center, Department of Orthopaedics, 2211 Lomas Boulevard, NE, Albuquerque, NM 87131 · 505-272-4107

George E. Omer, Jr. · Peripheral Nerve Surgery (Pediatric Hand Surgery, Reconstructive Surgery) · Carrie Tingley Hospital, University Hospital · University of New Mexico Medical Center, School of Medicine, Department of Orthopaedics, Ambulatory Care Center, Second Floor West, 2211 Lomas Boulevard, NE, Albuquerque, NM 87131-5296 · 505-272-4107

Charles Pribyl · General Hand Surgery (Microsurgery, Traumatic & Reconstructive Hand and Wrist Problems, Congenital Hand Deformities, General Orthopaedic Surgery) · University Hospital, VA Medical Center · University of New Mexico Health Sciences Center School of Medicine, Department of Orthopaedics, Ambulatory Care Center, Second Floor West, 2211 Lomas Boulevard, NE, Albuquerque, NM 87131-5296 · 505-272-4107

Santa Fe

Raphael I. Shapiro · General Hand Surgery (General Surgery) · St. Vincent Hospital, USPHS-IHS Santa Fe Hospital · Santa Fe Surgical Associates, 435 St. Michaels Drive, Suite B-202, Santa Fe, NM 87505 · 505-988-3975

INFECTIOUS DISEASE

Albuquerque

Frederick T. Koster · General Infectious Disease, AIDS (Tropical Diseases & Travel Medicine) · University of New Mexico Medical Center, Department of Internal Medicine, Division of Infectious Diseases, 2211 Lomas Boulevard, NE, Albuquerque, NM 87131-5271 · 505-277-5666

Gregory J. Mertz · Herpes Virus Infections · University Hospital · University of New Mexico Medical Center, Department of Infectious Disease, BRS-323, Albuquerque, NM 87131 · 505-277-8207

Santa Fe

Donald A. Romig · General Infectious Disease (AIDS, Travel Medicine, General Internal Medicine) · St. Vincent Hospital · 1482 St. Francis Drive, Suite C, Santa Fe, NM 87505 · 505-984-1981

INTERNAL MEDICINE (GENERAL)

Albuquerque

Frederick Hashimoto · University Hospital · University of New Mexico Health Sciences Center, Department of Internal Medicine, Ambulatory Care Center, Fifth Floor, 2211 Lomas Boulevard, NE, Albuquerque, NM 87106 · 505-272-2147

Patricia Kapsner · University of New Mexico Medical Center, Department of Medicine, 2211 Lomas Boulevard, NE, Albuquerque, NM 87131 · 505-272-2147

Glen H. Murata · VA Medical Center, General Internal Medicine, 2100 Ridgecrest Drive, SE, Mail Code 111, Albuquerque, NM 87108 · 505-256-2727

Ronald W. Quenzer · (General Infectious Diseases, Bone & Joint Infections) · University Hospital · University of New Mexico Medical Center, Department of Internal Medicine, Ambulatory Care Center, Fifth Floor, 2211 Lomas Boulevard, NE, Albuquerque, NM 87131-5271 · 505-272-2147

Richard H. Rubin · (General Geriatric Medicine, General Internal Medicine) · University Hospital · University of New Mexico Medical Center, Division of General Internal Medicine, Ambulatory Care Center, Fifth Floor, 2211 Lomas Boulevard, NE, Albuquerque, NM 87131 · 505-272-2147

Carolyn Voss · (Preoperative Risk Assessment, Hypertensive Disorders of Pregnancy) · University Hospital · University of New Mexico Medical Center, Division of General Internal Medicine, 2211 Lomas Boulevard, NE, Albuquerque, NM 87131-5271 · 505-272-2147

Los Alamos

Richard W. Honsinger · (General Allergy & Immunology) · Los Alamos Medical Center, St. Vincent Hospital (Santa Fe), University Hospital (Albuquerque) · Allergy & Asthma Associates, Los Alamos Medical Center, 3917 West Road, Los Alamos, NM 87544 · 505-662-4351

Santa Fe

Boudinot T. Atterbury · St. Vincent Hospital · St. Vincent Internal Medicine Associates, 435 St. Michaels Drive, Suite B-104, Santa Fe, NM 87505 · 505-988-5111

David A. Gonzales · 1650 Hospital Drive, Santa Fe, NM 87505 · 505-982-4276

MEDICAL ONCOLOGY & HEMATOLOGY

Albuquerque

James Liebmann · General Medical Oncology & Hematology (General Internal Medicine) · Presbyterian Hospital, St. Joseph Medical Center · New Mexico Oncology Hematology Consultants, 612 Encino Place, NE, Albuquerque, NM 87102 · 505-842-8171

Aroop Mangalik · General Medical Oncology & Hematology · University of New Mexico Medical Center, Cancer Research & Treatment Center, 900 Camino de Salud, NE, Albuquerque, NM 87131 · 505-277-8517

John H. Saiki · General Medical Oncology & Hematology · University of New Mexico Medical Center, Cancer Research & Treatment Center, 900 Camino de Salud, NE, Albuquerque, NM 87131 · 505-277-8740

Farmington

R. Graham Smith · General Medical Oncology & Hematology · San Juan Regional Cancer Center, 800 West Maple Street, Farmington, NM 87401 · 505-599-6259

Roswell

Gregory J. C. Yang · General Medical Oncology & Hematology · Cancer Center of Roswell, 405 West Country Club Road, Roswell, NM 88201 · 505-624-8723

Santa Fe

Timothy M. Lopez · General Medical Oncology & Hematology · St. Vincent Hospital · Santa Fe Hematology/Oncology, 465 St. Michaels Drive, Suite 101, Santa Fe, NM 87505 · 505-988-4493

NEPHROLOGY

Albuquerque

Richard F. Goldman · General Nephrology · Renal Medicine, 201 Cedar Street, SE, Suite 604, Albuquerque, NM 87106 · 505-242-2805

Antonia Harford · General Nephrology · University of New Mexico Medical Center, Department of Nephrology, 2211 Lomas Boulevard, NE, Albuquerque, NM 87131-5271 · 505-272-4750

Farmington

Mark C. Saddler · General Nephrology (Kidney Disease, Dialysis, Renal Hypertension) · San Juan Regional Medical Center · Four Corners Nephrology, 812 West Maple Street, Farmington, NM 87401-5620 · 505-326-6521

Santa Fe

Robert J. Kossman · General Nephrology · 1650 Hospital Drive, Suite 200, Santa Fe, NM 87505 · 505-982-4276

Paul J. Kovnat · General Nephrology · 1650 Hospital Drive, Suite 200, Santa Fe, NM 87505 · 505-982-4276

NEUROLOGICAL SURGERY

Albuquerque

John A. Anson · Vascular Neurological Surgery · University of New Mexico Medical Center, Division of Neurosurgery, 2211 Lomas Boulevard, NE, Albuquerque, NM 87131 · 505-272-3401

Edward C. Benzel · Spinal Surgery · University of New Mexico Medical Center, Department of Neurological Surgery, 2211 Lomas Boulevard, NE, Albuquerque, NM 87131 · 505-272-3401

Hal L. Hankinson · General Neurological Surgery (Skull-Base Surgery, Pituitary Surgery, Tumor Surgery, Spinal Surgery) · St. Joseph Medical Center, Presbyterian Hospital · Neurosurgical Associates, 522 Lomas Boulevard, NE, Albuquerque, NM 87102-2454 · 505-247-4253

Santa Fe

Erich P. Marchand · General Neurological Surgery · Neurological Surgery Association of Northern New Mexico, 531 Harkel Road, Suite D, Santa Fe, NM 87505 505-988-3233

Venkat I. Narayan · General Neurological Surgery · 1640 Hospital Drive, Santa Fe, NM 87505 · 505-820-1232

NEUROLOGY

Albuquerque

Douglas W. Barrett · General Neurology · Neurology Consultants, 201 Cedar Street, SE, Suite 700, Albuquerque, NM 87106 · 505-842-9554

Joseph M. Bicknell · General Neurology (Electromyography, Neuromuscular Disease) · University Hospital · University of New Mexico Health Sciences Center, Department of Neurology, 2211 Lomas Boulevard, NE, Albuquerque, NM 87131-5281 · 505-272-3342

Thomas J. Carlow · Neuro-Ophthalmology · Eye Associates of New Mexico and Southwest Colorado, 101 Hospital Loop, NE, Suite 103, Albuquerque, NM 87109 505-883-6800

Larry E. Davis · Infectious & Demyelinating Diseases (Multiple Sclerosis, Infectious Diseases) · VA Medical Center · VA Medical Center, Neurology Service, 2100 Ridgecrest Drive, SE, Mail Code 127, Albuquerque, NM 87108 · 505-256-2752

Corey C. Ford · Infectious & Demyelinating Diseases (Multiple Sclerosis, Magnetic Resonance Imaging) · University Hospital · University of New Mexico Health Sciences Center, Ambulatory Care Center, Second Floor, 915 Camino De Salud, NE, Albuquerque, NM 87131 · 505-272-3342

Donald F. Seelinger · General Neurology (Electromyography) · Presbyterian Hospital, St. Joseph Medical Center · 201 Cedar Road, SE, Suite 700, Albuquerque, NM 87106-4924 · 505-842-9554

Santa Fe

Michael Baten · General Neurology (Child Neurology, Epilepsy) · St. Vincent Hospital · Neurological Associates, 531 Harkel Road, Suite C, Santa Fe, NM 87505 · 505-983-8182

NEUROLOGY, CHILD

Albuquerque

Leslie A. Morrison · General Child Neurology · University of New Mexico Medical Center, Department of Neurology, 2211 Lomas Boulevard, NE, Albuquerque, NM 87131 · 505-272-3342

NUCLEAR MEDICINE

Albuquerque

Michael F. Hartshorne · General Nuclear Medicine · VA Medical Center, Department of Radiology, 2100 Ridgecrest Drive, SE, Albuquerque, NM 87108 · 505-256-2768

Frederick A. Mettler · General Nuclear Medicine, Radiation Accidents & Radiation Injury · University Hospital · University of New Mexico School of Medicine, 915 Camino de Salud, NE, Albuquerque, NM 87131 · 505-272-0011

OBSTETRICS & GYNECOLOGY

Albuquerque

Francisco Ampuero · Gynecologic Cancer · Presbyterian Professional Building, 201 Cedar Street, Suite 407, Albuquerque, NM 87106 · 505-843-7813

Luis Benjamin Curet · Maternal & Fetal Medicine (Diabetes in Pregnancy, Pre-Eclampsia, Substance Abuse in Pregnancy) · University Hospital · University of New Mexico Health Sciences Center, Department of Obstetrics & Gynecology, 2211 Lomas Boulevard, NE, Albuquerque, NM 87131-5286 · 505-272-6386

Maxine Dorin · General Obstetrics & Gynecology · University of New Mexico Medical Center, Department of Obstetrics & Gynecology, 2211 Lomas Boulevard, NE, Albuquerque, NM 87131 · 505-272-6370

Rebecca J. Shoden · General Obstetrics & Gynecology · 883 Lead Avenue, SE, Albuquerque, NM 87102 · 505-247-8820

Santa Fe

Lance J. Mikkelsen · General Obstetrics & Gynecology · 465 St. Michaels Drive, Suite 201, Santa Fe, NM 87505 · 505-988-9651

Cleveland H. Pardue III · General Obstetrics & Gynecology · 465 St. Michaels Drive, Suite 202, Santa Fe, NM 87505 · 505-984-0303

Deborah A. Vigil · General Obstetrics & Gynecology · 1651 Galisteo Road, SE, Suite Six, Santa Fe, NM 87505 · 505-983-8601

Laura D. Wolfswinkel · General Obstetrics & Gynecology (Operative Laparoscopy, Laser Surgery) · St. Vincent Hospital · Galisteo Ob-Gyn Associates, 539 Harkel Road, Suite C, Santa Fe, NM 87501 · 505-984-2300

OPHTHALMOLOGY

Albuquerque

Joe R. Cannon · Anterior Segment—Cataract & Refractive · Eye Associates, 806 Dr. Martin Luther King, Jr. Avenue, Albuquerque, NM 87102 · 505-842-6575

Mark T. Chiu · Medical Retinal Diseases (Uveitis, Vitreo-Retinal Surgery) · St. Joseph Hospital, Presbyterian Hospital, Lovelace Medical Center, Mercy Medical Center (Durango, CO) · Eye Associates of New Mexico and Southwestern Colorado, 806 Dr. Martin Luther King, Jr. Avenue, NE, Albuquerque, NM 87102 · 505-842-6575

Frank J. Mares · Glaucoma · Eye Associates, 101 Hospital Loop, Suite 103, Albuquerque, NM 87109 · 505-883-6800

Robert W. Reidy · (Retinal Diseases, Uveitis, Vitreo-Retinal Surgery) · St. Joseph Medical Center, Presbyterian Hospital, Lovelace Medical Center · Eye Associates of New Mexico and Southwestern Colorado, 806 Dr. Martin Luther King, Jr. Avenue, NE, Albuquerque, NM 87102 · 505-842-6575

Arthur J. Weinstein · Anterior Segment—Cataract & Refractive · St. Joseph Medical Center, Presbyterian Hospital, St. Vincent Hospital (Santa Fe), Los Alamos Medical Center (Los Alamos) · Eye Associates of New Mexico and Southwest Colorado, 806 Dr. Martin Luther King, Jr. Avenue, NE, Albuquerque, NM 87102 · 505-842-6575

ORTHOPAEDIC SURGERY

Albuquerque

Field Blevins · Shoulder Surgery, Sports Medicine/Arthroscopy (Knee Surgery) · University Hospital · University of New Mexico Health Sciences Center School of Medicine, Department of Orthopaedics, Ambulatory Care Center, Second Floor West, 2211 Lomas Boulevard, NE, Albuquerque, NM 87131-5296 · 505-272-4107

Thomas DeCoster · Trauma · University Hospital · University of New Mexico Health Sciences Center School of Medicine, Department of Orthopaedics, Ambulatory Care Center, Second Floor West, 2211 Lomas Boulevard, NE, Albuquerque, NM 87131-5296 · 505-272-4107

James C. Drennan · Pediatric Orthopaedic Surgery (Pediatric Foot Surgery, Neuromuscular Disorders, Congenital Anomalies, Foot & Ankle Surgery, Hip Surgery) · Carrie Tingley Hospital, University Hospital · University of New Mexico Health Sciences Center, Carrie Tingley Hospital, Department of Medical Affairs, 1127 University Boulevard, NE, Albuquerque, NM 87102-1715 · 505-272-5271

Richard Miller · Foot & Ankle Surgery · University of New Mexico Health Sciences Center School of Medicine, Department of Orthopaedics, Ambulatory Care Center, Second Floor West, 2211 Lomas Boulevard, NE, Albuquerque, NM 87131-5296 · 505-272-4107

John F. Ritterbusch · Pediatric Orthopaedic Surgery (Spinal Deformity, Scoliosis, Spinal Surgery, Sports Medicine/Arthroscopy) · Carrie Tingley Hospital, University Hospital · University of New Mexico Health Sciences Center, Department of Medical Affairs, 1127 University Boulevard, NE, Albuquerque, NM 87102-1715 · 505-272-5214

Dennis Rivero · Hip Surgery, Knee Surgery (Reconstructive Surgery) · University Hospital · University of New Mexico Health Sciences Center, Department of Orthopaedics, Ambulatory Care Center, Second Floor West, 2211 Lomas Boulevard, NE, Albuquerque, NM 87131-5296 · 505-272-4107

Samuel K. Tabet · Sports Medicine/Arthroscopy · New Mexico Orthopaedic Associates, 8300 Constitution Place, NE, Albuquerque, NM 87110 · 505-224-8280

Daniel Wascher · Sports Medicine/Arthroscopy · University Hospital · University of New Mexico Health Sciences Center School of Medicine, Department of Orthopaedics, Ambulatory Care Center, Second Floor West, 2211 Lomas Boulevard, NE, Albuquerque, NM 87131-5296 · 505-272-4107; 505-272-6300

Richard E. White, Jr. · Reconstructive Surgery (Hip, Knee) · New Mexico Center for Joint Replacement, Presbyterian Hospital · New Mexico Orthopaedic Associates, 415 Cedar Street, SE, Albuquerque, NM 87106 · 505-224-8200

Richard V. Worrell · Tumor Surgery · University Hospital, VA Medical Center · University of New Mexico Health Sciences Center School of Medicine, Department of Orthopaedics, Ambulatory Care Center, Second Floor West, 2211 Lomas Boulevard, NE, Albuquerque, NM 87131-5296 · 505-272-4107

Las Cruces

Edward R. Sweetser · General Orthopaedic Surgery (Sports Medicine/Arthroscopy, Knee Surgery, Reconstructive Surgery) · Memorial Medical Center · Las Cruces Orthopaedic Associates, 675 Avenida de Mesilla, P.O. Box 2243, Las Cruces, NM 88005 · 505-525-3535

Santa Fe

Jan Bear · General Orthopaedic Surgery · 1010 Calle Medico, Suite 10, Santa Fe, NM 87505 · 505-986-1440

David W. Caldwell · Spinal Surgery (General Orthopaedic Surgery) · St. Vincent Hospital · 465 St. Michaels Drive, Suite One, Santa Fe, NM 87505 · 505-986-1111

Steven Weiner · General Orthopaedic Surgery (Sports Medicine/Arthroscopy, Joint Replacement) · St. Vincent Hospital · 1630 Hospital Drive, Santa Fe, NM 87505-4772 · 505-982-5014

OTOLARYNGOLOGY

Albuquerque

Karl L. Horn · Otology (Surgery of the Ear, Skull-Base Surgery, Head & Neck Surgery, Pediatric Otolaryngology) · Presbyterian Hospital · Ear Associates, Presbyterian Professional Building, Suite 306, 201 Cedar Road, SE, Albuquerque, NM 87106 · 505-247-0301

Pamela J. Nicklaus · Pediatric Otolaryngology · University Hospital · University of New Mexico Health Sciences Center, Division of Otolaryngology, 2211 Lomas Boulevard, NE, Albuquerque, NM 87131-5341 · 505-272-6452

Santa Fe

David R. Brown · General Otolaryngology · Southwestern Ear, Nose & Throat Associates, 433 St. Michaels Drive, Santa Fe, NM 87505 · 505-982-4848

Paul W. Kaufman · General Otolaryngology · University Hospital (Albuquerque) Southwestern Ear, Nose & Throat Associates, 433 St. Michaels Drive, Santa Fe, NM 87505 · 505-982-4848

PATHOLOGY

Albuquerque

Elliott Foucar · General Pathology (Surgical Pathology, Dermatopathology, Gastrointestinal Pathology) · Presbyterian Hospital · Presbyterian Hospital, Department of Pathology, 1100 Central Avenue, Albuquerque, NM 87102 · 505-841-1259

M. Kathryn Foucar · Hematopathology · University Hospital · University of New Mexico Medical Center, Department of Hematopathology, 2211 Lomas Boulevard, NE, Albuquerque, NM 87106 · 505-843-2440

Mario Kornfeld · Neuropathology · University of New Mexico School of Medicine, Department of Pathology, 915 Stanford, NE, Albuquerque, NM 87131 · 505-277-9868

Santa Fe

Jack E. Zwemer · General Pathology · Santa Fe Pathology Services, 465 St. Michaels Drive, Suite 109, Santa Fe, NM 87505 · 505-820-5300

PEDIATRICS

Albuquerque

Jon M. Aase · (Dysmorphology, Medical Genetics) · University Hospital, Presbyterian Hospital · University of New Mexico School of Medicine, Department of Pediatrics, 2211 Lomas Boulevard, NE, Albuquerque, NM 87131-5296 · 505-243-5088

Dale C. Alverson · Neonatal-Perinatal Medicine · University of New Mexico Health Sciences Center, Department of Pediatrics, Division of Neonatology, 2211 Lomas Boulevard, NE, Albuquerque, NM 87131 · 505-272-3967

William Berman, Jr. · Pediatric Cardiology (General Pediatrics, Interventional Cardiac Catheterization) · University Hospital, Presbyterian Hospital, St. Joseph Medical Center, Plains Regional Medical Center-Clovis (Clovis) · Pediatric Cardiology Associates of New Mexico, 715 Dr. Martin Luther King, Jr. Avenue, NE, Suite 207, Albuquerque, NM 87102 · 505-848-3700

Carol L. Clericuzio · (Medical Genetics, Dysmorphology) · University of New Mexico Health Sciences Center, Department of Pediatrics, Division of Genetics and Dysmorphology, Ambulatory Care Center, Third Floor, 2211 Lomas Boulevard, NE, Albuquerque, NM 87131 · 505-272-6631

Marilyn H. Duncan · Pediatric Hematology-Oncology (Pediatric Oncology Homecare) · University Hospital · University of New Mexico Medical Center, Division of Pediatric Oncology, Ambulatory Care Center, Third Floor, 2211 Lomas Boulevard, NE, Albuquerque, NM 87131-5311 · 505-272-4461

Andrew Hsi · (Newborn Care, Care for Infants and Children Prenatally Exposed to Alcohol & Other Drugs) · University of New Mexico Health Sciences Center, Department of Pediatrics, 2211 Lomas Boulevard, NE, Albuquerque, NM 87131 505-272-5551

Robert Katz · Pediatric Critical Care · University of New Mexico Health Sciences Center, Department of Pediatrics, Division of Critical Care Medicine, 2211 Lomas Boulevard, NE, Third Floor, Albuquerque, NM 87131-5311 · 505-272-4358

Ellen D. Kaufman · Pediatric Endocrinology (Pediatric & Adolescent Diabetes) · Lovelace Medical Center · Lovelace Medical Center, Department of Endocrinology, 5400 Gibson Boulevard, SE, Albuquerque, NM 87108 · 505-262-7455

Shirley Murphy · Pediatric Pulmonology (Asthma) · University Hospital, Children's Hospital of New Mexico · University of New Mexico Medical Center, Ambulatory Care Center, Third Floor, 2211 Lomas Boulevard, NE, Albuquerque, NM 87131 · 505-272-5551

Gary Don Overturf · Pediatric Infectious Disease · University Hospital · University of New Mexico Medical Center, Ambulatory Care Center, 2211 Lomas Boulevard, NE, Albuquerque, NM 87131 · 505-272-5551

Lu-Ann Papile · Neonatal-Perinatal Medicine (Perinatal Brain Injury, Chronic Lung Disease, Intraventricular Hemorrhage) · University Hospital · University of New Mexico Health Sciences Center, Department of Pediatrics, Ambulatory Care Center, Third Floor West, 2211 Lomas Boulevard, NE, Albuquerque, NM 87131-5311 · 505-272-3967

Michael Radetsky · Pediatric Infectious Disease (Pediatric Critical Care, General Pediatrics) · Lovelace Medical Center · Lovelace Medical Center, Department of Pediatrics, 5400 Gibson Boulevard, SE, Albuquerque, NM 87108 · 505-262-7594

Edward L. Rose · Pediatric Gastroenterology · Pediatric Gastroenterology of New Mexico, 717 Encino Place, NE, Albuquerque, NM 87102 · 505-842-6601

Paul E. Stobie · Neonatal-Perinatal Medicine · Presbyterian Hospital · Neonatology Associates, 1100 Central Avenue, P.O. Box 26666, Albuquerque, NM 87125 · 505-841-1049

J. Deane Waldman · Pediatric Cardiology (Therapeutic Cardiac Catheterization, Pulmonary Hypertension in Children, Pediatric Cardiac Pathology) · University Hospital · University of New Mexico Medical Center, Children's Hospital Heart Center, 2211 Lomas Boulevard, NE, Albuquerque, NM 87131 · 505-272-3864

Stuart S. Winter · Pediatric Hematology-Oncology · University of New Mexico Health Sciences Center, Department of Pediatrics, Division of Pediatric Oncology, 2211 Lomas Boulevard, NE, Albuquerque, NM 87131-5311 · 505-272-4461

PEDIATRICS (GENERAL)

Alamogordo

Larry D. Starr · 1211 Eighth Street, Suite C, Alamogordo, NM 88310 · 505-434-1500

Nancy J. Starr · 1211 Eighth Street, Suite C, Alamogordo, NM 88310 · 505-434-1500

Albuquerque

David Allison · Lovelace Medical Center, Department of Pediatrics, 5400 Gibson Boulevard, SE, Albuquerque, NM 87108 · 505-262-7594

Manuel Archuleta · Presbyterian Family Health Care, 3436 Isleta Boulevard, SW, Albuquerque, NM 87105 · 505-224-7777

Carla Bloedel · Lovelace Medical Center, Pediatric Clinic, 5400 Gibson Boulevard, SE, Albuquerque, NM 87108 · 505-262-3219

Loretta M. Cordova de Ortega · (Developmental Disabilities, Asthma, Behavior Problems) · University Hospital · University of New Mexico Health Sciences Center, Department of Pediatrics, Ambulatory Care Center, Third Floor, 2211 Lomas Boulevard, NE, Albuquerque, NM 87131 · 505-272-2345

Clark Hansbarger · University of New Mexico Medical Center, Department of Pediatrics, 2211 Lomas Boulevard, NE, Albuquerque, NM 87106 · 505-272-6843

Hareen P. Kulasinghe · Albuquerque Pediatric Associates, 8308 Constitution Place, NE, Albuquerque, NM 87110 · 505-293-1333

Loretta L. McNamara · Presbyterian Hospital · Albuquerque Pediatric Associates, 8308 Constitution Place, NE, Albuquerque, NM 87110 · 505-293-1333

Irene J. Moody · Pediatric Associates, 3410 Indian School Road, NE, Albuquerque, NM 87106 · 505-265-7817

Thomas O. Rothfeld · Pediatric Associates, 3410 Indian School Road, NE, Albuquerque, NM 87106 · 505-265-7817

Stanley N. Stark · (Pediatric Hematology-Oncology, General Pediatrics) · Presbyterian Hospital, University of New Mexico Children's Hospital · Albuquerque Pediatric Associates, 8308 Constitution Place, NE, Albuquerque, NM 87110 · 505-293-1333

Mareth E. Williams · (Pulmonary Medicine) · University of New Mexico Medical Center, Department of Pediatrics, Ambulatory Care Center, Third Floor, 2211 Lomas Boulevard, NE, Albuquerque, NM 87131 · 505-272-2022

Linda R. Zipp · West Mesa Pediatrics, 4808 McMahon Boulevard, NW, Suite 16, Albuquerque, NM 87114 · 505-898-7898

Belen

Stephen Cohen · Presbyterian Hospital (Albuquerque) · Presbyterian Family Health Care, 609 South Christopher Road, Belen, NM 87002 · 505-864-5454

Carlsbad

J. Kent Raney · 2402 West Pierce Street, Suite 5A, Carlsbad, NM 88220 · 505-887-0530

Clovis

Richard W. Stamm · 120 West 21st Street, Clovis, NM 88101 · 505-769-2200

Farmington

James K. Fisk · Farmington Family Practice, 622 West Maple Street, Suite B, Farmington, NM 87401 · 505-327-4867

Preston B. Herrington · San Juan Regional Medical Center · Farmington Family Practice, 622 West Maple Street, Suite B, Farmington, NM 87401 · 505-327-4867

Las Cruces

Hernan Ciudad · First Step Pediatrics, 2450 South Telshor Boulevard, Las Cruces, NM 88011 · 505-521-7862

Maria G. Crawley · Lovelace Pediatrics, 2803 Doral Court, Las Cruces, NM 88001 · 505-522-4283

Robin Edward · First Step Pediatrics, 2450 South Telshor Boulevard, Las Cruces, NM 88011 · 505-521-7862

Jennifer Lichtenfels · Lovelace Pediatrics, 2803 Doral Court, Las Cruces, NM 88001 · 505-522-4283

Roberto Talamantes · 1250 Hillrise Circle, Las Cruces, NM 88001 · 505-521-1378

Las Vegas

George P. Bunch · (Child Safety) · Northeastern Regional Hospital · Las Vegas Clinic for Children and Youth, 501 Seventh Street, Las Vegas, NM 87701 · 505-425-3566

Los Alamos

John B. Neal · (Special Need Children, Neonatology, General Infectious Disease) Los Alamos Medical Center · Children's Clinic, Los Alamos Medical Center, Suite 128, 3917 West Road, Los Alamos, NM 87544 · 505-662-4234

Rio Rancho

Michael A. Nelson · Presbyterian Family Health Care, Section of Adolescent Health, 4100 High Resort Boulevard, NW, Rio Rancho, NM 87124-5900 · 505-823-8855

Richard D. Rolston · Lovelace Medical Center (Albuquerque), St. Joseph West Mesa Hospital · Lovelace Pediatrics, 3801 Southern Boulevard, Rio Rancho, NM 87124 · 505-896-8600

Roswell

Joseph Dean · (Pediatric Cardiology) · Eastern New Mexico Medical Center · BCA Medical Associates, 813 North Washington Street, Roswell, NM 88201 · 505-622-2606

William G. Liakos · BCA Medical Associates, 813 North Washington Street, Roswell, NM 88201 · 505-622-2606

Warren D. McKelvy · Eastern New Mexico Medical Center · BCA Medical Associates, 813 North Washington Street, Roswell, NM 88201 · 505-622-2606

Santa Fe

Edward Kleiner · Arroyo Chamiso Pediatric Center, 2025 Galisteo Street, Santa Fe, NM 87505 · 505-982-9844

Lawrence Shandler · Santa Fe Pediatrics, 1418 Luisa Street, Suite Five, Santa Fe, NM 87505 · 505-988-8024

Cheryl J. Whitman · Arroyo Chamiso Pediatric Center, 2025 Galisteo Street, Santa Fe, NM 87505 · 505-982-9844

Socorro

Leslie S. Johnson · Socorro General Hospital · Socorro Medical Associates, 1204 Highway 60, P.O. Box 1799, Socorro, NM 87801 · 505-835-0705

Taos

Charles W. Anderson · (Behavioral Pediatrics) · Holy Cross Hospital · Taos Clinic for Children and Youth, 123 Cruz Alta Road, Box 6134, Taos, NM 87571 · 505-758-8651

Loretta M. Ortiz y Pino · Holy Cross Hospital · Taos Clinic for Children and Youth, 123 Cruz Alta Road, Box 6134, Taos, NM 87571 · 505-758-8651

PHYSICAL MEDICINE & REHABILITATION

Albuquerque

Richard T. Radecki · General Physical Medicine & Rehabilitation (Pediatric Physical Medicine & Rehabilitation, Traumatic Brain Injury in Children and Young Adults, Spinal Cord Injury in Children and Young Adults, Limb Deficiencies in Children and Adults) · University Hospital, Carrie Tingley Hospital · Carrie Tingley Hospital, Division of Pediatrics, 1127 University Boulevard, Albuquerque, NM 87102-1715 · 505-272-4244

Santa Fe

Karyn R. Doddy · General Physical Medicine & Rehabilitation (Occupational Medicine) · St. Vincent Hospital · Rehabilitation Medicine Specialists, 435 St. Michaels Drive, Suite A 201, Santa Fe, NM 87505 · 505-983-9109

PLASTIC SURGERY

Albuquerque

Goesel Anson · General Plastic Surgery (Facial Aesthetic Surgery, Body Contouring, Breast Surgery) · Lovelace Medical Center, University Hospital · Lovelace Medical Center, Lovelace Cosmetic and Reconstructive Surgery, 5006 Gibson Boulevard, SE, Albuquerque, NM 87108 · 505-262-7777

Richard A. Gooding · General Plastic Surgery · 2207 San Pedro Park, NE, Albuquerque, NM 87110 · 505-884-4242

Michael G. Orgel · Peripheral Nerve Surgery · University of New Mexico Medical Center, Division of Plastic Surgery, 2211 Lomas Boulevard, NE, Albuquerque, NM 87131-5341 · 505-272-4264

Santa Fe

James F. Green, Jr. · General Plastic Surgery · 465 St. Michaels Drive, Suite 10, Santa Fe, NM 87505 · 505-988-2215

PSYCHIATRY

Albuquerque

Claudia Berenson · Child & Adolescent Psychiatry, Eating Disorders · University of New Mexico Children's Psychiatric Hospital, 1001 Yale Boulevard, NE, Albuquerque, NM 87131 · 505-843-2926

Michael Bogenschutz · Addiction Psychiatry · University of New Mexico Health Sciences Center, Mental Health Center, 2600 Marble Avenue, NE, Albuquerque, NM 87131 · 505-843-2397

Gregory Franchini · General Psychiatry · University of New Mexico Health Sciences Center, Department of Psychiatry, 2400 Tucker Avenue, NE, Fourth Floor, Room 470, Albuquerque, NM 87131-5326 · 505-277-5468

Debbie C. Gee · General Psychiatry (Child & Adolescent Psychiatry, Mood & Anxiety Disorders) · Memorial Hospital-Psychiatric Center of Albuquerque, Charter Heights Behavioral Health System · 7113 Prospect Place, NE, Albuquerque, NM 87110 · 505-837-9782 x4313

Rosemary S. Hunter · Eating Disorders, Child & Adolescent Psychiatry · 5728 Osuna Road, NE, Albuquerque, NM 87109 · 505-881-1123

Samuel J. Keith · Schizophrenia (Rehabilitation of Schizophrenia, Depression, Anxiety Disorders) · University of New Mexico Mental Health Center · University of New Mexico Medical Center, Department of Psychiatry, 2400 Tucker Avenue, NE, Albuquerque, NM 87131 · 505-277-0518

John Lauriello · General Psychiatry (Psychotic Disorders, Schizophrenia Research, Psychopharmacology Research) · University of New Mexico Health Sciences Center, Department of Psychiatry, 2400 Tucker Avenue, NE, Albuquerque, NM 87131-5326 · 505-277-4090

A. Lane Leckman · Addiction Psychiatry (Dissociative Disorders) · 7113 Prospect Place, NE, Albuquerque, NM 87110 · 505-883-5877

Teresita A. McCarty · General Psychiatry (General Hospital Psychiatry & Trauma) · University of New Mexico Health Sciences Center, Consultation Psychiatry, 2211 Lomas Boulevard, NE, Albuquerque, NM 87106 · 505-277-4763

Nancy K. Morrison · General Psychiatry · University of New Mexico Health Sciences Center, Department of Psychiatry, 2400 Tucker Avenue, NE, Albuquerque, NM 87131-5326 · 505-277-4517

H. George Nurnberg · General Psychiatry (Personality Disorders & Trauma, Mood & Anxiety Disorders, Psychopharmacology) · University of New Mexico Health Sciences Center, Mental Health Center, 2600 Marble Avenue, NE, Albuquerque, NM 87131-5456 · 505-272-4167

Allison Reeve · Neuropsychiatry · University of New Mexico Health Sciences Center, Department of Psychiatry, 2400 Tucker Avenue, NE, Albuquerque, NM 87131-5326 · 505-277-4091

Laura W. Roberts · General Psychiatry (Clinical Medical Ethics, Neuropsychiatry) · University of New Mexico Mental Health Center, University Hospital · University of New Mexico Medical Center, Department of Psychiatry, Family Practice Building, Fourth Floor, Room 411, 2400 Tucker Avenue, NE, Albuquerque, NM 87131-5326 · 505-277-2223

Sally K. Severino · General Psychiatry (Women's Psychiatry—Menstrual Cycle & Moods, Menopause) · University of New Mexico Medical Center, Department of Psychiatry, 2400 Tucker Avenue, NE, Albuquerque, NM 87131 · 505-277-2223

Peter Thompson · Psychopharmacology · University of New Mexico Medical Center, Department of Psychiatry, 2400 Tucker Avenue, NE, Albuquerque, NM 87131-5326 · 505-277-3892

E. H. Uhlenhuth · Mood & Anxiety Disorders, Psychopharmacology (General Psychiatry) · University Hospital · University of New Mexico Medical Center, Department of Psychiatry, Fourth Floor, 2400 Tucker Avenue, NE, Albuquerque, NM 87131 · 505-277-6265

Albert V. Vogel · General Psychiatry · University Hospital · University of New Mexico Medical Center, Office of Clinical Affairs, Family Practice Building, Room 172, 2400 Tucker Avenue, NE, Albuquerque, NM 87131-5121 · 505-277-0738

Cynthia C. Williams · Geriatric Psychiatry · University of New Mexico Medical Center, University of New Mexico Mental Health Center, 2600 Marble Avenue, NE, Albuquerque, NM 87131 · 505-843-2994

Joel Yager · Eating Disorders, Psychopharmacology (Mood & Anxiety Disorders, Marital Problems) · University of New Mexico Medical Center, Department of Psychiatry, 2400 Tucker Avenue, NE, Albuquerque, NM 87131-5326 · 505-277-4245

Santa Fe

John R. Evaldson · Child & Adolescent Psychiatry (Psychotherapy, General Psychiatry, Mood & Anxiety Disorders, Psychopharmacology) · 200 West DeVargas Street, Suite Three, Santa Fe, NM 87501 · 505-983-1887

Barbara J. Lampert · Mood & Anxiety Disorders (Trauma Spectrum Disorders, Psychopharmacology, Dissociative Disorders) · Pinon Hills Hospital · 400 Solona Street, Santa Fe, NM 87501 · 505-986-8224

Karl Ray · General Psychiatry · 2025 South Galisteo Road, Santa Fe, NM 87505 505-820-5335

PULMONARY & CRITICAL CARE MEDICINE

Santa Fe

Charles Riley · General Pulmonary & Critical Care Medicine (General Geriatric Medicine, General Internal Medicine, Exercise Physiology) · St. Vincent Hospital 465 St. Michaels Drive, Suite 104, Santa Fe, NM 87501 · 505-982-8338

RADIATION ONCOLOGY

Albuquerque

Kutub Khan · General Radiation Oncology · Radiation Oncology Associates, 601 Grand Avenue, Albuquerque, NM 87102 · 505-244-8229

Santa Fe

Ronda S. Fleck · General Radiation Oncology · St. Vincent Hospital, Cancer Treatment Center, 455 St. Michaels Drive, Santa Fe, NM 87505 · 505-820-5233

RADIOLOGY

Albuquerque

Stephen G. Babel · General Radiology (Interventional Radiology) · X-Ray Associates of New Mexico, 715 Dr. Martin Luther King, Jr. Avenue, NE, Suite 112, Albuquerque, NM 87102 · 505-842-8880

Blaine L. Hart · Pediatric Radiology (Neuroradiology, Pediatric Neuroradiology) University of New Mexico Medical Center, Department of Radiology, 915 Camino de Salud, NE, Albuquerque, NM 87131 · 505-272-2269

Robert W. Jahnke · Neuroradiology (Magnetic Resonance Imaging) · Lovelace Medical Center · Lovelace Medical Center, Department of Radiology, 5400 Gibson Boulevard, SE, Albuquerque, NM 87108 · 505-262-7115

Gregory Keck · General Radiology (Vascular & Interventional Radiology) · Lovelace Medical Center, Department of Radiology, 5400 Gibson Boulevard, SE, Albuquerque, NM 87108 · 505-262-7115

Michael N. Linver · General Radiology (Mammography, Nuclear Radiology) · St. Joseph Medical Center, St. Joseph Northeast Heights Hospital, St. Joseph West Mesa Hospital · X-Ray Associates of New Mexico, 715 Dr. Martin Luther King, Jr. Avenue, NE, Suite 112, Albuquerque, NM 87102 · 505-842-8880

James L. Lowry · General Radiology · X-Ray Associates of New Mexico, 715 Dr. Martin Luther King, Jr. Avenue, NE, Suite 112, Albuquerque, NM 87102 · 505-842-8880

William W. Orrison, Jr. · Neuroradiology (Magnetic Resonance Imaging) · University Hospital, New Mexico Regional Federal Medical Center · VA Medical Center, The New Mexico Institute of Neuroimaging, Building 49A, 2100 Ridgecrest Drive, SE, Mail Code 114M, Albuquerque, NM 87108 · 505-256-5711

Stuart B. Paster · General Radiology (Mammography) · X-Ray Associates of New Mexico, 715 Dr. Martin Luther King, Jr. Avenue, NE, Suite 112, Albuquerque, NM 87102 · 505-842-8880

Jesse Rael · Neuroradiology · University of New Mexico Medical Center, Department of Radiology, 915 Camino de Salud, NE, Albuquerque, NM 87131 · 505-272-2269

Robert D. Rosenberg · General Radiology (Mammography) · University of New Mexico Medical Center, Department of Radiology, 915 Camino de Salud, NE, Albuquerque, NM 87131 · 505-272-2269

Bruce Turlington · General Radiology (Magnetic Resonance Imaging) · Lovelace Medical Center, Department of Radiology, 5400 Gibson Boulevard, SE, Albuquerque, NM 87108 · 505-262-7115

Michael R. Williamson · General Radiology (Cross-Sectional Imaging, Magnetic Resonance Imaging, Nuclear Radiology) · University of New Mexico Medical Center, Department of Radiology, 915 Camino de Salud, NE, Albuquerque, NM 87131 · 505-272-2269

Susan L. Williamson · Pediatric Radiology · University of New Mexico Medical Center, Department of Radiology, 2211 Lomas Boulevard, NE, Albuquerque, NM 87106 · 505-272-0006

Keith G. Winterkorn · General Radiology (Interventional Radiology) · X-Ray Associates of New Mexico, 717 Encino Place, NE, Albuquerque, NM 87102 · 505-243-4788

William D. Zimmer · Magnetic Resonance Imaging (Computed Tomography, Ultrasound) · St. Joseph Medical Center · X-Ray Associates of New Mexico, 715 Dr. Martin Luther King, Jr. Avenue, NE, Suite 112, Albuquerque, NM 87102 · 505-842-8880

Los Alamos

David A. Williams · General Radiology · Los Alamos Medical Center, 3917 West Road, Los Alamos, NM 87544 · 505-662-4349

Santa Fe

Larry L. Cohen · General Radiology (Mammography) · Santa Fe Radiology, 465 St. Michaels Drive, Suite 113, Santa Fe, NM 87505 · 505-983-3357

RHEUMATOLOGY

Albuquerque

Arthur D. Bankhurst · General Rheumatology · University Hospital · University of New Mexico Health Sciences Center, Division of Rheumatology, 2211 Lomas Boulevard, NE, Albuquerque, NM 87131 · 505-272-4761

Willmer L. Sibbitt · General Rheumatology · University of New Mexico Health Sciences Center, Division of Rheumatology, 2211 Lomas Boulevard, NE, Albuquerque, NM 87131 · 505-272-4761

SURGERY

Albuquerque

Myriam J. Curet · General Surgery (Endoscopy, Laparoscopy, General Colon & Rectal Surgery, General Surgical Oncology) · University Hospital · University of New Mexico Health Sciences Center, Department of Surgery, 2211 Lomas Boulevard, NE, Albuquerque, NM 87131 · 505-272-6386

Mark Langsfeld · General Vascular Surgery · University of New Mexico Medical Center, Department of Surgery, Division of Peripheral Vascular Surgery, 2211 Lomas Boulevard, NE, Albuquerque, NM 87131-5341 · 505-272-5850

Brian G. Miscall · General Surgery (Endocrine Surgery, Gastroenterologic Surgery) · Presbyterian Hospital, St. Joseph Medical Center · Albuquerque Surgical Group, 718 Encino Place, NE, Albuquerque, NM 87102 · 505-247-3635

Don M. Morris · General Surgery (Breast Surgery, Gastroenterologic Surgery, Thyroid Surgery) · University Hospital, University of New Mexico Cancer Center University of New Mexico Medical Center, Department of Surgery, 2211 Lomas Boulevard, NE, Albuquerque, NM 87131-5341 · 505-272-4161

Ole A. Peloso · General Surgery (Laparoscopic Surgery, General Surgical Oncology, Phlebology) · Presbyterian Hospital, St. Joseph Medical Center · Albuquerque Surgical Group, 718 Encino Place, NE, Albuquerque, NM 87102 · 505-247-3635

Santa Fe

Gerald B. Demarest III · General Surgery (Surgical Critical Care, Burns, Trauma) St. Vincent Hospital, USPHS-IHS Santa Fe Hospital, University Hospital (Albuquerque), Lovelace Medical Center (Albuquerque) · Santa Fe Surgical Associates, 435 St. Michaels Drive, Suite B-202, Santa Fe, NM 87505 · 505-988-3975

Alfred J. Martin, Jr. · General Vascular Surgery · 1650 Hospital Drive, Suite 400, Santa Fe, NM 87505 · 505-982-6612

Susan A. Seedman · General Surgery (Breast Surgery, Laparoscopic Surgery) · 1691 Galisteo Street, Suite E, Santa Fe, NM 87505 · 505-988-9747

Joseph M. Smith · General Surgery · 465 St. Michaels Drive, Suite 209, Santa Fe, NM 87505 · 505-983-6651

SURGICAL ONCOLOGY

Albuquerque

Brian G. Miscall · General Surgical Oncology (Colon & Rectal Cancer, Breast Surgery) · Presbyterian Hospital, St. Joseph Medical Center · Albuquerque Surgical Group, 718 Encino Place, NE, Albuquerque, NM 87102 · 505-247-3635

Don M. Morris · General Surgical Oncology (Breast Cancer, Melanoma, Gastrointestinal Cancer) · University Hospital, University of New Mexico Cancer Center · University of New Mexico Medical Center, Department of Surgery, 2211 Lomas Boulevard, NE, Albuquerque, NM 87131-5341 · 505-272-4161

THORACIC SURGERY

Albuquerque

Stuart B. Pett, Jr. · General Thoracic Surgery · Lovelace Medical Center, Department of Cardiology, 5400 Gibson Boulevard, SE, Albuquerque, NM 87108 · 505-262-7451

Jorge A. Wernly · General Thoracic Surgery (Pediatric Cardiac Surgery, Adult Cardiothoracic Surgery, Pediatric Non-Cardiac Thoracic Surgery, Thoracic Oncological Surgery) · University Hospital, VA Medical Center, Lovelace Medical Center · University of New Mexico Medical Center, Department of Cardiothoracic Surgery, 2211 Lomas Boulevard, NE, Albuquerque, NM 87131 · 505-272-6901

UROLOGY

Albuquerque

Thomas A. Borden · Pediatric Urology, Urologic Oncology · University Hospital University of New Mexico Medical Center, Department of Surgery, Division of Urology, 2211 Lomas Boulevard, NE, Albuquerque, NM 87131 · 505-272-5504

Anthony Smith · General Urology (Transplantation, Urologic Oncology) · University of New Mexico Health Sciences Center, Department of Surgery, Division of Urology, Ambulatory Care Center, Second Floor, 2211 Lomas Boulevard, NE, Albuquerque, NM 87131 · 505-272-5504

Santa Fe

Steven C. Robeson · General Urology · 1630 Hospital Drive, Santa Fe, NM 87505 505-982-3534

NORTH DAKOTA

ALLERGY & IMMUNOLOGY

Fargo

Patrick J. Stoy · General Allergy & Immunology (General Pulmonary & Critical Care Medicine) · Meritcare Clinic, 737 North Broadway, Fargo, ND 58123 · 701-234-2524

Grand Forks

Robert A. Thompson · General Allergy & Immunology (Asthma) · United Hospital · Grand Forks Clinic, 1000 South Columbia Road, P.O. Box 6003, Grand Forks, ND 58206-6003 · 701-780-6420

Mandan

William B. Riecke · General Allergy & Immunology · Mandan Heart and Lung Clinic, 1006 East Main Street, Mandan, ND 58554 · 701-663-8600

ANESTHESIOLOGY

Bismarck

Hugh Carlson · General Anesthesiology · The Bismarck Heart & Lung Clinic, 311 North Ninth Street, P.O. Box 2698, Bismarck, ND 58502-2698 · 701-224-7500

Gary N. Johnson · General Anesthesiology · The Bismarck Heart & Lung Clinic, 311 North Ninth Street, P.O. Box 2698, Bismarck, ND 58502-2698 · 701-255-3234

Ronald Knutson · General Anesthesiology · The Bismarck Heart & Lung Clinic, 311 North Ninth Street, P.O. Box 2698, Bismarck, ND 58502-2698 · 701-224-7500

Matthew Layman · General Anesthesiology (Critical Care Medicine) · St. Alexius Medical Center · The Bismarck Heart & Lung Clinic, 311 North Ninth Street, P.O. Box 2698, Bismarck, ND 58502-2698 · 701-224-7500

Roger Loven · Critical Care Medicine · The Bismarck Heart & Lung Clinic, 311 North Ninth Street, P.O. Box 2698, Bismarck, ND 58502-2698 · 701-224-7500

Peter White · Critical Care Medicine · The Bismarck Heart & Lung Clinic, 311 North Ninth Street, P.O. Box 2698, Bismarck, ND 58502-2698 · 701-224-7500

Fargo

Robert A. Brunsvold · General Anesthesiology · Meritcare Medical Group, 737 North Broadway, Fargo, ND 58123 · 701-234-5621

Jayant S. Damle · General Anesthesiology (Pain Management) · Meritcare Health System · Meritcare Clinic, Department of Anesthesiology, 737 North Broadway, Fargo, ND 58123 · 701-234-6258

John K. Erie · General Anesthesiology · 2713 Twenty-Eighth Avenue, SW, Fargo, ND 58103-5044 · 701-280-3300

Panjini M. Sivanna · General Anesthesiology (Critical Care Medicine, Pain Management) · Meritcare Health System · Meritcare Medical Group, 737 North Broadway, Fargo, ND 58123 · 701-234-5621

Gustave E. Staahl · General Anesthesiology · Dakota Clinic, 1702 South University Drive, Fargo, ND 58103 · 701-280-4861

Grand Forks

Jitendra R. Parikh · General Anesthesiology · United Hospital · Anesthesia Associates, 2701 South Columbia Road, Suite 103, Grand Forks, ND 58208 · 701-746-8381

CARDIOVASCULAR DISEASE

Bismarck

Lisa Ann Abrahams · General Cardiovascular Disease (Interventional Cardiology, Heart Failure) · St. Alexius Medical Center · The Bismarck Heart & Lung Clinic, 311 North Ninth Street, P.O. Box 2698, Bismarck, ND 58502-2698 · 701-224-7500

Walter E. Frank · General Cardiovascular Disease (Pacemakers, Cardiac Catheterization) · Medcenter One, St. Alexius Medical Center · Medcenter One Health Care Systems, Quain & Ramstead Clinic, 222 North Seventh Street, P.O. Box 5505, Bismarck, ND 58506-5505 · 701-222-5202

Robert G. Oatfield · General Cardiovascular Disease · The Bismarck Heart & Lung Clinic, 311 North Ninth Street, P.O. Box 2698, Bismarck, ND 58502-2698 701-224-7500

Fargo

Donald B. Jenny · General Cardiovascular Disease · Dakota Clinic, 1702 South University Drive, P.O. Box 6001, Fargo, ND 58108-6001 · 701-280-3402

Craig R. Kouba · General Cardiovascular Disease · Meritcare Medical Group, 737 North Broadway, Fargo, ND 58123 · 701-234-2371

CLINICAL PHARMACOLOGY

Bismarck

Thomas D. Davis · St. Alexius Medical Center, 900 East Broadway, Bismarck, ND 58501 · 701-224-7182

Dan McPherson · St. Alexius Medical Center, 900 East Broadway, Bismarck, ND 58501 · 701-224-7261

Fargo

Richard D. Clarens · Family Practice Residency, 306 Fourth Street, North, Fargo, ND 58102 · 701-239-7111

COLON & RECTAL SURGERY

Bismarck

Douglas Berglund · General Colon & Rectal Surgery · Medcenter One · Medcenter One Health Care Systems, Quain & Ramstead Clinic, 222 North Seventh Street, P.O. Box 5505, Bismarck, ND 58506-5505 · 701-222-5219

Fargo

Brent E. Krantz · General Colon & Rectal Surgery · Meritcare Health System · Meritcare Medical Group, 737 North Broadway, Fargo, ND 58123 · 701-234-2251

Grand Forks

Mark B. Siegel · General Colon & Rectal Surgery · United Hospital · Grand Forks Clinic, 1000 South Columbia Road, P.O. Box 6003, Grand Forks, ND 58206-6003 · 701-780-6281

DERMATOLOGY

Bismarck

William E. Cornatzer, Jr. · Clinical Dermatology · 225 North Seventh Street, Suite B, Bismarck, ND 58501 · 701-224-1273

Denise Forte-Pathroff · Clinical Dermatology · Medcenter One, St. Alexius Medical Center · 225 North Seventh Street, Bismarck, ND 58501-4437 · 701-224-9643

Fargo

Lon D. Christianson · Clinical Dermatology (Aesthetic Surgery, Skin Cancer Surgery & Reconstruction, Acne, Aging Skin, Laser Surgery, Psoriasis) · Dakota Heartland Hospital · The Dermatology Clinic, 827 Twenty-Eighth Street, SW, Suite B, Fargo, ND 58103 · 701-280-2711

Paul R. Vandersteen · Clinical Dermatology · Meritcare Medical Group, 737 North Broadway, Fargo, ND 58123 · 701-234-2311

Grand Forks

Hector J. Gallego · Clinical Dermatology · Grand Forks Clinic, 1000 South Columbia Road, P.O. Box 6003, Grand Forks, ND 58206-6003 · 701-780-6201

ENDOCRINOLOGY & METABOLISM

Fargo

Juan M. Munoz · General Endocrinology & Metabolism · Meritcare Health System · Meritcare Medical Group, 737 North Broadway, Fargo, ND 58123 · 701-234-2245

Grand Forks

Casey J. Ryan · General Endocrinology & Metabolism · United Hospital · Grand Forks Clinic, 1000 South Columbia Road, P.O. Box 6003, Grand Forks, ND 58206-6003 · 701-780-6461

FAMILY MEDICINE

Bismarck

Deanna L. Carr · Mid Dakota Clinic, Kirkwood, 828 Kirkwood Mall, Bismarck, ND 58504 · 701-221-6490

John A. Erickstad · Mid Dakota Clinic, 401 North Ninth Street, Bismarck, ND 58501 · 701-221-6000

Jeffrey L. Orchard · (Attention Deficit Disorder) · St. Alexius Medical Center · Mid Dakota Clinic, 401 North Ninth Street, P.O. Box 5538, Bismarck, ND 58502 701-221-6045

Allen E. Wyman · Mid Dakota Clinic, 401 North Ninth Street, P.O. Box 5538, Bismarck, ND 58502 · 701-221-6408

Dickinson

Thomas R. Templeton · St. Joseph's Hospital & Health Center · Great Plains Clinic, 33 Ninth Street, West, Dickinson, ND 58601 · 701-225-6017

Dennis E. Wolf · Great Plains Clinic, 33 Ninth Street, West, Dickinson, ND 58601 · 701-225-6017

Fargo

David J. Glatt · Meritcare Southwest, 2701 Thirteenth Avenue, South, Fargo, ND 58103 · 701-234-3610

Russell J. Kuzel · Dakota Clinic, West Acres Shopping Center, 13th Avenue and Interstate 29, Fargo, ND 58103 · 701-298-6600

Grand Forks

Gary D. Kolle · United Hospital · Grand Forks Clinic, 1000 South Columbia Road, P.O. Box 6003, Grand Forks, ND 58206-6003 · 701-780-6506

William Stewart Mann · University of North Dakota Family Practice Center, 1200 South Columbia Road, Grand Forks, ND 58201 · 701-780-6800

Dale C. Moquist · Family Medicine Center in Med Park, 1380 South Columbia Road, Grand Forks, ND 58201 · 701-795-2000

Mandan

Dale A. Klein · Q & R Clinic, 910 Northwest 18th Street, Mandan, ND 58554 · 701-663-0010

Darwin K. Lange · Q & R Clinic, 910 Northwest 18th Street, Mandan, ND 58554 701-663-0010

GASTROENTEROLOGY

Bismarck

Joseph P. Moore · General Gastroenterology (Endoscopy, Pancreatic Disease) · Medcenter One Health Systems, 222 North Seventh Street, P.O. Box 5505, Bismarck, ND 58502 · 701-222-5219

Derek Oldenburger · General Gastroenterology · Mid Dakota Clinic, 401 North Ninth Street, P.O. Box 5538, Bismarck, ND 58506-5538 · 701-221-6034

Fargo

Michael T. Bader · General Gastroenterology · Dakota Clinic, 1702 South University Drive, Fargo, ND 58103 · 701-280-8573

Stephen Spellman · General Gastroenterology · Meritcare Medical Group, 737 North Broadway, Fargo, ND 58123 · 701-234-2525

Grand Forks

Steven H. Bollinger · General Gastroenterology · Grand Forks Clinic, 1000 South Columbia Road, P.O. Box 6003, Grand Forks, ND 58206-6003 · 701-780-6418

Anthony G. Chu · General Gastroenterology · Grand Forks Clinic, 1000 South Columbia Road, P.O. Box 6003, Grand Forks, ND 58206-6003 · 701-780-6399

GERIATRIC MEDICINE

Bismarck

Michael A. Spooner · (Dementia, Behavior Disorders in Dementia, General Geriatric Medicine) · Medcenter One, Department of Geriatric Services, 300 North Seventh Street, P.O. Box 5525, Bismarck, ND 58502-5525 · 701-224-6883

HAND SURGERY

Bismarck

Curtis A. Juhala · General Hand Surgery · St. Alexius Medical Center · Mid Dakota Clinic, 401 North Ninth Street, Bismarck, ND 58501 · 701-221-6000

Fargo

J. Donald Opgrande · General Hand Surgery (Reconstructive Surgery, Sports Medicine/Arthroscopy) · Dakota Heartland Hospital, Dakota Day Surgery, Meritcare Same Day Surgery · 2301 Twenty-Fifth Street, South, Suite G, Fargo, ND 58103 · 701-232-2848

Grand Forks

Robert H. Clayburgh · General Hand Surgery · Grand Forks Clinic, 1000 South Columbia Road, P.O. Box 6003, Grand Forks, ND 58206-6003 · 701-780-6112

INFECTIOUS DISEASE

Fargo

Robert R. Tight · General Infectious Disease · Meritcare Medical Group, 737 North Broadway, Fargo, ND 58123 · 701-234-2261

Grand Forks

James Hargreaves · General Infectious Disease (Infection Control, Hospital-Acquired Infections, Tropical Disease & Travel Medicine) · Grand Forks Clinic, 1000 South Columbia Road, P.O. Box 6003, Grand Forks, ND 58206-6003 · 701-780-6253

INTERNAL MEDICINE (GENERAL)

Bismarck

Mark A. Erickstad · Mid Dakota Clinic, 401 North Ninth Street, P.O. Box 5538, Bismarck, ND 58502 · 701-221-6066

Bruce M. Hetland · Mid Dakota Clinic, 401 North Ninth Street, Bismarck, ND 58501 · 701-221-6053

Gerry M. Lunn · Medcenter One Health Care Systems, Quain & Ramstead Clinic, 222 North Seventh Street, P.O. Box 5505, Bismarck, ND 58506-5505 · 701-222-5278

Steven J. Miller · Medcenter One Health Care Systems, Quain & Ramstead Clinic, 222 North Seventh Street, Bismarck, ND 58506 · 701-222-5384

Derek Oldenburger · Mid Dakota Clinic, 401 North Ninth Street, Bismarck, ND 58501-4507 · 701-221-6034

Dickinson

James Baumgartner · Great Plains Clinic, 33 Ninth Street, West, Dickinson, ND 58601 · 701-225-6017

Mark P. Hinrichs · Great Plains Clinic, 33 Ninth Street, West, Dickinson, ND 58601 · 701-225-6017

Bruce W. Olin · St. Joseph's Hospital & Health Center · Great Plains Clinic, 33 Ninth Street, West, Dickinson, ND 58601 · 701-225-6017

Fargo

Bruce G. Pitts · (General Internal Medicine, Critical Care Medicine) · Meritcare Health System · Meritcare Medical Group, 737 North Broadway, Fargo, ND 58123 · 701-234-2353

Janelle C. Sanda · Meritcare Medical Group, 737 North Broadway, Fargo, ND 58123 · 701-234-2000

Frank J. Sepe · (Pulmonary & Critical Care Medicine) · Meritcare Medical Group, 737 North Broadway, Fargo, ND 58123 · 701-234-2261

Grand Forks

Barbara J. Bollinger · Grand Forks Clinic, 1000 South Columbia Road, P.O. Box 6003, Grand Forks, ND 58206-6003 · 701-780-6570

James D. Brosseau · (Diabetes, General Geriatric Medicine, Epidemiology) · United Hospital · Grand Forks Clinic, 1000 South Columbia Road, Suite 3C, P.O. Box 6003, Grand Forks, ND 58206-6003 · 701-780-6202

MEDICAL ONCOLOGY & HEMATOLOGY

Bismarck

Ferdinand E. K. Addo · General Medical Oncology & Hematology (Cancer Prevention & Control) · Medcenter One, St. Alexius Medical Center · Medcenter One Health Care Systems, Quain & Ramstead Clinic, 222 North Seventh Street, P.O. Box 5505, Bismarck, ND 58502 · 701-222-5204

Bipin R. Amin · General Medical Oncology & Hematology · Mid Dakota Clinic, 401 North Ninth Street, Bismarck, ND 58501 · 701-221-6401

M. Roy Thomas · General Medical Oncology & Hematology (Breast Cancer) · St. Alexius Medical Center, Medcenter One · Mid Dakota Clinic, 401 North Ninth Street, P.O. Box 5538, Bismarck, ND 58502-5538 · 701-221-6068

Fargo

Paul S. Etzell · General Medical Oncology & Hematology · Roger Maris Cancer Center, 820 Fourth Street, North, Fargo, ND 58123 · 701-234-2397

Ralph Levitt · General Medical Oncology & Hematology · Roger Maris Cancer Center, 820 Fourth Street, North, Fargo, ND 58122 · 701-234-2397

Grand Forks

John Andrew Laurie · General Medical Oncology & Hematology · Grand Forks Clinic · Grand Forks Clinic, 1000 South Columbia Road, P.O. Box 6003, Grand Forks, ND 58206-6003 · 701-780-6000

Howard L. Russell · General Medical Oncology & Hematology · Grand Forks Clinic, 1000 South Columbia Road, P.O. Box 6003, Grand Forks, ND 58206-6003 701-780-6370

NEPHROLOGY

Bismarck

Robert E. Beach · General Nephrology · Mid Dakota Clinic, 401 North Main Street, P.O. Box 5538, Bismarck, ND 58506 · 701-221-6057

Earl J. Dunnigan · General Nephrology (Renal Transplantation) · St. Alexius Medical Center, Medcenter One · Mid Dakota Clinic, 401 North Ninth Street, P.O. Box 5538, Bismarck, ND 58506-5538 · 701-221-6035

Abel Tello · General Nephrology · Medcenter One Health Care Systems, Quain & Ramstead Clinic, 222 North Seventh Street, P.O. Box 5505, Bismarck, ND 58502 · 701-222-5204

Fargo

Thomas D. Ahlin · General Nephrology (Dialysis, Kidney Transplantation) · Meritcare Health System · Meritcare Medical Group, 737 North Broadway, Fargo, ND 58123 · 701-234-2261

Russell P. S. Knutson · General Nephrology (Dialysis, Kidney Disease) · Dakota Heartland Hospital · Dakota Clinic, 1702 South University Drive, P.O. Box 6001, Fargo, ND 58108-6001 · 701-280-3471

Grand Forks

Philip W. Marin · General Nephrology · Grand Forks Clinic, 1000 South Columbia Road, P.O. Box 6003, Grand Forks, ND 58206-6003 · 701-780-6211

NEUROLOGICAL SURGERY

Bismarck

Roger F. Kennedy · General Neurological Surgery · St. Alexius Medical Center, Physicians Services, 900 East Broadway, P.O. Box 997, Bismarck, ND 58502 · 701-224-7726

Mark S. Monasky · General Neurological Surgery (Pediatric Neurological Surgery, Spinal Surgery, Trauma, Tumor Surgery) · St. Alexius Medical Center, Medcenter One · St. Alexius Medical Center, Dakota Neurosurgical Associates, 900 East Broadway, P.O. Box 1114, Bismarck, ND 58502-1114 · 701-221-8297

Grand Forks

Stuart G. Rice · General Neurological Surgery · Grand Forks Clinic, 1000 South Columbia Road, P.O. Box 6003, Grand Forks, ND 58206-6003 · 701-780-6286

NEUROLOGY

Bismarck

Ralph T. Dunnigan, Jr. · General Neurology · St. Alexius Medical Center, Physicians Services, 900 East Broadway, P.O. Box 997, Bismarck, ND 58502 · 701-224-7058

James B. Ragland · General Neurology (Neuromuscular Disease) · St. Alexius Medical Center, Medcenter One · Regional Neurological Center, 810 East Rosser Avenue, Suite 305, Bismarck, ND 58501 · 701-222-1300

Chatree Wongjirad · General Neurology · St. Alexius Medical Center, Physicians Services, 900 East Broadway, Bismarck, ND 58501 · 701-224-7058

Fargo

Steven C. Julius · General Neurology · Dakota Clinic, 1702 South University Drive, Fargo, ND 58102 · 701-280-8549

Cynthia M. Knutson · General Neurology · Meritcare Health Systems, 700 First Avenue, South, Fargo, ND 58103 · 701-234-4036

Elliott D. Ross · Behavioral Neurology · VA Medical & Regional Office Center · University of North Dakota School of Medicine, Neuroscience Department, 1919 North Elm Street, Fargo, ND 58102 · 701-232-3241 x3554

Grand Forks

Norman T. Byers · General Neurology · Grand Forks Clinic, 1000 South Columbia Road, P.O. Box 6003, Grand Forks, ND 58206-6003 · 701-780-6432

Merle L. Teetzen · General Neurology · United Hospital, The Rehab Hospital · Medical Center Rehabilitation Hospital, 1300 Columbia Road, Grand Forks, ND 58201 · 701-780-2466

NEUROLOGY, CHILD

Bismarck

Siriwan Kriengkrairut · General Child Neurology (Epilepsy, Child Development) · St. Alexius Medical Center · St. Alexius Medical Center, Physicians Services, 900 East Broadway, Box 997, Bismarck, ND 58502-0997 · 701-224-7058

NUCLEAR MEDICINE

Fargo

Robert M. Arusell · General Nuclear Medicine · Roger Maris Cancer Center, 820 Fourth Street, North, Fargo, ND 58122 · 701-234-5126

OBSTETRICS & GYNECOLOGY

Bismarck

Jan Bury · General Obstetrics & Gynecology · St. Alexius Medical Center · Mid Dakota Clinic, 401 North Ninth Street, P.O. Box 5538, Bismarck, ND 58506-5538 701-221-6088

Robert J. Bury · General Obstetrics & Gynecology (Reproductive Surgery, Reproductive Endocrinology) · St. Alexius Medical Center · Mid Dakota Clinic, 401 North Ninth Street, P.O. Box 5538, Bismarck, ND 58506-5538 · 701-221-6459

Thomas Hutchens · General Obstetrics & Gynecology · Mid Dakota Clinic, 401 North Ninth Street, P.O. Box 5538, Bismarck, ND 58506-5538 · 701-221-6029

Jerry M. Obritsch · General Obstetrics & Gynecology · St. Alexius Medical Center, Medcenter One · Mid Dakota Clinic, 401 North Ninth Street, P.O. Box 5538, Bismarck, ND 58506-5538 · 701-221-6078

Robert K. Scarlet · General Obstetrics & Gynecology · Mid Dakota Clinic, 401 North Ninth Street, P.O. Box 5538, Bismarck, ND 58506-5538 · 701-221-6025

John M. Witt · General Obstetrics & Gynecology · St. Alexius Medical Center, Medcenter One · Mid Dakota Clinic, 401 North Ninth Street, P.O. Box 5538, Bismarck, ND 58506-5538 · 701-221-6019

Dickinson

Thomas F. Arnold · General Obstetrics & Gynecology · Dickinson Clinic, 938 Second Avenue, West, Dickinson, ND 58601 · 701-225-5183

Donn R. Slovachek · General Obstetrics & Gynecology · Dickinson Clinic, 938 Second Avenue, West, Dickinson, ND 58601 · 701-225-5183

Fargo

Steffen P. Christensen · Reproductive Endocrinology (Reproductive Surgery) · Meritcare Health System · Meritcare Medical Group, 737 North Broadway, Fargo, ND 58123 · 701-234-2698

Siri J. Fiebiger · General Obstetrics & Gynecology · Dakota Heartland Hospital Dakota Heartland Hospital, 1702 South University Drive, Fargo, ND 58103 · 701-280-3418

Grand Forks

Pamela R. Clancy · General Obstetrics & Gynecology · Grand Forks Clinic, 1000 South Columbia Road, P.O. Box 6003, Grand Forks, ND 58206-6003 · 701-780-6327

Gregory A. Gapp · General Obstetrics & Gynecology · United Hospital · Grand Forks Clinic, 1000 South Columbia Road, P.O. Box 6003, Grand Forks, ND 58206-6003 · 701-780-6000

Dean K. Midboe · General Obstetrics & Gynecology · United Hospital · Grand Forks Clinic, 1000 South Columbia Road, P.O. Box 6003, Grand Forks, ND 58206-6003 · 701-780-6329

OPHTHALMOLOGY

Bismarck

George H. Hilts III · General Ophthalmology · The Eye Specialists, 200 South Fifth Street, Bismarck, ND 58504 · 701-222-3937

Henry L. Reichert, Jr. · General Ophthalmology · The Eye Clinic of North Dakota, 620 North Ninth Street, Bismarck, ND 58501 · 701-255-4673

Charles R. Volk · Anterior Segment—Cataract & Refractive · The Eye Specialists, 200 South Fifth Street, Bismarck, ND 58504 · 701-222-3937

Fargo

David E. Grosz · General Ophthalmology (Anterior Segment—Cataract & Refractive, Glaucoma) · Dakota Heartland Hospital · Fercho Cataract & Eye Clinic, 100 Fourth Street, South, Suite 412, Fargo, ND 58103 · 701-235-0561

Max R. Johnson · Vitreo-Retinal Surgery · Retina Consultants, Pioneer Plaza, Suite 202, 101 North 10th Street, P.O. Box 1229, Fargo, ND 58107-1229 · 701-293-9791

Bruce A. Nelson · General Ophthalmology · 1702 South University Drive, Fargo, ND 58103 · 701-280-3364

C. Gary Pramhus · General Ophthalmology · Meritcare Health System, Dakota Heartland Hospital · Meritcare Medical Group, 737 North Broadway, Fargo, ND 58123 · 701-234-2305

Harold T. Rodenbiker, Jr. · (Anterior Segment—Cataract & Refractive, Corneal Diseases & Transplantation, Glaucoma) · Dakota Heartland Hospital · Fercho Cataract & Eye Clinic, 100 Fourth Street, South, Suite 412, Fargo, ND 58103 · 701-235-0561

Grand Forks

Gerald N. Gaul · General Ophthalmology · North Dakota Eye Clinic, 3035 De-Mers Avenue, Grand Forks, ND 58201 · 701-775-3151

Gary L. Karlstad · General Ophthalmology · The North Dakota Eye Clinic, 3035 DeMers Avenue, Grand Forks, ND 58201 · 701-775-3151

ORTHOPAEDIC SURGERY

Bismarck

Joseph W. Carlson · General Orthopaedic Surgery · The Bone and Joint Center, 810 East Rosser Avenue, P.O. Box 1397, Bismarck, ND 58502 · 701-222-8800

Charles P. Dahl · General Orthopaedic Surgery · The Bone and Joint Center, 810 East Rosser Avenue, P.O. Box 1397, Bismarck, ND 58502 · 701-222-8800

Ernest N. Godfread · General Orthopaedic Surgery · The Bone and Joint Center, 810 East Rosser Avenue, P.O. Box 1397, Bismarck, ND 58502 · 701-222-8800

Raymond S. Gruby · Knee Surgery · The Bone and Joint Center, 810 East Rosser Avenue, P.O. Box 1397, Bismarck, ND 58502 · 701-222-8800

Mark B. Hart · General Orthopaedic Surgery · The Bone and Joint Center, 810 East Rosser Avenue, P.O. Box 1397, Bismarck, ND 58502 · 701-222-8800

David H. Larsen · General Orthopaedic Surgery · The Bone and Joint Center, 810 East Rosser Avenue, P.O. Box 1397, Bismarck, ND 58502 · 701-222-8800

Fargo

Mark A. Lundeen · General Orthopaedic Surgery · Orthopaedic Associates, 2301 Twenty-Fifth Street, South, Suite A, Fargo, ND 58103 · 701-237-9712

Grand Forks

Brian T. Briggs · General Orthopaedic Surgery · Grand Forks Clinic, 1000 South Columbia Road, P.O. Box 6003, Grand Forks, ND 58206-6003 · 701-780-6112

Jeffrey F. Haasbeek · Pediatric Orthopaedic Surgery · United Hospital · Grand Forks Clinic, Department of Pediatric Orthopaedics, 1000 South Columbia Road, P.O. Box 6003, Grand Forks, ND 58206-6003 · 701-780-6131

OTOLARYNGOLOGY

Bismarck

Marcus M. Fiechtner · General Otolaryngology · Medcenter One, St. Alexius Medical Center · Fiechtner Ear, Nose & Throat Clinic, 225 North Seventh Street, Suite C, Bismarck, ND 58501 · 701-222-3368

Douglas Liepert · General Otolaryngology (Laser Surgery) · Medcenter One, St. Alexius Medical Center, University of Minnesota Hospital & Clinic · Medcenter One Health Care Systems, Quain & Ramstead Clinic, 222 North Seventh Street, P.O. Box 5505, Bismarck, ND 58506-5505 · 701-222-5283

Steven D. Spotts · General Otolaryngology · Ear, Nose & Throat Associates, 1605 East Capital Avenue, Bismarck, ND 58501-2102 · 701-258-6556

Fargo

James L. Frisk · General Otolaryngology · 100 South Fourth Street, Suite 302, Fargo, ND 58103 · 701-234-9063

James W. Nagle · General Otolaryngology · Meritcare Medical Group, 737 North Broadway, Fargo, ND 58123 · 701-234-2441

PATHOLOGY

Bismarck

Ward D. Fredrickson · General Pathology (Anatomic Pathology, Clinical Pathology, Cytopathology) · St. Alexius Medical Center · Pathology Consultants, 531 Airport Road, P.O. Box 2036, Bismarck, ND 58502-2036 · 701-224-7545

Dwight J. Hertz · General Pathology (Surgical Pathology, Cytology, Medical Informatics) · Medcenter One · Medcenter One, Quain & Ramstead Clinic, 222 North Seventh Street, P.O. Box 5505, Bismarck, ND 58506-5505 · 701-222-5496

John A. Hipp · General Pathology · St. Alexius Medical Center, 900 East Broadway, Bismarck, ND 58501-4586 · 701-222-2480

Michael J. Laszewski · General Pathology · St. Alexius Medical Center, 900 East Broadway, Bismarck, ND 58501-4586 · 701-222-2480

Grand Forks

A. Marvin Cooley · General Pathology · Grand Forks Clinic, 1000 South Columbia Road, P.O. Box 6003, Grand Forks, ND 58206-6003 · 701-780-5000

Timothy L. Weiland · General Pathology · United Pathology, 1200 South Columbia Road, Grand Forks, ND 58102 · 701-780-5358

PEDIATRICS

Bismarck

Joel T. Hardin · Pediatric Cardiology · Medcenter One, St. Alexius Medical Center, Trinity Medical Center (Minot), University of Minnesota Hospital & Clinic (Minneapolis, MN) · Medcenter One Health Systems, 300 North Seventh Street, P.O. Box 5525, Bismarck, ND 58502-5525 · 701-224-6970

Niran Kotrapu · Pediatric Cardiology · Mid Dakota Clinic, 401 North Ninth Street, P.O. Box 5538, Bismarck, ND 58506-5538 · 701-221-6077

Rudolph R. Roskos · Pediatric Hematology-Oncology · Medcenter One Health Systems, 300 North Seventh Street, Bismarck, ND 58502 · 701-224-6970

Charles Severn · Neonatal-Perinatal Medicine (General Pediatrics) · St. Alexius Medical Center · Neonatal Associates, 900 East Broadway, P.O. Box 5510, Bismarck, ND 58506-5510 · 701-224-7655

Fargo

Nathan L. Kobrinsky · Pediatric Hematology-Oncology · Roger Maris Cancer Center, 820 Fourth Street, North, Fargo, ND 58122 · 701-234-7544

PEDIATRICS (GENERAL)

Bismarck

Patricia S. Beach · St. Alexius Medical Center, Medcenter One · St. Alexius Medical Center, 900 East Broadway, Bismarck, ND 58501 · 701-221-6490

Ray C. Hippchen · Mid Dakota Clinic, 401 North Ninth Street, P.O. Box 5538, Bismarck, ND 58506-5538 · 701-221-6016

Kaye Obregon · St. Alexius Medical Center, Medcenter One · Mid Dakota Clinic, Kirkwood, 828 Kirkwood Mall, P.O. Box 5538, Bismarck, ND 58506-5538 701-221-6490

Dickinson

Brian O'Hara · (Pediatric Respiratory Diseases, Diabetes, Endocrinology, Pediatric Obesity) · Great Plains Clinic, 33 Ninth Street, West, Dickinson, ND 58601 701-225-6017

Fargo

Janet K. Tillisch · (Pediatric Oncology) · Dakota Heartland Hospital, Meritcare Health System · Dakota Clinic, 1702 South University Drive, Fargo, ND 58108 · 701-280-3491

Patrick J. Welle · Meritcare Clinic Southwest, 2701 Thirteenth Avenue, South, Fargo, ND 58103 · 701-234-3620

Grand Forks

Eric R. Lunn · Grand Forks Clinic, 1000 South Columbia Road, P.O. Box 6003, Grand Forks, ND 58206-6003 · 701-780-6110

James Van Looy · Grand Forks Clinic, 1000 South Columbia Road, P.O. Box 6003, Grand Forks, ND 58206-6003 · 701-780-6110

H. David Wilson · (Pediatric Infectious Disease) · United Hospital · University of North Dakota School of Medicine, 501 North Columbia Road, P.O. Box 9037, Grand Forks, ND 58202-9037 · 701-777-2520

PHYSICAL MEDICINE & REHABILITATION

Bismarck

Douglas K. Eggert · General Physical Medicine & Rehabilitation (Inpatient Rehabilitation, Stroke, Closed Head Injury, Electrodiagnostic Medicine) · Medcenter One · Medcenter One, 300 North Seventh Street, P.O. Box 5525, Bismarck, ND 58502 · 701-224-6140

Michael P. Martire · General Physical Medicine & Rehabilitation · Medcenter One, 300 North Seventh Street, P.O. Box 5525, Bismarck, ND 58502 · 701-224-6140

Bradley D. Root · (Electrodiagnostic Medicine, Musculoskeletal Medicine, Sports Medicine) · St. Alexius Medical Center · The Physical Medicine Clinic at St. Alexius Medical Center, 900 East Broadway, Box 997, Bismarck, ND 58502-0997 · 701-224-7993

Fargo

William N. Klava · General Physical Medicine & Rehabilitation (Electrodiagnostic Medicine, Pediatric Rehabilitation) · Meritcare Health System · Meritcare Rehabilitation Clinic, 736 North Broadway, Fargo, ND 58123 · 701-234-2203

Paul J. Lindquist · General Physical Medicine & Rehabilitation · Meritcare Rehabilitation Clinic, 736 North Broadway, Fargo, ND 58123 · 701-234-2203

Grand Forks

Donald F. Barcome · General Physical Medicine & Rehabilitation · Medical Center Rehabilitation Hospital, 1300 Columbia Road, Grand Forks, ND 58201 · 701-780-2465

Robert I. Cooper · General Physical Medicine & Rehabilitation · Medical Center Rehabilitation Hospital, 1300 Columbia Road, Grand Forks, ND 58201 · 701-780-2464

Genaro I. Tiongson · General Physical Medicine & Rehabilitation · Medical Center Rehabilitation Hospital, 1300 Columbia Road, Grand Forks, ND 58201 · 701-780-2473

PLASTIC SURGERY

Bismarck

Curtis A. Juhala · General Plastic Surgery · St. Alexius Medical Center · Mid Dakota Clinic, 401 North Ninth Street, Bismarck, ND 58501 · 701-221-6000

Fargo

Donald R. Lamb · General Plastic Surgery (Aesthetic Plastic Surgery, Hand Surgery, Microsurgery) · Dakota Heartland Hospital · Lamb Plastic Surgery Center, 100 Fourth Street, South, Suite 504, Fargo, ND 58103-1992 · 701-237-9592

PSYCHIATRY

Bismarck

G. Richard Athey · Addiction Psychiatry, Child & Adolescent Psychiatry · Archway Mental Health Services, 900 East Broadway, P.O. Box 5510, Bismarck, ND 58506 · 701-224-7300

Terry Max Johnson · General Psychiatry · St. Alexius Medical Center, Medcenter One · Archway Mental Health Services, 900 East Broadway, P.O. Box 5510, Bismarck, ND 58506 · 701-224-7300

Albert F. Samuelson · General Psychiatry · Archway Mental Health Services, 900 East Broadway, P.O. Box 5510, Bismarck, ND 58506 · 701-224-7300

Fargo

Ronald M. Burd · General Psychiatry · Meritcare Medical Group, 700 First Avenue, South, Fargo, ND 58101 · 701-234-4066

Grand Forks

Steven M. Hill · General Psychiatry · United Hospital · Center for Psychiatric Care, 3375 DeMers Avenue, P.O. Box 14545, Grand Forks, ND 58208-4545 · 701-780-1700

Jacob Kerbeshian · Child & Adolescent Psychiatry · Columbia Professional Park, 2812-B Seventeenth Avenue, South, Grand Forks, ND 58201-4048 · 701-780-5498

PULMONARY & CRITICAL CARE MEDICINE

Bismarck

James A. Hughes · General Pulmonary & Critical Care Medicine · The Bismarck Heart & Lung Clinic, 311 North Ninth Street, P.O. Box 2698, Bismarck, ND 58502-2698 · 701-224-7500

Tommy Ko · General Pulmonary & Critical Care Medicine · Medcenter One Health Care Systems, Quain & Ramstead Clinic, 222 North Seventh Street, P.O. Box 5505, Bismarck, ND 58506 · 701-222-5283

Craig J. Lambrecht · General Pulmonary & Critical Care Medicine (Emergency Medicine) · Medcenter One · Medcenter One, 300 North Seventh Street, P.O. Box 5525, Bismarck, ND 58506-5525 · 701-224-6150

Nicholas H. Neumann · General Pulmonary & Critical Care Medicine · The Bismarck Heart & Lung Clinic, 311 North Ninth Street, P.O. Box 2698, Bismarck, ND 58502-2698 · 701-224-7500

Benjamin Roller · (Critical Care Medicine only) · St. Alexius Medical Center, 900 East Broadway, Bismarck, ND 58501 · 701-224-7001

Grand Forks

Wayne R. Breitwieser · General Pulmonary & Critical Care Medicine (Bronchoscopy, Lung Infections, Asthma) · Grand Forks Clinic, 1000 South Columbia Road, P.O. Box 6003, Grand Forks, ND 58206-6003 · 701-780-6209

RADIATION ONCOLOGY

Bismarck

Jeffrey S. Brindle · General Radiation Oncology (Genito-Urinary Cancer, Brain Cancer) · Medcenter One, Department of Radiation Oncology, 300 North Seventh Street, P.O. Box 5525, Bismarck, ND 58501 · 701-224-6183

Glen Hyland · General Radiation Oncology · Medcenter One, Department of Radiation Oncology, 300 North Seventh Street, Bismarck, ND 58501 · 701-224-6183

Fargo

Robert M. Arusell · General Radiation Oncology · Roger Maris Cancer Center, 820 Fourth Street, North, Fargo, ND 58122 · 701-234-5126

Grand Forks

John W. Bollinger · General Radiation Oncology · Grand Forks Clinic, 1000 South Columbia Road, P.O. Box 6003, Grand Forks, ND 58206-6003 · 701-780-5860

RADIOLOGY

Bismarck

William H. Cain · General Radiology · Medcenter One Health Systems, 300 North Seventh Street, Bismarck, ND 58506 · 701-222-5200

W. Allen Hill · General Radiology (Nuclear Radiology) · Medcenter One Health Care Systems, Quain & Ramstead Clinic, 222 North Seventh Street, P.O. Box 5505, Bismarck, ND 58506-5505 · 701-222-5210

Bradley N. Meyer · General Radiology · Mid Dakota Clinic, 401 North Ninth Street, P.O. Box 5538, Bismarck, ND 58502 · 701-221-6013

Douglas R. Peterson · General Radiology · 810 East Rosser Avenue, Suite 201, Bismarck, ND 58501 · 701-224-7480

Fargo

Roger L. Gilbertson · General Radiology · Meritcare Medical Group, 720 North Fourth Street, Fargo, ND 58122 · 701-234-6960

Daniel Mickelson · General Radiology · Meritcare Medical Group, 737 North Broadway, Fargo, ND 58123 · 701-234-2406

Mark Ottmar · General Radiology · Meritcare Medical Group, 737 North Broadway, Fargo, ND 58123 · 701-234-2406

Grand Forks

Paul B. Jahn · General Radiology (Interventional Radiology) · Medical Center Rehabilitation Hospital, Invasive Radiology, 1300 Columbia Road, Grand Forks, ND 58206 · 701-780-5735

Gerald S. Smyser · Neuroradiology · United Hospital, 1200 South Columbia Road, Grand Forks, ND 58206 · 701-780-5246

RHEUMATOLOGY

Bismarck

James Lampman · General Rheumatology · St. Alexius Medical Center, Physicians Services, 900 East Broadway, P.O. Box 997, Bismarck, ND 58502 · 701-224-7960

Fargo

James R. Carpenter · General Rheumatology · Meritcare Health System · Meritcare Medical Center, 737 North Broadway, Fargo, ND 58123 · 701-234-2000

Grand Forks

James A. Lessard · General Rheumatology · Grand Forks Clinic, 1000 South Columbia Road, P.O. Box 6003, Grand Forks, ND 58206-6003 · 701-780-6228

SURGERY

Bismarck

Steven K. Hamar · General Vascular Surgery · Mid Dakota Clinic, 401 North Ninth Street, Bismarck, ND 58501 · 701-221-6046

Gaylord J. Kavlie · General Surgery · Mid Dakota Clinic, 401 North Ninth Street, Bismarck, ND 58501 · 701-221-6046

Fargo

Brent E. Krantz · General Surgery (Trauma, Endocrine Surgery) · Meritcare Health System · Meritcare Medical Group, 737 North Broadway, Fargo, ND 58123 · 701-234-2251

Stephen Stromstad · General Vascular Surgery · Meritcare Medical Group, 737 North Broadway, Fargo, ND 58123 · 701-234-2251

Grand Forks

Christian P. Schmidt · General Surgery (Gastroenterologic Surgery, General Surgical Oncology, Breast Surgery) · United Hospital · Grand Forks Clinic, 1000 South Columbia Road, P.O. Box 6003, Grand Forks, ND 58206-6003 · 701-780-6298

Mark B. Siegel · General Surgery (Endocrine Surgery, Breast Surgery) · United Hospital · Grand Forks Clinic, 1000 South Columbia Road, P.O. Box 6003, Grand Forks, ND 58206-6003 · 701-780-6281

Michael D. Traynor · General Surgery · United Hospital · Grand Forks Clinic, 1000 South Columbia Road, P.O. Box 6003, Grand Forks, ND 58206-6003 · 701-780-6280

SURGICAL ONCOLOGY

Fargo

Mark O. Jensen · General Surgical Oncology · Surgical Associates, Gateway Center, 300 Main Avenue, Fargo, ND 58103 · 701-237-3378

THORACIC SURGERY

Bismarck

A. Michael Booth · Adult Cardiothoracic Surgery (Coronary Bypass Surgery, Heart Valve Surgery, Pacemakers, Implantable Defibrillators, Adult and Pediatric

Thoracic Surgery, Adult Vascular Surgery, Surgery for Emphysema) · St. Alexius Medical Center · The Bismarck Heart & Lung Clinic, 311 North Ninth Street, P.O. Box 2698, Bismarck, ND 58502-2698 · 701-224-7500

David Holland · General Thoracic Surgery · Medcenter One, Quain & Ramstead Clinic, 222 North Seventh Street, P.O. Box 5505, Bismarck, ND 58506-5505 · 701-222-5300

Edward H. Williams · Adult Cardiothoracic Surgery (Coronary Bypass Surgery, General Thoracic Surgery, Thoracic Oncological Surgery) · St. Alexius Medical Center · The Bismarck Heart & Lung Clinic, 311 North Ninth Street, P.O. Box 2698, Bismarck, ND 58502-2698 · 701-224-7500

Grand Forks

Patrick M. Devig · General Thoracic Surgery · Grand Forks Clinic, 1000 South Columbia Road, P.O. Box 6003, Grand Forks, ND 58206-6003 · 701-780-6237

Kevin J. Tveter · General Thoracic Surgery · Grand Forks Clinic, 1000 South Columbia Road, P.O. Box 6003, Grand Forks, ND 58206-6003 · 701-780-6237

UROLOGY

Bismarck

Christopher J. Adducci · General Urology · Mid Dakota Clinic, 401 North Ninth Street, P.O. Box 5538, Bismarck, ND 58506-5538 · 701-221-6420

Henri P. Lanctin · General Urology (Endourology, Urologic Oncology) · Medcenter One Health Systems, 222 North Seventh Street, P.O. Box 5505, Bismarck, ND 58502 · 701-222-5219

Robert Pathroff · General Urology · Medcenter One, St. Alexius Medical Center, St. Joseph's Hospital & Health Center (Dickinson), West River Regional Medical Center (Hettinger) · 225 North Seventh Street, Suite B, Bismarck, ND 58501 · 701-224-9471

Fargo

Gregory J. Post · General Urology · Meritcare Clinic, 737 North Broadway, Desk 12, Fargo, ND 58123 · 701-234-2301

Grand Forks

Conrad D. Doce · General Urology · Grand Forks Clinic, 1000 South Columbia Road, P.O. Box 6003, Grand Forks, ND 58206-6003 · 701-780-6124

OKLAHOMA

ALLERGY & IMMUNOLOGY

Oklahoma City

John R. Bozalis · General Allergy & Immunology · Oklahoma Allergy & Asthma Clinic, 750 Northeast 13th Street, Oklahoma City, OK 73104 · 405-235-0040

Tulsa

David S. Hurewitz · General Allergy & Immunology · Allergy Clinic of Tulsa, 1727 South Utica Avenue, Tulsa, OK 74104-5397 · 918-743-6175

ANESTHESIOLOGY

Enid

S. Lynn Phillips · General Anesthesiology · 121 West Garriott Road, Suite B, Enid, OK 73701 · 405-242-3003

Oklahoma City

Robin L. Elwood · General Anesthesiology · University of Oklahoma Health Sciences Center, Department of Anesthesiology, 920 Stanton L. Young Boulevard, Suite 610, Oklahoma City, OK 73104 · 405-271-4351

Tulsa

John L. Aldridge · General Anesthesiology · Associated Anesthesiologists, 6839 South Canton Street, Tulsa, OK 74136 · 918-494-0612

Thomas D. Gillock · General Anesthesiology · Associated Anesthesiologists, 6839 South Canton Street, Tulsa, OK 74136 · 918-494-0612

CARDIOVASCULAR DISEASE

Enid

Nicholas Twidale · General Cardiovascular Disease (Interventional Cardiology) · 615 East Oklahoma Avenue, Suite 207, Enid, OK 73701 · 405-242-7938

Oklahoma City

Warren M. Jackman · Electrophysiology · University Hospital · University of Oklahoma Health Sciences Center, 920 Stanton L.Young Boulevard, Room 5SP300, P.O. Box 26901, Oklahoma City, OK 73190 · 405-271-8764

Ralph Lazzara · General Cardiovascular Disease (Cardiac Arrhythmias, Clinical Electrophysiology) · University Hospital, VA Medical Center · University of Oklahoma Health Sciences Center, 920 Stanton L. Young Boulevard, Oklahoma City, OK 73104 · 405-271-1353

Udho Thadani · General Cardiovascular Disease (Ischemic Heart Disease, Heart Failure) · University Hospital, VA Medical Center · University of Oklahoma Health Sciences Center, 920 Stanton L. Young Boulevard, Oklahoma City, OK 73104 · 405-271-4742

Thomas L. Whitsett · General Cardiovascular Disease (Peripheral Vascular Disease, Thromboembolic Disease, General Clinical Pharmacology) · University Hospital, Presbyterian Hospital · University of Oklahoma Health Sciences Center, University Hospital, 800 Northeast 13th Street, Oklahoma City, OK 73104 · 405-271-3119

Tulsa

Mark J. Friedman · General Cardiovascular Disease (Cardiac Catheterization, Echocardiography) · St. Francis Hospital · Springer Clinic, Cardiology Department, 6160 South Yale Avenue, Tulsa, OK 74136 · 918-497-3219

John M. Kalbfleisch · General Cardiovascular Disease · Cardiology of Tulsa, 6585 South Yale Avenue, Suite 800, Tulsa, OK 74136 · 918-494-8500

C. William McEntee · General Cardiovascular Disease · Cardiology of Tulsa, 6585 South Yale Avenue, Suite 800, Tulsa, OK 74136 · 918-494-8500

COLON & RECTAL SURGERY

Oklahoma City

Russell G. Postier · General Colon & Rectal Surgery (Gastroenterologic Surgery, General Surgery, Endocrine Surgery, General Vascular Surgery) · University Hospital, Children's Hospital of Oklahoma, VA Medical Center · University of Oklahoma Health Sciences Center, Department of Surgery, 920 Stanton L. Young Boulevard, Room SP310, Oklahoma City, OK 73104 · 405-271-7912

Tulsa

William C. Stone · General Colon & Rectal Surgery · Tulsa Colon & Rectal Surgery, 6565 South Yale Street, Suite 902, Tulsa, OK 74136 · 918-481-2788

DERMATOLOGY

Edmond

Michael D. John · Clinical Dermatology · 20 West 15th Street, Edmond, OK 73013 · 405-359-0551

Norman

Thomas D. Urice · Clinical Dermatology · 110 South Berry Road, Norman, OK 73069 · 405-321-5322

Oklahoma City

Mark Allen Everett · Clinical Dermatology (Dermatopathology) · Children's Hospital of Oklahoma, University Hospital · University of Oklahoma College of Medicine, Dermatology Clinic, 619 Northeast 13th Street, Oklahoma City, OK 73104 405-271-6112

Lela A. Lee · Cutaneous Immunology (Collagen Vascular Diseases) · University Hospital, VA Medical Center · Oklahoma University Health Sciences Center, Dermatology Clinic, 619 Northeast 13th Street, Oklahoma City, OK 73104 · 405-271-6112

Euan M. McMillan · Clinical Dermatology (Dermatopathology) · Mercy Doctors Tower, Suite 503, 4200 West Memorial Road, Oklahoma City, OK 73120-9328 · 405-752-1800

Thomas E. Nix · Clinical Dermatology · 1111 North Lee Street, Suite 249, Oklahoma City, OK 73103 · 405-236-5479

Mark S. Sullivan · Clinical Dermatology · 3433 Northwest 56th Street, Suite 880, Oklahoma City, OK 73112 · 405-947-0676

Dennis Allen Weigand · Clinical Dermatology (Dermatopathology, Dermatological Immunology) · VA Medical Center, University Hospital · University of Oklahoma College of Medicine, Dermatology Clinic, 619 Northeast 13th Street, Oklahoma City, OK 73104 · 405-271-6112

Tulsa

Vincent P. Barranco · Clinical Dermatology (Dermatopathology, Skin Cancer Surgery & Reconstruction) · St. John Medical Center, Hillcrest Medical Center · Tulsa Dermatology Clinic, 2121 East 21st Street, P.O. Box 52588, Tulsa, OK 74152-0588 · 918-749-2261

G. Pete Dosser · Clinical Dermatology · 6465 South Yale Avenue, Suite 522, Tulsa, OK 74136 · 918-492-8301

Lawrence J. Gregg · Clinical Dermatology (Aging Skin, Mucous Membrane Diseases) · St. John Medical Center, Hillcrest Medical Center · Tulsa Dermatology Clinic, 2121 East 21st Street, P.O. Box 52588, Tulsa, OK 74152 · 918-749-2261

Bernard N. Robinowitz · Clinical Dermatology · 6565 South Yale Avenue, Suite 508, Tulsa, OK 74136 · 918-492-8980

ENDOCRINOLOGY & METABOLISM

Enid

Daniel Dean Washburn · General Endocrinology & Metabolism (Diabetes, General Internal Medicine) · Springs Internal Medicine Associates, 615 East Oklahoma Avenue, Suite 208, Enid, OK 73701 · 405-242-3090

Oklahoma City

David C. Kem · General Endocrinology & Metabolism (Thyroid, Hypertension) University Hospital, Presbyterian Hospital · University of Oklahoma Health Sciences Center, 920 Stanton L. Young Boulevard, P.O. Box 26901, Oklahoma City, OK 73190 · 405-271-5896

Tulsa

Bill R. Sevier · General Endocrinology & Metabolism · Tulsa Internal Medicine, 1705 East 19th Street, Suite 603, Tulsa, OK 74104 · 918-747-2533

FAMILY MEDICINE

Bethany

Kenneth W. Whittington · Mercy Health Western Oaks, 7330 Northwest 23rd Street, Bethany, OK 73008 · 405-789-4150

Enid

Kurt S. Frantz · Springs Family Practice, 615 East Oklahoma Avenue, Suite 203, Enid, OK 73701 · 405-237-0403

David Matousek · St. Mary's Hospital, Bass Memorial Baptist Hospital · Parkview Family Practice, 330 South Fifth Street, Suite 202, Enid, OK 73701-5820 · 405-234-3320

J. Michael Pontious · (Ambulatory Research Networks, Rural Obstetrical Care, Rural HIV Care, General Family Practice) · Bass Memorial Baptist Hospital, St. Mary's Hospital · Enid Family Medicine Clinic, 620 South Madison, Suite 304, Enid, OK 73701 · 405-242-1300

Oklahoma City

James R. Barrett · The Family Medicine Center, 900 Northeast 10th Street, Oklahoma City, OK 73104 · 405-524-8540

Kenneth R. Smith · The Family Medicine Center, 900 Northeast 10th Street, Oklahoma City, OK 73104 · 405-524-8540

Michael L. Winzenread · 4200 West Memorial Road, Suite 612, Oklahoma City, OK 73120 · 405-755-1123

John Zubialde · Presbyterian Hospital, University Hospital, Children's Hospital of Oklahoma · The Family Medicine Center, Rose Clinic, 900 Northeast 10th Street, Oklahoma City, OK 73104 · 405-271-4311

GASTROENTEROLOGY

Oklahoma City

Paul N. Maton · General Gastroenterology (Peptic Disorders, Zollinger-Ellison Syndrome) · Presbyterian Hospital · Oklahoma Center for Digestive Medicine, 711 Stanton L. Young Boulevard, Suite 501, Oklahoma City, OK 73104 · 405-271-4044

Mark H. Mellow · Endoscopy (Endoscopic Laser Surgery) · Digestive Disease Specialists, 3366 Northwest Expressway, Suite 400, Oklahoma City, OK 73112 · 405-947-3545

Robert A. Rankin · General Gastroenterology (Endoscopy for Bleeding) · Baptist Medical Center of Oklahoma, Deaconess Hospital · Digestive Disease Specialists, 3366 Northwest Expressway, Suite 400, Oklahoma City, OK 73112 · 405-946-9929

Tulsa

Peter P. Aran · Hepatology (Liver Transplantation, Medical Outcomes Analysis) · St. Francis Hospital · Gastroenterology Specialists, 6565 South Yale Avenue, Suite 209, Tulsa, OK 74136 · 918-494-9433

GERIATRIC MEDICINE

Oklahoma City

Marie A. Bernard · University Hospital, VA Medical Center · VA Medical Center, 921 Northeast 13th Street (111R), Oklahoma City, OK 73104 · 405-270-0501 x5746

James W. Mold · (General Geriatric Medicine, General Family Practice) · University Hospital, Presbyterian Hospital · Family Medical Center, 900 Northeast 10th Street, Oklahoma City, OK 73104 · 405-271-4224

Tulsa

Insung Kim · (General Internal Medicine, Dementias, Alzheimer's Disease, Rehabilitation of the Elderly, Osteoporosis) · St. John Medical Center, Hillcrest Medical Center · University of Oklahoma College of Medicine—Tulsa, Department of Internal Medicine, 2808 South Sheridan Road, Tulsa, OK 74129-1077 · 918-838-4787

HAND SURGERY

Oklahoma City

Carlos A. Garcia-Moral · General Hand Surgery (Tumors of Hand & Forearm, Arthritis of the Hands) · Presbyterian Hospital, Baptist Medical Center of Oklahoma, Mercy Health Center · Oklahoma Hand Surgery Center, 3300 Northwest 56th Street, Suite 200, Oklahoma City, OK 73112-4401 · 405-945-4850

Tulsa

Perry D. Inhofe · Microsurgery (Peripheral Nerve Surgery) · St. Francis Hospital, St. John Hospital, Hillcrest Medical Center · Central States Orthopedic Specialists, Kelly Professional Building, Suite 1200, 6565 South Yale Avenue, Tulsa, OK 74136 · 918-481-7600

INFECTIOUS DISEASE

Oklahoma City

Douglas P. Fine · General Infectious Disease · University Hospital, Presbyterian Hospital, VA Medical Center · 920 Northeast 13th Street, Oklahoma City, OK 73104 · 405-271-7878

Ronald A. Greenfield · General Infectious Disease · VA Medical Center, University Hospital, Presbyterian Hospital · VA Medical Center, 921 Northeast 13th Street, Room 5A132 (111C), Oklahoma City, OK 73104 · 405-270-0501 x3284

Mark M. Huycke · General Infectious Disease · VA Medical Center · VA Medical Center, 921 Northeast 13th Street, Room 5A132 (111C), Oklahoma City, OK 73104 · 405-270-0501 x3284

Leonard N. Slater · General Infectious Disease · VA Medical Center · VA Medical Center, 921 Northeast 13th Street, Room 5A132 (111C), Oklahoma City, OK 73104 · 405-270-0501 x3284

Clifford G. Wlodaver · General Infectious Disease · Presbyterian Hospital · Oklahoma City Clinic, Department of Infectious Disease, 701 Northeast 10th Street, Oklahoma City, OK 73104 · 405-280-5463

Tulsa

Stanley Newton Schwartz · General Infectious Disease (Bone Infections, Chronic Fatigue Syndrome) · St. Francis Hospital · Kelly Professional Building, Suite 812, 6565 South Yale Avenue, Tulsa, OK 74136-8302 · 918-494-9486

INTERNAL MEDICINE (GENERAL)

Bartlesville

Thomas E. Riggs · (Pulmonary Medicine) · 226 Southeast DeBell Avenue, Bartlesville, OK 74006 · 918-333-6321

Edmond

Brian Levy · Oklahoma City Clinic, Department of Pediatrics, 200 North Bryant Street, Edmond, OK 73034 · 405-341-3623

Enid

Michael Z. Rickman · Enid Medical Associates, 427 East Cherokee Avenue, Enid, OK 73701 · 405-237-0322

David J. Shepherd, Jr. · Enid Medical Associates, 427 East Cherokee Avenue, Enid, OK 73701 · 405-237-0322

McAlester

Rhett Kern Jackson · McAlester Clinic, 1401 East Van Buren Street, McAlester, OK 74501 · 918-426-0240

Norman

John Krodel · Norman Regional Hospital · The Norman Clinic, 950 North Porter Avenue, Suite 300, Norman, OK 73071-6400 · 405-329-0121

Oklahoma City

Dewayne Andrews · (General Internal Medicine, Hypertension) · University Hospital · University of Oklahoma Health Sciences Center, 920 Stanton L. Young Boulevard, P.O. Box 26901, Oklahoma City, OK 73190 · 405-271-5882

Thomas C. Coniglione · St. Anthony Hospital, 1000 North Lee Street, Oklahoma City, OK 73102 · 405-272-6369

R. Timothy Coussons · Children's Hospital of Oklahoma · University of Oklahoma Health Sciences Center, Department of Internal Medicine, 920 Stanton L. Young Boulevard, P.O. Box 26901, Oklahoma City, OK 73190 · 405-271-5580

Susan Harmon · Medical Specialists, 711 Stanton L. Young Boulevard, Suite 406, Oklahoma City, OK 73104 · 405-232-0611

L. Scott Owen · Medical Specialists, 711 Stanton L. Young Boulevard, Suite 406, Oklahoma City, OK 73104 · 405-232-0611

Gerald B. Vannatta · Presbyterian Hospital · 711 Stanton L. Young Boulevard, Oklahoma City, OK 73104 · 405-235-6152

Tulsa

Richard A. Liebendorfer · 1919 South Wheeling Avenue, Suite 404, Tulsa, OK 74104 · 918-748-7520

Wallace Bond Love · (General Gastroenterology) · St. Francis Hospital · Warren Clinic, 6600 South Yale Avenue, Suite 750, Tulsa, OK 74136 · 918-491-5990

Joseph Lyndle Reese · 6585 South Yale Avenue, Suite 1150, Tulsa, OK 74136 · 918-494-9425

MEDICAL ONCOLOGY & HEMATOLOGY

Oklahoma City

Philip Comp · Disorders of Bleeding, Thrombosis · University Hospital · University Hospital, 800 Northeast 13th Street, Room EB400, Oklahoma City, OK 73126 · 405-271-6466

Kathy K. Dagg · General Medical Oncology & Hematology · Southwest Medical Center, Department of Hematology-Oncology, 4401 Southwestern Avenue, Oklahoma City, OK 73109 · 405-631-0919

Brian Vincent Geister · General Medical Oncology & Hematology (Breast Cancer, Lung Cancer, Gastrointestinal Cancer, Genito-Urinary Cancer, Leukemia, Lymphomas, Myeloma, Neuro-Oncology) · Baptist Medical Center of Oklahoma, Deaconess Hospital · Cancer Care Associates, 3366 Northwest Expressway, Suite 200, Oklahoma City, OK 73112-4414 · 405-945-4780

James N. George · Disorders of Bleeding, Thrombosis · University Hospital · University of Oklahoma Health Sciences Center, 920 Stanton L. Young Boulevard, P.O. Box 26901, Oklahoma City, OK 73190 · 405-271-4222

Ronald O. Gilcher · General Medical Oncology & Hematology (Blood Banking) The Oklahoma Blood Institute, 1001 North Lincoln Boulevard, Oklahoma City, OK 73104 · 405-297-5678

Tulsa

George W. Schnetzer III · General Medical Oncology & Hematology (Breast Cancer, Lung Cancer, Gastrointestinal Cancer) · St. Francis Hospital, Jane Phillips Medical Center (Bartlesville) · Cancer Care Associates, 6151 South Yale Avenue, Tulsa, OK 74136-1902 · 918-491-5800

Richard A. Shildt · General Medical Oncology & Hematology · The Fortune Cancer Center, 1705 East 19th Street, Suite 103, Tulsa, OK 74104 · 918-744-3180

NEPHROLOGY

Oklahoma City

Laura Ann Isaacs Rankin · General Nephrology · Nephrology Consultants, 3433 Northwest 56th Street, Suite 560, Oklahoma City, OK 73112 · 405-946-5307

Chris M. Sholer · General Nephrology · Plaza Medical Group, 3433 Northwest 56th Street, Suite 560, Oklahoma City, OK 73112 · 405-946-5307

LeRoy Southmayd III · General Nephrology (Transplantation Medicine, Dialysis) · Baptist Medical Center of Oklahoma, Deaconess Hospital, Bethany Health Center (Bethany), Mercy Health Center · Nephrology Consultants, 3433 Northwest 56th Street, Suite 560, Oklahoma City, OK 73112 · 405-946-5307

Tulsa

Robert M. Gold · General Nephrology (Dialysis, Kidney Transplantation, Acid Base Disorders) · St. Francis Hospital, St. John Medical Center, Hillcrest Medical Center · Tulsa Nephrology, 6585 South Yale Avenue, Suite 405, Tulsa, OK 74136 918-481-2760

NEUROLOGICAL SURGERY

Oklahoma City

L. Philip Carter · General Neurological Surgery (Vascular Neurological Surgery, Epilepsy Surgery) · University Hospital, Presbyterian Hospital, Children's Hospital of Oklahoma, VA Medical Center · University of Oklahoma Health Sciences Center, 920 Stanton L. Young Boulevard, Oklahoma City, OK 73190 · 405-271-4912

Mary K. Gumerlock · General Neurological Surgery (Brain Tumors, Cerebrovascular Disease, Pediatric Neurological Surgery) · University Hospital, VA Medical Center, Children's Hospital of Oklahoma, Presbyterian Hospital · University of Oklahoma Health Sciences Center, 920 Stanton L. Young Boulevard, Oklahoma City, OK 73104 · 405-271-4912

Donald D. Horton · Pediatric Neurological Surgery (Stereotactic Radiosurgery, Brain Tumors) · Baptist Medical Center of Oklahoma, Mercy Health Center, Children's Hospital of Oklahoma · 3366 Northwest Expressway, Suite 500D, Oklahoma City, OK 73112 · 405-271-4912; 405-345-4720

Donald F. Rhinehart · General Neurological Surgery · Oklahoma Neurological Surgery Clinic, 4140 West Memorial Road, Suite 300, Oklahoma City, OK 73120 405-748-3300

Tulsa

John A. Coates · General Neurological Surgery (Spinal Surgery) · St. Francis Hospital · Tulsa Neuromed, Warren Clinic, Suite 1315, 6600 South Yale Avenue, Tulsa, OK 74136 · 918-492-3500

NEUROLOGY

Enid

Rolfe D. Reitz · General Neurology · Northwest Neurology, 310 South Fourth Street, Enid, OK 73701 · 405-237-0093

Oklahoma City

John M. Banowetz · General Neurology · Medical Neurologists, 1211 North Shartel Street, Suite 1100, Oklahoma City, OK 73103 · 405-235-2661

James R. Couch, Jr. · Headache (Stroke, Electromyography) · University Hospital, Children's Hospital of Oklahoma, Presbyterian Hospital, VA Medical Center · University of Oklahoma Health Sciences Center, 920 Stanton L. Young Boulevard, Room 3SP203, P.O. Box 26901, Oklahoma City, OK 73190-3048 · 405-271-4113

Jeanne Ann F. King · General Neurology (Epilepsy) · University Hospital, Presbyterian Hospital · University of Oklahoma Health Sciences Center College of Medicine, Department of Neurology, 800 Northeast 13th Street, P.O. Box 26901, Oklahoma City, OK 73104 · 405-271-3635

Peggy J. Wisdom · General Neurology · VA Medical Center, 921 Northeast 13th Street, Oklahoma City, OK 73104 · 405-270-5140

Tulsa

Harvey J. Blumenthal · Headache · St. Francis Hospital · Neurological Associates of Tulsa, Kelly Professional Building, Suite 312, 6565 South Yale Avenue, Tulsa, OK 74136-8304 · 918-481-7711

Barbara A. Fries-Hastings · General Neurology · 1919 South Wheeling Avenue, Suite 707, Tulsa, OK 74104-5636 · 918-747-7517

John D. Hastings · General Neurology · 1919 South Wheeling Avenue, Suite 707, Tulsa, OK 74104-5636 · 918-747-7517

Randall M. Webb · General Neurology (Neurophysiology, Electromyography, Neuromuscular Disease, Stroke) · St. Francis Hospital · Neurological Associates of Tulsa, Kelly Professional Building, Suite 312, 6565 South Yale Avenue, Tulsa, OK 74136 · 918-481-7711

NEUROLOGY, CHILD

Oklahoma City

Julie T. Parke · General Child Neurology (Epilepsy, Neuromuscular Disease) · Children's Hospital of Oklahoma · University of Oklahoma Health Sciences Center, Neurologic Services, 920 Stanton L. Young Boulevard, Room 5SP400, Oklahoma City, OK 73104 · 405-271-6413

Sanford Schneider · General Child Neurology (Epilepsy, Developmental Delay) University Hospital, Children's Hospital of Oklahoma, Presbyterian Hospital · University of Oklahoma Health Sciences Center, 920 Stanton L. Young Boulevard, Room 5SP405, Oklahoma City, OK 73190-3048 · 405-271-4113

Tulsa

G. Steve Miller · General Child Neurology · Children's Medical Center, St. Francis Hospital, St. John Medical Center · Children's Medical Center, Child Neurology, 5300 East Skelley Avenue, Tulsa, OK 74135-6599 · 918-665-1300

Harley B. Morgan · General Child Neurology · Children's Medical Center, Child Neurology, 5300 East Skelley Avenue, Tulsa, OK 74135-6599 · 918-665-1300

OBSTETRICS & GYNECOLOGY

Enid

Ross Rumph · General Obstetrics & Gynecology · 620 South Madison Street, Suite 108, Enid, OK 73701 · 405-237-3677

Oklahoma City

J. Christopher Carey · Genital Dermatological Disease (Vulvar Disease) · University Hospital · University of Oklahoma Health Sciences Center, Department of Obstetrics & Gynecology, 920 Stanton L. Young Boulevard, Room 4SP700, Oklahoma City, OK 73104 · 405-271-7449

John I. Fishburne, Jr. · General Obstetrics & Gynecology (Obstetric Anesthesia) University Hospital · University Hospital, South Pavilion, Room 700, P.O. Box 26901, Oklahoma City, OK 73190 · 405-271-8787

Gilbert G. Haas, Jr. · Reproductive Endocrinology (Infertility, Endoscopic Surgery, Reproductive Immunology, Andrology) · University Hospital, Presbyterian Hospital · University Hospital, North Pavilion, Fourth Floor, P.O. Box 26901, Oklahoma City, OK 73190 · 405-271-8700

Robert S. Mannel · Gynecologic Cancer · University Hospital, Presbyterian Hospital, Baptist Medical Center of Oklahoma, Deaconess Hospital, Mercy Health Center · University of Oklahoma Health Sciences Center, Department of Obstetrics & Gynecology, 920 Stanton L. Young Boulevard, Oklahoma City, OK 73104 405-271-8707

William F. Rayburn · Maternal & Fetal Medicine · University Hospital, Presbyterian Hospital · University of Oklahoma Health Sciences Center, Department of Obstetrics & Gynecology, Section of Maternal-Fetal Medicine, 920 Stanton L. Young Boulevard, Oklahoma City, OK 73104 · 405-271-8711

Tulsa

Yew-Cheong Choo · Gynecologic Cancer (Pelvic Surgery) · St. Francis Hospital, St. John Medical Center, Hillcrest Medical Center, Cancer Treatment Center · 3020 South Harvard Avenue, Suite C, Tulsa, OK 74114 · 918-747-6100

Rhonda Badeen Lunn · General Obstetrics & Gynecology · St. Francis Hospital 6465 South Yale Avenue, Suite 815, Tulsa, OK 74136 · 918-481-2941

John M. Shane · Reproductive Endocrinology (Infertility, Menopausal Management, Reproductive Surgery) · St. John Medical Center · A Center for Women's Well-Being, 1705 East 19th Street, Suite 703, Tulsa, OK 74104-5418 · 918-748-7565

OPHTHALMOLOGY

Enid

Charles A. Lawrence · General Ophthalmology · Enid Eye Clinic, 615 East Oklahoma, Suite 101, Enid, OK 73701 · 405-233-4711

Oklahoma City

Hal D. Balyeat · Anterior Segment—Cataract & Refractive · Dean A. McGee Eye Institute, 608 Stanton L Young Boulevard, Oklahoma City, OK 73104 · 405-271-6060

Reagan H. Bradford, Jr. · Vitreo-Retinal Surgery · Presbyterian Hospital, St. Anthony Hospital · Dean A. McGee Eye Institute, Retinal Service, 608 Stanton L. Young Boulevard, Oklahoma City, OK 73104 · 405-271-1092

Bradley K. Farris · Neuro-Ophthalmology · Dean A. McGee Eye Institute, University Hospital, Presbyterian Hospital, St. Anthony Hospital · Dean A. McGee Eye Institute, 608 Stanton L. Young Boulevard, Oklahoma City, OK 73104 · 405-271-1091

Stephen R. Fransen · Medical Retinal Diseases · Dean A. McGee Eye Institute, 608 Stanton L. Young Boulevard, Oklahoma City, OK 73104 · 405-271-7521

Ronald M. Kingsley · Medical Retinal Diseases · Dean A. McGee Eye Institute, Retinal Service, 608 Stanton L. Young Boulevard, Oklahoma City, OK 73104 · 405-271-1092

James H. Little · Anterior Segment—Cataract & Refractive · Southwest Medical Center of Oklahoma · Southwest Eye Clinic, 1240 Southwest 44th Street, Oklahoma City, OK 73109 · 405-631-1527

Rebecca K. Morgan · Glaucoma · Presbyterian Hospital · Dean A. McGee Eye Institute, Retinal Service, 608 Stanton L. Young Boulevard, Oklahoma City, OK 73104-5040 · 405-271-1093

David W. Parke II · Medical Retinal Diseases (Vitreo-Retinal Surgery) · Presbyterian Hospital · Dean A. McGee Eye Institute, 608 Stanton L. Young Boulevard, Oklahoma City, OK 73104 · 405-271-4066

James M. Richard · Pediatric Ophthalmology · Dean A. McGee Eye Institute, 608 Stanton L. Young Boulevard, Oklahoma City, OK 73104-5040 · 405-271-6334

Mark H. Scott · Pediatric Ophthalmology · Dean A. McGee Eye Institute, 608 Stanton L. Young Boulevard, Oklahoma City, OK 73104-5040 · 405-271-7819

Gregory L. Skuta · Glaucoma · Presbyterian Hospital · Dean A. McGee Eye Institute, 608 Stanton L. Young Boulevard, Oklahoma City, OK 73104 · 405-271-7806

James Berry Wise · Glaucoma (Anterior Segment—Cataract & Refractive) · Baptist Medical Center of Oklahoma · 3435 Northwest 56th Street, Suite 1010, Oklahoma City, OK 73112 · 405-945-4747

Tulsa

Joseph F. Fleming · General Ophthalmology · The Eye Institute, 1717 South Utica Avenue, Suite 206, Tulsa, OK 74104 · 918-747-8644

Mark J. Weiss · General Ophthalmology (Glaucoma) · St. John Medical Center · The Eye Institute, 1717 South Utica Avenue, Suite 102, Tulsa, OK 74104 · 918-749-0123

ORTHOPAEDIC SURGERY

Enid

R. Kirk Fry · General Orthopaedic Surgery · Northwest Oklahoma Orthopaedic Clinic, 330 South Fifth Street, Suite 501, Enid, OK 73701 · 405-233-6707

Oklahoma City

William A. Grana · Sports Medicine/Arthroscopy · Presbyterian Hospital · Oklahoma Center for Athletes, 711 Stanton L. Young Boulevard, Suite 310, Oklahoma City, OK 73104 · 405-232-1208

Joseph A. Kopta · General Orthopaedic Surgery (Hip Surgery, Knee Surgery, Shoulder Surgery, Tumor Surgery) · University Hospital, Presbyterian Hospital · University of Oklahoma Health Sciences Center, 920 Stanton L. Young Boulevard, Suite 3SP520, P.O. Box 26901, Oklahoma City, OK 73190 · 405-271-4426

Mark S. Pascale · General Orthopaedic Surgery (Sports Medicine/Arthroscopy, Foot & Ankle Surgery, Hip Surgery, Knee Surgery, Shoulder Surgery) · Presbyterian Hospital · Oklahoma Orthopedics, 1000 North Lincoln Street, Suite 200, Oklahoma City, OK 73104 · 405-232-1208

J. Andy Sullivan · Pediatric Orthopaedic Surgery · University of Oklahoma Health Sciences Center, 920 Stanton L. Young Boulevard, P.O. Box 26901, Oklahoma City, OK 73190 · 405-271-5900

Tulsa

John B. Vosburgh · General Orthopaedic Surgery · Wheeling Medical Building, Suite 500, 1919 South Wheeling Avenue, Tulsa, OK 74104 · 918-748-7550

OTOLARYNGOLOGY

Oklahoma City

B. Hill Britton, Jr. · Otology (Neurotology) · University Hospital, Presbyterian Hospital · University of Oklahoma Health Sciences Center, 920 Stanton L. Young Boulevard, Room 3SP410, P.O. Box 26901, Oklahoma City, OK 73190 · 405-271-5504

Keith F. Clark · General Otolaryngology (Voice Disorders, Sinus & Nasal Surgery, Head & Neck Surgery, Laryngology, Pediatric Otolaryngology) · University Hospital, Presbyterian Hospital, Children's Hospital of Oklahoma, VA Medical Center, Vencor Hospital-Oklahoma City · University of Oklahoma Health Sciences Center, 920 Stanton L. Young Boulevard, Room 3SP410, P.O. Box 26901, Oklahoma City, OK 73190 · 405-271-5504

Jack Van Doren Hough · Otology/Neurotology · Baptist Medical Center of Oklahoma · Otologic Medical Clinic, Hough Ear Institute, 3400 Northwest 56th Street, Oklahoma City, OK 73112-4466 · 405-946-5563

Michael McGee · Otology/Neurotology · Baptist Medical Center of Oklahoma · Otologic Medical Clinic, Hough Ear Institute, 3400 Northwest 56th Street, Oklahoma City, OK 73112-4452 · 405-946-5563

Jesus Edilberto Medina · Head & Neck Surgery (Head & Neck Cancer) · University Hospital, Children's Hospital of Oklahoma, VA Medical Center, Presbyterian Hospital · University of Oklahoma Health Sciences Center, 920 Stanton L. Young Boulevard, Room 3SP410, P.O. Box 26901, Oklahoma City, OK 73190-3048 · 405-271-5504

Willard B. Moran · General Otolaryngology · Children's Hospital of Oklahoma · University of Oklahoma Health Sciences Center, 920 Stanton L. Young Boulevard, Room 3SP410, P.O. Box 26901, Oklahoma City, OK 73190 · 405-271-5504

Tulsa

Rollie E. Rhodes · General Otolaryngology · Eastern Oklahoma Ear, Nose & Throat, 5020 East 68th Street, Tulsa, OK 74136 · 918-492-3636

Roger E. Wehrs · Otology/Neurotology · St. Francis Hospital · Warren Medical Building, Suite 202, 6465 South Yale Avenue, Tulsa, OK 74136-7828 · 918-481-2753

David W. White · Otology/Neurotology · Eastern Oklahoma Ear, Nose & Throat, 5020 East 68th Street, Tulsa, OK 74136 · 918-492-3636

PATHOLOGY

Oklahoma City

Michael R. Harkey · General Pathology · Presbyterian Hospital, 700 Northeast 13th Street, Oklahoma City, OK 73104 · 405-271-8577

John H. Holliman · General Pathology · University of Oklahoma Health Sciences Center, Biomedical Sciences Building, Room 451, 940 Stanton L. Young Boulevard, Oklahoma City, OK 73104 · 405-271-2693

Jan V. Pitha · (Surgical Pathology, Autopsy Pathology) · VA Medical Center · VA Medical Center, 921 Northeast 13th Street, Room 4G102 (113), Oklahoma City, OK 73104 · 405-270-0501 x5339

Stan S. Shrago · General Pathology · Baptist Medical Center, Department of Pathology, 3300 Northwest Expressway, Oklahoma City, OK 73112 · 405-949-6840

Fred G. Silva II · General Pathology (Renal Pathology) · Biomedical Sciences Building, Room 451, 940 Stanton L. Young Boulevard, Oklahoma City, OK 73104 405-271-2422

Tulsa

William P. Illig · General Pathology · St. Francis Hospital · St. Francis Hospital, Department of Pathology, 6161 South Yale Avenue, Tulsa, OK 74136-1902 · 918-494-1420

PEDIATRICS

Oklahoma City

Piers R. Blackett · Pediatric Endocrinology (Diabetes) · Children's Hospital of Oklahoma · Children's Hospital of Oklahoma, Department of Pediatrics, 940 Northeast 13th Street, Room 2B251, Oklahoma City, OK 73104 · 405-271-6764

Harriet W. Coussons · (Developmental Pediatrics, Attention Deficit Hyperactivity Disorder, Spina Bifida, Developmental Disabilities) · Children's Hospital of Oklahoma, Department of Pediatrics, 1100 Northeast 13th Street, Oklahoma City, OK 73104 · 405-271-5700

Morris R. Gessouroun · Pediatric Critical Care (Respiratory Failure, Head Trauma, Asthma) · Children's Hospital of Oklahoma · Children's Hospital of Oklahoma, Department of Critical Care Medicine, 940 Northeast 13th Street, Room 6G230, Oklahoma City, OK 73104 · 405-271-5211

John E. Grunow · Pediatric Gastroenterology (General Pediatrics, Cystic Fibrosis) · Children's Hospital of Oklahoma · Children's Hospital of Oklahoma, Department of Gastroenterology & Nutrition, 940 Northeast 13th Street, Oklahoma City, OK 73104-5066 · 405-271-5884

Thomas L. Kuhls · Pediatric Infectious Disease · Children's Hospital of Oklahoma · Children's Hospital of Oklahoma, Section of Pediatric Infectious Disease, 940 Northeast 13th Street, Room 2B283, Oklahoma City, OK 73104 · 405-271-5703

Joe C. Leonard · Pediatric Hematology-Oncology · Children's Hospital of Oklahoma, 940 Northeast 13th Street, Room 2G567, Oklahoma City, OK 73104 · 405-271-6581

Mary Anne Wight McCaffree · Neonatal-Perinatal Medicine · Children's Hospital of Oklahoma, Columbia Presbyterian Hospital, Baptist Medical Center of Oklahoma · Children's Hospital of Oklahoma, Department of Pediatrics, 940 Northeast 13th Street, Room 2B307, P.O. Box 26901, Oklahoma City, OK 73190-3030 · 405-271-5215

Ruprecht Nitschke · Pediatric Hematology-Oncology · Children's Hospital of Oklahoma · Children's Hospital of Oklahoma, Department of Pediatrics, Division of Hematology-Oncology, 940 Northeast 13th Street, P.O. Box 26307, Oklahoma City, OK 73126 · 405-271-5311

Edward D. Overholt · Pediatric Cardiology · Children's Hospital of Oklahoma · Children's Hospital of Oklahoma, Department of Pediatric Cardiology, 940 Northeast 13th Street, Oklahoma City, OK 73104 · 405-271-4411

Joan Baxter K. Parkhurst · Pediatric Hematology-Oncology (Pediatric Cancer, Sickle Cell Disease) · Children's Hospital of Oklahoma, Department of Pediatrics, Division of Hematology-Oncology, 940 Northeast 13th Street, P.O. Box 26307, Oklahoma City, OK 73126 · 405-271-5311

Roger E. Sheldon · Neonatal-Perinatal Medicine (Children with Special Healthcare Needs, Technology-Dependent Children) · Children's Hospital of Oklahoma, University Hospital, Presbyterian Hospital · Children's Hospital of Oklahoma, Department of Pediatrics, 940 Northeast 13th Street, Room 2B307, Oklahoma City, OK 73104 · 405-271-5215

Kent E. Ward · Pediatric Cardiology · Children's Hospital of Oklahoma, Department of Pediatric Cardiology, 940 Northeast 13th Street, Oklahoma City, OK 73104 · 405-271-4411

James E. Wenzl · Pediatric Nephrology (Dialysis, Kidney Transplantation, Hypertension in Children & Adolescents) · Children's Hospital of Oklahoma · Children's Hospital of Oklahoma, 940 Northeast 13th Street, Suite 2B287, P.O. Box 26901, Oklahoma City, OK 73190 · 405-271-4409

PEDIATRICS (GENERAL)

Edmond

Kelly G. Stephen · Oklahoma City Clinic, Department of Pediatrics, 200 North Bryant Street, Edmond, OK 73034 · 405-341-3623

Enid

William H. Simon · Northwest Pediatrics, 409 East Cherokee Avenue, Enid, OK 73701 · 405-234-7070

Oklahoma City

Shirley Ella Dearborn · Central Oklahoma Medical Group, Department of Pediatrics, 3330 Northwest 56th Street, Suite 400, Oklahoma City, OK 73112 · 405-942-6620

Thomas A. Lera, Jr. · Children's Hospital of Oklahoma · Children's Hospital of Oklahoma, 940 Northwest 13th Street, Room 1B805, P.O. Box 26307, Oklahoma City, OK 73126 · 405-271-4790

Kendall Lane Stanford · Children's Hospital of Oklahoma, Department of Pediatrics, 940 Northeast 13th Street, Room 1B339, Oklahoma City, OK 73104 · 405-271-4407

John H. Stuemky · (Pediatric Emergency Medicine, Abused Children, General Pediatrics) · Children's Hospital of Oklahoma, University Hospital, Presbyterian Hospital, St. Anthony Hospital, O'Donoghue Rehabilitation Institute · Children's Hospital of Oklahoma, Department of Pediatrics, 940 Northeast 13th Street, Room 1B1303, Oklahoma City, OK 73104 · 405-271-4407

Terrence L. Stull · (Infectious Disease) · Children's Hospital of Oklahoma, 940 Northeast 13th Street, Room 2B300, Oklahoma City, OK 73104 · 405-271-4401

Tulsa

J. Perry Ward · Warren Clinic Pediatrics, 6565 South Yale Avenue, Suite 704, Tulsa, OK 74136 · 918-494-9400

PHYSICAL MEDICINE & REHABILITATION

Oklahoma City

Donald R. Chadwell · General Physical Medicine & Rehabilitation (Pain Management, Musculoskeletal, Electrodiagnostic Medicine, Electromyography, Stroke) · HealthSouth Rehabilitation Hospital · HealthSouth Rehabilitation Hospital, 700 Northwest Seventh Street, Oklahoma City, OK 73102 · 405-236-3131 x1182

PLASTIC SURGERY

Oklahoma City

Robert T. Buchanan · General Plastic Surgery · St. Anthony North Center, 6201 North Santa Fe, Suite 2000, Oklahoma City, OK 73118 · 405-879-7935

J. Michael Kelly · General Plastic Surgery (Facial Aesthetic Surgery, Breast Surgery, Body Contouring) · Baptist Medical Center of Oklahoma, Mercy Health Center · Oklahoma Plastic Surgeons, 3301 Northwest 63rd Street, Oklahoma City, OK 73116 · 405-842-9732

Norman S. Levine · General Plastic Surgery · University of Oklahoma Health Sciences Center, Section of Plastic Surgery, 920 Stanton L. Young Boulevard, P.O. Box 26901, 4SP220, Oklahoma City, OK 73190 · 405-271-4864

Paul Silverstein · General Plastic Surgery (Burn Care & Reconstruction, Body Contouring, Breast Surgery, Facial Aesthetic Surgery, Laser Surgery & Birthmarks) · Baptist Medical Center of Oklahoma, Mercy Health Center, Presbyterian Hospital · Oklahoma Plastic Surgeons, 3301 Northwest 63rd Street, Oklahoma City, OK 73116 · 405-842-9732

Tulsa

John M. Clark · General Plastic Surgery · Plastic Surgery Associates of Tulsa, 6585 South Yale Avenue, Suite 1020, Tulsa, OK 74136 · 918-481-2900

Eugene Bradley Garber, Jr. · General Plastic Surgery · St. John Medical Center 1784 South Utica Avenue, Tulsa, OK 74104 · 918-745-2117

Palmer R. Ramey, Jr. · (Facial Aesthetic Surgery, Laser Surgery & Birthmarks, Body Contouring, Breast Surgery, Microsurgery, Pediatric Plastic Surgery, Reconstructive Surgery) · St. Francis Hospital, St. John Medical Center · Plastic Surgery

Associates of Tulsa, 6585 South Yale Avenue, Suite 1020, Tulsa, OK 74136 · 918-481-2900

PSYCHIATRY

Oklahoma City

Gordon H. Deckert · General Psychiatry (Mood & Anxiety Disorders) · University Hospital · University of Oklahoma Health Sciences Center, Department of Psychiatry and Behavioral Sciences, South Pavilion, Suite 5SP520, 920 Stanton L. Young Boulevard, Oklahoma City, OK 73104 · 405-271-4488

Betty Pfefferbaum · Child & Adolescent Psychiatry · Children's Hospital of Oklahoma · University of Oklahoma Health Sciences Center, 920 Stanton L. Young Boulevard, Suite 5SP139, Oklahoma City, OK 73104 · 405-271-4219

PULMONARY & CRITICAL CARE MEDICINE

Oklahoma City

Gary T. Kinasewitz · General Pulmonary & Critical Care Medicine (Pulmonary Vascular Disease) · University Hospital · University of Oklahoma Health Sciences Center, 920 Stanton L. Young Boulevard, Room 3SP400, P.O. Box 26901, Oklahoma City, OK 73190 · 405-271-6173

Donald Robert McCaffree · General Pulmonary & Critical Care Medicine · VA Medical Center, University Hospital · VA Medical Center, 921 Northeast 13th Street, Oklahoma City, OK 73104 · 405-271-6173

Tulsa

Richard M. Bregman · General Pulmonary & Critical Care Medicine (Sleep Medicine) · St. Francis Hospital · Pulmonary Medicine Associates, 6585 South Yale Avenue, Suite 650, Tulsa, OK 74136 · 918-494-9288

RADIATION ONCOLOGY

Midwest City

Carl R. Borgardus · General Radiation Oncology · Cancer Treatment Center of Oklahoma, 230 North Midway Boulevard, Midwest City, OK 73110 · 405-733-2230

Oklahoma City

Clinton Amos Medbery III · General Radiation Oncology (Gynecologic Cancer, Lymphomas) · Presbyterian Hospital · Southwest Radiation Oncology, 700 Northeast 13th Street, Oklahoma City, OK 73104-5070 · 405-271-6445

Elizabeth J. Syzek · General Radiation Oncology · University Hospital, Department of Radiation Therapy, 800 Northeast 13th Street, BNP 603, P.O. Box 26307, Oklahoma City, OK 73126 · 405-271-5641

RADIOLOGY

Enid

Jonathan Ross Vanhooser · General Radiology · Radiology Associates, 405 East Cherokee, Enid, OK 73701 · 405-234-2878

Oklahoma City

Carol V. Sheldon · General Radiology · Oklahoma City Clinic, Department of Radiology, 701 Northeast 10th Street, Oklahoma City, OK 73104 · 405-280-5723

Timothy L. Tytle · General Radiology · University of Oklahoma Health Sciences Center, Department of Radiological Sciences, 940 Northeast 13th Street, P.O. Box 26901, Oklahoma City, OK 73190 · 405-271-5125

Clark Anderson Ward · General Radiology · Oklahoma City Clinic, 701 Northeast 10th Street, Oklahoma City, OK 73104 · 405-280-5700

Thomas Wallace White · General Radiology · Oklahoma City Clinic, Department of Radiology, 701 Northeast 10th Street, Oklahoma City, OK 73104 · 405-280-5503

Tulsa

Steven B. Leonard · Neuroradiology · St. Francis Hospital, Department of Radiology, 6161 South Yale Avenue, Tulsa, OK 74136 · 918-494-1600

RHEUMATOLOGY

Oklahoma City

John B. Harley · General Rheumatology (Systemic Lupus Erythematosus, Sjogren's Syndrome, Rheumatoid Arthritis) · University Hospital · University of Oklahoma Health Sciences Center, 825 Northeast 13th Street, Oklahoma City, OK 73104 · 405-271-7768

Morris Reichlin · General Rheumatology · University Hospital, Presbyterian Hospital · Oklahoma Medical Research Foundation, Arthritis & Immunology Program, 825 Northeast 13th Street, Room MS-24, Oklahoma City, OK 73104 · 405-271-7766

Ira N. Targoff · General Rheumatology (Myositis) · University Hospital, VA Medical Center · University of Oklahoma Health Sciences Center, 825 Northeast 13th Street, Room MS-24, Oklahoma City, OK 73104 · 405-271-7395

Elizabeth Taylor-Albert · General Rheumatology · University of Oklahoma Health Sciences Center, 825 Northeast 13th Street, Oklahoma City, OK 73104 · 405-271-7061

Tulsa

Lawrence A. Jacobs · General Rheumatology · St. Francis Hospital · Rheumatology Associates, 5555 East 71st Street, Suite 7100, Tulsa, OK 74136 · 918-491-9007

SURGERY

Enid

David M. Selby · General Surgery · 620 South Madison Street, Suite 109, Enid, OK 73701 · 405-242-1090

Oklahoma City

Alan B. Hollingsworth · Breast Surgery (Breast Pathology) · University Hospital, Presbyterian Hospital · University of Oklahoma Health Sciences Center, 920 Stanton L. Young Boulevard, Room 3SP101, Oklahoma City, OK 73104 · 405-271-7867

M. Alex Jacocks · General Surgery (General Vascular Surgery) · University Hospital, VA Medical Center · University of Oklahoma Health Sciences Center, Department of Surgery, 920 Stanton L. Young Boulevard, P.O. Box 26901, Oklahoma City, OK 73190 · 405-271-8096

David W. Tuggle · Pediatric Surgery (Surgical Critical Care, Trauma) · Children's Hospital of Oklahoma, Columbia-Presbyterian Medical Center, Mercy Health Center · Children's Hospital of Oklahoma, Section of Pediatric Surgery, 940 Northeast 13th Street, Room 2B204, Oklahoma City, OK 73104 · 405-271-5922

William P. Tunell · Pediatric Surgery · Children's Hospital of Oklahoma · Children's Hospital of Oklahoma, Section of Pediatric Surgery, 940 Northeast 13th Street, Room 2B204, Oklahoma City, OK 73104 · 405-271-5922

Tulsa

C. T. Thompson · General Surgery (General Surgical Oncology, Breast Surgery, Endocrine Surgery) · St. Francis Hospital · Surgical Associates, Warren Professional Building, Suite 915, 6465 South Yale Avenue, Tulsa, OK 74136 · 918-481-4800

THORACIC SURGERY

Oklahoma City

Ronald C. Elkins · Adult Cardiothoracic Surgery (Ross Procedure, Pediatric Cardiac Surgery, Esophageal Surgery) · University Hospital · University of Oklahoma Health Sciences Center, Department of Thoracic Surgery, 920 Stanton L. Young Boulevard, Room 4SP250, Oklahoma City, OK 73104 · 405-271-5789

Tulsa

Charles M. Berry · Adult Cardiothoracic Surgery · St. Francis Hospital, St. John Medical Center, Hillcrest Medical Center · Cardiac Surgery of Tulsa, William Medical Building, Suite 1250, 6585 South Yale Avenue, Tulsa, OK 74136-8325 · 918-481-2929

Spencer H. Brown, Jr. · General Thoracic Surgery (Cardiac Surgery) · Cardiac Surgery of Tulsa, William Medical Building, Suite 1250, 6585 South Yale Avenue, Tulsa, OK 74136 · 918-481-2929

UROLOGY

Enid

Jerry B. Blankenship · General Urology · Enid Urology Associates, Springs Medical Building, Suite 202, 615 East Oklahoma Avenue, Enid, OK 73701 · 405-233-3230

Oklahoma City

James S. Archer · Urologic Oncology · 711 Stanton L. Young Boulevard, Suite 707, Oklahoma City, OK 73104 · 405-235-4600

Daniel J. Culkin · General Urology · University of Oklahoma Health Sciences Center, 920 Stanton L. Young Boulevard, P.O. Box 26901, Oklahoma City, OK 73190 · 405-271-6900

Donald B. Halverstadt · General Urology (Pediatric Urology, Transplantation) · Children's Hospital of Oklahoma, Columbia Presbyterian Hospital · 711 Stanton L. Young Boulevard, Suite 707, Oklahoma City, OK 73104-5080 · 405-235-3506

Richard E. Herlihy · General Urology · Oklahoma City Clinic, 701 Northeast 10th Street, Oklahoma City, OK 73104 · 405-280-5700

Tulsa

Robert R. Bruce · General Urology (Prostate Cancer, Incontinence, Impotence) St. Francis Hospital, Broken Arrow Medical Center · Associated Urologists, Warren Professional Building, Suite 704, 6465 South Yale Avenue, Tulsa, OK 74136-7850 · 918-491-5700

Edward O. Nonweiler · General Urology (Urologic Oncology, Stone Disease) · St. Francis Hospital · Associated Urologists, Warren Professional Building, Suite 704, 6465 South Yale Avenue, Tulsa, OK 74136 · 918-491-5700

Michael B. Smith · General Urology · Associated Urologists, Warren Professional Building, Suite 704, 6465 South Yale Avenue, Tulsa, OK 74136 · 918-491-57000

SOUTH DAKOTA

ADDICTION MEDICINE

Rapid City

Jeffrey Knowles · General Addiction Medicine · 2218 Jackson Boulevard, Suite Eight, Rapid City, SD 57702 · 605-348-7859

ALLERGY & IMMUNOLOGY

Sioux Falls

Lowell J. Hyland · General Allergy & Immunology · Sioux Valley Hospital, McKennan Hospital, Weiner Memorial (Marshall, MN), Prairie Lakes Health Care Center (Watertown), St. Mary's Hospital (Pierre), Huron Regional (Huron) High Plains Asthma and Allergy Clinic, 1800 South Summit, Sioux Falls, SD 57103 · 605-336-3939

ANESTHESIOLOGY

Rapid City

Robert Allen · General Anesthesiology · Neurosurgical & Spinal Surgery Associates, 2805 Fifth Street, Suite 110, Rapid City, SD 57709 · 605-341-2424

Ben J. Howard · General Anesthesiology · West River Anesthesiology Consultants, 710 Saint Ann Street, P.O. Box 1560, Rapid City, SD 57709 · 605-343-1333

Sioux Falls

Edward F. Anderson · General Anesthesiology (Critical Care Medicine, Pain Management) · Sioux Valley Hospital · Anesthesia Physicians, 1201 South Euclid Avenue, Suite 212, Sioux Falls, SD 57105-0412 · 605-336-6376

Scott R. Atchison · General Anesthesiology · Anesthesia Physicians, 1201 South Euclid Avenue, Suite 212, Sioux Falls, SD 57105 · 605-338-5488

Thomas J. Christopherson · General Anesthesiology · Sioux Valley Hospital · Anesthesia Physicians, 1201 South Euclid Avenue, Suite 212, Sioux Falls, SD 57105 · 605-338-5488

Gary A. Halma · General Anesthesiology (Ambulatory Surgery Anesthesia, Pediatric Anesthesiology) · Anesthesia Physicians, 1201 South Euclid Avenue, Suite 212, Sioux Falls, SD 57105 · 605-338-5488

Steve E. Kunkel · General Anesthesiology · Anesthesia Physicians, 1201 South Euclid Avenue, Suite 212, Sioux Falls, SD 57105 · 605-338-5488

CARDIOVASCULAR DISEASE

Rapid City

Samuel J. Durr · General Cardiovascular Disease · Cardiology Associates, 2880 Fifth Street, Rapid City, SD 57701 · 605-399-4300

Sioux Falls

Paul L. Carpenter · General Cardiovascular Disease (Cardiac Catheterization, Pacemakers) · McKennan Hospital, Sioux Valley Hospital · North Central Heart Institute, 911 East 20th Street, Suite 305, Sioux Falls, SD 57105 · 605-331-5394

Jerry L. Moench · General Cardiovascular Disease · North Central Heart Institute, 1100 South Euclid Avenue, Sioux Falls, SD 57105 · 605-331-5394

Lloyd E. Solberg · General Cardiovascular Disease · North Central Heart Institute, 1100 South Euclid Avenue, P.O. Box 5009, Sioux Falls, SD 57117-5009 · 605-331-5394

CLINICAL PHARMACOLOGY

Rapid City

James J. Scherrer · Intramed Infusion Therapy, 2100 South Seventh Street, Suite 252, Rapid City, SD 57701 · 605-348-6796

COLON & RECTAL SURGERY

Rapid City

J. R. Bedingfield · General Colon & Rectal Surgery · Rapid City Medical Center, 728 Columbus Street, P.O. Box 6020, Rapid City, SD 57709-6020 · 605-342-3280

Michael J. Statz · General Colon & Rectal Surgery · Rapid City Medical Center, 728 Columbus Street, P.O. Box 6020, Rapid City, SD 57709-6020 · 605-342-3280

Sioux Falls

Eric S. Rolfsmeyer · General Colon & Rectal Surgery (Colon & Rectal Cancer) · Sioux Valley Hospital, McKennan Hospital · Surgical Associates, 1201 South Euclid Avenue, Suite 201, Sioux Falls, SD 57105-0483 · 605-336-1593

DERMATOLOGY

Rapid City

Marc E. Boddicker · Clinical Dermatology (Skin Cancer Surgery & Reconstruction, Liposuction, Laser Surgery) · Rapid City Regional Hospital · 2929 Fifth Street, Suite 250, Rapid City, SD 57701 · 605-342-3280

Sioux Falls

Marc A. Green · Clinical Dermatology · Central Plains Clinic, 1100 East 21st Street, Sioux Falls, SD 57105 · 605-331-3400

Dennis D. Knutson · Clinical Dermatology · Dermatology Associates, 1201 South Euclid Avenue, Suite 310, Sioux Falls, SD 57105 · 605-336-3400

James R. McGrann · Clinical Dermatology · Dermatology Associates, 1201 South Euclid Avenue, Suite 310, Sioux Falls, SD 57105 · 605-336-3400

EATING DISORDERS

Sioux Falls

Kenneth P. Aspaas · General Eating Disorders · Internal Medicine, 1201 South Euclid Avenue, Suite 610, Sioux Falls, SD 57105 · 605-339-3677

ENDOCRINOLOGY & METABOLISM

Rapid City

Stephen N. Haas · General Endocrinology & Metabolism (Thyroid) · Rapid City Regional Hospital · University Physicians Clinic, 3625 Fifth Street, Rapid City, SD 57701 · 605-341-3140

Sioux Falls

J. Michael McMillin · General Endocrinology & Metabolism (Thyroid, Diabetes) Sioux Valley Hospital, McKennan Hospital · Diabetes and Endocrine Clinic of the Sioux Empire, 1320 South Minnesota Avenue, Suite 102, Sioux Falls, SD 57105 605-334-8387

FAMILY MEDICINE

Rapid City

Steven E. Waltman · Black Hills Family Practice, 902 Columbus Avenue, Rapid City, SD 57701 · 605-348-2273

Alvin E. Wessel · Black Hills Family Practice, 902 Columbus Avenue, Rapid City, SD 57701 · 605-348-2273

Sioux Falls

Richard W. Friess · (General Family Practice, General Obstetrics & Gynecology) Sioux Valley Hospital, McKennan Hospital · Family Practice Physicians, 3401 West 49th Street, Sioux Falls, SD 57106 · 605-333-1850

Gregory L. Magnuson · (Obstetrics, Preventive Medicine, General Family Practice, General Cardiovascular Disease, Clinical Dermatology, Obesity, Diabetes) · Sioux Valley Hospital · Medical Arts Center, 1212 West 18th Street, Sioux Falls, SD 57104-4699 · 605-336-0910

Patricia Peters · McGreevy Clinic, 1200 South Seventh Street, Sioux Falls, SD 57105 · 605-336-2140

Craig J. Uthe · Family Practice Physicians, 3401 West 49th Street, Sioux Falls, SD 57106 · 605-333-1850

Jerry L. Walton · (General Surgery) · Sioux Valley Hospital, McKennan Hospital Family Practice Physicians, 1621 South Minnesota Avenue, Sioux Falls, SD 57105 605-333-1800

Spearfish

Gregory D. Hewitt · Queen City Medical Center, 1420 North 10th Street, Spearfish, SD 57783 · 605-642-2775

GASTROENTEROLOGY

Rapid City

Robert F. Gibson · General Gastroenterology · Rapid City Medical Center, 728 Columbus Street, P.O. Box 6020, Rapid City, SD 57709-6020 · 605-342-3280

Sioux Falls

John Barker · General Gastroenterology (Inflammatory Bowel Disease, Hepatology) · McKennan Hospital, Sioux Valley Hospital · 111 West 39th Street, Sioux Falls, SD 57105-5794 · 605-331-4050

GERIATRIC MEDICINE

Rapid City

David E. Sandvik · University Physicians Clinic, 3625 Fifth Street, Rapid City, SD 57701 · 605-341-3140

HAND SURGERY

Rapid City

David H. Lang · General Hand Surgery · Black Hills Orthopaedics, 2805 Fifth Street, Suite 120, Rapid City, SD 57701 · 605-341-1414

Robert J. Schutz · General Hand Surgery · Black Hills Plastic and Reconstructive Surgery, 715 Saint Francis Street, Rapid City, SD 57701 · 605-343-7208

Sioux Falls

Robert E. Van Demark, Jr. · General Hand Surgery (Hip Surgery, Knee Surgery) Sioux Valley Hospital, McKennan Hospital · Van Demark Bone and Joint Clinic, 911 East 20th Street, Suite 400, Sioux Falls, SD 57105 · 605-335-3707

INFECTIOUS DISEASE

Rapid City

J. M. Keegan · General Infectious Disease · Rapid City Medical Center, 728 Columbus Street, P.O. Box 6020, Rapid City, SD 57709-6020 · 605-342-3280

Sioux Falls

Wendall W. Hoffman · General Infectious Disease · Central Plains Clinic, 1100 East 21st Street, Sioux Falls, SD 57105 · 605-331-3487

INTERNAL MEDICINE (GENERAL)

Aberdeen

John R. Fritz · Internal Medicine Associates, Physicians Plaza, Suite 101, 201 South Lloyd Street, Aberdeen, SD 57401 · 605-225-8800

Arlin M. Myrmoe · 310 Eighth Avenue NW, Suite 205, Aberdeen, SD 57401 · 605-229-2077

Rapid City

Jeanne Bennett · University Physicians Clinic, 3625 Fifth Street, Rapid City, SD 57701 · 605-341-3140

Robert K. Johnson · University Physicians Clinic, 3625 Fifth Street, Rapid City, SD 57701 · 605-341-3140

H. Streeter Shining · Rapid City Regional Hospital · University Physicians Clinic, 3625 Fifth Street, Rapid City, SD 57701 · 605-341-3140

Douglas M. Traub · University Physicians Clinic, 3625 Fifth Street, Rapid City, SD 57701 · 605-341-3140

Sioux Falls

Kenneth P. Aspaas · (Eating Disorders) · Internal Medicine, 1201 South Euclid Avenue, Suite 610, Sioux Falls, SD 57105 · 605-339-3677

Leonard M. Gutnik · (Cardiovascular Medicine, Vascular Disease) · Central Plains Clinic · Central Plains Clinic, 1100 East 21st Street, Sioux Falls, SD 57105 605-331-3118

William O. Rossing · (General Geriatric Medicine, Preventive Care, Health Screening) · Sioux Valley Hospital, McKennan Hospital · Internal Medicine, 1201 South Euclid Avenue, Suite 610, Sioux Falls, SD 57105 · 605-339-3677

Jerel Edward Tieszen · Central Plains Clinic, 1100 East 21st Street, Sioux Falls, SD 57105 · 605-335-2727

MEDICAL ONCOLOGY & HEMATOLOGY

Rapid City

Larry P. Ebbert · General Medical Oncology & Hematology · Cancer Care Institute, 353 Fairmont Boulevard, Rapid City, SD 57701 · 605-341-8901

Paul Steven Johnson · General Medical Oncology & Hematology · Cancer Care Institute, 353 Fairmont Boulevard, Rapid City, SD 57701 · 605-341-8901

Sioux Falls

Michael S. McHale · General Medical Oncology & Hematology · University Physicians, 1018 West 18th Street, Sioux Falls, SD 57104 · 605-331-3834

NEPHROLOGY

Rapid City

Fredric M. Birch · General Nephrology · University Physicians Clinic, 3625 Fifth Street, Rapid City, SD 57701 · 605-341-3140

Sioux Falls

Edward Thaddeus Zawada, Jr. · General Nephrology (General Clinical Pharmacology, General Geriatric Medicine) · Sioux Valley Hospital, McKennan Hospital, Sioux Falls VA Hospital · University Physicians Clinic, 3701 West 49th Street, Sioux Falls, SD 57106 · 605-361-8872

NEUROLOGICAL SURGERY

Rapid City

Edward L. Seljeskog · General Neurological Surgery · Neurosurgical & Spinal Surgery Associates, 2805 Fifth Street, Suite 110, Rapid City, SD 57701 · 605-341-2424

Larry L. Teuber · General Neurological Surgery · Rapid City Regional Hospital Neurosurgical & Spinal Surgery Associates, 2805 Fifth Street, Suite 110, Rapid City, SD 57701 · 605-341-2424

Sioux Falls

Gonzalo M. Sanchez · General Neurological Surgery · Neurosurgical Associates, 1201 South Euclid Avenue, Suite 304, Sioux Falls, SD 57105 · 605-335-8470

NEUROLOGY

Rapid City

Robert C. Finley · General Neurology · Black Hills Neurology, 2929 Fifth Street, Suite 240, Rapid City, SD 57701 · 605-341-3770

Matthew E. Simmons · General Neurology · Rapid City Regional Hospital · Black Hills Neurology, 2929 Fifth Street, Suite 240, Rapid City, SD 57701 · 605-341-3770

Sioux Falls

Jerome W. Freeman · General Neurology · Neurology Associates, 1200 South Euclid Avenue, Suite 304, Sioux Falls, SD 57105 · 605-332-1610

Harlan Payne · General Neurology · Neurology Associates, 911 East 20th Street, Suite 205, Sioux Falls, SD 57105 · 605-335-0844

NUCLEAR MEDICINE

Sioux Falls

Frederick C. Lovrien · General Nuclear Medicine · Nuclear Imaging, 109 South Petro Avenue, Sioux Falls, SD 57107 · 605-330-9060

OBSTETRICS & GYNECOLOGY

Rapid City

Jeffrey L. Bendt · General Obstetrics & Gynecology (High-Risk Obstetrics) · Rapid City Regional Hospital · Obstetrics & Gynecology Associates, 1010 Ninth Street, Rapid City, SD 57701 · 605-343-9224

Raymond G. Burnett · General Obstetrics & Gynecology · Obstetrics & Gynecology Associates, 1010 Ninth Street, Rapid City, SD 57701 · 605-343-9224

Sioux Falls

Robert J. George · General Obstetrics & Gynecology · Sioux Valley Hospital, McKennan Hospital · 1201 South Euclid Avenue, Suite 204, Sioux Falls, SD 57105 · 605-357-7700

Shirley Yeh Kunkel · General Obstetrics & Gynecology · Sioux Valley Hospital, McKennan Hospital · 1201 South Euclid Avenue, Suite 204, Sioux Falls, SD 57105 · 605-336-3873

Dean L. Madison · General Obstetrics & Gynecology · Sioux Valley Hospital · 1201 South Euclid Avenue, Suite 204, Sioux Falls, SD 57105 · 605-336-3873

Milton G. Mutch, Jr. · General Obstetrics & Gynecology (Reproductive Surgery, Laparoscopic Surgery) · Sioux Valley Hospital · 1201 South Euclid Avenue, Suite 201, Sioux Falls, SD 57105 · 605-336-3873

William J. Watson · Maternal & Fetal Medicine · Sioux Valley Hospital, McKennan Hospital · 1201 South Euclid Avenue, Suite 501, Sioux Falls, SD 57105 605-336-3873

OPHTHALMOLOGY

Aberdeen

Curt A. Wischmeier · General Ophthalmology (Vitreo-Retinal Surgery, Anterior Segment—Cataract & Refractive) · St. Luke's Midland Regional Medical Center Ophthalmology Associates, 507 Professional Arts Plaza, Aberdeen, SD 57401 · 605-226-2108

Rapid City

Scott G. Eccarius · General Ophthalmology · 2001 Seventh Street, Rapid City, SD 57701 · 800-368-3596

John J. Herlihy · General Ophthalmology (Anterior Segment—Cataract & Refractive, Vitreo-Retinal Surgery) · Rapid City Regional Hospital, Lookout Memorial Hospital (Spearfish), Chadron Community Hospital (Chadron, NE), Gordon Memorial Hospital (Gordon, NE), Southern Hills General Hospital (Hot Springs) Black Hills Eye Associates, 705 Columbus Street, Rapid City, SD 57701 · 605-343-2020

Sioux Falls

Byron T. Hohm · General Ophthalmology · Ophthalmology Limited, 1200 South Euclid Avenue, Suite 204, Sioux Falls, SD 57105 · 605-336-6295

Michael W. Pekas · General Ophthalmology · Central Plains Clinic, 1100 East 21st Street, Sioux Falls, SD 57105 · 605-331-3220

Richard T. Tschetter · General Ophthalmology · Ophthalmology Limited, 1200 South Euclid Avenue, Suite 204, Sioux Falls, SD 57105 · 605-336-6294

ORTHOPAEDIC SURGERY

Rapid City

Dale R. Anderson · General Orthopaedic Surgery · Rapid City Regional Hospital 725 Indiana Street, Rapid City, SD 57701-5484 · 605-341-1122

Sioux Falls

Gail M. Benson · General Orthopaedic Surgery · Midwest Orthopaedics Center, 911 East 20th Street, Suite 700, Sioux Falls, SD 57105 · 605-336-1573

Walter O. Carlson · General Orthopaedic Surgery (Pediatric Orthopaedic Surgery, Spinal Surgery) · McKennan Hospital, Sioux Valley Hospital · Midwest Orthopaedics Center, 911 East 20th Street, Suite 700, Sioux Falls, SD 57105 · 605-336-1573

Joseph R. Cass · General Orthopaedic Surgery · Midwest Orthopaedics Center, 911 East 20th Street, Suite 700, Sioux Falls, SD 57105 · 605-336-1573

OTOLARYNGOLOGY

Aberdeen

Thomas G. Bunker · General Otolaryngology · St. Luke's Midland Regional Medical Center · Physicians Plaza, Suite 260, 201 South Lloyd Street, Aberdeen, SD 57401 · 605-225-1420

Rapid City

Gary L. Carlson · General Otolaryngology · 2929 Fifth Street, Suite 220, Rapid City, SD 57701 · 605-348-0020

Sioux Falls

Paul A. Cink · General Otolaryngology · North Central Head and Neck Clinic, 1201 South Euclid Avenue, Suite 401, Sioux Falls, SD 57105 · 605-338-8008

PATHOLOGY

Rapid City

John Barlow · General Pathology · Clinical Lab, 2805 Fifth Street, Rapid City, SD 57701 · 605-343-2267

Sioux Falls

Barry T. Pitt-Hart · General Pathology · LCM Pathologists, 1212 South Euclid Avenue, Sioux Falls, SD 57105 · 605-339-1212

PEDIATRICS

Sioux Falls

Jerome Blake · (Developmental Pediatrics) · The South Dakota Children's Specialty Clinic, 1100 South Euclid Avenue, P.O. Box 5039, Sioux Falls, SD 57117-5039 · 605-333-7169

PEDIATRICS (GENERAL)

Aberdeen

Juan R. Chavier · Aberdeen Pediatrics, Physicians Plaza, Suite 205E, 201 South Lloyd Street, Aberdeen, SD 57401 · 605-225-1500

Rapid City

Samuel L. Mortimer · Black Hills Pediatrics, 2905 Fifth Street, Rapid City, SD 57701 · 605-341-7337

Donald E. Oliver · Black Hills Pediatrics, 2905 Fifth Street, Rapid City, SD 57701 · 605-348-5910

Martin S. Spahn · Black Hills Pediatrics, 2905 Fifth Street, Rapid City, SD 57701 605-341-7337

Sioux Falls

Terry A. Lang · Sioux Valley Hospital, McKennan Hospital, Children's Care Hospital School · Pediatric Specialists of Sioux Falls, 1201 South Euclid Avenue, Suite 407, Sioux Falls, SD 57104 · 605-357-7800

Brent A. Willman · Central Plains Clinic, 1100 East 21st Street, Sioux Falls, SD 57105 · 605-331-3230

PHYSICAL MEDICINE & REHABILITATION

Rapid City

Dwight K. Caughfield · General Physical Medicine & Rehabilitation (Electrodiagnostic Medicine, Musculoskeletal Medicine & Back Pain) · Rapid City Regional Hospital, Black Hills Rehabilitation Hospital · 2908 Fifth Street, Suite 327, Rapid City, SD 57701 · 605-399-1330

Steven K. Goff · General Physical Medicine & Rehabilitation · 2908 Fifth Street, Suite 327, Rapid City, SD 57701 · 605-399-1330

Sioux Falls

Dong S. Cho · General Physical Medicine & Rehabilitation (Electrodiagnostic Medicine) · McKennan Hospital, Sioux Valley Hospital · 911 East 20th Street, Suite 200, Sioux Falls, SD 57105 · 605-334-4547

Myung J. Cho · General Physical Medicine & Rehabilitation · 3934 South Western Avenue, Sioux Falls, SD 57105 · 605-339-7524

PLASTIC SURGERY

Rapid City

Robert J. Schutz · General Plastic Surgery · Black Hills Plastic and Reconstructive Surgery, 715 Saint Francis Street, Rapid City, SD 57701 · 605-343-7208

Sioux Falls

Vaughn H. Meyer · General Plastic Surgery · Plastic Surgery Associates of South Dakota, 911 East 20th Street, Suite 602, Sioux Falls, SD 57105 · 605-335-3349

David J. Witzke · General Plastic Surgery (Skin Cancer Surgery & Reconstruction) · McKennan Hospital, Sioux Valley Hospital, Royal C. Johnson Veterans Hospital, Dakota Hospital (Vermillion), Sacred Heart Hospital (Yankton) · Plastic Surgery Associates of South Dakota, 911 East 20th Street, Suite 602, Sioux Falls, SD 57105 · 605-335-3349

PSYCHIATRY

Rapid City

Stephen P. Manlove · General Psychiatry · The Manlove Psychiatric Group, 809 South Street, Rapid City, SD 57701 · 605-348-8000

Sioux Falls

David W. Bean · General Psychiatry (Mood & Anxiety Disorders) · Psychiatry Associates, 4009 West 49th Street, Suite 308, Sioux Falls, SD 57106 · 605-361-7264

William C. Fuller · General Psychiatry · Psychiatry Associates, 4009 West 49th Street, Suite 308, Sioux Falls, SD 57106 · 605-361-7264

PULMONARY & CRITICAL CARE MEDICINE

Rapid City

Stephen L. Calhoon · General Pulmonary & Critical Care Medicine · Rapid City Medical Center, 728 Columbus Street, P.O. Box 6020, Rapid City, SD 57709-6020 · 605-342-3280

William J. Howard · General Pulmonary & Critical Care Medicine · Rapid City Medical Center, 728 Columbus Street, P.O. Box 6020, Rapid City, SD 57709-6020 · 605-342-3280

James McCafferty · General Pulmonary & Critical Care Medicine · Rapid City Medical Center, 728 Columbus Street, P.O. Box 6020, Rapid City, SD 57709-6020 · 605-342-3280

Elmo J. Rosario · General Pulmonary & Critical Care Medicine · Rapid City Medical Center, 728 Columbus Street, P.O. Box 6020, Rapid City, SD 57709-6020 · 605-342-3280

Sioux Falls

Brian Hurley · General Pulmonary & Critical Care Medicine (Sleep Disorders) · Sioux Valley Hospital, McKennan Hospital · Central Plains Clinic, 1201 South Euclid Avenue, Suite 507, Sioux Falls, SD 57105 · 605-331-3464

David A. Thomas · General Pulmonary & Critical Care Medicine · Central Plains Clinic, 1201 South Euclid Avenue, Suite 507, Sioux Falls, SD 57105 · 605-331-3464

RADIATION ONCOLOGY

Rapid City

Ronald G. Drummond · General Radiation Oncology · Cancer Care Institute, 353 Fairmont Boulevard, Rapid City, SD 57701 · 605-341-3360

Daniel M. Tackett · General Radiation Oncology · Cancer Care Institute, 353 Fairmont Boulevard, Rapid City, SD 57701 · 605-341-3360

RADIOLOGY

Rapid City

Timothy R. Frost · General Radiology · Rapid City Regional Hospital, Radiology Department, 353 Fairmont Boulevard, Rapid City, SD 57701 · 605-341-8200

Thomas L. Krafka · General Radiology · Rapid City Regional Hospital, Radiology Department, 353 Fairmont Boulevard, Rapid City, SD 57701 · 605-341-8200

Dennis E. Nesbit · General Radiology · Rapid City Regional Hospital, Radiology Department, 353 Fairmont Boulevard, Rapid City, SD 57701 · 605-341-8200

Sioux Falls

Marshall L. Brewer · General Radiology · Medical X-Ray Center, 1417 South Minnesota Avenue, Sioux Falls, SD 57105 · 605-336-0515

Thomas M. Cink · General Radiology (Chest Imaging & Diagnosis, Breast Imaging & Diagnosis) · Sioux Valley Hospital · Medical X-Ray Center, 1417 South Minnesota Avenue, Sioux Falls, SD 57105 · 605-336-0515

Daryl R. Wierda · General Radiology · Medical X-Ray Center, 1417 South Minnesota Avenue, Sioux Falls, SD 57105 · 605-336-0515

RHEUMATOLOGY

Rapid City

James A. Engelbrecht · General Rheumatology · Dakota Regional Medical Center, 2929 Fifth Street, Suite 230, Rapid City, SD 57701 · 605-341-5272

Cynthia A. Weaver · General Rheumatology · Rapid City Regional Hospital · Dakota Regional Medical Center, 2929 Fifth Street, Suite 230, Rapid City, SD 57701 · 605-341-5272

Sioux Falls

P. James Eckhoff, Jr. · General Rheumatology (Childhood Rheumatic Diseases, Osteoporosis) · Sioux Valley Hospital, McKennan Hospital · Central Plains Clinic, 1100 East 21st Street, Sioux Falls, SD 57105-1002 · 605-331-3485

SURGERY

Aberdeen

Alvin J. Janusz · General Surgery · Physicians Plaza, Suite E202, 201 South Lloyd Street, Aberdeen, SD 57401 · 605-229-1367

Rapid City

J. R. Bedingfield · General Vascular Surgery · Rapid City Medical Center, 728 Columbus Street, P.O. Box 6020, Rapid City, SD 57709-6020 · 605-342-3280

Michael J. Statz · General Vascular Surgery · Rapid City Medical Center, 728 Columbus Street, P.O. Box 6020, Rapid City, SD 57709-6020 · 605-342-3280

Sioux Falls

Donald B. Graham · General Surgery (Laparoscopic Surgery, Surgery for Morbid Obesity, Breast Surgery) · Sioux Valley Hospital, McKennan Hospital · Surgical Associates, 1201 South Euclid Avenue, Suite 201, Sioux Falls, SD 57105 · 605-336-1593

Peter J. O'Brien · General Surgery (Gastroenterologic Surgery, Trauma) · Sioux Valley Hospital · Surgical Associates, 1201 South Euclid Avenue, Suite 201, Sioux Falls, SD 57105-0483 · 605-336-1593

Gregory A. Schultz · General Vascular Surgery (Endovascular Surgery, General Surgery) · Sioux Valley Hospital, McKennan Hospital · Surgical Associates, 1201 South Euclid Avenue, Suite 201, Sioux Falls, SD 57105 · 605-336-1593

THORACIC SURGERY

Sioux Falls

Lewis C. Ofstein · General Thoracic Surgery · North Central Heart Institute, 1100 South Euclid Avenue, Sioux Falls, SD 57105 · 605-331-5394

James R. Reynolds · General Thoracic Surgery (Adult Cardiothoracic Surgery, Thoracic Oncological Surgery) · Sioux Valley Hospital, McKennan Hospital · North Central Heart Institute, 1100 South Euclid Avenue, P.O. Box 5009, Sioux Falls, SD 57117-5009 · 605-331-5394

Tommy Ray Reynolds · General Thoracic Surgery · North Central Heart Institute, 1100 South Euclid Avenue, P.O. Box 5009, Sioux Falls, SD 57117-5009 · 605-331-5394

UROLOGY

Aberdeen

Karl H. Kosse · General Urology · 1440 Northwest 15th Avenue, Aberdeen, SD 57401 · 605-229-1602

Rapid City

Gerald W. Butz · General Urology (Pediatric Urology, Female Urology) · Rapid City Regional Hospital · Black Hills Urology, 2051 Seventh Street, Rapid City, SD 57701 · 605-348-4100

Sioux Falls

R. C. Johnson · General Urology · Urology Specialists, 1200 South Euclid Avenue, Room 312, Sioux Falls, SD 57105 · 605-336-0635

TEXAS

ADDICTION MEDICINE

Beaumont

Jackson T. Achilles · General Addiction Medicine · 2497 Liberty Street, Beaumont, TX 77702 · 409-838-1116

Houston

Terry Aubrey Rustin · General Addiction Medicine (Forensic Medicine, Group Psychotherapy) · St. Joseph Hospital, Harris County Psychiatric Center, Hermann Hospital, West Oaks Hospital · Houston Recovery Campus, 4514 Lyons, Houston, TX 77020 · 713-678-2069

San Antonio

J. Thomas Pate · General Addiction Medicine · 3701 West Commerce Street, San Antonio, TX 78207 · 210-434-0531

ALLERGY & IMMUNOLOGY

Amarillo

Constantine Khalil Saadeh · General Allergy & Immunology · Texas Tech University Health Sciences Center, Department of Internal Medicine, 1400 Wallace Boulevard, Amarillo, TX 79106 · 806-354-5497

Kent K. Sorajja · (Dermatology) · Amarillo Hospital District-Northwest Texas Hospital, High Plains Baptist Hospital · 1900 Coulter Drive, Suite D, Amarillo, TX 79106 · 806-359-5461

Austin

Robert David Cook · General Allergy & Immunology · Seton Medical Center, St. David's Healthcare Center, Brackenridge Hospital, Children's Hospital of Austin Central Texas Allergy & Asthma Center, 4150 North Lamar Boulevard, Austin, TX 78756 · 512-467-0978

William Charles Howland III · General Allergy & Immunology (Adult and Pediatric Allergy & Immunology) · St. David's Healthcare Center, Brackenridge Hospital, Seton Medical Center, Seton Northwest Hospital, Austin Diagnostic Medical Center, South Austin Medical Center · Allergy Center of Austin, 3807 Spicewood Springs Road, Suite 200, Austin, TX 78759 · 512-345-7635

Julius Henry Van Bavel · General Allergy & Immunology (Adult and Pediatric Allergy & Immunology, Clinical Drug Research, Immunodeficiency) · Austin Diagnostic Medical Center · Allergy Associates of Austin Diagnostic Clinic, 1510 West 34th Street, P.O. Box 85111, Austin, TX 78708-5111 · 512-454-5821

Thurman Ray Vaughan · General Allergy & Immunology (Asthma, Food Hypersensitivity) · Seton Medical Center, St. David's Healthcare Center, Brackenridge Hospital · Austin Allergy Associates, 715 West 34th Street, Austin, TX 78705 · 512-458-9191

Beaumont

Krishna Devaru Bhat · General Allergy & Immunology (Adult and Pediatric Allergy & Immunology, Asthma, Cystic Fibrosis, Lung Infections) · 2627 Laurel Street, Beaumont, TX 77702-2204 · 409-835-5382

William Arthur Fawcett IV · General Allergy & Immunology (Immunotherapy, Adult, Pediatric, Immunodeficiency) · St. Elizabeth Hospital, Baptist Hospital Beaumont, St. Mary Hospital (Port Arthur), Beaumont Regional Medical Center 3030 North Street, Suite 450, Beaumont, TX 77702-1541 · 409-892-7090

Brenham

Ernest Neal Charlesworth · General Allergy & Immunology (Allergic Skin Disease) · Trinity Community Medical Center of Brenham · Brenham Clinic, 600 North Park, Brenham, TX 77833 · 210-836-6153

College Station

David R. Weldon · General Allergy & Immunology · Columbia Medical Center, St. Joseph Regional Health Center (Bryan) · Scott & White Clinic, Department of Allergy, 1600 University Drive, East, College Station, TX 77840 · 409-691-3636

Dallas

Gary Neil Gross · General Allergy & Immunology (Asthma, Sinus Disease) · Presbyterian Hospital of Dallas, Baylor University Medical Center · Dallas Allergy and Asthma Center, 5499 Glen Lakes Drive, Suite 100, Dallas, TX 75231-4383 · 214-691-1330

Rebecca Sue Gruchalla · General Allergy & Immunology (Antibiotic Drug Allergy, Sulfonamide Drug Reactions in AIDS Patients, Pediatric Inner City Asthma) · Parkland Memorial Hospital, Zale Lipshy University Hospital · University of Texas-Southwestern Medical Center at Dallas, 5323 Harry Hines Boulevard, Dallas, TX 75235-8859 · 214-648-3004

Donald A. Kennerly · General Allergy & Immunology (Asthma) · Parkland Memorial Hospital, Zale Lipshy University Hospital, Children's Medical Center of Dallas · University of Texas-Southwestern Medical Center at Dallas, Department of Internal Medicine, Division of Allergy, 5323 Harry Hines Boulevard, Dallas, TX 75235-8859 · 214-648-3004

William Raymond Lumry · General Allergy & Immunology (Asthma Treatment & Prevention, Nasal Allergy) · Presbyterian Hospital of Dallas · 9900 North Central Parkway, Suite 525, Dallas, TX 75231 · 214-691-3001

Michael E. Ruff · General Allergy & Immunology (Asthma, Pediatric Allergy/ Asthma) · Presbyterian Hospital of Dallas · Dallas Allergy Clinic, 5499 Glen Lakes Drive, Suite 100, Dallas, TX 75231 · 214-691-1330

Richard L. Wasserman · General Allergy & Immunology (Immunodeficiency/ Recurrent Infection, Asthma, Food Allergy) · Medical City Dallas, Children's Medical Center of Dallas · 7777 Forest Lane, Suite C-706, Dallas, TX 75230 · 214-788-8877

Dickinson

Susan Louise Andrew · General Allergy & Immunology · Clear Lake Regional Medical Center (Webster), Alvin Medical Center (Alvin), Mainland Center Hospital (Texas City) · Mainland Allergy Clinic, 914 FM 517 West, Dickinson, TX 77539-4224 · 713-337-1512

Fort Worth

Robert Jean Rogers · General Allergy & Immunology (Adult and Pediatric Allergy & Immunology, Asthma) · Cook Children's Medical Center · Fort Worth Allergy & Asthma Associates, 5929 Lovell Avenue, Fort Worth, TX 76107 · 817-731-7511

Normand Francis Tremblay · General Allergy & Immunology (Adult and Pediatric Allergy & Immunology) · Cook Children's Medical Center · Fort Worth Allergy & Asthma Associates, 5929 Lovell Avenue, Fort Worth, TX 76107 · 817-377-8457

Susan Rudd Wynn · General Allergy & Immunology (Adult and Pediatric Allergy & Immunology) · Cook Children's Medical Center, Harris Methodist-Southwest Fort Worth Allergy & Asthma Associates, 5929 Lovell Avenue, Fort Worth, TX 76107-5129 · 817-731-7511

Galveston

Rafeul Alam · General Allergy & Immunology · University of Texas Medical Branch Hospitals · University of Texas Medical Branch, Clinical Sciences Building, Room 409, Ninth And Market Streets, Route R-G62, Galveston, TX 77555-0762 · 409-772-8993

Armond S. Goldman · Immunodeficiency (Pediatric, Infant Nutrition, General Allergy & Immunology) · University of Texas Medical Branch Hospitals · University of Texas Medical Branch, Division of Pediatric Immunology/Allergy, 301 University Boulevard, Galveston, TX 77555 · 409-772-2658

J. Andrew Grant, Jr. · General Allergy & Immunology (Allergic Mechanisms, Novel Therapies for Allergies) · University of Texas Medical Branch Hospitals · University of Texas Medical Branch, Clinical Sciences Building, Room 409, 301 University Boulevard, Galveston, TX 77555-0762 · 409-772-3411

Frank C. Schmalstieg · General Allergy & Immunology (Pediatric Allergy & Immunology) · University of Texas Medical Branch, Division of Pediatric Immunology/Allergy, 301 University Boulevard, Galveston, TX 77555-0369 · 409-772-2658

Harlingen

William Robert McKenna · General Allergy & Immunology (Asthma, Multiple and Massive Bee Stings) · Valley Baptist Medical Center · 1713 Treasure Hills Boulevard, Suite 1B, Harlingen, TX 78550-8912 · 210-425-9240

Houston

Robert Burgess Bressler · General Allergy & Immunology (Adult Allergy & Immunology, Clinical & Lab Immunology, Immunodeficiency, Asthma, Immunotherapy, Cancer Biotherapy) · Methodist Hospital, St. Luke's Episcopal Hospital · Baylor College of Medicine, One Baylor Plaza, Mail Code FBRN B567, Houston, TX 77030 · 713-790-5310

Abraham H. Eisen · General Allergy & Immunology (Pediatric Allergy & Immunology) · Memorial Hospital-Southwest · 7500 Beechnut Street, Suite 290, Houston, TX 77074 · 713-988-2222

Linda J. Gorin · General Allergy & Immunology (Adult and Pediatric Allergy & Immunology, Asthma, Sinusitis, Pediatric Rheumatology) · Texas Children's Hospital · 902 Frostwood Drive, Suite 256, Houston, TX 77024 · 713-973-9424

I. Celine Hanson · General Allergy & Immunology (Pediatric AIDS, Childhood Immunizations, Immunodeficiency) · Texas Children's Hospital · Texas Children's Hospital, Department of Allergy/Immunology, 6621 Fannin Street, Mail Code 1-3291, Houston, TX 77030 · 713-770-1319

James Jay Herman · General Allergy & Immunology (Adult and Pediatric Allergy & Immunology) · Texas Children's Hospital, Cypress Fairbanks Medical Center 11301 Fallbrook Drive, Suite 300, Houston, TX 77065-4237 · 713-890-7007

Leonard S. Hoffman · General Allergy & Immunology · Hermann Hospital · Allergy & Asthma Center, 909 Frostwood Drive, Suite 155, Houston, TX 77024-2304 · 713-973-0051

David Paul Huston · Immunodeficiency (Allergy, Asthma, Autoimmunity, General Allergy & Immunology) · Methodist Hospital · Baylor Internal Medicine Consultants, 6550 Fannin Street, Suite 1101, Houston, TX 77030 · 713-790-5310

Glenn B. Kline · General Allergy & Immunology · Hermann Hospital · Allergy Associates of Houston, 909 Frostwood Drive, Suite 155, Houston, TX 77024-2304 713-973-0051

Jean G. Marcoux · General Allergy & Immunology (Pediatric Allergy & Immunology, Asthma in Adults and Children) · Memorial Hospital-Memorial City · Allergy & Asthma Center, 909 Frostwood Drive, Suite 207, Houston, TX 77024 713-827-7222

Gailen D. Marshall, Jr. · General Allergy & Immunology (Adult and Pediatric Allergy & Immunology, Clinical & Lab Immunology, Immunodeficiency) · Hermann Hospital, Lyndon B. Johnson General Hospital · University of Texas Medical School at Houston, 6431 Fannin Street, Room 4.044, Houston, TX 77030 · 713-792-4175

Jack Bernard Mazow · General Allergy & Immunology (Asthma, Adult) · Methodist Hospital · Methodist Hospital, 6550 Fannin Street, Suite 1804, Houston, TX 77030-2714 · 713-790-0571

Kristin Ann Moore · General Allergy & Immunology (Asthma, Sinus Disease, Adult, Pediatric, Pregnancy) · Methodist Hospital, Texas Children's Hospital · Allergy & Asthma Associates, 7505 Fannin Street, Suite 515, Houston, TX 77054 713-797-0045

Kurt Ralph Peters · General Allergy & Immunology (Adult and Pediatric Allergy & Immunology, Chronic Sinus Disease) · St. Luke's Episcopal Hospital, Texas Children's Hospital, Methodist Hospital · Allergy & Asthma Associates, 7505 Fannin Street, Suite 515, Houston, TX 77054 · 713-797-0045

Howard M. Rosenblatt · (Asthma, Pediatric Immunodeficiency, Clinical & Lab Immunology, Pediatric Transplantation) · Texas Children's Hospital · Texas Children's Hospital, Department of Allergy/Immunology, 6621 Fannin Street, Mail Code 1-3291, Houston, TX 77030 · 713-770-1319

William Thomas Shearer · Immunodeficiency (AIDS, Pediatric Infectious Disease, Clinical & Lab Immunology, General Allergy & Immunology) · Texas Children's Hospital · Texas Children's Hospital, Department of Allergy/Immunology, 6621 Fannin Street, Mail Code 1-3291, Houston, TX 77030 · 713-770-1319

Thomas Richard Woehler · General Allergy & Immunology · Memorial Hospital-Memorial City · Allergy & Asthma Associates, 909 Frostwood Drive, Suite 135, Houston, TX 77024 · 713-461-6711

Kingwood

Claude Larose · General Allergy & Immunology (Adult and Pediatric Allergy & Immunology) · Northeast Medical Center Hospital (Humble) · Houston Northeast Allergy, 22999 US Highway 59, Suite 290, Kingwood, TX 77339 · 713-348-3321

Lackland Air Force Base

Theodore Monroe Freeman · General Allergy & Immunology · Wilford Hall Medical Center · Wilford Hall Medical Center, Department of Allergy & Immunology, 2200 Bergquist Drive, Suite One, Lackland Air Force Base, TX 78236-5300 · 210-670-7147

Lubbock

Jitra S. Anuras · General Allergy & Immunology (Asthma, Immunodeficiency) · University Medical Center · Texas Tech University Health Sciences Center, Department of Internal Medicine, 3601 Fourth Street, Lubbock, TX 79430 · 806-743-3150

Suzanne A. Beck · General Allergy & Immunology (Pediatric Allergy & Immunology) · Allergy & Asthma Clinic of West Texas, 4102 Twenty-Second Place, Lubbock, TX 79410 · 806-799-4192

Robert J. Mamlok · General Allergy & Immunology (Adult and Pediatric Allergy & Immunology, Immunodeficiency) · Lubbock Methodist Hospital, St. Mary of the Plains Hospital, University Medical Center · Allergy & Asthma Associates, 3606 Twenty-First Street, Suite 311, Lubbock, TX 79410-1225 · 806-795-4391

Midland

John D. Bray · General Allergy & Immunology · 606-B North Kent Street, Midland, TX 75959 · 915-686-8658

Stephen Wiesenfeld · General Allergy & Immunology · 2407 Louisiana Avenue West, Midland, TX 79701 · 915-683-2718

Missouri City

Lewis A. Brown · General Allergy & Immunology (Pediatric and Adult Allergy & Immunology, Pediatric and Adult Asthma, Immunodeficiency) · Texas Children's Hospital (Houston), West Houston Medical Center (Houston), Columbia Fort Bend Medical Center, Memorial Hospital-Southwest (Houston) · Southwest Allergy Associates, 5819 Highway Six South, Suite 330, Missouri City, TX 77459 713-499-9505

Lawrence R. Shirley · General Allergy & Immunology (Adult and Pediatric Allergy & Immunology) · Southwest Allergy Associates, 5819 Highway Six South, Suite 330, Missouri City, TX 77459 · 713-499-9505

Odessa

Puthalath K. Raghuprasad · General Allergy & Immunology · Allergy & Asthma Center, 2400 East Eighth Street, Odessa, TX 79761 · 915-332-5533

San Antonio

Joseph David Diaz · General Allergy & Immunology (Adult and Pediatric Allergy & Immunology) · Santa Rosa Health Care · Allergy, Asthma & Immunology Associates of South Texas, 2414 Babcock Road, Suite 109, San Antonio, TX 78229 210-616-0882

Victor Armando Estrada · General Allergy & Immunology (Adult and Pediatric Allergy & Immunology) · Santa Rosa Children's Hospital, Southwest Texas Methodist Hospital, Northeast Baptist Hospital · 14615 San Pedro Avenue, Suite 250, San Antonio, TX 78232 · 210-490-2051

Robert Lee Jacobs · General Allergy & Immunology (Environmental & Occupational Allergy) · Southwest Texas Methodist Hospital · 8279 Fredericksburg Road, San Antonio, TX 78229 · 210-614-3923

Naynesh R. Kamani · Immunodeficiency (Pediatric Immunology, Bone Marrow Transplantation, Clinical & Lab Immunology) · Santa Rosa Children's Hospital Santa Rosa Children's Hospital, Bone Marrow Transplant Unit, 519 West Houston Street, San Antonio, TX 78207-3108 · 210-704-3458

Daniel Alberto Ramirez · General Allergy & Immunology · 7940 Floyd Curl Drive, Suite 670, San Antonio, TX 78229 · 210-692-0634

Temple

George W. Brasher · General Allergy & Immunology (Pediatric Allergy & Immunology, Childhood Asthma) · Scott & White Memorial Hospital & Clinic · Scott & White Memorial Hospital, Department of Allergy & Immunology, 2401 South 31st Street, Temple, TX 76508-0001 · 817-724-2111

Texarkana

Donald C. Fournier · General Allergy & Immunology · Medical Arts Hospital, St. Michael Health Care Center, Wadley Regional Medical Center · Ark-La-Tex Allergy, Asthma & Immunology, 2435 College Drive, Suite Five, Texarkana, TX 75501-2784 · 903-793-3161

The Woodlands

Enrique Tadeo Quintero · General Allergy & Immunology (Asthma, Pediatric Allergy) · Memorial Hospital-The Woodlands, Medical Center Hospital (Conroe), Houston Northwest Medical Center (Houston) · Allergy and Asthma Associates, 1001 Medical Plaza Drive, Suite 240, The Woodlands, TX 77380 · 713-364-1001

Tyler

Jack R. Harris · General Allergy & Immunology · Trinity Mother Frances Health Care Center · Allergy Clinic, 1128 Medical Drive, Tyler, TX 75701 · 903-593-8273

Robert B. Klein · General Allergy & Immunology · University of Texas Health Center-Tyler, US Highway 271 and State Highway 155, P.O. Box 2003, Tyler, TX 75710-2003 · 903-877-7226

Christopher J. Wrenn · General Allergy & Immunology · Trinity Mother Frances Health Care Center · Allergy Clinic, 1128 Medical Drive, P.O. Box 130789, Tyler, TX 75713 · 903-593-8273

Waco

N. J. Amar · General Allergy & Immunology · Hillcrest Baptist Medical Center, Providence Health Center · Central Texas Allergy Clinic, 405 Londonderry Drive, Suite 103, Waco, TX 76712-7999 · 817-751-1144

ANESTHESIOLOGY

Amarillo

Thomas D. Easley · General Anesthesiology · Amarillo Anesthesia Consultants, 1901 Medical Park Plaza, Suite 1059, Amarillo, TX 79106 · 806-356-2770

David N. McDonald · General Anesthesiology · 301 Amarillo Boulevard, West, Amarillo, TX 79107 · 806-372-2303

Robert W. Paige · General Anesthesiology · 6103 Amarillo Boulevard, West, Suite B, Amarillo, TX 79106-1901 · 806-359-3161

T. Bruce Pistocco · General Anesthesiology · Amarillo Hospital District-Northwest Texas Hospital · Northwest Texas Hospital, Department of Anesthesiology, P.O. Box 1110, Amarillo, TX 79175 · 806-354-1744

Austin

Joseph Payne Annis · General Anesthesiology · Austin Anesthesiology Group, 2911 Medical Arts Street, Suite One, Austin, TX 78705-3329 · 512-478-1655

Carolyn G. Biebas · General Anesthesiology · St. David's Healthcare Center · Austin Anesthesiology Group, 2911 Medical Arts Street, Suite One, Austin, TX 78705-3329 · 512-478-1655

Joe D. Kocks, Jr. · General Anesthesiology · Austin Anesthesiology Group, 2911 Medical Arts Street, Suite One, Austin, TX 78705-3329 · 512-478-1655

James P. McMichael · (Anesthesia for Cardiovascular Surgery, Regional Anesthesia, Obstetric Anesthesia) · Seton Medical Center, Brackenridge Hospital · Capitol Anesthesiology Association, 3705 Medical Parkway, Suite 570, Austin, TX 78705 512-454-2554

Thomas Miller · General Anesthesiology · Austin Anesthesiology Group, 2911 Medical Arts Street, Suite One, Austin, TX 78705-3329 · 512-478-1655

Robert Wayne Porter · General Anesthesiology · Brackenridge Hospital · Capitol Anesthesiology Association, 3705 Medical Parkway, Suite 570, Austin, TX 78705 512-454-2554

Catherine L. Scholl · General Anesthesiology · Austin Anesthesiology Group, 2911 Medical Arts Street, Suite One, Austin, TX 78705-3329 · 512-478-1655

Beaumont

Joseph S. Marino · General Anesthesiology · Anesthesia Associates, 2929 Calder Avenue, Suite 212, Beaumont, TX 77702-1830 · 409-838-5214

Michael James McCredie · General Anesthesiology · Anesthesia Associates, 2929 Calder Avenue, Suite 212, Beaumont, TX 77702-1830 · 409-838-5214

Todd Whitney McKenney · General Anesthesiology · St. Elizabeth Hospital · Anesthesia Associates, 2929 Calder Avenue, Suite 212, Beaumont, TX 77702-1830 · 409-838-5214

Carlos B. Ortiz · General Anesthesiology (Adult Cardiovascular, Neuroanesthesia, Pediatric Anesthesiology, Cardiothoracic Anesthesiology, Orthopaedic Procedures) · St. Elizabeth Hospital, Baptist Hospital Beaumont, Beaumont Regional Medical Center · Anesthesia Associates, 2929 Calder Avenue, Suite 212, P.O. Box 5587, Beaumont, TX 77726 · 409-838-5214

David C. Powell · General Anesthesiology · Anesthesia Associates, 2929 Calder Avenue, Suite 212, Beaumont, TX 77702-1830 · 409-838-5214

Corpus Christi

James A. Arnold · Pediatric Anesthesiology · 1415 Third Street, Suite 208, P.O. Box 331667, Corpus Christi, TX 78463-1667 · 512-883-6211

Thomas P. Helms · Pediatric Anesthesiology · Spohn Hospital · 1415 Third Street, Suite 208, P.O. Box 331667, Corpus Christi, TX 78463-1667 · 512-883-6211

Paul R. Hummell · General Anesthesiology · Spohn Hospital · 1415 Third Street, Suite 203, P.O Box 331717, Corpus Christi, TX 78404 · 512-884-4872

Sandra L. McCutchon · Pediatric Anesthesiology · Spohn Hospital, Bay Area Medical Center, Doctors Regional Medical Center · 1415 Third Street, Suite 203, Corpus Christi, TX 78404 · 512-884-2602

John J. Navar · General Anesthesiology · 1415 Third Street, Suite 208, P.O. Box 331667, Corpus Christi, TX 78463-1667 · 512-883-6211

Mary Dahlen Peterson · Pediatric Anesthesiology, Critical Care Medicine · Driscoll Children's Hospital · Anesthesiology Associates, 3533 South Alameda Street, Corpus Christi, TX 78411-1721 · 512-850-5449

Bruce Douglas Taylor · Pediatric Anesthesiology (Pediatric Intensive Care, Pediatric Cardiovascular) · Driscoll Children's Hospital · Driscoll Children's Hospital, Department of Anesthesiology, 3533 South Alameda Street, P.O. Box 6530, Corpus Christi, TX 78466-6530 · 512-850-5445

Dallas

Vincent H. Bradley · General Anesthesiology · Medical City Hospital of Dallas, Building C, Suite 700, 7777 Forest Lane, Dallas, TX 75230 · 214-788-6218

James Grady Crosland · Pediatric Anesthesiology (Craniofacial Anesthesiology) · Medical City Dallas Hospital · Medical City Dallas Hospital, Building B, Suite 236, 7777 Forest Lane, Dallas, TX 75230-2509 · 214-934-3388

Adolph H. Giesecke, Jr. · General Anesthesiology (Complications of Anesthesia, Critical Care Medicine, Obstetric Anesthesia, Orthopaedic Procedures) · Parkland Memorial Hospital · University of Texas-Southwestern Medical Center at Dallas, Department of Anesthesiology, 5323 Harry Hines Boulevard, Dallas, TX 75235-9068 · 214-590-7254

Robert F. Hainsworth · Pain (Pain Management) · Baylor University Medical Center · Baylor Center for Pain Management, Wadley Tower, Suite 360, 3600 Gaston Avenue, Dallas, TX 75246 · 214-820-7246

Frances Connally Morriss · Pediatric Anesthesiology (Pediatric Critical Care, Anesthesia for Pediatric Liver Transplant) · Children's Medical Center of Dallas Children's Medical Center of Dallas, 1935 Motor Street, Dallas, TX 75235-7794 214-640-2399

Robert I. Parks, Jr. · General Anesthesiology (Cardiovascular, Transplantation, Neuroanesthesia) · Baylor University Medical Center · 3600 Gaston Avenue, Suite 654, Dallas, TX 75246-1908 · 214-824-2851

Michael A. Ramsay · General Anesthesiology (Cardiovascular, Neonatal, Transplantation) · Baylor University Medical Center · Baylor University Medical Center, Department of Anesthesiology, 3500 Gaston Avenue, Dallas, TX 75246 · 214-820-3296

El Paso

Thomas R. Navar, Jr. · General Anesthesiology · Anesthesia Consultants, 1800 North Mesa Street, Suite 2D, El Paso, TX 79902 · 915-533-3474

Lynn W. Neill · General Anesthesiology · Anesthesia Consultants, 1800 North Mesa Street, Suite 2D, El Paso, TX 79902 · 915-533-3474

Luis F. Vigil · General Anesthesiology · 12150 East Cliff Drive, Suite 3-G, El Paso, TX 79902 · 915-543-2336

Fort Worth

Lyndon John Busch · Pediatric Anesthesiology · Cook Children's Medical Center Cook Children's Medical Center, 801 Seventh Avenue, Fort Worth, TX 76104-2796 · 817-885-4054

Charles C. Coffee · General Anesthesiology · All Saints Episcopal Hospital-Fort Worth · 1701 River Run, Suite 200, P.O. Box 100459, Fort Worth, TX 76185 · 817-878-9620

Laura K. Diaz · Pediatric Anesthesiology (Pediatric Cardiovascular) · Cook Children's Medical Center · Cook Children's Medical Center, Department of Anesthesia, 801 Seventh Avenue, Fort Worth, TX 76104-2796 · 817-885-4054

Mark Alan Frankel · General Anesthesiology · 1701 River Run, Suite 200, P.O. Box 100459, Fort Worth, TX 76185 · 817-878-9620

James D. Harper · General Anesthesiology (Cardiothoracic Anesthesiology, Obstetric Anesthesia) · Harris Methodist-Fort Worth, Harris Methodist-Southwest · 1301 Pennsylvania Avenue, P.O. Box 9480, Fort Worth, TX 76147 · 817-877-5056

H. Kennon Hughens · General Anesthesiology (Cardiothoracic Anesthesiology) · All Saints Episcopal Hospital-Fort Worth (Fort Worth) · All Saints Episcopal Hospital-Fort Worth, 1400 Eighth Avenue, Fort Worth, TX 76104 · 817-570-3216

Jeffrey W. Jordan · Cardiothoracic Anesthesiology · Harris Methodist-Fort Worth, Harris Methodist-Southwest · Harris Methodist-Fort Worth, 1301 Pennsylvania Avenue, Fort Worth, TX 76104 · 817-882-2000

Edward M. Sankary · General Anesthesiology · 1701 Pennsylvania Avenue, Fort Worth, TX 76104 · 817-334-0530

Glen R. Wyant · Pediatric Anesthesiology · Cook Children's Medical Center · Cook Children's Medical Center, 801 Seventh Avenue, Fort Worth, TX 76104-2796 · 817-885-4054

Galveston

James Frederick Arens · Cardiothoracic Anesthesiology · University of Texas Medical Branch, Administration Building, Room 5.118, 301 University Boulevard, Galveston, TX 77555-0138 · 409-772-5403

Robert V. Johnston · General Anesthesiology (Critical Care Medicine, Pain Management) · University of Texas Medical Branch Hospitals · University of Texas Medical Branch, Department of Anesthesiology, 301 University Boulevard, Room 0591, Galveston, TX 77555-0591 · 409-772-8555

Donald S. Prough · Critical Care Medicine · University of Texas Medical Branch Hospitals · University of Texas Medical Branch, Department of Anesthesiology, 301 University Boulevard, Suite 2A, E-91, Galveston, TX 77555-0591 · 409-772-2965

Daneshvari R. Solanki · General Anesthesiology (Orthopaedic Procedures, Obstetric Anesthesia, Pain Management) · University of Texas Medical Branch Hospitals · University of Texas Medical Branch, Department of Anesthesiology, 301 University Boulevard, Room 0591, Galveston, TX 77555-0591 · 409-772-1221

Harry K. Wallfisch · Critical Care Medicine (Neuroanesthesia, General Anesthesiology) · University of Texas Medical Branch Hospitals, Shriners Hospital for Crippled Children Galveston Burn Unit · University of Texas Medical Branch, Department of Anesthesiology, 301 University Boulevard, Suite 2A, E-91, Galveston, TX 77555-0591 · 409-772-5663

Houston

William Allan Alexander · Cardiothoracic Anesthesiology (Transesophageal Echocardiography, Pediatric Cardiovascular, Adult Cardiovascular) · Texas Heart Institute, St. Luke's Episcopal Hospital · Texas Heart Institute, Department of Cardiovascular Anesthesiology, 6720 Bertner Avenue, Suite 0520, P.O. Box 20345, Houston, TX 77225-0345 · 713-791-2666

John Travis Algren · Pediatric Anesthesiology (Pediatric Critical Care, Pain Management) · Texas Children's Hospital · Texas Children's Hospital, 6621 Fannin Street, Mail Code 2-1495, Houston, TX 77030 · 713-770-5800

Steven J. Allen · Critical Care Medicine · Hermann Hospital · Hermann Hospital, 6411 Fannin Street, Houston, TX 77030-1597 · 713-792-5566 x1018

Sudha A. Bidani · Pediatric Anesthesiology · Texas Children's Hospital · Greater Houston Anesthesia Group, 5615 Kirby Drive, Suite 850, Houston, TX 77005 · 713-791-3152

William Frank Childres · General Anesthesiology (Cardiovascular, Neuroanesthesia) · Baylor College of Medicine, 6550 Fannin Street, Suite 1003, Houston, TX 77030 · 713-798-7356

John Robert Cooper, Jr. · Cardiothoracic Anesthesiology (Complications of Anesthesia, Pediatric Cardiovascular) · Texas Heart Institute, St. Luke's Episcopal Hospital, Texas Children's Hospital · Texas Heart Institute, Division of Cardiovascular Anesthesiology, 6720 Bertner Avenue, Suite O520, Mail Code 1-226, P.O. Box 20345, Houston, TX 77225-0345 · 713-791-2666

Lewis A. Coveler · Pediatric Anesthesiology (Trauma Anesthesiology, General Anesthesiology) · Ben Taub General Hospital · Baylor College of Medicine, Department of Anesthesiology, Smith Tower, Room 1003, 6550 Fannin Street, Houston, TX 77030 · 713-793-2860

Patrick E. Curling · Cardiothoracic Anesthesiology · Methodist Hospital · Baylor College of Medicine, 6550 Fannin Street, Suite 1003, Houston, TX 77030 · 713-798-8073

Burdett S. Dunbar · Pediatric Anesthesiology · Texas Children's Hospital · Texas Children's Hospital, 6621 Fannin Street, Mail Code 2-1495, Houston, TX 77030 · 713-770-5800

Nancy Lee Glass · Pediatric Anesthesiology (General Anesthesiology) · Texas Children's Hospital · Texas Children's Hospital, Department of Anesthesiology, 6621 Fannin Street, Suite 310, Mail Code 2-1495, Houston, TX 77030 · 713-770-5800

Jeffrey Katz · General Anesthesiology (Neuroanesthesia) · Hermann Hospital · University of Texas Medical School at Houston, Department of Anesthesiology, 6431 Fannin Street, Room 5.020, Houston, TX 77030 · 713-792-5566 x1022

Mary B. Neal · General Anesthesiology · St. Luke's Episcopal Hospital · 7550 Fannin Street, Houston, TX 77054 · 713-797-9123

Betty P. Stephenson · General Anesthesiology (Ambulatory Anesthesiology [Day Surgery Patients]) · Memorial Hospital-Southwest · 7777 Southwest Freeway, Suite 425, Houston, TX 77074 · 713-772-5212

Alan S. Tonnesen · Critical Care Medicine (Adult Respiratory Distress Syndrome) · Hermann Hospital · University of Texas Medical School at Houston, Department of Anesthesiology, 6431 Fannin Street, Room 5020, Houston, TX 77030 · 713-792-5566 x1014

Longview

Aaron K. Calodney · Pain · Longview Regional Hospital · 707 Hollybrook Medical Park Building, Fifth Floor, Longview, TX 75608 · 903-758-6520

Steven R. Ford · Critical Care Medicine (Cardiothoracic Anesthesiology) · Good Shepherd Medical Center · 701 East Marshall Avenue, Suite 208, Longview, TX 75601 · 903-236-2705

Lubbock

Jon M. Badgwell · Pediatric Anesthesiology · University Medical Center · Texas Tech University Health Sciences Center, Department of Anesthesiology, 3601 Fourth Street, Lubbock, TX 79430 · 806-743-2981

Byron L. Brown · General Anesthesiology · Lubbock Methodist Hospital · Lubbock Methodist Hospital, Department of Anesthesiology, 3508 Twenty-Second Place, Lubbock, TX 79410 · 806-799-2093

Bonny Carter · Obstetric Anesthesia · University Medical Center · Texas Tech University Health Sciences Center, Department of Anesthesiology, 3601 Fourth Street, Lubbock, TX 79430 · 806-743-2981

Eaon Cockings · Pediatric Anesthesiology (Orthopaedic Procedures, General Anesthesiology) · University Medical Center · Texas Tech University Health Sciences Center, Department of Anesthesiology, 3601 Fourth Street, Room 1C-282, Lubbock, TX 79430 · 806-743-2920

George Ronald Heinrich · Hepatic Disease · University Medical Center · Texas Tech University Health Sciences Center, Department of Anesthesiology, 3601 Fourth Street, Lubbock, TX 79430 · 806-743-2981

Margaret U. Leicht · (Ambulatory Care) · St. Mary of the Plains Hospital · 3809 Twenty-Second Street, Lubbock, TX 79410 · 806-793-8801

Gabor B. Racz · Pain (Chronic Pain Management) · University Medical Center · Texas Tech University Health Sciences Center, Department of Anesthesiology, 3601 Fourth Street, Room 1C282, Lubbock, TX 79430 · 806-743-3112

Stanley F. Thornton · Pediatric Anesthesiology · Lubbock Methodist Hospital · 3508 Twenty-Second Street, Lubbock, TX 79410 · 806-793-8801

L. Ray Wilson, Jr. · Cardiothoracic Anesthesiology · Lubbock Methodist Hospital Southwest Cardiovascular Surgery Associates, 3420 Twenty-Second Place, Lubbock, TX 79410 · 806-792-8185

Midland

Edward L. Carter · General Anesthesiology · Memorial Hospital & Medical Center, Department of Anesthesiology, 2200 West Illinois Street, Midland, TX 79701 · 915-685-1111

Chester Klunick · General Anesthesiology · Memorial Hospital & Medical Center, Department of Anesthesiology, 2200 West Illinois Street, Midland, TX 79701 915-685-1616

Pasadena

Johan K. Trautmann · General Anesthesiology · Bayshore Medical Center · 3222 Burke Street, Suite 104, Pasadena, TX 77504 · 713-944-5151

San Angelo

Vayden F. Stanley · General Anesthesiology · 107 North Main Street, San Angelo, TX 76903-3619 · 915-655-0601

San Antonio

Elizabeth Alice Colonna · General Anesthesiology · Baptist Medical Center, Southwest Texas Methodist Hospital, Metropolitan Hospital, Northeast Methodist Hospital, Nix Health Care System, Women's & Children's Hospital, Santa Rosa Health Care, Santa Rosa Northwest Hospital, San Antonio Community Hospital, South Texas Ambulatory Surgery Hospital · 4207 Gardendale Street, Suite B102, San Antonio, TX 78229 · 210-614-6061

Mark E. Crum · General Anesthesiology (Adult Cardiovascular) · Southwest Texas Methodist Hospital · Tejas Anesthesia, 7711 Louis Pasteur Drive, Suite 504, San Antonio, TX 78229 · 210-615-1187

James Albert Davenport · General Anesthesiology · 7711 Louis Pasteur Drive, Suite 502, San Antonio, TX 78229 · 210-696-0076

Ralph Fernand Erian · Critical Care Medicine (Cardiothoracic Anesthesiology, Adult Cardiovascular, General Anesthesiology) · University Hospital-South Texas Medical Center, Audie L. Murphy Memorial Veterans Hospital · University of Texas Health Science Center at San Antonio, Department of Anesthesiology, 7703 Floyd Curl Drive, San Antonio, TX 78284-7838 · 210-567-4501

Cora C. Felts · Pediatric Anesthesiology · Southwest Texas Methodist Hospital · 234 San Pedro Avenue, San Antonio, TX 78205 · 210-226-3000

Joseph R. Furman · Pediatric Anesthesiology · Santa Rosa Children's Hospital Anesthesia Practice Group, 1017 North Main Street, Suite 225, San Antonio, TX 78212 · 210-224-1021

Ramon Gonzalez, Jr. · General Anesthesiology · Southwest Texas Methodist Hospital · Tejas Anesthesia, 7711 Louis Pasteur Drive, Suite 504, San Antonio, TX 78229 · 210-615-1187

William H. Hadnott · General Anesthesiology · Nix Health Care System · 414 Navarro Street, Suite 905, San Antonio, TX 78205 · 210-226-0056

Mark A. Harle · General Anesthesiology · 7711 Louis Pasteur Drive, Suite 502, San Antonio, TX 78229 · 210-696-0076

Brian Boru Harrington · General Anesthesiology · Northeast Baptist Hospital · Northeast Anesthesiology Associates, 8800 Village Drive, Suite 203, San Antonio, TX 78217 · 210-654-1464

Rosemary Hickey · Neuroanesthesia (General Anesthesiology) · University Hospital-South Texas Medical Center · University of Texas Health Science Center at San Antonio, Department of Anesthesiology, 7703 Floyd Curl Drive, San Antonio, TX 78284-7838 · 210-567-4501

Robert Lee Howard · General Anesthesiology · Northeast Baptist Hospital · Northeast Anesthesiology Associates, 8800 Village Drive, Suite 203, San Antonio, TX 78217 · 210-654-1464

Scott Eugene Kercheville · General Anesthesiology (Adult Cardiovascular, Cardiothoracic Anesthesiology, Critical Care Medicine) · Southwest Texas Methodist Hospital, San Antonio Community Hospital, St. Luke's Baptist Hospital · Tejas Anesthesia, 7711 Louis Pasteur Drive, Suite 504, San Antonio, TX 78229 · 210-615-1187

Gary G. Loudermilk · General Anesthesiology · Tejas Anesthesia, 7711 Louis Pasteur Drive, Suite 504, San Antonio, TX 78229 · 210-615-1187

Joseph John Naples · Cardiothoracic Anesthesiology (Adult Cardiovascular, Transplantation Anesthesiology) · University Hospital-South Texas Medical Center · University of Texas Health Science Center at San Antonio, Department of Anesthesiology, 7703 Floyd Curl Drive, San Antonio, TX 78284-7838 · 210-567-6214

Trevor Gordon Pollard · Pediatric Anesthesiology · Methodist Healthcare System, Baptist Memorial Healthcare System, Santa Rosa Health Care · Tejas Anesthesia, Oak Hills Medical Building, Suite 504, 7711 Louis Pasteur Drive, San Antonio, TX 78229 · 210-615-1187

Stephen Frederick Rabke · General Anesthesiology (Orthopaedic Procedures) · Santa Rosa Northwest Hospital, Southwest Texas Methodist Hospital, St. Luke's Baptist Hospital, San Antonio Community Hospital, South Texas Ambulatory Surgery Hospital · 7711 Louis Pasteur Drive, Suite 502, San Antonio, TX 78229 · 210-696-0076

Somayaji Ramamurthy · Pain (Pain Management) · University Hospital-South Texas Medical Center · University of Texas Health Science Center at San Antonio, Department of Anesthesiology, 7703 Floyd Curl Drive, San Antonio, TX 78284-7838 · 210-567-4543

Deborah K. Rasch · Pediatric Anesthesiology · University Hospital-South Texas Medical Center · University of Texas Health Science Center at San Antonio, Department of Anesthesiology, 7703 Floyd Curl Drive, San Antonio, TX 78284-7838 · 210-567-4536

John S. Richardson · Cardiothoracic Anesthesiology · Metropolitan Hospital · Tejas Anesthesia, 7711 Louis Pasteur Drive, Suite 504, San Antonio, TX 78229 · 210-615-1187

James N. Rogers · Pain Management, Neuroanesthesia (Regional Anesthesia) · University Hospital-South Texas Medical Center · University of Texas Health Science Center at San Antonio, Department of Anesthesiology, 7703 Floyd Curl Drive, San Antonio, TX 78284-7838 · 210-567-4543

Steven Glen Schuleman · General Anesthesiology · Tejas Anesthesia, 7711 Louis Pasteur Drive, Suite 504, San Antonio, TX 78229 · 210-615-1187

Tod B. Sloan · Neuroanesthesia · University Hospital-South Texas Medical Center · University of Texas Health Science Center at San Antonio, Department of Anesthesiology, 7703 Floyd Curl Drive, San Antonio, TX 78284-7838 · 210-567-4493

Dale Edward Solomon · Critical Care Medicine (Cardiothoracic Anesthesiology) University Hospital-South Texas Medical Center · University of Texas Health Science Center at San Antonio, Department of Anesthesiology, 7703 Floyd Curl Drive, San Antonio, TX 78284-7838 · 210-567-4516

Dawn Elaine Webster · Pediatric Anesthesiology · Methodist Healthcare System, Women's & Children's Hospital, Santa Rosa Children's Hospital · Tejas Anesthesia, 7711 Louis Pasteur Drive, Suite 504, San Antonio, TX 78229 · 210-615-1187

Margaret A. Wilson · General Anesthesiology · Tejas Anesthesia, 7711 Louis Pasteur Drive, Suite 504, San Antonio, TX 78229 · 210-615-1187

Alan D. Zablocki · General Anesthesiology · Methodist Healthcare System, Baptist Memorial Healthcare System, Santa Rosa Health Care, Metropolitan Hospital, Nix Health Care System · Tejas Anesthesia, 7711 Louis Pasteur Drive, Suite 504, San Antonio, TX 78229 · 210-615-1187

Temple

R. Dennis Bastron · General Anesthesiology · Scott & White Memorial Hospital & Clinic · Scott & White Memorial Hospital, Department of Anesthesiology, 2401 South 31st Street, Temple, TX 76508-0001 · 817-724-2407

T. Keller Matthews III · General Anesthesiology · Scott & White Memorial Hospital & Clinic · Scott & White Memorial Hospital, Department of Anesthesiology, 2401 South 31st Street, Temple, TX 76508-0001 · 817-724-2407

Charles H. McLeskey · General Anesthesiology (Geriatric Anesthesiology) · Scott & White Memorial Hospital & Clinic · Scott & White Memorial Hospital, Department of Anesthesiology, 2401 South 31st Street, Temple, TX 76508-0001 · 817-724-4528

Frank J. Villamaria · General Anesthesiology (Adult Cardiovascular, Cardiothoracic Anesthesiology) · Scott & White Memorial Hospital & Clinic · Scott & White Memorial Hospital, Department of Anesthesiology, 2401 South 31st Street, Temple, TX 76508-0001 · 817-724-2407

Tyler

H. Don Smith · General Anesthesiology (Adult Cardiovascular, Cardiothoracic Anesthesiology) · University of Texas Health Center-Tyler, Department of Anesthesiology, US Highway 271 and State Highway 155, P.O. Box 2003, Tyler, TX 75710-2003 · 903-877-7116

Victoria

John William Hodges · General Anesthesiology · Detar Hospital · Victoria Anesthesiology Associates, 1501 East Mockingbird Lane, Suite 220, Victoria, TX 77904 · 512-573-2481

Waco

Nelson D. De Staffany · General Anesthesiology · Providence Health Center · Providence Health Center, Department of Anesthesiology, 405 Londonderry Drive, Suite 105, Waco, TX 76712-7999 · 817-776-0266

Benjamin Wiseman · General Anesthesiology · Providence Health Center · Providence Health Center, Department of Anesthesiology, 405 Londonderry Drive, Suite 105, Waco, TX 76712-7999 · 817-776-0266

CARDIOVASCULAR DISEASE

Amarillo

R. Lowell Chaffin · General Cardiovascular Disease · Amarillo Diagnostic Clinic, 6700 West Ninth Street, Amarillo, TX 79106-1701 · 806-358-3171

John Robert Logsdon · General Cardiovascular Disease · Amarillo Diagnostic Clinic, 6700 West Ninth Street, Amarillo, TX 79106-1701 · 806-358-3171

Joel C. Osborn · General Cardiovascular Disease · Amarillo Diagnostic Clinic, 6700 West Ninth Street, Amarillo, TX 79106-1701 · 806-353-2138

Austin

David Saul Abrams · General Cardiovascular Disease · Austin Heart, 1301 West 38th Street, Suite 300, Austin, TX 78705 · 512-206-3600

James Nelson Black · General Cardiovascular Disease · Seton Medical Center · Austin Heart, 1301 West 38th Street, Suite 300, Austin, TX 78705 · 512-206-3600

James Philip Goolsby, Jr. · General Cardiovascular Disease · Austin Heart, 1301 West 38th Street, Suite 300, Austin, TX 78705 · 512-206-3600

William Edwards McCarron · General Cardiovascular Disease · Austin Diagnostic Medical Center, 12221 MoPac Expressway North, P.O. Box 85075, Austin, TX 78708-5075 · 512-459-1111

David L. Morris · General Cardiovascular Disease · Austin Heart, 1301 West 38th Street, Suite 300, Austin, TX 78705 · 512-206-3600

William A. Robinson, Jr. · General Cardiovascular Disease · Austin Heart, 1301 West 38th Street, Suite 300, Austin, TX 78705 · 512-206-3600

George Piper Rodgers · General Cardiovascular Disease · St. David's Healthcare Center · Austin Heart, 1301 West 38th Street, Suite 300, Austin, TX 78705 · 512-206-3600

Michael G. Watkins · General Cardiovascular Disease · Austin Cardiovascular Associates, 1301 West 38th Street, Suite 605, Austin, TX 78705 · 512-458-1006

Beaumont

Alfred Bernard Brady, Jr. · General Cardiovascular Disease · St. Elizabeth Hospital, Beaumont Regional Medical Center · 2900 North Street, Suite 100, Beaumont, TX 77702 · 409-892-7118

Timothy Kelly Colgan · General Cardiovascular Disease (Cardiac Catheterization, Angioplasty, Echocardiography) · St. Elizabeth Hospital, Baptist Hospital Beaumont, Beaumont Regional Medical Center · 2955 Harrison Street, Suite 207, Beaumont, TX 77702 · 409-899-5757

Thomas R. Lombardo · General Cardiovascular Disease (Invasive and Interventional Cardiology) · St. Elizabeth Hospital, Baptist Hospital Beaumont, Beaumont Regional Medical Center · 2955 Harrison Street, Suite 304, Beaumont, TX 77702 409-892-1192

Robert Leldon Sweet · General Cardiovascular Disease (Critical Care Medicine) St. Elizabeth Hospital · 3345 Plaza 10 Drive, Suite E, Beaumont, TX 77707-2508 409-838-2626

College Station

W. Richard Cashion · General Cardiovascular Disease (Cardiac Catheterization, Angioplasty, Nuclear Cardiology, Pacemakers) · Columbia Medical Center, St. Joseph Regional Health Center (Bryan) · Cashion Cardiology, 1605 Rock Prairie Road, Suite 310, College Station, TX 77845 · 409-764-1474

Corpus Christi

Joseph Garcia · General Cardiovascular Disease · Spohn Hospital · Coastal Cardiology, 613 Elizabeth Street, Suite 402, Corpus Christi, TX 78404-2223 · 512-887-2900

Raymond H. Graf, Jr. · General Cardiovascular Disease · Coastal Cardiology, 613 Elizabeth Street, Suite 402, Corpus Christi, TX 78404-2223 · 512-887-2900

Paul W. Heath · General Cardiovascular Disease (Invasive Cardiology, Clinical Cardiac Electrophysiology) · Spohn Hospital, Doctors Regional Medical Center, Memorial Medical Center, Bay Area Medical Center · Cardiology Associates of Corpus Christi, 1521 South Staples Street, Suite 704, Corpus Christi, TX 78404-3155 · 512-888-8271

William D. Jack II · General Cardiovascular Disease · Spohn Hospital · Cardiology Associates of Corpus Christi, 1521 South Staples Street, Suite 704, Corpus Christi, TX 78404-3155 · 512-888-8271

Jackson E. Ormand, Jr. · General Cardiovascular Disease · Spohn Hospital, Doctors Regional Medical Center, Bay Area Medical Center, Memorial Medical Center · Cardiology Associates of Corpus Christi, 1521 South Staples Street, Suite 704, Corpus Christi, TX 78404-3155 · 512-888-8271

Dallas

L. David Hillis · Cardiac Catheterization · Parkland Memorial Hospital, Zale Lipshy University Hospital · University of Texas-Southwestern Medical Center at Dallas, Department of Internal Medicine, 5323 Harry Hines Boulevard, Dallas, TX 75235-9047 · 214-590-8879

Vernon P. H. Horn · General Cardiovascular Disease · St. Paul Medical Center · Texas Cardiology, 5939 Harry Hines Boulevard, Suite 630, Dallas, TX 75235 · 214-879-6450

John Walton Hyland · General Cardiovascular Disease · Baylor University Medical Center · The Heart Place, 411 North Washington Street, Suite 2200, Dallas, TX 75246 · 214-841-2000

Stephen Bryce Johnston · General Cardiovascular Disease (Cardiac Catheterization, Pacemakers) · Baylor University Medical Center · Texas Cardiology Consultants, 712 North Washington Street, Dallas, TX 75246 · 214-824-8721

Craig Riggs Malloy · Magnetic Resonance Imaging (General Cardiovascular Disease, Heart Failure) · VA Medical Center · University of Texas-Southwestern Medical Center at Dallas, Department of Radiology, 5801 Forest Park Road, Dallas, TX 75235-9085 · 214-648-5886

Ronald Michael Peshock · Magnetic Resonance Imaging · Zale Lipshy University Hospital, Parkland Memorial Hospital · Mary Nell & Ralph B. Rogers Magnetic Resonance Center, 5801 Forest Park Road, Dallas, TX 75235 · 214-648-5800

C. Venkata S. Ram · General Cardiovascular Disease (Hypertension) · St. Paul Medical Center, Parkland Memorial Hospital · University of Texas-Southwestern Medical Center at Dallas, Department of Internal Medicine, 5323 Harry Hines Boulevard, Dallas, TX 75235-8899 · 214-648-3111

James H. Shelton · General Cardiovascular Disease (Cardiac Catheterization, Nuclear Cardiology, Angioplasty) · Baylor University Medical Center · Baylor University Medical Center, 3600 Gaston Avenue, Suite 851, Dallas, TX 75246 · 214-826-6044

R. Barrett Steelman · General Cardiovascular Disease (Coronary Artery Disease, Valvular Heart Disease, Congenital Heart Disease in the Adult) · Presbyterian Hospital of Dallas · North Texas Heart Center, 8230 Walnut Hill Lane, Suite 220, Dallas, TX 75231 · 214-361-3300

Christopher R. C. Wyndham · Electrophysiology · Presbyterian Hospital of Dallas, Medical City Dallas Hospital, Medical Center of Plano (Plano), Presbyterian Hospital of Plano (Plano) · North Texas Heart Center, 8230 Walnut Hill Lane, Suite 220, Dallas, TX 75231 · 214-361-3300

El Paso

George J. Di Donna · General Cardiovascular Disease · Providence Memorial Hospital · 1700 Curie Drive, Suite 5100, El Paso, TX 79902-2905 · 915-544-2972

Dorothy D. Ekery · General Cardiovascular Disease · Texas Tech University Health Sciences Center, Department of Internal Medicine, 4800 Alberta Avenue, El Paso, TX 79905 · 915-545-6617

David C. Gough · General Cardiovascular Disease · El Paso Cardiology Consultants, 1733 Curie Drive, Suite 305, El Paso, TX 79902 · 915-545-2995

Melvin J. Spicer · Nuclear Cardiology · Providence Memorial Hospital, Department of Cardiology, 2001 North Oregon Street, El Paso, TX 79902 · 915-577-7100

Michael T. Traylor · General Cardiovascular Disease · Border Cardiology, 10555 Vista del Sol, Suite 120, El Paso, TX 79925 · 915-593-5813

Stanley C. Wagner · General Cardiovascular Disease · El Paso Cardiology Consultants, 1733 Curie Drive, Suite 305, El Paso, TX 79902-2909 · 915-545-2995

Fort Sam Houston

Joe Marshall Moody, Jr. · General Cardiovascular Disease (Clinical Exercise Testing) · Brooke Army Medical Center · Brooke Army Medical Center, Cardiology Service, 3851 Roger Brooke Drive, Mail Code MSCHE-MDC, Fort Sam Houston, TX 78234-6200 · 210-916-2913

Fort Worth

John L. Durand · General Cardiovascular Disease (Invasive and Interventional Cardiology) · Consultants in Cardiology, 750 Eighth Avenue, Suite 600, Fort Worth, TX 76104-2500 · 817-336-4433

Phil Lobstein · General Cardiovascular Disease · 1650 West Rosedale Street, Suite 201, Fort Worth, TX 76104 · 817-335-4344

Kenneth Wade McBride · Electrophysiology · Consultants in Cardiology, 750 Eighth Avenue, Fort Worth, TX 76104 · 817-336-4433

Billie Raymond Pugh, Jr. · General Cardiovascular Disease · Consultants in Cardiology, 750 Eighth Avenue, Suite 600, Fort Worth, TX 76104-2500 · 817-336-4433

William S. Vance, Jr. · General Cardiovascular Disease (Cardiac Catheterization, Echocardiography) · Harris Methodist-Fort Worth, Harris Methodist-Southwest, All Saints Episcopal Hospital-Fort Worth, Plaza Medical Center · Consultants in Cardiology, 750 Eighth Avenue, Suite 600, Fort Worth, TX 76104-2500 · 817-336-4433

Galveston

Marschall S. Runge · General Cardiovascular Disease · University of Texas Medical Branch, Division of Cardiology, 301 University Boulevard, Galveston, TX 77555-0553 · 409-772-1631

Barry F. Uretsky · Heart Failure (Interventional Cardiology) · University of Texas Medical Branch, Division of Cardiology, 301 University Boulevard, Galveston, TX 77555-0553 · 409-772-1631

Harlingen

Garner F. Klein · General Cardiovascular Disease · Valley Diagnostic Clinic, 2200 Haine Drive, Harlingen, TX 78550-8599 · 210-425-7200

Houston

Christie M. Ballantyne · General Cardiovascular Disease (Lipids, Prevention of Cardiovascular Disease) · Methodist Hospital · Methodist Hospital, Department of Medicine, 6565 Fannin Street, Mail Stop A-601, Houston, TX 77030 · 713-790-5800

Charles H. Caplan · General Cardiovascular Disease · Cardiology Associates of Houston, 909 Frostwood Drive, Suite 323, Houston, TX 77024 · 713-467-0605

Gary Merrill Coleman · General Cardiovascular Disease · Houston Northwest Medical Center, Memorial Hospital-The Woodlands (The Woodlands), Tomball Regional Hospital (Tomball) · 800 Peakwood Drive, Suite 8A, Houston, TX 77090 · 713-440-5321

Patrick J. Cook · General Cardiovascular Disease (Cardiac Catheterization, Transplantation Medicine) · St. Luke's Episcopal Hospital, Methodist Hospital Medical Clinic of Houston, 1707 Sunset Boulevard, Houston, TX 77005 · 713-526-5511

Francisco Fuentes · General Cardiovascular Disease · Hermann Hospital · University of Texas Medical School at Houston, 6431 Fannin Street, Room 1.246, Houston, TX 77030 · 713-794-4128

Efrain Garcia · General Cardiovascular Disease (Clinical Exercise Testing, Cardiac Catheterization) · St. Luke's Episcopal Hospital, Texas Heart Institute · 6624 Fannin Street, Suite 2480, Houston, TX 77030-2336 · 713-529-5530

K. Lance Gould · Cardiac Positron Emission Tomography (PET), Nuclear Cardiology (Reverse Treatment for Coronary Heart Diseases) · Hermann Hospital · University of Texas Medical School at Houston, Medical School Building, 6431 Fannin Street, Room 4.258, Houston, TX 77030 · 713-792-5185

Bruce S. Lachterman · General Cardiovascular Disease · Northwest Houston Cardiovascular Associates, 800 Peakwood Drive, Suite 8A, Houston, TX 77090 · 713-440-5321

Mark E. Lambert · General Cardiovascular Disease (Echocardiography, Heart Failure) · Memorial Hospital-Southwest · Memorial Hospital-Southwest, Department of Cardiology, 7737 Southwest Freeway, Suite 780, Houston, TX 77074 · 713-988-9512

John J. Mahmarian · Nuclear Cardiology · Methodist Hospital · 6550 Fannin Street, Mail Code SM 1246, Houston, TX 77030 · 713-793-1891

Ronald P. Mahoney · General Cardiovascular Disease · Memorial Hospital-Southwest · Diagnostic Cardiology, 7777 Southwest Freeway, Suite 420, Houston, TX 77074 · 713-776-9500

Edward Krauss Massin · General Cardiovascular Disease (Heart Failure, Transplantation) · St. Luke's Episcopal Hospital · Cardiology Consultants of Houston, 6624 Fannin Street, Suite 2310, Houston, TX 77030 · 713-796-2668

Akira Nishikawa · General Cardiovascular Disease · Hermann Hospital, St. Joseph Hospital · Advanced Cardiac Care Associates, 12121 Richmond Avenue, Suite 211, Houston, TX 77082 · 713-558-0400

Craig Murdoch Pratt · General Cardiovascular Disease · Methodist Hospital · Baylor College of Medicine, 6535 Fannin Street, Mail Stop F-905, Houston, TX 77030 · 713-790-3102

Miguel A. Quiñones · Echocardiography · Methodist Hospital · Baylor College of Medicine, 6550 Fannin Street, Suite SM 677, Houston, TX 77030 · 713-790-2783

Albert E. Raizner · General Cardiovascular Disease (Interventional, Cardiac Catheterization, Angioplasty) · Methodist Hospital · Smith Tower, Suite 2021, 6550 Fannin Street, Houston, TX 77030 · 713-790-9125

Robert Roberts · General Cardiovascular Disease (Heart Failure) · Methodist Hospital · Methodist Hospital, 6550 Fannin Street, Mail Stop SM677, Houston, TX 77030 · 713-790-4864

David A. Samuels · General Cardiovascular Disease (Interventional) · Methodist Hospital · Houston Cardiology Associates, 6560 Fannin Street, Suite 1654, Houston, TX 77030 · 713-790-0841

Mark J. M. Schnee · General Cardiovascular Disease (Angioplasty) · St. Luke's Episcopal Hospital · Cardiology Consultants of Houston, 6624 Fannin Street, Suite 2310, Houston, TX 77030 · 713-796-2668

Mario S. Verani · Nuclear Cardiology (Clinical Exercise Testing, General Cardiovascular Disease) · Methodist Hospital · Methodist Hospital, 6535 Fannin Street, Mail Stop F-905, Houston, TX 77030 · 713-790-3385

James T. Willerson · General Cardiovascular Disease · Texas Heart Institute · University of Texas Medical School at Houston, 6431 Fannin Street, Room 1.150, Houston, TX 77030 · 713-792-5075

William L. Winters, Jr. · General Cardiovascular Disease (Echocardiography) · Methodist Hospital · Baylor College of Medicine, 6550 Fannin Street, Suite 1025, Houston, TX 77030 · 713-798-8770

William A. Zoghbi · Echocardiography (General Cardiovascular Disease) · Methodist Hospital · Methodist Hospital, 6550 Fannin Street, Mail Stop SM 677, Houston, TX 77030 · 713-790-4342

Longview

Rodney L. Henry · General Cardiovascular Disease (Cardiac Catheterization) · Good Shepherd Medical Center, Longview Regional Hospital · Longview Cardiology, 402 North Seventh Street, Longview, TX 75601 · 903-757-5804

Lubbock

James C. Buell · General Cardiovascular Disease (Heart Failure, Peripheral Vascular Disease) · University Medical Center · 3502 Ninth Street, Suite 420, Lubbock, TX 79415 · 806-743-1501

Howard Perrin Hurd II · General Cardiovascular Disease (Interventional Therapy, Heart Failure, Lipid Abnormalities, Endocarditis, Nuclear Cardiology, Vascular & Interventional) · Lubbock Methodist Hospital · Cardiology Associates of Lubbock, 3514 Twenty-First Street, Lubbock, TX 79407 · 806-792-5105

Midland

Bart R. Mayron · General Cardiovascular Disease · Permian Cardiology, 2401 West Wall Street, Midland, TX 79701-6315 · 915-683-2723

Michael S. Miller · General Cardiovascular Disease · Memorial Hospital & Medical Center · Permian Cardiology, 2401 West Wall Street, Midland, TX 79701-6315 · 915-683-2723

San Angelo

Denver C. Marsh, Jr. · General Cardiovascular Disease (Clinical Exercise Testing, Pacemakers) · Shannon Medical Center-Harris Street, Shannon Medical Center-St. John's Campus · Shannon Clinic, 2030 Pulliam Street, Suite Eight, P.O. Box 268, San Angelo, TX 76905-5157 · 915-653-5997

San Antonio

Steven Roderick Bailey · (Interventional Cardiology, Stents, Rotoblator, Intervascular Ultrasound, Peripheral Vascular Disease, Cardiac Catheterization, Transplantation Medicine) · University Hospital-South Texas Medical Center, Baptist Hospital Medical Center, Santa Rosa Northwest Hospital · University of Texas Health Science Center at San Antonio, Department of Medicine, Division of Cardiology, 7703 Floyd Curl Drive, San Antonio, TX 78284-7872 · 210-567-4601

Gregory Lane Freeman · General Cardiovascular Disease · University Hospital-South Texas Medical Center · University of Texas Health Science Center at San Antonio, Department of Medicine, Division of Cardiology, 7703 Floyd Curl Drive, San Antonio, TX 78284-7872 · 210-567-4601

David McCall · General Cardiovascular Disease (Clinical Exercise Testing, Heart Failure) · University Hospital-South Texas Medical Center · University of Texas Health Science Center at San Antonio, Department of Medicine, Division of Cardiology, 7703 Floyd Curl Drive, San Antonio, TX 78284-7872 · 210-567-4600

Robert Anthony O'Rourke · General Cardiovascular Disease · University Hospital-South Texas Medical Center · University of Texas Health Science Center at San Antonio, Department of Medicine, Division of Cardiology, 7703 Floyd Curl Drive, San Antonio, TX 78284-7872 · 210-617-5100

Sumanth Damodar Prabhu · General Cardiovascular Disease (Heart Failure, Echocardiography) · University Hospital-South Texas Medical Center · University of Texas Health Science Center at San Antonio, Department of Medicine, Division of Cardiology, 7703 Floyd Curl Drive, San Antonio, TX 78284-7872 · 210-567-4602

John Nathaniel Sanderson · General Cardiovascular Disease · Southwest Texas Methodist Hospital · 4330 Medical Drive, Suite 550, San Antonio, TX 78229 · 210-615-1234

Hector Raul Villasenor · General Cardiovascular Disease · 401 North San Saba, San Antonio, TX 78207 · 210-223-7500

Temple

Troy H. Williams · General Cardiovascular Disease · Scott & White Memorial Hospital · Scott & White Memorial Hospital, Department of Cardiology, 2401 South 31st Street, Temple, TX 76508-0001 · 817-724-2111

Tyler

David A. Hector · General Cardiovascular Disease (Cardiac Catheterization, Pacemakers, Clinical Exercise Testing) · University of Texas Health Center-Tyler · University of Texas Health Center-Tyler, US Highway 271 and State Highway 155, P.O. Box 2003, Tyler, TX 75710-2003 · 903-877-7230

Robert M. Payne · General Cardiovascular Disease (Cardiac Catheterization, Clinical Exercise Testing) · University of Texas Health Center-Tyler · University of Texas Health Center-Tyler, US Highway 271 and State Highway 155, P.O. Box 2003, Tyler, TX 75710-2003 · 903-877-7371

Clyde F. Sanford III · General Cardiovascular Disease (Heart Failure, Critical Care Medicine) · Trinity Mother Frances Health Care Center · Trinity Cardiology, 619 South Fleishel Avenue, Suite 101, Tyler, TX 75701-2066 · 903-595-5514

Waco

Wayne Falcone · General Cardiovascular Disease · Waco Cardiology Associates, 6901 Medical Parkway, P.O. Box 2089, Waco, TX 76703 · 817-756-8571

Jose M. Garrido · General Cardiovascular Disease · 6901 Medical Parkway, P.O. Box 2589, Waco, TX 76702-2589 · 817-751-4790

Charles A. Shoultz, Jr. · General Cardiovascular Disease · Waco Cardiology Associates, 6901 Medical Parkway, P.O. Box 2089, Waco, TX 76703 · 817-756-8571

CLINICAL PHARMACOLOGY

Galveston

Donald J. Di Pette · (Hypertension) · University of Texas Medical Branch Hospitals · University of Texas Medical Branch, 301 University Drive, Route 0566, Galveston, TX 77550 · 409-772-4182

Houston

James L. Pool · (Lipid Hypertension) · Methodist Hospital · Methodist Hospital, 6536 Fannin Street, Mail Stop F-504, Houston, TX 77030 · 713-790-3261

Addison A. Taylor · (Hypertension) · Baylor College of Medicine, 6535 Fannin Street, Mail Stop F-504, Houston, TX 77030 · 713-790-3261

San Antonio

Michael Jamieson · (Hypertension) · University Hospital-South Texas Medical Center · University of Texas Health Science Center at San Antonio, Division of Clinical Pharmacology, 7703 Floyd Curl Drive, Room 5.4 MCD, San Antonio, TX 78284 · 210-567-8505

Alexander M. M. Shepherd · (Hypertension) · University Hospital-South Texas Medical Center, Audie L. Murphy Memorial Veterans Hospital · University of Texas Health Science Center at San Antonio, Division of Clinical Pharmacology, 7703 Floyd Curl Drive, San Antonio, TX 78284 · 210-567-8505

Michael Skinner · (Hypertension, Hyperlipidemia, Drug Abuse Problems) · University Hospital-South Texas Medical Center · University of Texas Health Science Center at San Antonio, Division of Clinical Pharmacology, 7703 Floyd Curl Drive, Room 5.4 MCD, San Antonio, TX 78284 -6205 · 210-567-8505

COLON & RECTAL SURGERY

Austin

David C. Fleeger · General Colon & Rectal Surgery (Colon & Rectal Cancer, Inflammatory Bowel Disease, Anorectal Surgery) · St. David's Healthcare Center, Seton Medical Center, South Austin Medical Center, Brackenridge Hospital ·

Austin Colon & Rectal Clinic, 4208 Medical Parkway, Austin, TX 78756 · 512-452-9551

John Stewart Mangione · General Colon & Rectal Surgery · Seton Medical Center · 6818 Austin Center Boulevard, Suite 205, Austin, TX 78731 · 512-418-1755

William G. Robertson III · (Anal Incontinence, Colon & Rectal Cancer, Inflammatory Bowel Disease) · Seton Medical Center, St. David's Healthcare Center, HealthSouth Surgical Hospital · 6818 Austin Center Boulevard, Suite 205, Austin, TX 78731 · 512-418-1755

Beaumont

Matthew M. Sooudi · General Colon & Rectal Surgery · St. Elizabeth Hospital, Beaumont Regional Medical Center · 3210 Medical Center Drive, Beaumont, TX 77701-4627 · 409-838-0135

Corpus Christi

Truman F. Appel · General Colon & Rectal Surgery · Spohn Hospital, Bay Area Medical Center, Doctors Regional Medical Center · 1521 South Staples Street, Suite 602, Corpus Christi, TX 78404-3154 · 512-884-4197

Fred B. Brackett · General Colon & Rectal Surgery (Colon & Rectal Cancer, Colonoscopy) · Spohn Hospital, Memorial Medical Center, Doctors Regional Medical Center, Bay Area Medical Center · 613 Elizabeth Street, Suite 612, Corpus Christi, TX 78404 · 512-883-3831

Dallas

Randall W. Crim · General Colon & Rectal Surgery, Colon & Rectal Cancer · St. Paul Medical Center · Texas Colon & Rectal Surgeons, 5939 Harry Hines Boulevard, Suite 315, Dallas, TX 75235 · 214-661-3575

R. D. Dignan · General Colon & Rectal Surgery (Constipation, Colon & Rectal Cancer, Inflammatory Bowel Disease) · Baylor University Medical Center · Baylor University Medical Center, 3600 Gaston Avenue, Suite 1209, Dallas, TX 75246-1802 · 214-824-2573

Philip J. Huber, Jr. · General Colon & Rectal Surgery, Colon & Rectal Cancer · Parkland Memorial Hospital, Zale Lipshy University Hospital · University of Texas-Southwestern Medical Center at Dallas, Department of General Surgery, 5323 Harry Hines Boulevard, Dallas, TX 75235-9031 · 214-648-3749

Robert Morris Jacobson · General Colon & Rectal Surgery (Colitis, Inflammatory Bowel Disease, Colon Cancer, Constipation) · Baylor University Medical Center, Medical City Dallas Hospital, Doctors Hospital of Dallas, Mary Shiels Hospital · 3409 Worth Street, Suite 500, Dallas, TX 75246 · 214-824-1730

Warren E. Lichliter · General Colon & Rectal Surgery (Oncology) · Baylor University Medical Center · North Texas Colon & Rectal, 3409 Worth Street, Suite 500, Dallas, TX 75246 · 214-823-2107

Floyd Clark Odom · General Colon & Rectal Surgery (Colon & Rectal Cancer, Anorectal Disease, Colonoscopy) · Presbyterian Hospital of Dallas · Texas Colon & Rectal Surgeons, 8220 Walnut Hill Lane, Suite 205, Dallas, TX 75231 · 214-739-5758

Fort Worth

Stephen Fitzgerald · General Colon & Rectal Surgery (Colon & Rectal Cancer, Inflammatory Bowel Disease) · Harris Methodist-Fort Worth, All Saints Episcopal Hospital-Fort Worth, Plaza Medical Center · 1556 West Magnolia Street, Fort Worth, TX 76104 · 817-336-2971

Paul Ross Senter · General Colon & Rectal Surgery · 1307 Eighth Avenue, Suite 602, Fort Worth, TX 76102-4140 · 817-926-5576

Britton R. West · General Colon & Rectal Surgery (Colon & Rectal Cancer) · All Saints Episcopal Hospital-Fort Worth, Harris Methodist-Fort Worth · 1556 West Magnolia Street, Fort Worth, TX 76104-4106 · 817-336-1063

Houston

Harold Randolph (Randy) Bailey · General Colon & Rectal Surgery, Colon & Rectal Cancer · Hermann Hospital, Methodist Hospital, Park Plaza Hospital, The Woman's Hospital of Texas · Colon & Rectal Clinic, Smith Tower, Suite 2307, 6550 Fannin Street, Houston, TX 77030-2717 · 713-790-9250

Donald R. Butts · General Colon & Rectal Surgery · Houston Northwest Medical Center · Colon & Rectal Clinic, 800 Peakwood Drive, Suite 2C, Houston, TX 77090 · 713-440-7495

Ernest Max · General Colon & Rectal Surgery · Methodist Hospital · Colon & Rectal Clinic, Smith Tower, Suite 2307, 6550 Fannin Street, Houston, TX 77030-2717 · 713-790-9250

Gary B. Skakun · General Colon & Rectal Surgery · Park Plaza Hospital, Methodist Hospital, Diagnostic Center Hospital, Memorial Hospital-Southeast · Colon & Rectal Clinic, Smith Tower, Suite 2307, 6550 Fannin Street, Houston, TX 77030 · 713-790-9250

Lubbock

Clint E. Chambers · General Colon & Rectal Surgery · Lubbock Methodist Hospital · 3506 Twenty-First Street, Suite 601, Lubbock, TX 79410 · 806-795-4357

Midland

Guillermo E. Brachetta · General Colon & Rectal Surgery · 2300 West Michigan Avenue, Midland, TX 79701 · 915-687-0181

San Antonio

William E. Bode · General Colon & Rectal Surgery (Colon & Rectal Cancer, Inflammatory Bowel Disease) · St. Luke's Baptist Hospital, Southwest Texas Methodist Hospital, Santa Rosa Northwest Hospital, Baptist Medical Center · Colon and Rectal Surgical Associates of San Antonio, Medical Center Tower One, Suite 101, 7950 Floyd Curl Drive, San Antonio, TX 78229 · 210-614-0880

Raul Ramos · General Colon & Rectal Surgery · Baptist Medical Center, Santa Rosa Health Care, Santa Rosa Northwest Hospital, San Antonio Community Hospital · Colon and Rectal Surgical Associates of San Antonio, Medical Center Tower One, Suite 101, 7950 Floyd Curl Drive, San Antonio, TX 78229-3916 · 210-614-0880

Randall David Rogers · General Colon & Rectal Surgery (Laser Surgery, Colon & Rectal Cancer) · Metropolitan Hospital, Southwest Texas Methodist Hospital, Baptist Medical Center, North Central Baptist Hospital, Northeast Baptist Hospital, Santa Rosa Health Care, Nix Health Care System · Metropolitan Professional Building, Suite 265, 1303 McCullough Avenue, San Antonio, TX 78212 · 210-224-0402

Daniel Rosenthal · General Colon & Rectal Surgery (Early Diagnosis of Colorectal Cancer) · Baptist Medical Center, Southwest Texas Methodist Hospital · 8711 Village Drive, Suite 320, San Antonio, TX 78218 · 210-655-0844

DERMATOLOGY

Abilene

Earl G. Cockerell · Clinical Dermatology (Aging Skin, Skin Cancer Surgery & Reconstruction) · Abilene Regional Medical Center, Hendrick Medical Center · 598 Westwood Drive, Suite 103, Abilene, TX 79603 · 915-672-8525

Amarillo

Turner M. Caldwell III · Clinical Dermatology · Amarillo Hospital District-Northwest Texas Hospital · High Plains Dermatology Center, 4302 Wolflin Avenue, Amarillo, TX 79106-5959 · 806-355-9866

Randal E. Posey · (Acne, Radiotherapy, Psychodermatology) · High Plains Baptist Hospital · High Plains Dermatology Center, 4302 Wolflin Avenue, Amarillo, TX 79106-5959 · 806-355-9866

Larry C. Roberts · Clinical Dermatology · High Plains Baptist Hospital · High Plains Dermatology Center, 4302 Wolflin Avenue, Amarillo, TX 79106-5959 · 806-355-9866

Jack Douglas Waller · Clinical Dermatology · St. Anthony's Hospital · High Plains Dermatology Center, 4302 Wolflin Avenue, Amarillo, TX 79106-5959 · 806-355-9866

Austin

R. John Fox, Jr. · Clinical Dermatology · Brackenridge Hospital · 2911 Medical Arts Street, Suite Three, Austin, TX 78705 · 512-476-9195

Michael Taylor Jarratt · Clinical Dermatology · Seton Medical Center · 8140 Mopac Expressway North, Building Three, Suite 116, Austin, TX 78759 · 512-345-3599

Eugene P. Schoch, Jr. · Clinical Dermatology (Skin Cancer Surgery, Radiation Therapy for Skin Cancer) · Brackenridge Hospital · 2911 Medical Arts Street, Suite Three, Austin, TX 78705 · 512-476-9195

Baytown

William R. Holder · Clinical Dermatology · 2802 Garth Road, Suite 109, Baytown, TX 77521 · 713-425-9375

Beaumont

Weldon Edward Collins · Clinical Dermatology · 2929 Calder Avenue, Suite 204, Beaumont, TX 77702 · 409-835-1333

William A. Gilmore · Clinical Dermatology · 3110 Fannin Street, Beaumont, TX 77701-7702 · 409-833-7458

Gary E. Vaughn · Clinical Dermatology · 3155 Stagg Drive, Suite 203, Beaumont, TX 77701 · 409-833-0017

Bedford

Gene Patrick Ream · Clinical Dermatology (Skin Cancer, Acne) · Harris Methodist-HEB · Harris Euless Bedford Professional Place, 1604 Hospital Parkway, Suite 307, Bedford, TX 76022 · 817-571-5879

Corpus Christi

Carmen C. Casas · Clinical Dermatology · 5756 South Staples Street, Suite J-1, Corpus Christi, TX 78413 · 512-994-1001

Mary Cathleen Cole-Perez · Clinical Dermatology · 5920 Saratoga Boulevard, Suite 400, Corpus Christi, TX 78414 · 512-993-7546

Beverly L. Held · Clinical Dermatology · Spohn Hospital, Doctors Regional Medical Center · 5756 South Staples Street, Suite J2, Corpus Christi, TX 78413-3782 512-993-3190

Dallas

Paul R. Bergstresser · Cutaneous Immunology, Photobiology · Parkland Memorial Hospital, Zale Lipshy University Hospital, St. Paul Medical Center · University of Texas-Southwestern Medical Center at Dallas, 5323 Harry Hines Boulevard, Dallas, TX 75235-9069 · 214-648-2203

Clay J. Cockerell · Dermatopathology (Clinical Dermatology, Cutaneous Lymphomas, HIV Infection, AIDS, Melanoma, Clinicopathologic Correlation) · Zale Lipshy University Hospital, Parkland Memorial Hospital, Methodist Medical Center, Baylor University Medical Center, Presbyterian Hospital of Dallas, St. Paul Medical Center · Freeman-Cockerell Dermatopathology Laboratories, 2330 Butler Street, Suite 115, Dallas, TX 75235 · 214-638-2222

Ponciano D. Cruz, Jr. · Contact Dermatitis (Cutaneous Immunology, Dermatological Immunology, Photobiology) · Aston Center Clinic, The University of Texas—Southwestern Medical Center at Dallas, Department of Dermatology, 5323 Harry Hines Boulevard, Dallas, TX 75235-7200 · 214-648-2203

Phillip James Eichhorn · Clinical Dermatology (Contact Dermatitis, Connective Tissue Diseases) · St. Paul Medical Center, VA Medical Center · 1851 Prairie View, Suite E, Dallas, TX 75235 · 214-630-9331

Robert G. Freeman · Dermatopathology · Parkland Memorial Hospital · Freeman-Cockerell Dermatopathology Labs, 2330 Butler Street, Suite 115, Dallas, TX 75235 · 214-638-2222

James H. Herndon, Jr. · General Dermatology · Presbyterian Hospital of Dallas Dermatology Center of Dallas, 8230 Walnut Hill Lane, Suite 500, Dallas, TX 75231-4404 · 214-739-5821

Karen R. Houpt · Clinical Dermatology (Psoriasis) · Zale Lipshy University Hospital, St. Paul Medical Center, Parkland Memorial Hospital, Children's Medical Center of Dallas · University of Texas-Southwestern Medical Center at Dallas, 5323 Harry Hines Boulevard, Dallas, TX 75235-9069 · 214-648-2203

Daniel M. Ingraham · Hair (Hair Transplantation) · Baylor University Medical Center, Baylor Hair Research & Treatment Center · Baylor University Medical Center, Baylor Hair Research & Treatment Center, 3600 Gaston Avenue, Dallas, TX 75246 · 214-820-4247

Carolyn B. Lyde · General Dermatology (Leprosy) · University of Texas-Southwestern Medical Center at Dallas, Department of Dermatology, 5323 Harry Hines Boulevard, Dallas, TX 75235 · 214-648-2203

M. Alan Menter · Psoriasis · Baylor University Medical Center, Baylor Psoriasis Center · Texas Dermatology Associates, 5925 Forest Lane, Suite 110, Dallas, TX 75230 · 214-826-8390

Dennis E. Newton · Clinical Dermatology (Laser Surgery, Aesthetic Surgery, Skin Cancer Surgery & Reconstruction, Aging Skin) · RHD Memorial Medical Center · Professional Plaza Three, Suite 304, 10 Medical Parkway, Dallas, TX 75234 · 214-243-4530

Amit G. Pandya · Clinical Dermatology (Blistering Disorders, Pigmentary Disorders, Cutaneous Lymphomas, Laser Surgery) · Zale Lipshy University Hospital, Parkland Memorial Hospital · University of Texas-Southwestern Medical Center at Dallas, Department of Dermatology, 5323 Harry Hines Boulevard, Dallas, TX 75235-7200 · 214-648-2203

Lynne Jeanine Roberts · Pediatric Dermatology (Laser Surgery [Adult & Pediatric], Aesthetic Surgery) · Parkland Memorial Hospital, Children's Medical Center of Dallas, Medical City Dallas Hospital · Medical City Dallas Hospital, Building C, Suite 737, 7777 Forest Lane, Dallas, TX 75230 · 214-788-8822

Laura L. Sears · General Dermatology · Baylor University Medical Center · Baylor University Medical Center, 3600 Gaston Avenue, Suite 1051, Dallas, TX 75246-1910 · 214-824-2087

Jerald L. Sklar · Clinical Dermatology (Skin Cancer Surgery & Reconstruction, Laser Surgery) · Baylor University Medical Center · Baylor University Medical Center, Department of Dermatology, 3600 Gaston Avenue, Suite 1051, Dallas, TX 75246-1910 · 214-824-2087

Richard D. Sontheimer · Cutaneous Immunology, Clinical Dermatology (Dermatological Immunology, Rheumatic Skin Disease [including Lupus]) · Parkland Memorial Hospital, Children's Medical Center of Dallas, Zale Lipshy University Hospital, St. Paul Medical Center · University of Texas-Southwestern Medical Center at Dallas, Department of Dermatology, 5323 Harry Hines Boulevard, Dallas, TX 75235-9069 · 214-648-3436; 214-648-2203

Lori D. Stetler · Clinical Dermatology (Laser Surgery, Cosmetic Dermatology) · Medical City Dallas Hospital, Presbyterian Hospital of Dallas, Parkland Memorial Hospital · Medical City Dallas Hospital, Building C, Suite 737, 7777 Forest Lane, Dallas, TX 75230 · 214-788-8855

R. Stan Taylor · Skin Cancer Surgery & Reconstruction · Zale Lipshy University Hospital · University of Texas-Southwestern Medical Center at Dallas, 5323 Harry Hines Boulevard, Dallas, TX 75235-9069 · 214-648-8085

David A. Whiting · Hair (Dermatopathology, Pediatric Dermatology) · Baylor University Medical Center · Baylor University Medical Center, 3600 Gaston Avenue, Suite 1051, Dallas, TX 75246 · 214-824-2087

El Paso

David F. Butler · Clinical Dermatology · Sierra Medical Center · Southwest Dermatology, 1600 Medical Center Drive, Suite 218, El Paso, TX 79902 · 915-533-6880

Peter S. Herman · Clinical Dermatology (Photosensitivity, Contact Allergic Dermatitis) · Providence Memorial Hospital, Columbia Medical Center-West, Sierra Medical Center · Dermatology Center of El Paso, 2100 North Mesa Drive, El Paso, TX 79902-3312 · 915-544-3800

Clinton R. King · Clinical Dermatology · 10657 Vista Del Sol, Suite A, El Paso, TX 79936 · 915-598-3943

Michael Homer Simpson · Clinical Dermatology · Providence Memorial Hospital 1501 Arizona Avenue, Suite 1A, El Paso, TX 79902-5007 · 915-544-3254

Fort Worth

Philip W. Giles · Clinical Dermatology · Harris Methodist-Fort Worth · 800 Hemphill Street, Fort Worth, TX 76104-3107 · 817-335-6155

C. Leroy Goodman · Clinical Dermatology · 800 Eighth Avenue, Suite 236, Fort Worth, TX 76104 · 817-335-4549

James Douglas Maberry · Clinical Dermatology · 1200 West Rosedale Street, Fort Worth, TX 76104-4454 · 817-336-8131

Douglas Scott Miller · Clinical Dermatology (Psoriasis, Photobiology) · Harris Methodist-Fort Worth · 1307 Eighth Avenue, Suite 505, Fort Worth, TX 76104 · 817-927-2332

Robin A. Roberts · Clinical Dermatology · 800 Fifth Avenue, Suite 519, Fort Worth, TX 76104-7302 · 817-336-3376

Danny R. Thomas · Clinical Dermatology · 800 Fifth Avenue, Suite 519, Fort Worth, TX 76104 · 817-335-3487

Galveston

Sharon Smith Raimer · Pediatric Dermatology · University of Texas Medical Branch Hospitals · University of Texas Medical Branch, Department of Dermatology, 301 University Boulevard, Galveston, TX 77550-0518 · 409-772-7210

Ramon L. Sanchez · Dermatopathology · University of Texas Medical Branch Hospitals · University of Texas Medical Branch, Department of Dermatology, 301 University Boulevard, Galveston, TX 77550-0783 · 409-772-1911

Edgar Benton Smith · Clinical Dermatology (Fungal Infections) · University of Texas Medical Branch Hospitals · University of Texas Medical Branch, Department of Dermatology, 301 University Boulevard, Galveston, TX 77550-0783 · 409-772-7210

Houston

Samuel F. Bean · Clinical Dermatology (Blistering Disorders, Oral Disease, Mucous Membrane Diseases) · Park Plaza Hospital, Diagnostic Center Hospital · 1200 Binz Street, Suite 990, Houston, TX 77004 · 713-523-8200

Fred F. Castrow II · Clinical Dermatology · Memorial Hospital-Southwest · 7777 Southwest Freeway, Suite 448, Houston, TX 77074-1808 · 713-774-7433

Marvin E. Chernosky · Clinical Dermatology · Hermann Hospital · 6410 Fannin Street, Suite 703, Houston, TX 77030 · 713-790-9270

C. William Doubleday · Clinical Dermatology (Acne, Pediatric Dermatology) · St. Luke's Episcopal Hospital · 515 Post Oak Boulevard, Suite 535, Houston, TX 77027 · 713-627-1776

Madeleine Duvic · Psoriasis, Cutaneous Lymphomas (Cell Lymphomas, Skin Cancer, Cutaneous Immunology) · University of Texas-M. D. Anderson Cancer Center, Hermann Hospital, St. Luke's Episcopal Hospital · University of Texas Medical School at Houston, Department of Dermatology, 6655 Travis Street, Suite 820, Houston, TX 77030 · 713-792-5115 x1158

Jan Frederic Fuerst · Clinical Dermatology · 909 Frostwood Drive, Suite 311, Houston, TX 77024 · 713-468-7033

Adelaide A. Hebert · Pediatric Dermatology · Hermann Hospital, University of Texas-M. D. Anderson Cancer Center · University of Texas Medical School at Houston, Department of Dermatology, 6431 Fannin Street, Room 1.204, Houston, TX 77030 · 713-792-5115 x1159

Robert E. Jordon · Cutaneous Immunology (Blistering Disorders, Dermatological Immunology, Clinical Dermatology) · Hermann Hospital · University of Texas Medical School at Houston, Department of Dermatology, 6431 Fannin Street, Room 1.204, Houston, TX 77030 · 713-792-5115 x1165

Moise L. Levy · Pediatric Dermatology (Laser Surgery & Birthmarks, Inherited Skin Diseases) · Texas Children's Hospital · Texas Children's Hospital, 6621 Fannin Street, Suite 700, Houston, TX 77030 · 713-770-3720

Donald W. Owens · Clinical Dermatology (Dermatopathology, Photobiology) · St. Luke's Episcopal Hospital · Woodway Clinic, 5757 Woodway Drive, Suite 110, Houston, TX 77057 · 713-783-7960

Theodore Rosen · Clinical Dermatology · Methodist Hospital · Baylor College of Medicine, 6560 Fannin Street, Suite 802, Houston, TX 77030-2706 · 713-798-6131

John K. Stern · Clinical Dermatology · 7500 Beechnut Street, Suite 350, Houston, TX 77074 · 713-988-8442

John E. Wolf, Jr. · Clinical Dermatology (Psoriasis, Aging Skin) · Methodist Hospital · Baylor College of Medicine, 6560 Fannin Street, Suite 802, Houston, TX 77030-2706 · 713-798-6131

Lubbock

William H. Radentz · Clinical Dermatology · Texas Tech University Health Sciences Center, Department of Dermatology, 3516 Twenty-Second Place, Lubbock, TX 79410 · 806-796-7193

Ronald P. Rapini · Clinical Dermatology, Dermatopathology (Skin Cancer Surgery) · University Medical Center · Texas Tech University Health Sciences Center, Department of Dermatology, 3601 Fourth Street, Room 4A117, Lubbock, TX 79430 · 806-743-2456

Farah Shah · Pediatric Dermatology · Texas Tech University Health Sciences Center, Department of Dermatology, 3601 Fourth Street, Lubbock, TX 79430 · 806-743-1842

Barbara H. Way · Clinical Dermatology (Psoriasis, Contact Dermatitis) · St. Mary of the Plains Hospital, Lubbock Methodist Hospital · 4102 Twenty-Fourth Street, Suite 201, Lubbock, TX 79410 · 806-797-1892

McAllen

Richard C. Newton · Clinical Dermatology · 216 Lindberg Street, McAllen, TX 78501 · 210-631-2501

Oscar Sotelo · Clinical Dermatology · 301 North Main Street, Suite One, McAllen, TX 78501-4632 · 210-682-1591

Midland

Louis B. Barkley, Jr. · Clinical Dermatology (Acne, Aging Skin, Skin Cancer Surgery) · Memorial Hospital & Medical Center · 1300 West Wall Street, Midland, TX 79701 · 915-683-6281

Odessa

Robert L. Chappell, Jr. · Clinical Dermatology · Medical Center Hospital · 2487 East Eleventh Street, Odessa, TX 79761-4232 · 915-333-6603

Donald O. Naylor · Clinical Dermatology · 404 North Washington Street, Odessa, TX 79761 · 915-332-0169

Pasadena

Lawrence Maurice Joseph · Clinical Dermatology · 3801 Vista, Suite 340, Pasadena, TX 77504 · 713-941-6598

Richardson

Hein Johan Ter Poorten · Clinical Dermatology (Acne, Skin Cancer Surgery & Reconstruction) · Parkland Memorial Hospital (Dallas), Baylor Medical Center-Richardson · 375 Municipal Drive, Suite 226, Richardson, TX 75080 · 214-234-3123

San Antonio

Richard L. DeVillez · Hair (Hair Disorders) · Audie L. Murphy Memorial Veterans Hospital, University Hospital-South Texas Medical Center · University of Texas Health Science Center at San Antonio, Department of Medicine, Division of Dermatology, 7703 Floyd Curl Drive, San Antonio, TX 78284-7876 · 210-567-4887

Scott C. Duncan · Clinical Dermatology (Cosmetic Surgery, Hair Transplantation, Laser Surgery) · Southwest Texas Methodist Hospital · 4499 Medical Drive, Suite 316, San Antonio, TX 78229 · 210-692-0601

Eric Werner Kraus · Contact Dermatitis (Superficial Fungal Infections, Photoprotection) · University Hospital-South Texas Medical Center · University of Texas Health Science Center at San Antonio, Department of Medicine, Division of Dermatology, 7703 Floyd Curl Drive, San Antonio, TX 78284-7876 · 210-567-4885

Bobby L. Limmer · Hair, Aesthetic Surgery (Hair Transplantation, Chemical Peel, Dermabrasion, Scar Removal) · One Medical Park, Suite 210, 14615 San Pedro Avenue, San Antonio, TX 78232 · 210-496-9929

Byron Lee Limmer · Clinical Dermatology (Dermatologic Surgery, Liposuction, Mohs Micrographic Surgery) · One Medical Park, Suite 210, 14615 San Pedro Avenue, San Antonio, TX 78232-4316 · 210-496-9929

Robert L. Magnon · Clinical Dermatology · 1303 McCullough Avenue, Suite 525, San Antonio, TX 78212 · 210-225-2769

Gregory Wilkins Thompson · Clinical Dermatology · Baptist Medical Center · 14615 San Pedro Avenue, Suite 200, San Antonio, TX 78232 · 210-494-5192

Charles Sparks Thurston · Clinical Dermatology (Vitiligo) · Santa Rosa Health Care · 343 West Houston Street, Suite 909, San Antonio, TX 78205 · 210-222-0376

Sherman

Donald F. Fincher · Clinical Dermatology (Aging Skin, Skin Cancer Surgery) · Wilson N. Jones Memorial Hospital, Texoma Medical Center (Denison), Columbia Medical Center (Sherman) · Texoma Dermatology Clinic, 3403 Loy Lake Road, Sherman, TX 75090 · 903-892-2126

Mark D. Koone · Clinical Dermatology (Skin Cancer, Wound Healing) · Wilson N. Jones Memorial Hospital · Texoma Dermatology Clinic, 3403 Loy Lake Road, Sherman, TX 75090 · 903-892-2126

Roy E. Spencer · Clinical Dermatology (Skin Cancer, Acne) · Texoma Medical Center (Denison) · Texoma Dermatology Clinic, 3403 Loy Lake Road, Sherman, TX 75090 · 903-892-2126

Temple

David D. Barton · Clinical Dermatology (Pediatric Dermatology, Psoriasis) · Scott & White Memorial Hospital · Scott & White Memorial Hospital, Department of Dermatology, 2401 South 31st Street, Temple, TX 76508-0001 · 817-724-2391

Delma P. Posey · Clinical Dermatology · Scott & White Memorial Hospital · Scott & White Memorial Hospital, Department of Dermatology, 2401 South 31st Street, Temple, TX 76508-0001 · 817-724-2391

Tyler

Dannise Beckley · Clinical Dermatology · University of Texas Health Center-Tyler, US Highway 271 and State Highway 155, P.O. Box 2003, Tyler, TX 75710-2003 · 903-877-7213

Robert E. Rossman · Clinical Dermatology · 1301 Doctors Drive, Tyler, TX 75701 · 903-593-8381

Waco

Sandra Gardere · Clinical Dermatology (Psoriasis, Acne, Phlebology/Sclerotherapy) · Hillcrest Baptist Medical Center · Dermatology & Plastic Surgery Association, 3115 Pine Avenue, Suite 908, Waco, TX 76708 · 817-752-2575

Thomas Henry Jackson, Jr. · Clinical Dermatology · Providence Health Center 1607 Lake Success Drive, Waco, TX 76710-2985 · 817-776-1390

James W. Mason · Clinical Dermatology · Hillcrest Baptist Medical Center · 3115 Pine Avenue, Suite 806, Waco, TX 76708 · 817-753-0841

Wichita Falls

Thomas E. Taylor · Clinical Dermatology (Skin Malignancies) · Red River Hospital, Bethania Regional Health Care Center, Wichita General Hospital · 1500 Brook Avenue, Wichita Falls, TX 76301-5688 · 817-766-4365

EATING DISORDERS

Temple

Susan M. P. Nickel · General Eating Disorders · Scott & White Memorial Hospital & Clinic · Scott & White Memorial Hospital, Department of Pediatrics, 2401 South 31st Street, Temple, TX 76508-0001 · 817-724-3109

ENDOCRINOLOGY & METABOLISM

Amarillo

Leonard E. Dodson · (Eating Disorders, Nutrition) · Amarillo Diagnostic Clinic, 6700 West Ninth Street, Amarillo, TX 79106 · 806-358-3171

Austin

Thomas Craig Blevins · (Cholesterol, Diabetes, Osteoporosis) · Austin Diagnostic Medical Center · Austin Diagnostic Medical Center, 12221 MoPac Expressway North, P.O. Box 85075, Austin, TX 78708-5075 · 512-901-4005

Beaumont

Robert Cameron Hood · General Endocrinology & Metabolism · Endocrinology Associates of Southeast Texas, 740 Hospital Drive, Suite Two, Beaumont, TX 77701-4629 · 409-835-9834

Yugal K. Maheshwari · General Endocrinology & Metabolism · 2194-B Eastex Freeway, Beaumont, TX 77703-4939 · 409-899-2750

Jose Ortiz · General Endocrinology & Metabolism (Diabetes, Thyroid) · Baptist Hospital Beaumont, St. Elizabeth Hospital, Beaumont Regional Medical Center Endocrinology Associates of Southeast Texas, 740 Hospital Drive, Suite Two, Beaumont, TX 77701-4629 · 409-835-9834

Corpus Christi

Melissa Ann Wilson · General Endocrinology & Metabolism · 3301 South Alameda Street, Suite 401, Corpus Christi, TX 78411-1871 · 512-854-3300

Dallas

Daniel W. Foster · Diabetes · Parkland Memorial Hospital, Zale Lipshy University Hospital · University of Texas-Southwestern Medical Center at Dallas, 5323 Harry Hines Boulevard, Dallas, TX 75235-9060 · 214-648-3486

James E. Griffin III · General Endocrinology & Metabolism (Thyroid, Reproductive Endocrinology) · Parkland Memorial Hospital, Zale Lipshy University Hospital · University of Texas-Southwestern Medical Center at Dallas, 5323 Harry Hines Boulevard, Dallas, TX 75235-8857 · 214-648-3494

Norman M. Kaplan · Hypertension · Zale Lipshy University Hospital, Parkland Memorial Hospital · University of Texas-Southwestern Medical Center at Dallas, 5323 Harry Hines Boulevard, Dallas, TX 75235-8899 · 214-648-2103

Charles Pak · General Endocrinology & Metabolism (Bone Disease, Renal Stones, Osteoporosis) · Zale Lipshy University Hospital, Parkland Memorial Hospital · University of Texas-Southwestern Medical Center at Dallas, 5323 Harry Hines Boulevard, Dallas, TX 75235 · 214-648-2100

Philip Raskin · Diabetes · Diabetes Clinic, University Diabetes Treatment Center/Parkland Memorial Hospital, VA Medical Center, Zale Lipshy University Hospital, Presbyterian Hospital of Dallas, Medical City Dallas Hospital · University of Texas-Southwestern Medical Center at Dallas, 5323 Harry Hines Boulevard, Dallas, TX 75235-8858 · 214-648-2017

Richard A. Sachson · Diabetes (General Endocrinology & Metabolism, Neuroendocrinology, Thyroid, Osteoporosis) · Presbyterian Hospital of Dallas · Endocrine Associates of Dallas, 5480 La Sierra Drive, Dallas, TX 75231 · 214-363-5535

Jean D. Wilson · Neuroendocrinology (Reproductive Endocrinology) · Parkland Memorial Hospital, Zale Lipshy University Hospital · University of Texas-Southwestern Medical Center at Dallas, Department of Internal Medicine, 5323 Harry Hines Boulevard, Dallas, TX 75235-8857 · 214-648-3494

El Paso

Irene R. Chiucchini · General Endocrinology & Metabolism · 10500 Vista Del Sol, Suite B-79925, El Paso, TX 79936 · 915-590-3777

Gerald S. Kidd II · General Endocrinology & Metabolism (Diabetes, Thyroid) · Columbia Medical Center-West, Sierra Medical Center, Providence Memorial Hospital, Columbia Medical Center-East · Southwest Endocrine Consultants, 1201 Schuster Building, Suite Seven, El Paso, TX 79902-4646 · 915-533-5486

Robert Lindley Young · Thyroid (Diabetes, General Endocrinology & Metabolism) · Columbia Medical Center-West, Providence Memorial Hospital, Sierra Medical Center · Southwest Endocrinology Consultants, 1201 Schuster Building, Suite Seven, El Paso, TX 79902-4646 · 915-533-5486

Fort Worth

R. Lee Forshay · General Endocrinology & Metabolism · Harris Methodist-Fort Worth · Medical Clinic of North Texas, 1325 Pennsylvania Avenue, Suite 200, Fort Worth, TX 76104 · 817-878-5200

David B. Wilson · General Endocrinology & Metabolism · Harris Methodist-Fort Worth · Medical Clinic of North Texas, 1325 Pennsylvania Avenue, Suite 200, Fort Worth, TX 76104 · 817-878-5200

Galveston

O. Bryan Holland · General Endocrinology & Metabolism (Hypertension) · University of Texas Medical Branch Hospitals · University of Texas Medical Branch, Department of Endocrinology, 301 University Boulevard, Galveston, TX 77555 · 409-772-1176

Houston

Glenn Ross Cunningham · Neuroendocrinology (Male Reproductive Endocrinology, Androgen Deficiency, General Endocrinology & Metabolism, Thyroid, Diabetes) · Methodist Hospital, VA Medical Center · VA Medical Center, 2002 Holcombe Boulevard, Mail Code 151, Houston, TX 77030-4211 · 713-794-7566

Keith E. Friend · General Endocrinology & Metabolism (Pituitary Tumors) · University of Texas-M. D. Anderson Cancer Center, 1515 Holcombe Boulevard, Box 15, Houston, TX 77030 · 713-792-2840

Robert F. Gagel · General Endocrinology & Metabolism (Endocrine Tumors, Metabolic Bone Disease, Neuroendocrinology, Thyroid, Disorders of Calcium Metabolism) · University of Texas-M. D. Anderson Cancer Center · University of Texas-M. D. Anderson Cancer Center, 1515 Holcombe Boulevard, Box 15, Houston, TX 77030 · 713-792-2840

Alan J. Garber · Diabetes · Methodist Hospital · Baylor College of Medicine, 6550 Fannin Street, Suite 1045, Houston, TX 77030 · 713-790-4768

Antonio M. Gotto, Jr. · General Endocrinology & Metabolism (Lipids [Cardiology], Atherosclerosis) · 6550 Fannin Street, Suite 1423, Houston, TX 77030 · 713-790-3267

Dale J. Hamilton · General Endocrinology & Metabolism (Diabetes) · Cypress Fairbanks Medical Center · 11302 Fallbrook Drive, Suite 301, Houston, TX 77065 · 713-890-5658

Lawrence Edward Mallette · Paget's Disease (Osteoporosis, Hyperparathyroidism) · VA Medical Center · VA Medical Center, 2002 Holcombe Boulevard, Mail Code 111, Houston, TX 77211 · 713-794-7151

Shahla Nader · General Endocrinology & Metabolism (Reproductive Endocrinology, Diabetes) · Hermann Hospital · University of Texas Medical School at Houston, 6410 Fannin Street, Suites 350 & 1400, Houston, TX 77030 · 713-792-5360

Sheldon Rubenfeld · Thyroid · Methodist Hospital, St. Luke's Episcopal Hospital · 7515 South Main Street, Suite 475, Houston, TX 77030 · 713-795-5750

Rena V. Sellin · Thyroid (Thyroid Cancer, Estrogen Replacement, Menopause, Breast Cancer, Growth Disorders, Late Effects, Pediatric Cancer) · University of Texas-M. D. Anderson Cancer Center · University of Texas-M. D. Anderson Cancer Center, 1515 Holcombe Boulevard, Box 15, Houston, TX 77030 · 713-792-2840

Longview

James W. Sawyer · General Endocrinology & Metabolism · Longview Regional Hospital · 701 East Marshall Avenue, Suite 310, Longview, TX 75601 · 903-236-7090

McAllen

Robert L. Hatcher · General Endocrinology & Metabolism · VA Outpatient Clinic, 2101 South Second Street, McAllen, TX 78503 · 210-618-7100

Odessa

James K. Burks · General Endocrinology & Metabolism · Texas Tech Medical Group, 800 West Fourth Street, Odessa, TX 79763 · 915-563-0146

San Antonio

Laura Sand Akright · General Endocrinology & Metabolism · 8711 Village Drive, Suite 305, San Antonio, TX 78217 · 210-650-3360

Richard Arthur Becker · Thyroid · Santa Rosa Health Care · Endocrinology-Nuclear Medicine Associates, 1303 McCullough Avenue, Suite 374, San Antonio, TX 78212-5609 · 210-223-5483

Karen Shipp Black · General Endocrinology & Metabolism (Osteoporosis, Thyroid Disease, Pituitary Disease, Calcium Disorders, Neuroendocrinology) · Santa Rosa Health Care, Southwest Texas Methodist Hospital, St. Luke's Baptist Hospital, Women's & Children's Hospital · Endocrinology-Nuclear Medicine Associates, 1303 McCullough Avenue, Suite 374, San Antonio, TX 78212-5609 · 210-223-5483

Ralph Anthony De Fronzo · General Endocrinology & Metabolism (Diabetic Kidney Disease, Electrolyte & Acid-Base Disorders, General Nephrology, General Internal Medicine) · University Hospital-South Texas Medical Center · University of Texas Health Science Center at San Antonio, Department of Medicine, Diabetes Division, 7703 Floyd Curl Drive, San Antonio, TX 78284-7886 · 210-567-6691

Dianne A. Fetchick · General Endocrinology & Metabolism · University Hospital-South Texas Medical Center · 8711 Village Drive, Suite 305, San Antonio, TX 78217 · 210-650-3360

Theresa Ann Guise · General Endocrinology & Metabolism (Osteoporosis, Thyroid) · University Health System · University of Texas Health Science Center at San Antonio, Department of Medicine, Division of Endocrinology, 7703 Floyd Curl Drive, San Antonio, TX 78284-7877 · 210-567-1952; 210-567-4900

Edward A. Kohl · General Endocrinology & Metabolism · University Hospital-South Texas Medical Center · 4499 Medical Drive, Suite 245, San Antonio, TX 78229 · 210-616-0789

Gregory Robert Mundy · General Endocrinology & Metabolism (Bone Disease) Audie L. Murphy Memorial Veterans Hospital · University of Texas Health Science Center at San Antonio, Department of Medicine, Division of Endocrinology, 7703 Floyd Curl Drive, San Antonio, TX 78284-7877 · 210-567-4900

Charles A. Reasner II · General Endocrinology & Metabolism (Diabetes, Lipids, Thyroid) · University Hospital-South Texas Medical Center · University of Texas Health Science Center at San Antonio, Department of Medicine, Division of Endocrinology, 7703 Floyd Curl Drive, San Antonio, TX 78284-7877 · 210-567-1952

Harry L. Uy · General Endocrinology & Metabolism (Thyroid, Bone, Pituitary) · University Hospital-South Texas Medical Center, Audie L. Murphy Memorial Veterans Hospital · University of Texas Health Science Center at San Antonio, Department of Medicine, Division of Endocrinology, 7703 Floyd Curl Drive, San Antonio, TX 78284-7877 · 210-567-4900

Temple

Veronica Kelly Piziak · General Endocrinology & Metabolism (Women's Health, Osteoporosis, Diabetes) · Scott & White Memorial Hospital & Clinic · Scott & White Memorial Hospital, Department of Medicine, Division of Endocrinology, 2401 South 31st Street, Temple, TX 76508-0001 · 817-724-2111

Tyler

Larry M. Wiertz · General Endocrinology & Metabolism · Trinity Mother Frances Health Care Center, East Texas Medical Center · 1040 South Fleishel Avenue, Suite Four, Tyler, TX 75701 · 903-595-5228

Waco

Meera Amar · General Endocrinology & Metabolism (Diabetes Mellitus, Thyroid) · Providence Health Center, Hillcrest Baptist Medical Center · 405 Londonderry Drive, Suite 103, Waco, TX 76712 · 817-751-4923

FAMILY MEDICINE

Abilene

George Dawson · Abilene Family Practice, 1210 North 18th Street, Abilene, TX 79606 · 915-673-8309

Amarillo

Richard H. Bechtol · (Sports Medicine) · St. Anthony's Hospital, Amarillo Hospital District-Northwest Texas Hospital · 1900 South Coulter Drive, Suite P, Amarillo, TX 79106 · 806-353-4328

David G. Carruth · High Plains Baptist Hospital, Amarillo Hospital District-Northwest Texas Hospital · Amarillo Family Physicians Clinic, 6842 Plum Creek Drive, Amarillo, TX 79124 · 806-359-4701

Robert Cotton · 2300 West Seventh Street, Amarillo, TX 79106 · 806-376-5552

Donald A. Frank · (General Family Practice, Medical Treatment of Drug Abusers, Geriatric Medicine) · High Plains Baptist Hospital · 5211 West Ninth Street, Suite 205, Amarillo, TX 79106-4149 · 806-359-8583

Jerry Lynn Kirkland · High Plains Baptist Hospital · 1901 Medical Park Plaza, Suite 1048, Amarillo, TX 79106-2107 · 806-356-2705

Austin

Mary E. Bartz · 900 East 30th Street, Suite 300, Austin, TX 78705 · 512-476-6555

Michael Bruce Bogdanovich · (Sports Medicine, Dermatology) · The Austin Regional Clinic at Far West, 6835 Austin Center Boulevard, P.O. Box 26726, Austin, TX 78755-0726 · 512-346-6611

Cynthia C. Brinson · (HIV in Women, General Family Practice) · Brackenridge Hospital, St. David's Healthcare Center, Christopher House · Blackstock Family Health Center, 4614 North IH-35, Austin, TX 78751 · 512-458-9176

David Courtney Carter · (Preventive Care, General Pediatrics, Adolescent Medicine, HIV Disease) · South Austin Medical Center, Brackenridge Hospital · 621 Radam Lane, Austin, TX 78745 · 512-442-5566

Walter T. Caven, Jr. · (Pediatrics) · Travis Physician Associates, 12007 Technology Boulevard, Austin, TX 78727 · 512-258-5337

Donald R. Counts · (Preventive Medicine, Weight Management, Acupuncture, Alternative Medicine) · 2905 San Gabriel Street, Suite 306, Austin, TX 78705 · 512-474-2772

Mark C. Dawson · 5716-B Highway 290 West, Suite 111, Austin, TX 78735 · 512-892-5881

Jill A. Grimes · 631 West 38th Street, Austin, TX 78705 · 512-453-3542

James S. Hahn · 631 West 38th Street, Austin, TX 78705 · 512-459-3177

David G. Joseph · 621 Radam Lane, Austin, TX 78745 · 512-442-5566

Paul David Keinarth · St. David's Healthcare Center, Seton Medical Center · Austin Family Care Center, 4315 Guadalupe Street, Suite 200, Austin, TX 78751 512-459-3204

Jacqueline Marie Kerr · (Hispanic Health, Diabetes, Adolescent Medicine, Women's Health) · Seton Medical Center · Seton East Community Clinic, 2811 East Second Street, Austin, TX 78702 · 512-385-4114

Steve Margolin · 4315 Guadalupe Street, Suite 200, Austin, TX 78751 · 512-459-3204

William J. Moran · 4315 Guadalupe Street, Suite 200, Austin, TX 78751 · 512-459-3204

Gary Wayne Piefer · Travis Physician Associates, 12007 Technology Boulevard, Austin, TX 78727 · 512-335-9825

Robert Raley · Family Care—Northwest Hills, 8014 Mesa Drive, Austin, TX 78731 · 512-323-4960

Beaumont

Maria S. Blahey · (Depression, Type II Diabetes, Attention Deficit Disorder, Attention Deficit Hyperactivity Disorder, General Family Practice) · St. Elizabeth Hospital, Baptist Hospital Beaumont, Beaumont Regional Medical Center · 3155 Stagg Drive, Suite 227, Beaumont, TX 77701 · 409-835-6109

Ronald Eger · 740 Hospital Drive, Beaumont, TX 77701 · 409-832-1688

Charles A. Evans · (Diabetes, Preventive Medicine, General Family Practice) · St. Elizabeth Hospital, Baptist Hospital Beaumont, Beaumont Regional Medical Center · 3155 Stagg Drive, Suite 227, Beaumont, TX 77701 · 409-838-4632

Bryan

Nancy W. Dickey · (Obstetrics, Adolescent Medicine) · St. Joseph Regional Health Center, Columbia Medical Center (College Station) · 1301 Memorial Drive, Bryan, TX 77802 · 409-862-4465

Comanche

Forrest A. Eisenrich · Comanche Family Medical Clinic, 1507 North Austin Street, Comanche, TX 76442 · 915-356-7537

Corpus Christi

Francisco A. Acebo · 2601 Hospital Boulevard, Suite 201, Corpus Christi, TX 78405 · 512-887-4541

J. Robert Cone · (Sports and Wilderness Medicine) · 3560 South Alameda Street, Corpus Christi, TX 78411-1722 · 512-854-4828

Richard C. Davis · 5920 Saratoga Boulevard, Suite 320, Corpus Christi, TX 78414 512-985-0085

Mark A. Dodson · Family Practice Associates, 3301 South Alameda Street, Corpus Christi, TX 78411-1829 · 512-857-2900

Jonathan E. Martin · Family Practice Associates, 3301 South Alameda Street, Suite 201, Corpus Christi, TX 78411 · 512-852-8231

Dallas

Michael Steven de Larios · (Diabetes, Clinical Dermatology, General Surgery) · Baylor University Medical Center · 2801 Lemmon Avenue, West, Suite 310, Dallas, TX 75204 · 214-720-0264

Richard Leon Grandjean · (Families with Young Children, Minor Surgery, Preventive Medicine) · Baylor University Medical Center · 9323 Garland Road, Suite 207, Dallas, TX 75218 · 214-327-3333

Perry E. Gross · Baylor University Medical Center · Baylor University Medical Center, 3600 Gaston Avenue, Suite 454, Dallas, TX 75246 · 214-823-2166

Kevin Charles Oeffinger · Zale Lipshy University Hospital, St. Paul Medical Center · University of Texas-Southwestern Medical Center at Dallas, 5323 Harry Hines Boulevard, Dallas, TX 75235 · 214-648-7840

Shelley Roaten, Jr. · Zale Lipshy University Hospital, St. Paul Medical Center, Parkland Memorial Hospital · University of Texas-Southwestern Medical Center at Dallas, 5323 Harry Hines Boulevard, Dallas, TX 75235-9067 · 214-648-7840

T. Theodore Teel · Baylor University Medical Center · 2514 South Buckner Boulevard, Dallas, TX 75227 · 214-381-1187

El Paso

Rogelio Gonzalez, Jr. · (Industrial Injuries, Allergic Rhinitis, Minor Surgery) · Columbia Medical Center-East · Family Medicine Associates, 10555 Vista Del Sol, Suite 200, El Paso, TX 79925 · 915-594-1033

Kathryn V. Horn · Mesa Hills Medical Clinic, 700 South Mesa Hills Drive, El Paso, TX 79912 · 915-584-0051

Barbara M. Reeves · Providence Memorial Hospital · University Family Practice Associates, 125 West Hague Road, Suite 550, El Paso, TX 79902 · 915-533-6435

Fort Worth

Geoffrey Barst · (General Family Practice, General Pediatrics) · Harris Methodist-Fort Worth, Harris Methodist-Southwest, Plaza Medical Center, Cook Children's Medical Center, All Saints Episcopal Hospital-Fort Worth, All Saints Hospital-Cityview · 6316 Rufe Snow Drive, Fort Worth, TX 76148 · 817-281-3627

Barbara Ann Birdwell · Harris Methodist-Fort Worth · Health Partners, 4760 Barwick Drive, Suite C, Fort Worth, TX 76132 · 817-370-9200

Mark R. Dambro · Harris Methodist-Fort Worth · Texas Health Care, 1650 West Rosedale Street, Suite 307, Fort Worth, TX 76104 · 817-877-4411

Robert H. Lilli · Harris Methodist-Southwest · Texas Health Care, 6100 Harris Parkway, Suite 250, Fort Worth, TX 76132 · 817-346-5111

William S. Lorimer III · Texas Health Care, 6601 Dan Danciger Street, Suite 100, Fort Worth, TX 76133 · 817-294-2531

James A. Murphy · All Saints Episcopal Hospital-Fort Worth · 1201 Eighth Avenue, Suite B, Fort Worth, TX 76104 · 817-335-8479

Galveston

Edgar F. Jones III · St. Mary's Hospital · Galveston Family Health Associates, 3828 Ursuline Street, Galveston, TX 77550 · 409-765-6391

Donald Eugene Nease, Jr. · University of Texas Medical Branch Hospitals · University of Texas Medical Branch, Department of Family Medicine, 301 University Boulevard, Galveston, TX 77555-0853 · 409-772-3125

Angela J. Shepherd · Galveston Family Health Associates, 3828 Ursuline Street, Galveston, TX 77550 · 409-765-6391

Stephen J. Spann · University of Texas Medical Branch Hospitals · University of Texas Medical Branch, Department of Family Medicine, 301 University Boulevard, Galveston, TX 77555-0853 · 409-772-3125

Jeffrey R. Steinbauer · University of Texas Medical Branch Hospitals · University of Texas Medical Branch, Department of Family Medicine, 301 University Boulevard, Galveston, TX 77550 · 409-772-5819

Barbara L. Thompson · (Geriatric Medicine) · University of Texas Medical Branch Hospitals · Family Medical Clinic, 415 Texas Avenue, Galveston, TX 77555-0853 · 409-772-3126

Garland

Carl Edward Couch · Baylor Medical Center-Garland · Family Medical Center, 530 Clara Barton Boulevard, Garland, TX 75042 · 214-272-6561

Seth Bailey Cowan · Baylor Medical Center-Garland · Family Health Care Associates, 3232 Broadway Boulevard, Garland, TX 75043 · 214-864-0252

Houston

Stuart A. Bergman · Kelsey-Seybold Medical, 6624 Fannin Street, 20th Floor, Houston, TX 77030 · 713-791-8700

Jane E. Corboy · Methodist Hospital, St. Luke's Episcopal Hospital, Park Plaza Hospital, Texas Children's Hospital · Baylor College of Medicine, Department of Family Medicine, 1200 Binz Street, Suite 100, Houston, TX 77004 · 713-285-1800

Clive K. Fields · Village Family Practice, 9055 Katy Freeway, Suite 200, Houston, TX 77024 · 713-461-2915

Harold J. Fields · (Addictive Disorders, Obesity) · Spring Branch Medical Center, Memorial Healthcare System, Memorial Hospital-Memorial City, St. Luke's Episcopal Hospital, Twelve Oaks Hospital · 9055 Katy Freeway, Suite 200, Houston, TX 77024 · 713-461-2915

Grant C. Fowler · (Preventive Medicine, Office Procedures, Deliveries) · Hermann Hospital · University of Texas-Hermann Center of Family Practice, 6410 Fannin Street, Suite 250, Houston, TX 77030 · 713-704-5600

Leslie Julian Garb · Bellaire Hospital · Family & General Practice Associates, 5420 Dashwood Road, Suite 100, Houston, TX 77081 · 713-664-0719

Roland A. Goertz · (Medical Management) · Hermann Hospital · OneCare, 6424 Fannin Street, Houston, TX 77030 · 713-704-8100

Edward Lee Langston · Memorial Family Medical Center, 7737 Southwest Freeway, Houston, TX 77074 · 713-776-5320

Karen Maness · (General Pediatrics, Women's Healthcare) · Memorial Hospital-Memorial City, West Houston Medical Center, Hermann Hospital, Memorial Hospital-Southwest, Bellaire Hospital · Family & General Practice, 909 Dairy Ashford, Suite 215, Houston, TX 77079 · 713-493-1971

Susan Maria Miller · (HIV/AIDS, Public Health) · Methodist Hospital, St. Luke's Episcopal Hospital · Baylor College of Medicine, Department of General Internal Medicine, 6550 Fannin Street, Mail Stop 1200, Houston, TX 77030 · 713-790-3321

Les Nowitz · Family & General Practice Associates, 6699 Chimney Rock, Suite 103, Houston, TX 77081 · 713-664-0719

Robert E. Rakel · (Depression, Colon Cancer, Anxiety Disorders) · Methodist Hospital, St. Luke's Episcopal Hospital · Baylor College of Medicine, Department of Family Medicine, 5510 Greenbriar Street, Suite 266, Houston, TX 77005-2646 · 713-798-7788

John C. Rogers · (Clinical Prevention) · Texas Children's Hospital, St. Luke's Episcopal Hospital, Methodist Hospital, Park Plaza Hospital · Baylor College of Medicine, Department of Family Medicine, 5510 Greenbriar Street, First Floor, Houston, TX 77005-2646 · 713-798-7744

Joseph Segel · 909 Dairy Ashford, Suite 215, Houston, TX 77079 · 713-493-1971

Robert C. Vanzant · Memorial Hospital-Memorial City · Memorial Hospital-Memorial City, Department of Medicine, 920 Frostwood Drive,Suite 214, Houston, TX 77024 · 713-932-6288

Lubbock

Richard Van Ness Homan · (Sports Medicine, Geriatric Medicine, General Family Practice) · University Medical Center · Texas Tech University Health Sciences Center, Department of Family Medicine, 3601 Fourth Street, Lubbock, TX 79430 · 806-743-2757

Charles Alvin Jones · University Medical Center · University Medical Center, Department of Family Medicine, 602 Indiana Avenue, Lubbock, TX 79415-3364 806-743-1177

Round Rock

Don Baker Cauthen · Scott & White Clinic · Scott & White Clinic, Department of Family Medicine, One Chisholm Trail, Suite 200, Round Rock, TX 78681 · 512-310-3000

San Antonio

Michael Gerard Blanchett · Santa Rosa Health Care, Santa Rosa Children's Hospital, Baptist Medical Center · Barrio Comprehensive Family Health Center, 1102 Barclay Street, San Antonio, TX 78207-7197 · 210-434-0513

Javier Cerda Bocanegra · 1616 Callaghan Road, San Antonio, TX 78228 · 210-435-1218

Kevin Patrick Comfort · 8711 Village Drive, Suite 325, San Antonio, TX 78217 210-637-0000

Lynne Marie Diamond · 4318 Woodcock Street, Suite 120, San Antonio, TX 78228 · 210-735-5225

David Guerrero · Holy Cross Family Practice, 590 North General McMullen Street, Suite One, San Antonio, TX 78228 · 210-433-2334

Kimberly Koester Heller · 4318 Woodcock Street, Suite 120, San Antonio, TX 78228 · 210-735-5225

Gordon Travis Hill, Jr. · 8500 Village Drive, Suite 302, San Antonio, TX 78217 210-650-3933

Curtis Scott Horn · 303 West Sunset, Suite 101, San Antonio, TX 78209 · 210-824-5201

W. Ross Lawler · University Hospital-South Texas Medical Center · University of Texas Health Science Center at San Antonio, Department of Family Practice, 7703 Floyd Curl Drive, San Antonio, TX 78284-7794 · 210-567-4550

Erwin Richard Lochte III · Southwest Texas Methodist Hospital · Diagnostic Clinic of San Antonio, 5282 Medical Drive, Suite 510, San Antonio, TX 78229 · 210-615-1300

James C. Martin · (Lipid Disorders, Preventive Health) · Northeast Baptist Hospital · Health Texas, 7300 Blanco Road, Suite 301, San Antonio, TX 78216 · 210-344-3021

Carlos A. Moreno · University Hospital-South Texas Medical Center · University of Texas Health Science Center at San Antonio, Department of Family Practice, 7703 Floyd Curl Drive, San Antonio, TX 78284-7794 · 210-567-4553

Cheryl Hacker Mueller · San Antonio Community Hospital · 2829 Babcock Road, Suite 236A, San Antonio, TX 78229 · 210-614-8088

Francis William Mueller · Methodist Healthcare System, St. Luke's Baptist Hospital, San Antonio Community Hospital, Santa Rosa Northwest Hospital · 2829 Babcock Road, Suite 236A, San Antonio, TX 78229 · 210-614-8088

Horacio Rafael Ramirez · 9179 Grisom Road, San Antonio, TX 78251 · 210-680-8081

Janet P. Realini · (Contraception, Women's Health, Epidemiology) · University Hospital-South Texas Medical Center · University of Texas Health Science Center at San Antonio, Department of Family Practice, 7703 Floyd Curl Drive, San Antonio, TX 78284-7794 · 210-270-3920

George Merritt Richmond, Jr. · Metropolitan Family Practice, 1303 McCullough Avenue, Suite GL60, San Antonio, TX 78212 · 210-227-9214

Abelardo Rodriguez · Northeast Baptist Hospital · 8527 Village Drive, Suite 200, San Antonio, TX 78217 · 210-653-2693

Charles Martin Sawyer · Diagnostic Clinic of San Antonio, 4647 Medical Drive, San Antonio, TX 78229 · 210-615-1300

Karen Sue Shimotsu · North Blanco Family Physicians, 14855 Blanco Road, Suite 204, San Antonio, TX 78216 · 210-493-5330

Bernard Karl Weiner · (Geriatric Medicine) · Southwest Texas Methodist Hospital · Jefferson Medical Center, 929 Manor Drive, San Antonio, TX 78228-3295 210-735-9151

Sugar Land

Mickey V. Bush · Colony Medical Center, 4415 Highway Six South, Sugar Land, TX 77478 · 713-494-1234

The Woodlands

Gary Mueck · Woodlands Family Practice, 1055 Evergreen Circle, The Woodlands, TX 77380 · 713-363-3560

Waco

Glen R. Couchman · Scott & White Clinic, 7700 Fish Pond Road, Waco, TX 76710 · 817-741-4444

Keith D. Horner · 405 Londonderry Drive, Suite 303, Waco, TX 76712 · 817-776-4341

John Richard Jackson · Hillcrest Baptist Medical Center · Hillcrest Medical Clinic, 3312 Hillcrest Drive, Waco, TX 76708 · 817-752-4641

John D. Kosarek · 201 Old Hewitt Road, Waco, TX 76712 · 817-776-5430

David L. Lockhart · Hillcrest Baptist Medical Center · Hillcrest Medical Clinic, 3312 Hillcrest Drive, Waco, TX 76708 · 817-752-4641

Samuel Warren Ralston · Hillcrest Baptist Medical Center · Hillcrest Medical Clinic, 1001 Huwitt Drive, Waco, TX 76712 · 817-666-7888

Reginald B. Schleider · Waco Family Medicine, 405 Londonderry Drive, Suite 100, Waco, TX 76712 · 817-751-4971

John W. Speckmiear · 201 Old Hewitt Road, Waco, TX 76712 · 817-776-5430

GASTROENTEROLOGY

Amarillo

Martin I. Cohen · General Gastroenterology (Gastroenterologic Cancer, Inflammatory Bowel Disease) · High Plains Baptist Hospital, St. Anthony's Hospital, Amarillo Hospital District-Northwest Texas Hospital · Amarillo Diagnostic Clinic, 6700 West Ninth Street, Amarillo, TX 79106 · 806-358-3171

Thomas L. Johnson · (Endoscopy, Gastroenterologic Cancer, Hepatology) · St. Anthony's Hospital, Amarillo Hospital District-Northwest Texas Hospital · Amarillo Diagnostic Clinic, 6700 West Ninth Street, Amarillo, TX 79106-1701 · 806-358-3171

Jake C. Lennard, Jr. · General Gastroenterology (Hepatology, Biliary Disease) · St. Anthony's Hospital, High Plains Baptist Hospital · Amarillo Diagnostic Clinic, 6700 West Ninth Street, Amarillo, TX 79106 · 806-358-3171

Leslie E. Reese · General Gastroenterology (Endoscopy, Inflammatory Bowel Disease) · St. Anthony's Hospital, High Plains Baptist Hospital, Amarillo Hospital District-Northwest Texas Hospital · Amarillo Diagnostic Clinic, 6700 West Ninth Street, Amarillo, TX 79106-1701 · 806-358-3171

Austin

Rashad E. Dabaghi · General Gastroenterology · 1910 West 35th Street, Austin, TX 78703-1324 · 512-454-4588

Robert L. Frachtman · General Gastroenterology (Biliary Tract Endoscopy, Esophageal Manometry) · Austin Diagnostic Medical Center · Austin Diagnostic Medical Center, 12221 MoPac Expressway North, P.O. Box 85075, Austin, TX 78708-5075 · 512-901-4007

George Edward Kitzmiller · General Gastroenterology · Austin Diagnostic Medical Center · Austin Diagnostic Medical Center, 12221 MoPac Expressway North, P.O. Box 85075, Austin, TX 78708-5075 · 512-901-1000

Craig H. Lubin · General Gastroenterology · Brackenridge Hospital, St. David's Healthcare Center, Seton Medical Center · 1910 West 35th Street, Austin, TX 78703 · 512-454-4588

Stephen James Utts · General Gastroenterology · 4310 James Casey Street, Suite B-1, Austin, TX 78745 · 512-448-4344

George Willeford III · Gastrointestinal Motility · 1910 West 35th Street, Austin, TX 78703 · 512-454-4588

Beaumont

Phillip L. Chaney · General Gastroenterology · Southeast Texas Gastroenterology Associates, 950 North 11th Street, Beaumont, TX 77702 · 409-898-4471

Wallace Combs II · General Gastroenterology · Southeast Texas Gastroenterology Associates, 950 North 11th Street, Beaumont, TX 77702 · 409-898-4471

Joseph William Holland, Jr. · General Gastroenterology · St. Elizabeth Hospital Southeast Texas Gastroenterology Associates, 2900 North Street, Suite 200, Beaumont, TX 77702-1540 · 409-898-4471

Conroe

Ralph P. Pearce · General Gastroenterology · 500 Medical Center Boulevard, Suite 218, Conroe, TX 77304 · 409-756-4429

Corpus Christi

Daniel Acosta · General Gastroenterology · 1301 Ocean Drive, Corpus Christi, TX 78404 · 512-884-2858

Jose M. Duran · General Gastroenterology (Endoscopy, Esophageal Disease) · Memorial Medical Center, Spohn Hospital, Bay Area Medical Center, Doctors Regional Medical Center · 2222 Morgan Street, Suite 111, Corpus Christi, TX 78405 · 512-883-6623

Richard R. Evans · General Gastroenterology · 1301 Ocean Drive, Corpus Christi, TX 78404 · 512-884-2858

Dallas

Burton Combes · Hepatology (Primary Biliary Cirrhosis, Autoimmune Liver Disease, Liver Disease in Pregnancy) · The University of Texas-Southwestern Medical Center, Parkland Memorial Hospital, Zale Lipshy University Hospital · University of Texas-Southwestern Medical Center at Dallas, 5323 Harry Hines Boulevard, Dallas, TX 75235-8887 · 214-648-3440

Jeffrey Steven Crippin · Hepatology (Liver Transplantation) · Baylor University Medical Center · Baylor University Medical Center, Liver Service, Three Truett Tower, 3500 Gaston Avenue, Dallas, TX 75246-2017 · 214-820-6896

Daniel Carl DeMarco · General Gastroenterology (Liver Transplantation, Endoscopic Ultrasonography, Small Bowel Transplantation) · Baylor University Medical Center · Baylor University Medical Center, 3500 Gaston Avenue, Dallas, TX 75246-2017 · 214-820-2232

Mark Feldman · Peptic Disorders, Endoscopy · VA Medical Center · VA Medical Center, Medical Service, 4500 South Lancaster Road, Mail Code 111, Dallas, TX 75216 · 214-376-5451 x5344

John S. Fordtran · Inflammatory Bowel Disease, Peptic Disorders (General Gastroenterology) · Baylor University Medical Center · Baylor University Medical Center, Gastrointestinal Research, One Truett Tower, Room 1230, 3500 Gaston Avenue, Dallas, TX 75246 · 214-820-2672

J. Kent Hamilton, Jr. · Endoscopy · Baylor University Medical Center · Baylor University Medical Center, Truett Tower, Third Floor, 3500 Gaston Avenue, Dallas, TX 75246-4017 · 214-820-2232

William M. Lee · Hepatology (Chronic Hepatitis, Acute Liver Failure) · Zale Lipshy University Hospital · University of Texas-Southwestern Medical Center at Dallas, Department of Gastroenterology, Liver Unit, 5323 Harry Hines Boulevard, Dallas, TX 75235-8887 · 214-648-3323

Peter Mayer Loeb · Endoscopy (Hepatology, Pancreatic Disease, Gall Bladder and Biliary Disease) · Presbyterian Hospital of Dallas · Dallas Digestive Disease Associates, 8230 Walnut Hill Lane, Suite 408, Dallas, TX 75231-4403 · 214-345-7398

Willis C. Maddrey · Hepatology · Zale Lipshy University Hospital · University of Texas-Southwestern Medical Center at Dallas, Office of the Executive Vice-President for Clinical Affairs, 5323 Harry Hines Boulevard, Dallas, TX 75235-8570 · 214-648-2024

Walter L. Peterson, Jr. · Endoscopy · VA Medical Center · VA Medical Center, 4500 South Lancaster Road, Mail Code 111B1, Dallas, TX 75216-7191 · 214-371-6441

Daniel Earl Polter · General Gastroenterology · Baylor University Medical Center Baylor University Medical Center, 3500 Gaston Avenue, Dallas, TX 75246-2017 214-820-2232

Charles T. Richardson · General Gastroenterology (Peptic Disorders, Esophageal Disease) · Baylor University Medical Center · Texas Digestive Disease Consultants, 3409 Worth Street, Dallas, TX 75246 · 214-820-2266

Allen W. Rubin · Hepatology (Inflammatory Bowel Disease, Endoscopy, Esophageal Disease, General Gastroenterology, Pancreatic Disease, Peptic Disorders) · St. Paul Medical Center · University of Texas-Southwestern Medical Center at Dallas, St. Paul Medical Building, 5939 Harry Hines Boulevard, Dallas, TX 75235-6243 · 214-879-6900

Lawrence R. Schiller · Gastrointestinal Motility (Diarrheal Disease, Anorectal Motility Disorders, Peptic Disorders, Malabsorption) · Baylor University Medical Center · Baylor University Medical Center, Department of Internal Medicine, 3500 Gaston Avenue, Dallas, TX 75246 · 214-820-2671

Dwain Louis Thiele · Hepatology · Parkland Memorial Hospital · University of Texas-Southwestern Medical Center at Dallas, 5323 Harry Hines Boulevard, Dallas, TX 75235-8887 · 214-648-3440

Denison

Ronald M. Barkley · Gastrointestinal Motility · 105 Memorial Drive, Suite 103, Denison, TX 75020 · 903-465-2761

El Paso

Tej Pratap Gupta · General Gastroenterology (Endoscopy, Hepatology) · Thomason Hospital, Sierra Medical Center, Providence Memorial Hospital, Columbia Medical Center-East, Columbia Medical Center-West · 1733 Curie Drive, Suite 200, El Paso, TX 79902 · 915-534-2500

Jesus Antonio Hernandez · General Gastroenterology · Thomason Hospital, William Beaumont Army Medical Center · Texas Tech University Health Sciences Center, Department of Internal Medicine, 4800 Alberta Avenue, El Paso, TX 79905-2708 · 915-545-6618

Alan J. Karp · General Gastroenterology (Liver & Biliary Tract Disease, Inflammatory Bowel Disease) · Providence Memorial Hospital, Sierra Medical Center, Columbia Medical Center-West, Columbia Medical Center-East · 125 West Hague Road, Suite 590, El Paso, TX 79902 · 915-532-1620

John Melvin Tune · General Gastroenterology · 125 West Hague Road, Suite 590, El Paso, TX 79902 · 915-532-1620

Marc J. Zuckerman · (Irritable Bowel Syndrome, Endourology, Hepatology) · Thomason Hospital · Texas Tech University Health Sciences Center, Department of Internal Medicine, 4800 Alberta Avenue, El Paso, TX 79905 · 915-533-3020

Fort Worth

Desmond B. Corbett · Gastrointestinal Motility · 724 Pennsylvania Avenue, Fort Worth, TX 76104-2221 · 817-335-2487

Galveston

Sheila E. Crowe · Inflammatory Bowel Disease (Peptic Ulcer Disease, Gastrointestinal Food Allergies) · University of Texas Medical Branch Hospitals · University of Texas Medical Branch, Division of Gastroenterology, 301 University Boulevard, Room 0764, Galveston, TX 77555-0764 · 409-772-1501

Don W. Powell · General Gastroenterology · University of Texas Medical Branch, Department of Internal Medicine, Division of Gastroenterology, 301 University Boulevard, Room 0567, Galveston, TX 77555-0567 · 409-772-9891

Roger D. Soloway · Hepatology · University of Texas Medical Branch, Division of Gastroenterology, 301 University Boulevard, Galveston, TX 77555-0764 · 409-772-1501

Steven A. Weinman · Hepatology · University of Texas Medical Branch, Division of Gastroenterology, 301 University Boulevard, Room 0764, Galveston, TX 77555-0764 · 409-772-1501

Houston

Philip S. Bentlif · Inflammatory Bowel Disease (General Gastroenterology, Endoscopy) · St. Luke's Episcopal Hospital · Medical Clinic of Houston, 1707 Sunset Boulevard, Houston, TX 77005 · 713-526-5511

Robert E. Davis · General Gastroenterology (Endoscopy, Hepatology) · Gastroenterology Consultants, 7777 Southwest Freeway, Suite 708, Houston, TX 77074 713-776-1074

David Y. Graham · Peptic Disorders (Inflammatory Bowel Disease) · VA Medical Center · VA Medical Center, 2002 Holcombe Boulevard, Houston, TX 77030-4211 · 713-794-7280

Alfred Joe Hernandez, Jr. · General Gastroenterology · Park Plaza Hospital · 1200 Binz Street, Suite 650, Houston, TX 77004 · 713-520-6007

Frank L. Lanza · Endoscopy (Gastroenterologic Cancer, Inflammatory Bowel Disease) · Memorial Hospital-Southwest, Rosewood Medical Center · 2500 Fondren Street, Suite 250, Houston, TX 77063 · 713-977-9095

Bernard Levin · Gastroenterologic Cancer · University of Texas-M. D. Anderson Cancer Center · University of Texas-M. D. Anderson Cancer Center, 1515 Holcombe Boulevard, Box 203, Houston, TX 77030 · 713-792-3900

Patrick Michael Lynch · Gastroenterologic Cancer (Endoscopy) · University of Texas-M. D. Anderson Cancer Center · University of Texas-M. D. Anderson Cancer Center, 1515 Holcombe Boulevard, Box 78, Houston, TX 77030-4009 · 713-792-2828

John R. Mathias · Gastrointestinal Motility (Small Intestinal Motility, Functional Bowel Disease, Irritable Bowel Syndrome) · The Woman's Hospital of Texas · Columbia Woman's Hospital of Texas, 7600 Fannin Street, Houston, TX 77054 · 409-772-1501

Isaac Raijman · Endoscopy (Pancreatobiliary Endoscopy, Expandable Endopyosthesis, Esophageal Disease, Pancreatic Disease) · Hermann Hospital, University of Texas-M. D. Anderson Cancer Center, St. Luke's Episcopal Hospital, Methodist Hospital · 6414 Fannin Street, Suite G-125, Houston, TX 77030 · 713-704-5910

Jim Taub Schwartz · General Gastroenterology · Methodist Hospital · Baylor College of Medicine, Department of Gastroenterology, 6550 Fannin Street, Suite SM1122, Houston, TX 77030 · 713-790-2171

Joseph H. Sellin · Inflammatory Bowel Disease (Bicarbonate Transport by Intestinal Epithelia, Evaluation of Chronic Diarrhea, General Gastroenterology) · Hermann Hospital, Lyndon B. Johnson General Hospital, Methodist Hospital, St. Joseph Hospital · Digestive Disease Center, 6414 Fannin Street, Suite 125, Houston, TX 77030 · 713-792-5422

John R. Stroehlein · Gastroenterologic Cancer (Gastrointestinal Endoscopy, Functional Disorders of the GI Tract) · Hermann Hospital · University of Texas Medical School at Houston, 6431 Fannin Street, Room 4.234, Houston, TX 77030 713-792-5422

J. Guillermo Trabanino · Endoscopy (Peptic Disorders, General Gastroenterology) · Memorial Hospital-Southwest · Gastroenterology Consultants, 7777 Southwest Freeway, Suite 708, Houston, TX 77074 · 713-776-1074

Jose A. Fernando Urrutia · Endoscopy · 6624 Fannin Street, Suite 2590, Houston, TX 77030 · 713-796-0035

Ray Alan Verm · Endoscopy (Esophageal Disease, Gastrointestinal Motility) · Methodist Hospital · 6560 Fannin Street, Suite 1625, Houston, TX 77030 · 713-791-1800

George E. Whalen · General Gastroenterology (Inflammatory Bowel Disease, Colitis, Crohn's Disease, Gastrointestinal Motility) · Memorial Hospital-Southwest, St. Luke's Episcopal Hospital · 7737 Southwest Freeway, Suite 860, Houston, TX 77074 · 713-988-7188

Karen Lee Woods · Endoscopy · Methodist Hospital · Baylor College of Medicine, 6550 Fannin Street, Suite 1122, Houston, TX 77030 · 713-790-2171

Lubbock

David S. Hodges · Gastrointestinal Motility (Endoscopy, Biliary Disease) · University Medical Center · Texas Tech University Health Sciences Center, Department of Internal Medicine, 3601 Fourth Street, Lubbock, TX 79430 · 806-743-3155

Mark E. Mailliard · Hepatology (General Gastroenterology) · Texas Tech University Health Sciences Center, Department of Internal Medicine, 3601 Fourth Street, Lubbock, TX 79430 · 806-743-3150

Justin McCarthy · Endoscopy (Pancreas, Biliary) · Southwest Gastroenterology Associates, 3702 Twenty-First Street, Suite 201, Lubbock, TX 79410 · 800-685-8251

William Anderson Shaver · (Screening for Gastrointestinal Cancers, Therapeutic Endoscopy, Care of Terminally Ill and Dying Patients) · St. Mary of the Plains Hospital, Lubbock Methodist Hospital · Southwest Gastroenterology Associates, 3702 Twenty-First Street, Suite 201, Lubbock, TX 79410 · 800-685-8251; 806-799-3644

Eugene A. Trowers · Endoscopy (Ultrasound) · Texas Tech University Health Sciences Center, Department of Internal Medicine, 3601 Fourth Street, Lubbock, TX 79430 · 806-743-3150

Midland

R. P. Sarva · General Gastroenterology · 2201 West Tennessee Avenue, Midland, TX 79701 · 915-685-0053

Plano

Markus Goldschmiedt · Endoscopy (Pancreas, Biliary, Inflammatory Bowel Disease, Gastrointestinal Tumors) · Medical Center of Plano · 1600 Coit Road, Suite 401, Plano, TX 75075 · 214-867-0019

San Antonio

H. Leonard Bentch · General Gastroenterology (Nutrition) · Southwest Texas Methodist Hospital, St. Luke's Baptist Hospital, San Antonio Community Hospital · Gastroenterology Clinic of San Antonio, Medical Center Tower II, Suite 1050, 7940 Floyd Curl Drive, San Antonio, TX 78229 · 210-615-8308

Delbert Lee Chumley · General Gastroenterology (Hepato-Biliary Endoscopy, Pancreatic Disorders) · Southwest Texas Methodist Hospital, San Antonio Community Hospital, St. Luke's Baptist Hospital · Gastroenterology Consultants of San Antonio, 8214 Wurzbach Road, San Antonio, TX 78229-3374 · 210-614-1234

Alonzo John Drummond · General Gastroenterology (Hepatology, Inflammatory Bowel Disease, Pancreatic Disorders) · Baptist Medical Center, North Central Baptist Hospital, Metropolitan Hospital · Gastroenterology Associates, Madison Square Medical Building, Suite 608, 311 Camden Street, San Antonio, TX 78215 210-222-1347; 210-490-0202

Fred Henry Goldner · General Gastroenterology · Southwest Texas Methodist Hospital, San Antonio Community Hospital, Baptist Memorial Healthcare System, Santa Rosa Northwest Hospital · Gastroenterology Consultants of San Antonio, 8214 Wurzbach Road, San Antonio, TX 78229-3374 · 210-614-1234

Gerald Ira Green · General Gastroenterology (Inflammatory Bowel Disease, Hepatology) · Baptist Medical Center, North Central Baptist Hospital, Metropolitan Hospital, Santa Rosa Health Care · Gastroenterology Associates, Madison Square Medical Building, Suite 608, 311 Camden Street, San Antonio, TX 78215 · 210-222-1347

Glenn Weston W. Gross · Hepatology (Endoscopy, Pancreatic Disease) · University Hospital-South Texas Medical Center, Audie L. Murphy Memorial Veterans Hospital · University of Texas Health Science Center at San Antonio, Department of Medicine, Division of Gastroenterology & Nutrition, 7703 Floyd Curl Drive, San Antonio, TX 78284-7878 · 210-567-4880

Ernesto Guerra, Jr. · General Gastroenterology · 520 East Euclid Avenue, San Antonio, TX 78212 · 210-271-0606

Steven Eric Hearne · General Gastroenterology · San Antonio Digestive Disease Consultants, 1804 Northeast Loop 410, Suite 101, San Antonio, TX 78217 · 210-828-8400

Lawrence Joel Hoberman · General Gastroenterology · Southwest Texas Methodist Hospital · 7950 Floyd Curl Drive, Suite 801, San Antonio, TX 78229 · 210-692-0707

Patrick Allen Masters · General Gastroenterology · Gastroenterology Consultants of San Antonio, 8214 Wurzbach Road, San Antonio, TX 78229-3374 · 210-614-1234

Victor Stanley Ostrower · Hepatology (General Gastroenterology) · 7940 Floyd Curl Drive, Suite 1050, San Antonio, TX 78229 · 210-615-8308

Richard Luis Otero · General Gastroenterology · 520 East Euclid Avenue, San Antonio, TX 78212 · 210-271-0606

Charles Randall · General Gastroenterology (Gastrointestinal Malignancies, Helicobacter Pylori/Peptic Ulcers, Esophageal Disease) · Methodist Healthcare System, St. Luke's Baptist Hospital, San Antonio Community Hospital, Hill Country Memorial Hospital (Fredericksburg) · 7940 Floyd Curl Drive, Suite 1050, San Antonio, TX 78229 · 210-615-8308

Steven Schenker · Hepatology (General Gastroenterology, Pancreatic Disease) · University of Texas Health Science Center at San Antonio, Audie L. Murphy Memorial Veterans Hospital · University of Texas Health Science Center at San Antonio, Department of Medicine, Division of Gastroenterology & Nutrition, 7703 Floyd Curl Drive, San Antonio, TX 78284-7878 · 210-567-4878

Kermit Vincent Speeg, Jr. · General Gastroenterology · Audie L. Murphy Memorial Veterans Hospital, University Hospital-South Texas Medical Center · University of Texas Health Science Center at San Antonio, Department of Medicine, Division of Gastroenterology & Nutrition, 7703 Floyd Curl Drive, San Antonio, TX 78284-7878 · 210-567-4878

David L. Stump · General Gastroenterology (Chronic Hepatitis, Pancreatitis, Biliary Tract Disease) · Methodist Healthcare System, St. Luke's Baptist Hospital Gastroenterology Clinic of San Antonio, Medical Center Tower II, Suite 1050, 7940 Floyd Curl Drive, San Antonio, TX 78229 · 210-615-8308

John Thomas Swann · General Gastroenterology · Gastroenterology Consultants of San Antonio, 8214 Wurzbach Road, San Antonio, TX 78229-3374 · 210-614-1234

Joycelyn Marie Theard · General Gastroenterology · 8527 Village Drive, Suite 207, San Antonio, TX 78217 · 210-656-3070

San Marcos

Edward F. Coles · (Inflammatory Bowel Disease, Esophageal Disease, Biliary Disease) · Central Texas Medical Center, McKenna Memorial Hospital (New Braunfels), Guadalupe Valley Hospital (Seguin) · Gastroenterology of San Marcos & New Braunfels, 1305 Wonderworld Drive, Suite 200, San Marcos, TX 78666 · 512-754-8676

Temple

Kim Steven Culp · General Gastroenterology · Scott & White Memorial Hospital Scott & White Memorial Hospital, Department of Gastroenterology, 2401 South 31st Street, Temple, TX 76508-0001 · 817-724-2489

Walter P. Dyck · General Gastroenterology (Pancreatic Disease, Inflammatory Bowel Disease) · Scott & White Memorial Hospital & Clinic · Scott & White Memorial Hospital, Department of Gastroenterology, 2401 South 31st Street, Temple, TX 76508-0001 · 817-724-2237

Gene D. LeSage · General Gastroenterology · Scott & White Memorial Hospital Scott & White Memorial Hospital, Department of Gastroenterology, 2401 South 31st Street, Temple, TX 76508-0001 · 817-724-2489

Tyler

Gary D. Boyd · General Gastroenterology · East Texas Medical Center, Trinity Mother Frances Health Care Center · Tyler Digestive Disease Associates, Physicians' Office Building, Suite 407, 701 Olympic Plaza, Tyler, TX 75701 · 903-592-2611

David K. Teegarden · Gastrointestinal Motility · Trinity Clinic, 910 East Houston Street, Suite 550, Tyler, TX 75702 · 903-595-5101

Waco

Daniel W. Bell · General Gastroenterology · 3115 Pine Avenue, Suite 101, Waco, TX 76708-3234 · 817-754-0099

James W. Boss · General Gastroenterology · Waco Medical Group, 2911 Herring Avenue, Suite 211, Waco, TX 76708 · 817-755-4400

Edward D. Carpenter · Gastrointestinal Motility (Endoscopy, Inflammatory Bowel Disease) · Providence Health Center · Providence Health Center, 6901 Medical Parkway, P.O. Box 2589, Waco, TX 76702-2589 · 817-751-4000

Edward D. Contreras · General Gastroenterology (Hepatology) · Providence Health Center, Hillcrest Baptist Medical Center · Waco Gastroenterology Associates, 6901 Medical Parkway, P.O. Box 2589, Waco, TX 76702-2589 · 817-754-0099

Thomas F. Eastwood · General Gastroenterology · Waco Gastroenterology, 6901 Medical Parkway, P.O. Box 2589, Waco, TX 76702-2589 · 817-751-4717

James E. Gray · General Gastroenterology · Hillcrest Baptist Medical Center · Central Texas Gastroenterology Consultants, 2911 Herring Avenue, Suite 211, Waco, TX 76708 · 817-755-4480

Ned Snyder III · General Gastroenterology (Hepatology) · Providence Health Center, Hillcrest Baptist Medical Center · Waco Gastroenterology, Medical Parkway, P.O. Box 2589, Waco, TX 76702 · 817-751-4717

Wichita Falls

Ricky Yuen-Yau Ho · Gastrointestinal Motility · Wichita General Hospital · Clinics of North Texas, 501 Midwestern Parkway, Wichita Falls, TX 76307-7521 · 817-766-3551

GERIATRIC MEDICINE

Amarillo

Ted M. Nicklaus · High Plains Baptist Hospital · 11 Medical Drive, Amarillo, TX 79106-4138 · 806-355-9741

Beaumont

Linda S. Cabrera · Senior Health Center, 810 Hospital Drive, Suite 200, Beaumont, TX 77701 · 409-833-6565

George Ellis Thomas · Internal Medicine Diagnostic, 2965 Harrison Street, Suite 312, P.O. Box 5757, Beaumont, TX 77726 · 409-898-2994

Corpus Christi

Andres Bonelli · 1415 Third Street, Suite 211, Corpus Christi, TX 78404 · 512-882-1917

Dallas

Craig Douglas Rubin · (Osteoporosis, Geriatric Assessment, Dementia) · Parkland Memorial Hospital, Zale Lipshy University Hospital, St. Paul Medical Center · University of Texas-Southwestern Medical Center at Dallas, Department of Internal Medicine, 5323 Harry Hines Boulevard, Dallas, TX 75235-8889 · 214-648-2992

El Paso

Kathryn V. Horn · Mesa Hills Medical Clinic, 700 South Mesa Hills Drive, El Paso, TX 79912 · 915-584-0051

Fort Worth

Kendra L. Jensen Belfi · Fort Worth Clinic, 1221 West Lancaster Avenue, Fort Worth, TX 76102-4511 · 817-336-7191

Galveston

James S. Goodwin · (General Geriatric Medicine, Geriatric Rheumatology) · University of Texas Medical Branch Hospitals · University of Texas Medical Branch, Division of Geriatric Medicine, 301 University Boulevard, Suite 0460, Galveston, TX 77555-0460 · 409-772 -1987

Patsy Koeppe · (General Internal Medicine, Endocrinology) · University of Texas Medical Branch Hospitals, Turner Geriatric Center · University of Texas Medical Branch, Division of Geriatric Medicine, 301 University Boulevard, Room 0460, Galveston, TX 77555-0460 · 409-772-1987

Houston

Paul D. Garcia · MacGregor Medical Association, Department of Geriatrics, 8100 Greenbriar Street, Suite 250, Houston, TX 77054 · 713-741-2273

Lillian G. Howard · General Geriatric Medicine (General Family Practice, Sports Physicals, Preventive Health Issues) · Memorial Hospital-Northwest, Cypress Fairbanks Medical Center · Memorial Hospital-Northwest, Department of Geriatric Medicine, 1631 North Loop West, Suite 530, Houston, TX 77008 · 713-869-2020; 713-345-9955

Robert J. Luchi · Methodist Hospital, VA Medical Center · Baylor College of Medicine, Geriatric Medicine Associates, 6550 Fannin Street, Suite 1153, Houston, TX 77030 · 713-798-3967

Alan K. Schultz · General Geriatric Medicine (Geriatric Neuropsychology, General Family Medicine) · Memorial Hospital-Southwest · Memorial Geriatric Evaluation and Resource Center, 7737 Southwest Freeway, Suite 425, Houston, TX 77074 · 713-776-5100

Joseph Trumble · Methodist Hospital · Baylor College of Medicine, Geriatric Medicine Associates, 6550 Fannin Street, Suite 1153, Houston, TX 77030 · 713-798-3967

Lubbock

Charles Alvin Jones · University Medical Center · University Medical Center, Department of Family Medicine, 602 Indiana Avenue, Lubbock, TX 79415-3364 806-743-1177

San Antonio

Meghan B. Gerety · (Long-Term Care) · Audie L. Murphy Memorial Veterans Hospital · Audie L. Murphy Memorial Veterans Hospital, 7400 Merton Minter Boulevard, Mail Code 11C6, San Antonio, TX 78284 · 210-617-5300 x5407

Michael Steven Katz · (Geriatric Endocrinology) · Audie L. Murphy Memorial Veterans Hospital · Audie L. Murphy Memorial Veterans Hospital, 7400 Merton Minter Boulevard, Mail Code GRECC 182, San Antonio, TX 78284 · 210-617-5197

Michael J. Lichtenstein · General Geriatric Medicine (Home Care, Hospice) · Audie L. Murphy Memorial Veterans Hospital, University Hospital-South Texas Medical Center · University of Texas Health Science Center at San Antonio, University Clinic, 4502 Medical Drive, San Antonio, TX 78229 · 210-567-2777

Rowland Sanchez Reyna · (Cardiology, Diabetes, Preventive Medicine) · Santa Rosa Health Care, Baptist Medical Center · Health Texas Medical Group, 215 East Quincy Street, Suite 500, San Antonio, TX 78215 · 210-223-1600

Bernard Karl Weiner · Southwest Texas Methodist Hospital · Jefferson Medical Center, 929 Manor Drive, San Antonio, TX 78228-3295 · 210-735-9151

HAND SURGERY

Amarillo

Louise Ferland · General Hand Surgery (General Plastic Surgery, Facial Aesthetic Surgery, Laser Surgery, Cosmetic and Reconstructive Breast Surgery) · St. Anthony's Hospital, High Plains Baptist Hospital, Amarillo Hospital District-Northwest Texas Hospital, Columbia Panhandle Surgical Hospital, Crown of Texas Surgical Hospital · 722 North Polk Street, Amarillo, TX 79107 · 806-345-4245

John C. Kelleher, Jr. · General Hand Surgery (Peripheral Nerve Surgery, Reconstructive Surgery) · High Plains Baptist Hospital · Panhandle Plastic Surgery, 1810 Coulter Drive, Amarillo, TX 79106-1777 · 806-358-8731

Austin

Susan K. Adler · General Hand Surgery · 3705 Medical Parkway, Suite 350, Austin, TX 78705 · 512-458-4224

Don Emery Johnson · General Hand Surgery · South Austin Medical Center · 4207 James Casey Street, Suite 109, Austin, TX 78745-1192 · 512-443-3933

Gary Neil Pamplin · General Hand Surgery · 3705 Medical Parkway, Suite 530, Austin, TX 78705 · 512-459-4249

Robert M. Walters · General Hand Surgery · 3705 Medical Parkway, Suite 520, Austin, TX 78705 · 512-451-0211

Beaumont

Curtis M. Baldwin, Jr. · Reconstructive Surgery, Microsurgery · Southeast Texas Plastic Surgery, 2965 Harrison Street, Suite 315, Beaumont, TX 77702-1150 · 409-899-1277

John Taylor · General Hand Surgery (Upper Extremities) · Beaumont Bone & Joint Clinic, 3650 Laurel Street, Beaumont, TX 77707-2216 · 409-838-0346

Corpus Christi

David Parker · General Hand Surgery · Orthopaedic Associates, 3301 South Alameda Street, Suite 101, Corpus Christi, TX 78411 · 512-854-0811

Dallas

Peter R. Carter · Pediatric Orthopaedic Surgery (Reconstruction of Scaphoid Fracture, Pediatric Hand Problems, Digital Radius Fractures) · Baylor University Medical Center, Texas Scottish Rite Hospital for Children · 2731 Lemmon Avenue, East, Suite 300, Dallas, TX 75204 · 214-528-4185

Marybeth Ezaki · Pediatric Orthopaedic Surgery · Texas Scottish Rite Hospital for Children · Texas Scottish Rite Hospital for Children, Department of Orthopaedics, 2222 Welborn Street, Dallas, TX 75219 · 214-521-3168

El Paso

Mark T. Buchman · (Peripheral Nerve Surgery, Microsurgery) · Thomason Hospital, Providence Memorial Hospital, Columbia Medical Center · Texas Tech University Health Sciences Center, Department of Orthopaedics, 4800 Alberta Avenue, El Paso, TX 79905-2709 · 915-545-6750

Fort Worth

Robert E. Bunata · General Hand Surgery · 801 West Terrell Avenue, Fort Worth, TX 76104 · 817-877-3179

Larry Earl Reaves · General Hand Surgery (Adult, Pediatric) · Harris Methodist-Fort Worth · 800 Eighth Avenue, Suite 606, Fort Worth, TX 76104-2605 · 817-335-4755

Luiz Carlos Toledo · General Hand Surgery (General Orthopaedic Surgery, Peripheral Nerve Surgery) · Harris Methodist-Southwest · 6100 Harris Parkway, Suite 140, Fort Worth, TX 76132-4107 · 817-346-5555

William J. Van Wyk · General Hand Surgery · 803 West Terrell Avenue, Fort Worth, TX 76104 · 817-877-3113

B. J. Wroten · General Hand Surgery · All Saints Episcopal Hospital-Fort Worth, Harris Methodist-Fort Worth · 801 West Terrell Avenue, Fort Worth, TX 76104-3155 · 817-877-3177

Houston

James B. Bennett · General Hand Surgery · Methodist Hospital, Texas Orthopedic Hospital, St. Luke's Episcopal Hospital · Fondren Orthopaedic Group, 7401 South Main Street, Houston, TX 77030 · 713-799-2300

Benjamin E. Cohen · General Hand Surgery (Reconstructive Surgery) · St. Joseph Hospital · Cohen & Cronin Clinic Association, 1315 Calhoun Street, Suite 920, Houston, TX 77002 · 713-951-0400

Gerard T. Gabel · General Hand Surgery · Baylor College of Medicine, Department of Orthopaedic Surgery, 6550 Fannin Street, Suite 2625, Houston, TX 77030 · 713-790-2927

David H. Hildreth · (Reconstructive Microsurgery) · Methodist Hospital, St. Luke's Episcopal Hospital, St. Joseph Hospital, Diagnostic Center Hospital, Hermann Hospital · Baylor College of Medicine, Department of Orthopaedic Surgery, 6550 Fannin Street, Suite 2625, Houston, TX 77030 · 713-790-3703

Fred B. Kessler · General Hand Surgery (Reconstructive Surgery, Peripheral Nerve Surgery) · St. Luke's Episcopal Hospital, Texas Children's Hospital · St. Luke's Episcopal Hospital, Hand Surgical Associates, Medical Towers, Suite 2730, 6624 Fannin Street, Houston, TX 77030 · 713-795-4950

David M. Lichtman · General Hand Surgery (Wrist Surgery) · Methodist Hospital, St. Luke's Episcopal Hospital, Ben Taub General Hospital, Texas Children's Hospital · Baylor College of Medicine, 6550 Fannin Street, Suite 2625, Houston, TX 77030 · 713-793-7616

Saleh Mousa Shenaq · Peripheral Nerve Surgery, Microsurgery (Congenital, Reconstruction) · Methodist Hospital, Texas Children's Hospital, St. Luke's Hospital, The Institute for Rehabilitation & Research · Texas Medical Center-Baylor College of Medicine, Scurlock Tower, Suite 800, 6560 Fannin Street, Houston, TX 77030 · 713-798-6310

Lubbock

Eugene Jean Dabezies · General Hand Surgery (Arthritis Surgery, Trauma) · University Medical Center · Texas Tech University Health Sciences Center, 3601 Fourth Street, Room 1A113, Lubbock, TX 79430 · 806-743-2465

Midland

David J. Mallams · General Hand Surgery · 2000 West Cuthbert Street, Midland, TX 79701 · 915-682-9869

San Antonio

Fred Goodwin Corley · General Hand Surgery (Shoulder Surgery, Elbow Surgery, Orthopaedic Trauma) · University Hospital-South Texas Medical Center · University of Texas Health Science Center at San Antonio, Department of Orthopaedics, 7703 Floyd Curl Drive, San Antonio, TX 78264-7774 · 210-567-5125

James Harold Dobyns · Reconstructive Surgery (Congenital) · University Hospital-South Texas Medical Center · The Hand Center of San Antonio, 7940 Floyd Curl Drive, Suite 900, San Antonio, TX 78229 · 210-614-7025

David P. Green · General Hand Surgery · Baptist Medical Center · The Hand Center of San Antonio, 7940 Floyd Curl Drive, Suite 900, San Antonio, TX 78229 210-614-7025

Eugene Thomas O'Brien · Elbow Surgery · The Hand Center of San Antonio, 7940 Floyd Curl Drive, Suite 900, San Antonio, TX 78229-3906 · 210-614-7025

William C. Pederson · Reconstructive Surgery · Baptist Medical Center · The Hand Center of San Antonio, 7940 Floyd Curl Drive, Suite 900, San Antonio, TX 78229-3906 · 210-614-7025

Temple

Wallace E. Lowry, Jr. · General Hand Surgery (General Orthopaedic Surgery) · Scott & White Memorial Hospital & Clinic · Scott & White Memorial Hospital, Department of Orthopaedic Surgery, 2401 South 31st Street, Temple, TX 76508-0001 · 817-724-2749

Waco

Bill H. Berryhill · General Hand Surgery · 7003 Woodway Drive, Suite 304, Waco, TX 76712 · 817-776-0310

INFECTIOUS DISEASE

Amarillo

Joseph T. Carlisle · General Infectious Disease · Amarillo Diagnostic Clinic, 6700 West Ninth Street, Amarillo, TX 79106 · 806-358-3171

Austin

Jack Bissett · General Infectious Disease (HIV, AIDS, Transplantation Infections) · Seton Medical Center · Austin Infectious Disease Consultants, 1301 West 38th Street, Suite 404, Austin, TX 78705 · 512-459-0301

Earl Bertram Matthew · General Infectious Disease · Brackenridge Hospital · Central Texas Medical Foundation, Brackenridge Hospital, 601 East 15th Street, Austin, TX 78701 · 512-480-1862

Beaumont

Frank J. Baker · General Infectious Disease · St. Elizabeth Hospital · Infectious Disease Associates, 2955 Harrison Street, Suite 107, Beaumont, TX 77702-1155 · 409-892-6099

Corpus Christi

Michael Glen Bullen · General Infectious Disease · 1521 South Staples Street, Suite 404, Corpus Christi, TX 78404-3150 · 512-887-0075

Dallas

Jack A. Barnett · General Infectious Disease · Methodist Medical Center, 1441 Beckley Avenue, Dallas, TX 75203 · 214-947-2351

Edward Leo Goodman · General Infectious Disease (Granulomatous Infections, Hospital-Acquired Infections, Antibiotic Utilization) · Presbyterian Hospital of Dallas · 8210 Walnut Hill Lane, Suite 700, Dallas, TX 75231 · 214-691-8306

Clark R. Gregg · General Infectious Disease (Hospital-Acquired Infections, Fungus Infections) · VA Medical Center · VA Medical Center, 4500 South Lancaster Road, Mail Code 111D, Dallas, TX 75216-7167 · 214-376-5451

Robert W. Haley · Hospital-Acquired Infections (Epidemiology and Preventive Medicine) · University of Texas-Southwestern Medical Center at Dallas, Department of Internal Medicine, Division of Epidemiology, 5323 Harry Hines Boulevard, Dallas, TX 75235-8874 · 214-648-3075

James P. Luby · General Infectious Disease (Infections of the Central Nervous System, Sexually Transmitted Diseases, Clinical Virology) · Parkland Memorial Hospital, Zale Lipshy University Hospital · University of Texas-Southwestern Medical Center at Dallas, Department of Internal Medicine, Division of Infectious Disease, 5323 Harry Hines Boulevard, Dallas, TX 75235-9113 · 214-648-3480

Robert S. Munford · General Infectious Disease (Sepsis & Septic Shock) · Parkland Memorial Hospital · University of Texas-Southwestern Medical Center at Dallas, Department of Internal Medicine, Division of Infectious Disease, 5323 Harry Hines Boulevard, Dallas, TX 75235-9113 · 214-648-3480

Perry G. Pate · General Infectious Disease (AIDS, Hospital-Acquired Infections) St. Paul Hospital, Irving Hospital · ID Associates, 5939 Harry Hines Boulevard, Suite 545, Dallas, TX 75235 · 214-879-2387

Jay Philip Sanford · General Infectious Disease (Tropical Disease & Travel Medicine) · Parkland Memorial Hospital, Zale Lipshy University Hospital · Antimicrobial Therapy, 5910 North Central Expressway, Suite 1955, Dallas, TX 75206 · 214-750-5783

Steven M. Seidenfeld · General Infectious Disease · Medical City Dallas Hospital 12200 Park Central Drive, Suite 220, Dallas, TX 75251 · 214-661-5550

Paul M. Southern · General Infectious Disease (Parasitology, Tropical Disease & Travel Medicine) · Zale Lipshy University Hospital · University of Texas-Southwestern Medical Center at Dallas, Department of Pathology, 5323 Harry Hines Boulevard, Dallas, TX 75235-9060 · 214-648-3587

William Levin Sutker · General Infectious Disease (AIDS, Endocarditis) · Baylor University Medical Center · North Texas Infectious Diseases Consultants, 3409 Worth Street, Suite 710, Dallas, TX 75246 · 214-823-2533

El Paso

W. Lee Hand · General Infectious Disease · Thomason Hospital · Texas Tech University Health Sciences Center, Department of Internal Medicine, 4800 Alberta Avenue, El Paso, TX 79905 · 915-545-6627

Hoi Ho · General Infectious Diseases (Hospital-Acquired Infections, Tropical Disease & Travel Medicine) · Thomason Hospital · Texas Tech University Health Sciences Center, Department of Internal Medicine, 4800 Alberta Avenue, El Paso, TX 79905 · 915-545-6633

Abraham C. Verghese · AIDS (Pneumonia, General Infectious Disease, Lung Infections) · Thomason Hospital · Texas Tech University Health Sciences Center, Department of Internal Medicine, 4800 Alberta Avenue, El Paso, TX 79905 · 915-545-6623

Fort Worth

Daniel J. Barbaro · General Infectious Disease · 1350 South Main Street, Suite 1300, Fort Worth, TX 76104 · 817-877-3442

James Allen Reinarz · General Infectious Disease · John Peter Smith Hospital · John Peter Smith Hospital, Department of Medicine, 1500 South Main Street, Fort Worth, TX 76104 · 817-927-1395

Steven B. Sotman · General Infectious Disease · 1350 South Main Street, Suite 1300, Fort Worth, TX 76104 · 817-877-3442

Galveston

Jon T. Mader · General Infectious Disease (Bone Infections, Anaerobic Infections, Surgical Infections) · University of Texas Medical Branch Hospitals · University of Texas Medical Branch, Hyperbaric Facility, 301 University Boulevard, Room 1.100, Galveston, TX 77555-1115 · 409-772-1307

C. Glen Mayhall · Hospital-Acquired Infections (Hospital Epidemiology, General Infectious Diseases) · University of Texas Medical Branch Hospitals · University of Texas Medical Branch, Division of Infectious Diseases, Route 0835, 301 University Boulevard, Galveston, TX 77555-0835 · 409-747-0229

Richard B. Pollard · AIDS (Herpes Virus Infections, Toxoplasmosis) · University of Texas Medical Branch Hospitals · University of Texas Medical Branch, Department of Internal Medicine, Division of Infectious Disease, 301 University Boulevard, Galveston, TX 77555-0835 · 409-772-4979

Harlingen

Abraham G. Miranda · General Infectious Disease · 2121 Pease Street, Suite 1G, Harlingen, TX 78550 · 210-428-5604

Houston

Gerald P. Bodey · Cancer & Infections, Fungal Infections · University of Texas-M. D. Anderson Cancer Center · University of Texas-M. D. Anderson Cancer Center, Department of Medical Specialties, 1515 Holcombe Boulevard, Box 47, Houston, TX 77030 · 713-792-6830

Ricardo Bolivar-Briceno · General Infectious Disease (Hospital-Acquired Infections) · Houston Northwest Medical Center, Northeast Medical Center Hospital (Humble), Columbia Kingwood Medical Center (Kingwood) · 800 Peakwood Drive, Suite 2F, Houston, TX 77090 · 713-893-4376

Major William Bradshaw · General Infectious Disease (Endocarditis, Tropical Disease & Travel Medicine) · Methodist Hospital · Methodist Hospital, 6565 Fannin Street, Room 979, Mail Stop 910, Houston, TX 77030-2730 · 713-790-2507

Thomas R. Cate · Respiratory Infections · Ben Taub General Hospital · Baylor College of Medicine, Influenza Research Center, One Baylor Plaza, Room 628E, Houston, TX 77030-2397 · 713-798-4469

Robert Barnard Couch · (Virus Infections, Respiratory Infections) · Ben Taub General Hospital · Baylor College of Medicine, Department of Microbiology & Immunology, One Baylor Plaza, Room 205A, Houston, TX 77030 · 713-798-4474

Rabih Darouiche · General Infectious Disease (Infections Associated with Spinal Cord Injury) · VA Medical Center · VA Medical Center, 2002 Holcombe Boulevard, Room 4B-370, Houston, TX 77030 · 713-794-7384

Herbert L. DuPont · Tropical Disease & Travel Medicine, Diarrhea · St. Luke's Episcopal Hospital, Hermann Hospital, Methodist Hospital · St. Luke's Episcopal Hospital, 6720 Bertner Avenue, Room P-153, Mail Code 1-164, Houston, TX 77030 · 713-791-4122

Charles Derwin Ericsson · Tropical Disease & Travel Medicine (General Infectious Disease, Hospital-Acquired Infections) · Hermann Hospital · University of Texas Medical School at Houston, Division of Infectious Disease, 6431 Fannin Street, Room 1.729, Houston, TX 77030 · 713-794-4255

Victor Fainstein · Transplantation Infections (Bone Marrow Transplantation, Cancer & Transplantations, AIDS, Fungal Infections) · Methodist Hospital, St. Luke's Episcopal Hospital · 6560 Fannin Street, Suite 1540, Houston, TX 77030 713-799-9997

Joseph Clayton Gathe, Jr. · AIDS (General Infectious Disease, Hospital-Acquired Infections) · Park Plaza Hospital, St. Luke's Episcopal Hospital, Methodist Hospital, St. Joseph Hospital, Twelve Oaks Hospital · 1200 Binz Street, Suite 120, Houston, TX 77004 · 713-526-9821

Layne O. Gentry · Transplantation Infections, Bone Infections (Heart) · St. Luke's Episcopal Hospital · St. Luke's Episcopal Hospital, 6720 Bertner Avenue, Mail Code 2-233, Houston, TX 77030 · 713-791-4888

Stephen B. Greenberg · Respiratory Infections (AIDS, Virology) · Ben Taub General Hospital · Ben Taub General Hospital, Department of Infectious Disease, 1504 Taub Loop, Houston, TX 77030 · 713-798-4775

Richard J. Hamill · Fungal Infections (AIDS) · VA Medical Center · VA Medical Center, Infectious Disease Section, 2002 Holcombe Boulevard, Mail Code 111G, Houston, TX 77030-4211 · 713-794-7384

Richard L. Harris · General Infectious Disease (Epidemiology, Infection Control) Methodist Hospital · Methodist Hospital, 6565 Fannin Street, Room 979, Mail Stop 910, Houston, TX 77030 · 713-790-2507

Philip C. Johnson III · General Infectious Disease (General Internal Medicine, AIDS, Fungal Infections, Transplantation Infections) · Hermann Hospital, Lyndon B. Johnson General Hospital · University of Texas Houston Health Science Center, 6431 Fannin Street, Room MSB 1.122, P.O. Box 20708, Houston, TX 77030 · 713-792-8347

Marcia Ann Kielhofner · General Infectious Disease (Endocarditis, Hospital-Acquired Infections, Transplantation Infections) · St. Luke's Episcopal Hospital Houston Infectious Disease Associates, St. Luke's Medical Tower, Suite 1410, 6624 Fannin Street, Houston, TX 77030 · 713-791-4882

Barbara Elizabeth Murray · General Infectious Disease · University of Texas Medical School at Houston, Department of Infectious Disease, 6431 Fannin Street, Room 1.729, Houston, TX 77030 · 713-792-4988

Daniel M. Musher · General Infectious Disease (Bacterial Infections) · VA Medical Center · VA Medical Center, Infectious Disease Section, 2002 Holcombe Boulevard, Houston, TX 77030-4211 · 713-794-7384

John H. Rex · Fungal Infections (Hospital-Acquired Infections, Cancer & Infections) · Hermann Hospital · University of Texas Medical School at Houston, Department of Infectious Diseases, 6431 Fannin Street, Room JFB 1.728, Houston, TX 77030 · 713-792-4929

Kenneth V. I. Rolston · Cancer & Infections · University of Texas-M. D. Anderson Cancer Center · University of Texas-M. D. Anderson Cancer Center, Department of Medical Specialties, 1515 Holcombe Boulevard, Box 47, Houston, TX 77030 · 713-792-6830

Tobias Samo · General Infectious Disease (AIDS, Viral Infections) · Methodist Hospital · Infectious Disease Associates of Houston, 6550 Fannin Street, Suite 1540, Houston, TX 77030 · 713-799-9997

Terry K. Satterwhite · General Infectious Disease (Tuberculosis, Hospital-Acquired Infections) · Hermann Hospital · Hermann Hospital, 6411 Fannin Street, One Cullen, Houston, TX 77030-1501 · 713-704-3700

Edward Joel Septimus · General Infectious Disease (Hospital-Acquired Infections, Bone Infections, Travel Medicine) · Memorial Healthcare System · Infectious Disease Consultants, 7777 Southwest Freeway, Suite 740, Houston, TX 77074 · 713-777-7751

William Terry Siebert · General Infectious Disease (AIDS, Osteomyelitis) · St. Joseph Hospital · Medical Place One, Suite 1710, 1315 Calhoun Avenue, Houston, TX 77002 · 713-757-7475

Carl Victor Vartian · General Infectious Disease · Infectious Disease Consultants, 7777 Southwest Freeway, Suite 740, Houston, TX 77074 · 713-777-7751

Temple W. Williams, Jr. · Endocarditis (Fungal Infections, Postoperative Infections) · Methodist Hospital · Methodist Hospital, 6565 Fannin Street, Room 979, Mail Stop 910, Houston, TX 77030 · 713-790-2507

Edward J. Young · General Infectious Disease (Brucellosis) · VA Medical Center VA Medical Center, Infectious Disease Section, 2002 Holcombe Boulevard, Houston, TX 77030-4211 · 713-794-7384

Barry J. Zeluff · Transplantation Infections (General Infectious Disease, Hospital-Acquired Infections) · St. Luke's Episcopal Hospital · Houston Infectious Disease Associates, St. Luke's Medical Tower, Suite 1410, 6624 Fannin Street, Houston, TX 77030 · 713-791-4882

Lubbock

Thomas C. Butler · General Infectious Disease (Lung, Urinary Tract, Skin, HIV) Texas Tech University Health Sciences Center, Department of Internal Medicine, 3601 Fourth Street, Lubbock, TX 79430 · 806-743-3155

Dennis Efren Duriex · General Infectious Disease · Consultants in Infectious Disease, 4404 Nineteenth Street, Suite C, Lubbock, TX 79490 · 806-795-8150

Clark M. Kerr · General Infectious Disease (Clinical Mycology, Osteomyelitis, Outpatient Infusion Therapy) · Lubbock Methodist Hospital, St. Mary of the Plains Hospital · Consultants in Infectious Diseases, 4404 Nineteenth Street, Suite C, Lubbock, TX 79407 · 806-795-8150

Robert Kimbrough · (Fungal Infections, Endocarditis, Bone Infections) · University Medical Center · Texas Tech University Health Sciences Center, Department of Internal Medicine, 3601 Fourth Street, Lubbock, TX 79430 · 806-743-3155

San Antonio

Carl Michael Berkowitz · General Infectious Disease · Infectious Disease Consultants, 8042 Wurzbach Road, Suite 280, San Antonio, TX 78229-3856 · 210-614-8100

Luis Alfredo Cisneros · General Infectious Disease · Santa Rosa Health Care · 343 West Houston Street, Suite 808, San Antonio, TX 78205 · 210-224-9616

John R. Graybill · Fungal Infections · Audie L. Murphy Memorial Veterans Hospital · Audie L. Murphy Memorial Veterans Hospital, 7400 Merton Minter Boulevard, Mail Code 111F, San Antonio, TX 78284-5700 · 210-617-5111

Charles Jay Lerner · General Infectious Disease (Travel Medicine) · Infectious Disease Consultants, 8042 Wurzbach Road, Suite 280, San Antonio, TX 78229-3856 · 210-614-8100

Jan E. Evans Patterson · Hospital-Acquired Infections (Antibody-Resistant Bacteria, Fungal Infections) · University Hospital-South Texas Medical Center, Audie L. Murphy Memorial Veterans Hospital · University of Texas Health Science Center at San Antonio, Department of Medicine, Division of Infectious Disease, 7703 Floyd Curl Drive, San Antonio, TX 78284-7881 · 210-567-4823

Thomas Frost Patterson · AIDS, Fungal Infections · University Hospital-South Texas Medical Center · University of Texas Health Science Center at San Antonio, Department of Medicine, Division of Infectious Disease, 7703 Floyd Curl Drive, San Antonio, TX 78284-7881 · 210-567-4823

Patricia Kay Sharkey · AIDS · University Hospital-South Texas Medical Center University of Texas Health Science Center at San Antonio, Department of Medicine, Division of Infectious Disease, 7703 Floyd Curl Drive, San Antonio, TX 78284-7881 · 210-567-4823

Jean Alice Smith · AIDS (Anti-Viral Therapy, Herpes Virus Infections, General Infectious Disease) · University Hospital-South Texas Medical Center, Audie L. Murphy Memorial Veterans Hospital · University of Texas Health Science Center at San Antonio, Department of Medicine, Division of Infectious Disease, 7703 Floyd Curl Drive, San Antonio, TX 78284-7881 · 210-567-4823

Richard E. Thorner · General Infectious Disease · Southwest Texas Methodist Hospital · Infectious Disease Consultants, 8042 Wurzbach Road, Suite 280, San Antonio, TX 78229-3856 · 210-614-8100

Temple

Douglas Lee Hurley · General Infectious Disease · Scott & White Memorial Hospital · Scott & White Memorial Hospital, Department of Infectious Disease, 2401 South 31st Street, Temple, TX 76508-0001 · 817-724-2983

Tyler

Richard James Wallace, Jr. · Respiratory Infections (Micobacterial Infections) · University of Texas Health Center-Tyler · University of Texas Health Center-Tyler, US Highway 271 and State Highway 155, P.O. Box 2003, Tyler, TX 75710-2003 · 903-877-7680

Waco

A. Scott Lea · General Infectious Disease · Hillcrest Baptist Medical Center, Providence Health Center · Waco Infectious Disease Associates, 2911 Herring Avenue, Suite 203, Waco, TX 76708-3243 · 817-755-4450

E. Farley Verner · General Infectious Disease · Hillcrest Baptist Medical Center, Providence Health Center · Waco Infectious Disease Associates, 2911 Herring Avenue, Suite 203, Waco, TX 76708 · 817-755-4450

INTERNAL MEDICINE (GENERAL)

Alvin

Robert D. DeWitt · Alvin Medical Center, Clear Lake Regional Medical Center (Webster), Memorial Hospital-Southeast (Houston) · One Medic Lane, Alvin, TX 77511 · 713-331-0082; 713-331-7062

Amarillo

Rita Cherni-Smith · High Plains Baptist Hospital · 11 Medical Drive, Amarillo, TX 79106 · 806-355-9741

John R. Pierce, Jr. · High Plains Baptist Hospital · 11 Medical Drive, Amarillo, TX 79106-4138 · 806-355-9741

H. Wayne Smith · Amarillo Diagnostic Clinic, 6700 West Ninth Street, Amarillo, TX 79106-1701 · 806-358-3171

Robert S. Urban · High Plains Baptist Hospital · 11 Medical Drive, Amarillo, TX 79106-4138 · 806-355-9741

Austin

Ace Hill Alsup III · Austin Internal Medicine Associates, 3407 Glenview Avenue, Austin, TX 78703 · 512-459-3149

Richard Davis De Behnke · South Austin Diagnostic Clinic, 4315 James Casey Street, Austin, TX 78745 · 512-441-5096

Nancy Thorne Foster · 1301 West 38th Street, Suite 402, Austin, TX 78705 · 512-459-6503

Laura J. Guerrero · Austin Diagnostic Clinic, 3508 Far West Boulevard, Austin, TX 78731 · 512-459-1111

Jerry Lynn Hood · (Hypertension, Diabetes, Elevated Cholesterol) · South Austin Medical Center · South Austin Diagnostic Clinic, 4315 James Casey Street, Austin, TX 78745 · 512-441-5096

Isabel Vreeland Hoverman · Seton Medical Center · Austin Internal Medicine Associates, 3407 Glenview Avenue, Austin, TX 78703 · 512-459-3149

William Cleveland Lockett · South Austin Diagnostic Clinic, 4315 James Casey Street, Austin, TX 78745 · 512-441-5096

Philip J. Maple · Austin Diagnostic Medical Center, 12221 MoPac Expressway North, P.O. Box 85075, Austin, TX 78758 · 512-901-1000

John Robert Marietta · Austin Diagnostic Medical Center, 12221 MoPac Expressway North, P.O. Box 85075, Austin, TX 78708-5075 · 512-459-1111

Sheldon L. Markowitz · Capitol Medical Clinic, 1301 West 38th Street, Suite 601, Austin, TX 78705 · 512-454-5171

Michael D. Martin · Austin Diagnostic Medical Center, 12221 MoPac Expressway North, P.O. Box 85075, Austin, TX 78708-5075 · 512-901-4009

Thomas S. McHorse · (General Gastroenterology) · Seton Medical Center · 1301 West 38th Street, Suite 402, Austin, TX 78705 · 512-459-6503

Kenneth W. Mitchell · Austin Diagnostic Medical Center, 12221 MoPac Expressway North, P.O. Box 85075, Austin, TX 78758 · 512-901-1000

Roy Scott Ream · Seton Medical Center, St. David's Healthcare Center · Austin Internal Medicine Associates, 3407 Glenview Avenue, Austin, TX 78703 · 512-459-3149

Frank E. Robinson · Seton Medical Center · Austin Internal Medicine Associates, 3407 Glenview Avenue, Austin, TX 78703 · 512-459-3149

Robert C. Stern · Austin Diagnostic Clinic, 3508 Far West Boulevard, Austin, TX 78731 · 512-459-1111

Beaumont

Bertron Travis Brown · 2955 Harrison Street, Suite 300, Beaumont, TX 77702-1157 · 409-898-8440

Bruce W. Brown · 3570 College Street, Beaumont, TX 77702-1157 · 409-833-4433

Daniel James Harmon · St. Elizabeth Hospital · 2900 North Street, Suite 315, Beaumont, TX 77702-1541 · 409-899-2764

Santos M. Soberon · (General Geriatric Medicine, Nutrition, Primary Care) · Internal Medicine Diagnostic, 2965 Harrison Street, Suite 312, Beaumont, TX 77702 · 409-898-2994

George Ellis Thomas · Internal Medicine Diagnostic, 2965 Harrison Street, Suite 312, Beaumont, TX 77702 · 409-898-2994

Dwight M. Toups · 3570 College Street, Beaumont, TX 77701 · 409-833-4433

Corpus Christi

Cecil Martindale Bourne · (General Cardiovascular Disease, Osteoporosis) · Bay Area Medical Center, Doctors Regional Medical Center, Spohn Hospital · Thomas Spann Clinic, 7121 South Padre Island Drive, Suite 300, Corpus Christi, TX 78412 · 512-886-4158

Glenn Lamar Bugay · Spohn Hospital · Gulf Coast Medical Clinic, 613 Elizabeth Street, Suite 701, Corpus Christi, TX 78404 · 512-888-4262

John Robert Pettigrove · (Pulmonary Disease) · Spohn Hospital, Bay Area Medical Center · Thomas Spann Clinic, 7121 South Padre Island Drive, Suite 300, Corpus Christi, TX 78412 · 512-844-6005

John Richard Porter · Gulf Coast Medical Clinic, 613 Elizabeth Street, Suite 701, Corpus Christi, TX 78404 · 512-888-4262

Dallas

William Mark Armstrong · Baylor University Medical Center · 3434 Swiss Avenue, Suite 420, Dallas, TX 75204 · 214-828-5020

Robert King Bass · (Cardiology, Gastroenterology, Endocrinology) · Presbyterian Hospital of Dallas · 3330 Douglas Avenue, Dallas, TX 75219 · 214-526-8808

John Wayne Burnside · (Difficult Diagnostic Problems, Addictions) · Zale Lipshy University Hospital, Parkland Memorial Hospital · University of Texas-Southwestern Medical Center at Dallas, 5323 Harry Hines Boulevard, Dallas, TX 75235-9005 · 214-648-2097

Michael Chiu · (Sexually Transmitted Diseases) · Parkland Memorial Hospital, Zale Lipshy University Hospital · University of Texas-Southwestern Medical Center at Dallas, Department of Internal Medicine, 5323 Harry Hines Boulevard, Dallas, TX 75235-8889 · 214-648-2992

Robert Reed Click, Jr. · Zale Lipshy University Hospital · University of Texas-Southwestern Medical Center at Dallas, 5323 Harry Hines Boulevard, Dallas, TX 75235-9124 · 214-648-3100

Leonard J. Comess · Doctors Hospital of Dallas · 1000 Emerald Isle, Suite 118, Dallas, TX 75218 · 214-321-6485

M. Scott Daniel · Presbyterian Hospital of Dallas · North Texas Internist, 8335 Walnut Hill Lane, Suite 120, Dallas, TX 75231 · 214-368-6424

Robert Lee Fine · (Preventive Medicine, Geriatrics) · Baylor University Medical Center · 3434 Swiss Avenue, Suite 430, Dallas, TX 75204 · 214-828-5030

Philip Goodman · Presbyterian Hospital of Dallas · 7150 Greenville Avenue, Suite 650, Dallas, TX 75231 · 214-369-3613

Robert Joseph Haddox · St. Paul Medical Center · 1000 Emerald Isle, Suite 118, Dallas, TX 75218 · 214-321-6485

Allen Maulsby Jones · (General Internal Medicine) · Baylor University Medical Center · 3434 Swiss Avenue, Suite 320, Dallas, TX 75246 · 214-821-1720

R. Ellwood Jones · (Liver Disease, General Internal Medicine) · Baylor University Medical Center · 3434 Swiss Avenue, Dallas, TX 75204 · 214-828-5060

Arnold H. Kassanoff · (General Cardiovascular Disease, General Internal Medicine) · Presbyterian Hospital of Dallas · Cardiology & Internal Medicine Associates, 7150 Greenville Avenue, Suite 650, Dallas, TX 75231-5193 · 214-369-3613

Lynne M. Kirk · (Geriatric Medicine) · Parkland Memorial Hospital, Zale Lipshy University Hospital · University of Texas-Southwestern Medical Center at Dallas, 5323 Harry Hines Boulevard, Dallas, TX 75235-9005 · 214-648-3433

Paul Ewing Madeley · (General Cardiovascular Disease) · Baylor University Medical Center · 3434 Swiss Avenue, Suite 430, Dallas, TX 75204 · 214-828-5030

Russell Lionel Martin, Jr. · (Cardiovascular Disease, Hypertension) · Baylor University Medical Center · 3434 Swiss Avenue, Suite 320, Dallas, TX 75204 · 214-828-5060

Paul Muncy · (Diabetes, Hypercholesterolemia, Sports Medicine) · Baylor University Medical Center · 3434 Swiss Avenue, Suite 420, Dallas, TX 75204 · 214-828-5020

Paul Arnold Neubach · Baylor University Medical Center · 3434 Swiss Avenue, Suite 410, Dallas, TX 75204 · 214-828-5010

Stuart Frederick Owen · (Health Maintenance Issues, Risk Factor Control, Diabetes Mellitus, General Internal Medicine) · Baylor University Medical Center · 3600 Gaston Avenue, Suite 1004, Dallas, TX 75246 · 214-827-7600

Murray Pizette · Doctors Hospital of Dallas · 1000 Emerald Isle, Suite 118, Dallas, TX 75218-3949 · 214-321-6485

Irving David Prengler · (Inpatient Acute Hospital Care, Disease Prevention & Health Maintenance) · Baylor University Medical Center · Texas Primary Care Associates, 3600 Gaston Avenue, Suite 550, Dallas, TX 75246-1808 · 214-821-1177

W. Gary Reed · Zale Lipshy University Hospital, Parkland Memorial Hospital · University of Texas-Southwestern Medical Center at Dallas, 5323 Harry Hines Boulevard, Dallas, TX 75235-8889 · 214-648-2992

Albert Dee Roberts, Jr. · (General Nephrology, General Internal Medicine) · Zale Lipshy University Hospital · University of Texas-Southwestern Medical Center at Dallas, 5323 Harry Hines Boulevard, Dallas, TX 75235-8889 · 214-648-8897

Joseph Martin Rothstein · Baylor University Medical Center · Baylor University Medical Center, 3600 Gaston Avenue, Suite 1004, Dallas, TX 75246 · 214-827-7600

Walter Nathaniel Skinner · 8230 Walnut Hill Lane, Suite 804, Dallas, TX 75231 214-363-6217

Neal Lawrence Sklaver · (Headaches, Primary Care, General Internal Medicine) Presbyterian Hospital of Dallas · Medical Specialists Associated, 5461 La Sierra Drive, Dallas, TX 75231-4198 · 214-692-8541

Randlow Smith, Jr. · 3434 Swiss Avenue, Suite 330, Dallas, TX 75204 · 214-828-5070

Paul Arthur Tobolowsky · Medical City Dallas Hospital · Dallas Diagnostic Association, Building C, Suite 300, 7777 Forest Lane, Dallas, TX 75230 · 214-991-6000

Martin Earl True, Jr. · (General Cardiology, General Gastroenterology, General Infectious Disease) · Presbyterian Hospital of Dallas · 8210 Walnut Hill Lane, Suite 505, Dallas, TX 75231 · 214-369-8101

Paul Douglas Wade · 5939 Harry Hines Boulevard, Suite 930, Dallas, TX 75235 214-630-6222

Kenneth L. Walgren · St. Paul Medical Center · 5959 Harry Hines Boulevard, Suite 402, Dallas, TX 75235 · 214-630-7866

Frederick D. Winter, Jr. · Baylor University Medical Center · 3434 Swiss Avenue, Suite 410, Dallas, TX 75204 · 214-828-5010

Kathleen Rae Zeller · Parkland Memorial Hospital · Dallas Diagnostic Association, 7777 Forest Lane, Suite C300, Dallas, TX 75230 · 214-991-6000

El Paso

Luis G. Guerra · Providence Memorial Hospital, Columbia Medical Center-West, Columbia Medical Center-East, Sierra Medical Center · 1501 North Mesa, Third Floor, El Paso, TX 79902 · 915-532-1587

Fort Worth

Teresa W. Boydston · Harris Methodist-Fort Worth · Medical Clinic of North Texas, 1651 West Rosedale Street, Suite 200, Fort Worth, TX 76104 · 817-334-1400

Charles Anthony Carlton · Texas Health Care, 1650 West Magnolia Street, Fort Worth, TX 76104-4009 · 817-926-2561

James Steven Childers · Harris Methodist-Fort Worth · Fort Worth Clinic, 1221 West Lancaster Avenue, Fort Worth, TX 76102-4511 · 817-336-7191

N. Alan Davenport · Texas Health Care, 1650 West Magnolia Street, Fort Worth, TX 76104-4009 · 817-926-2571

James E. Davidson · Medical Clinic of North Texas, 1651 West Rosedale Street, Suite 200, Fort Worth, TX 76104 · 817-334-1400

Craig Lee Dearden · 1000 Ninth Avenue, Suite C, Fort Worth, TX 76104-3906 817-332-3039

Stephen Eppstein · Medical Clinic of North Texas, 1651 West Rosedale Street, Suite 200, Fort Worth, TX 76104 · 817-334-1400

Curtis R. Evans · Texas Health Care, 6100 Harris Parkway, Suite 355, Fort Worth, TX 76132 · 817-346-5488

Edward R. Nelson, Jr. · Medical Clinic of North Texas, 1651 West Rosedale Street, Suite 200, Fort Worth, TX 76104 · 817-334-1400

James Fulton Parker · Texas Health Care, 6100 Harris Parkway, Suite 355, Fort Worth, TX 76132 · 817-346-5488

Richard E. Penny · Medical Clinic of North Texas, 6100 Harris Parkway, Suite 345, Fort Worth, TX 76132 · 817-346-5960

James C. Readinger · Harris Methodist-Southwest, All Saints Hospital-Cityview Medical Clinic of North Texas, 6100 Harris Parkway, Suite 345, Fort Worth, TX 76132 · 817-346-5960

Brian Culwell Rutledge · 1650 West Magnolia Street, Suite 104, Fort Worth, TX 76104-4009 · 817-926-7991

Robert L. Ward · Medical Clinic of North Texas, 6100 Harris Parkway, Suite 345, Fort Worth, TX 76132 · 817-346-5960

Richard D. Wilson · Medical Clinic of North Texas, 1325 Pennsylvania Avenue, Suite 200, Fort Worth, TX 76104 · 817-878-5200

Galveston

Thomas A. Blackwell · University of Texas Medical Branch, Department of Internal Medicine, 301 University Boulevard, Room 0570, Galveston, TX 77555-0570 · 409-772-2653

Eugene Boisaubin · John Sealy Hospital · University of Texas Medical Branch, Department of Internal Medicine, John Sealy Annex, Room 4.156, 301 University Boulevard, Galveston, TX 77555-0572 · 409-747-1820

Elisha L. Brownfield · (Preventive Medicine, General Internal Medicine, Women's Health) · University of Texas Medical Branch Hospitals · University of Texas Medical Branch, Department of Internal Medicine, John Sealy Annex, Room 4.156, 301 University Boulevard, Galveston, TX 77555-0572 · 409-772-5275

Kirk A. Calhoun · University of Texas Medical Branch, Department of Internal Medicine, 301 University Boulevard, Galveston, TX 77555-0569 · 409-772-1145

Benjamin Clyburn · University of Texas Medical Branch, Department of Internal Medicine, 301 University Boulevard, Room 0570, Galveston, TX 77555-0570 · 409-772-2653

Donald J. Di Pette · (Hypertension) · University of Texas Medical Branch Hospitals · University of Texas Medical Branch, 301 University Drive, Route 0566, Galveston, TX 77550 · 409-772-4182

Aaron Fradkin · (Geriatric Medicine) · University of Texas Medical Branch Hospitals · Coastal Medical Associates, 1701 Tremont, Galveston, TX 77550-2532 · 409-765-8180

Karen Hansen · Gulf Coast Medical Group, 1501 Broadway Avenue, Galveston, TX 77550 · 409-764-6332

Nasir Hussain · (General Internal Medicine, Ambulatory Care Education, Medical Management, Managed Care) · John Sealy Hospital, University of Texas Medical Branch Hospitals · University of Texas Medical Branch, Department of Internal Medicine, Division of General Medicine, 301 University Boulevard, Galveston, TX 77555-0566 · 409-772-4183

Michelle Mercatante · (General Internal Medicine, General Geriatric Medicine) John Sealy Hospital, University of Texas Medical Branch Hospitals, St. Mary's Hospital · Family Health Centers, Galveston Internal Medicine Associates, McLarty Clinic, 501 Holiday Drive, Galveston, TX 77555 · 409-765-1488

James S. Newman · Gulf Coast Medical Group, 1501 Broadway Avenue, Galveston, TX 77550 · 409-764-6332

Paul A. Remmers · (Medical Education [Ambulatory], General Addiction Medicine, General Internal Medicine) · University of Texas Medical Branch Hospitals University of Texas Medical Branch, Department of Internal Medicine, 301 University Boulevard, Galveston, TX 77555-0572 · 409-772-5275

Alice J. Speer · University of Texas Medical Branch, Department of Internal Medicine, 301 University Boulevard, Room 0772, Galveston, TX 77555-0772 · 409-772-3115

Houston

Keith Aldinger · (Endocrinology, Diabetes) · St. Joseph Hospital, Park Plaza Hospital, Hermann Hospital · Memorial Sisters of Charity, 1315 Calhoun Street, Suite 1605, Houston, TX 77002 · 713-756-8890

John M. Bergland III · (Bronchial Asthma, Chronic Obstructive Airway Disease, Pulmonary Tumors) · St. Luke's Episcopal Hospital, Methodist Hospital · Medical Clinic of Houston, 1707 Sunset Boulevard, Houston, TX 77005 · 713-526-5511

Richard W. Blakely · Hermann Hospital · Houston Medical Associates, 1200 Binz Street, Suite 1495, Houston, TX 77004 · 713-529-0543

David Braden · Two K Chelsey Road, Houston, TX 77006 · 713-523-3654

Joseph David Bybee · Medical Clinic of Houston, 1707 Sunset Boulevard, Houston, TX 77005-1713 · 713-526-5511

Marie N. Cepero · 6410 Fannin Street, Houston, TX 77030 · 713-790-1010

Laura Ann Colletti · 6410 Fannin Street, Suite 500, Houston, TX 77030 · 713-704-4700

Clifford Clark Dacso · (General Geriatric Medicine, General Infectious Disease) Methodist Hospital, THC Houston, Cypress Fairbanks Medical Center, St. Luke's Episcopal Hospital · Baylor College of Medicine, 6550 Fannin Street, Suite 1100, Houston, TX 77030 · 713-790-3321

John Eichelberger · Medical Clinic of Houston, 1707 Sunset Boulevard, Houston, TX 77005 · 713-526-5511

Mark Farnie · University Texas General Medicine Clinic, 6410 Fannin Street, Suite 500, Houston, TX 77053 · 713-792-5075

Michael J. Feltovich · 6560 Fannin Street, Room 1408, Houston, TX 77030 · 713-790-2651

Michael J. Gordon · (Cardiology) · Park Plaza Hospital · 1200 Binz Street, Suite 290, Houston, TX 77004 · 713-523-4222

James M. Gray · (Hypertension) · 1213 Hermann Drive, Suite 610, Houston, TX 77004 · 713-524-8286

Carlos R. Hamilton, Jr. · Medical Clinic of Houston, 1707 Sunset Boulevard, Houston, TX 77005 · 713-526-5511

J. Bernard Hicks · (Renal Hypertension, Preoperative Consultation) · Methodist Hospital, St. Luke's Episcopal Hospital · Medical Clinic of Houston, 1707 Sunset Boulevard, Houston, TX 77005 · 713-526-5511

Richard A. Jackson · Methodist Hospital · Associates in Medicine, 6560 Fannin Street, Suite 1860, Houston, TX 77030 · 713-797-1087

Philip C. Johnson III · (AIDS, Fungal Infections, Transplantation Infections, General Internal Medicine) · Hermann Hospital, Lyndon B. Johnson General Hospital · University of Texas Medical School at Houston, 6410 Fannin Street, Suite 500, Houston, TX 77030 · 713-704-4700

Robert Johnston · Medical Clinic of Houston, 1707 Sunset Boulevard, Houston, TX 77005 · 713-526-5511

Peter H. Jones · (Lipids) · Methodist Hospital, Department of Medicine, 6565 Fannin Street, Mail Stop A-601, Houston, TX 77030 · 713-790-5800

William A. Lent · Park Plaza Hospital, Methodist Hospital, St. Luke's Episcopal Hospital, Hermann Hospital · Internal Medicine Specialists, 1200 Binz Street, Suite 930, Houston, TX 77004 · 713-526-5606

William Rugeley Livesay · (Cardiovascular Disease, Cerebral Vascular Disease, General Medicine Diagnostic Problems, General Internal Medicine) · St. Luke's Episcopal Hospital · Medical Clinic of Houston, 1707 Sunset Boulevard, Houston, TX 77005-1713 · 713-526-5511

David H. Miller · (General Internal Medicine, General Infectious Disease, Clinical Dermatology, General Neurology) · Methodist Hospital, St. Luke's Episcopal Hospital · 6550 Fannin Street, Suite 2339, Houston, TX 77030 · 713-795-4847

James E. Muntz · (Hemostasis, Thrombosis, Peri-Operative Medical Treatment) Methodist Hospital, St. Luke's Episcopal Hospital, Hermann Hospital, Texas Orthopedic Hospital · Baylor College of Medicine, Smith Tower, Suite 2339, 6550 Fannin Street, Houston, TX 77030 · 713-795-4847

Benjamin F. Orman · Methodist Hospital · Medical Clinic of Houston, 1707 Sunset Boulevard, Houston, TX 77005-1713 · 713-526-5511

Edwin M. Ory · Medical Clinic of Houston, 1707 Sunset Boulevard, Houston, TX 77005 · 713-526-5511

James L. Pool · (Hypertension) · Methodist Hospital · Methodist Hospital, 6536 Fannin Street, Mail Stop F-504, Houston, TX 77030 · 713-790-3261

John A. Posey, Jr. · (Preventive Medicine, Hypertension, Diabetes Mellitus) · St. Luke's Episcopal Hospital, Methodist Hospital · 6624 Fannin Street, Suite 2360, Houston, TX 77030-2335 · 713-795-5702

H. Irving Schweppe, Jr. · St. Luke's Episcopal Hospital, Department of Internal Medicine, 6720 Bertner Avenue, Mail Code 1-192, Houston, TX 77030 · 713-791-4050

Nicholas P. Sollenne III · Methodist Hospital · Medical Clinic of Houston, 1707 Sunset Boulevard, Houston, TX 77005 · 713-526-5511

H. Keith Stonecipher · 1213 Hermann Drive, Suite 870, Houston, TX 77004 · 713-528-6394

John Robert Strawn · St. Luke's Episcopal Hospital, Methodist Hospital · Medical Clinic of Houston, 1707 Sunset Boulevard, Houston, TX 77005-1713 · 713-526-5511

Susan M. Vogel · Hermann Hospital · 1315 Calhoun Street, Suite 1605, Houston, TX 77002 · 713-704-0450

Martin Ray White · (Hematology) · Medical Clinic of Houston, 1707 Sunset Boulevard, Houston, TX 77005-1713 · 713-526-5511

Irving

Richard Coleman Johnston · St. Paul Medical Center (Dallas) · 5100 North O'Connor Road, Suite 200, Irving, TX 75039 · 214-556-1616

Lackland Air Force Base

Richard Edward Hannigan · Wilford Hall Medical Center · Wilford Hall Medical Center, 2200 Bergquist Drive, Suite One, Lackland Air Force Base, TX 78236-5300 · 210-670-5333

Lubbock

Vernon C. Farthing, Jr. · University Medical Center · 3502 Ninth Street, Suite 170, Lubbock, TX 79415 · 806-762-8461

Philip J. Galasso · University Medical Center · Texas Tech University Health Sciences Center, Department of Internal Medicine, 3601 Fourth Street, Lubbock, TX 79430 · 806-743-3155

Wayne Karaki · Texas Tech University Health Sciences Center, Department of Internal Medicine, 3601 Fourth Street, Lubbock, TX 79430 · 806-743-3155

D. Dale Little · Lubbock Methodist Hospital · Lubbock Diagnostic Clinic, 3506 Twenty-First Street, Suite 202, Lubbock, TX 79410 · 806-788-8045

Brenda S. Morrow · Lubbock Methodist Hospital, St. Mary of the Plains Hospital Lubbock Diagnostic Clinic, 3506 Twenty-First Street, Suite 203, Lubbock, TX 79410 · 806-788-8060

James R. Partin · Lubbock Methodist Hospital · Lubbock Diagnostic Clinic, 3506 Twenty-First Street, Suite 203, Lubbock, TX 79410 · 806-788-8045

N. Scott Robins · St. Mary of the Plains Hospital, Lubbock Methodist Hospital Medical Arts Clinic, 4102 Twenty-Fourth Street, Suite 100, Lubbock, TX 79410 806-788-1111

W. Brad Snodgrass · Lubbock Diagnostic Clinic, 3506 Twenty-First Street, Suite 302, Lubbock, TX 79410 · 806-788-8100

Midland

William M. Hibbitts · 2201 West Tennessee Avenue, Midland, TX 79701 · 915-683-5631

San Antonio

John C. Anes · 1303 McCullough Avenue, Suite 560, San Antonio, TX 78212 · 210-223-9617

Charles George Briseno · Nix Health Care System · San Antonio Medical Associates, 703 Nix Professional Building, San Antonio, TX 78205-2522 · 210-224-4811

Charles Richard Clemons · Diagnostic Clinic of San Antonio, 4647 Medical Drive, P.O. Box 29249, San Antonio, TX 78284-3100 · 210-615-1300

Emanuel P. De Noia · Southwest Texas Methodist Hospital, St. Luke's Baptist Hospital, San Antonio Community Hospital · 5282 Medical Drive, Suite 614, San Antonio, TX 78229 · 210-614-0062

Andrew Kemper Diehl · (Gallbladder Diseases) · University Hospital-South Texas Medical Center · University of Texas Health Science Center at San Antonio, Department of Medicine, Division of General Medicine, 7703 Floyd Curl Drive, San Antonio, TX 78284-7879 · 210-270-3941

Richard Burks Ferguson · 8530 Village Drive, San Antonio, TX 78217 · 210-657-4241

George Almond Ford III · Diagnostic Clinic of San Antonio, 5282 Medical Drive, Suite 316, San Antonio, TX 78229 · 210-616-3769

Robert B. Goff, Jr. · 7210 Louis Pasteur Drive, Suite 100, San Antonio, TX 78229 210-614-4000

James Ernest Goral · Diagnostic Clinic of San Antonio, 4647 Medical Drive, San Antonio, TX 78229 · 210-615-1300

Mark Henderson · University Hospital-South Texas Medical Center · University of Texas Health Science Center at San Antonio, Department of Medicine, Division of General Medicine, 7703 Floyd Curl Drive, San Antonio, TX 78284-7879 · 210-567-4808

Timothy Jones · University of Texas Health Science Center at San Antonio, University Clinic, 7703 Floyd Curl Drive, San Antonio, TX 78284-7870 · 210-567-4808

Daniel Juarez · 1303 McCullough Avenue, Suite 560, San Antonio, TX 78212 · 210-223-9617

Bradley Basch Kayser · (General Geriatric Medicine) · 7210 Louis Pasteur Drive, Suite 100, San Antonio, TX 78229 · 210-614-4000

John Conrad Klahn · (General Cardiovascular Disease, General Geriatric Medicine) · Northeast Baptist Hospital, Northeast Methodist Hospital · 8601 Village Drive, Suite 100, San Antonio, TX 78217 · 210-654-6352

John Sidney Matlock · Diagnostic Clinic of San Antonio, 4647 Medical Drive, San Antonio, TX 78229 · 210-615-1300

Richard S. Reyna · Baptist Medical Center · Health Texas Medical Group, 215 East Quincy Street, Suite 500, San Antonio, TX 78215 · 210-223-1600

Rowland Sanchez Reyna · (General Geriatric Medicine) · Santa Rosa Health Care, Baptist Medical Center · Health Texas Medical Group, 215 East Quincy Street, Suite 500, San Antonio, TX 78215 · 210-223-1600

Edward R. Sargent · Diagnostic Clinic of San Antonio, 4647 Medical Drive, San Antonio, TX 78229 · 210-615-1300

Paul Heermans Smith, Jr. · Northeast Baptist Hospital · 5307 Broadway, Suite 207, San Antonio, TX 78209 · 210-824-3291

Mark Lee Thornton · 1303 McCullough Avenue, Suite 560, San Antonio, TX 78212 · 210-223-9617

Tony Milton Toledo · Metropolitan Hospital · Internal Medicine Associates, 1303 McCullough Avenue, Suite 600, San Antonio, TX 78212 · 210-225-2551

Randall Mark Vanover · Northeast Methodist Hospital, Northeast Baptist Hospital · 12709 Toepperwein Road, Suite 201, San Antonio, TX 78233 · 210-650-9669

Clyde W. Wagner, Jr. · (General Internal Medicine, General Cardiovascular Disease, General Endocrinology & Metabolism) · Nix Health Care System, Metropolitan Hospital, Baptist Medical Center · Internal Medicine Associates, 1303 McCullough Avenue, Suite 600, San Antonio, TX 78212 · 210-225-2551

Gordon D. Willey · 4499 Medical Drive, Suite 105, San Antonio, TX 78229 · 210-616-0851

Jerald Winakur · (General Geriatric Medicine) · 7210 Louis Pasteur Drive, Suite 100, San Antonio, TX 78229 · 210-614-4000

Temple

John R. Bowling · Scott & White Memorial Hospital · Scott & White Memorial Hospital, Department of Internal Medicine, 2401 South 31st Street, Temple, TX 76508-0001 · 817-724-2974

Phillip T. Cain · Scott & White Memorial Hospital, Department of Internal Medicine, 2401 South 31st Street, Temple, TX 76508-0001 · 817-724-4309

Richard H. Jesse · Scott & White Memorial Hospital · Scott & White Memorial Hospital, Department of Internal Medicine, 2401 South 31st Street, Temple, TX 76508-0001 · 817-724-2111

Kathy B. Kimmey · (Breast Cancer Prevention, Long-Term Follow-up of Breast Cancer Survivors, Women's Health) · Scott & White Memorial Hospital & Clinic Scott & White Memorial Hospital, Department of Internal Medicine, 2401 South 31st Street, Temple, TX 76508-0001 · 817-724-2973

Bruce D. Koehler · Scott & White Memorial Hospital, Department of Internal Medicine, 2401 South 31st Street, Temple, TX 76508-0001 · 817-724-2973

Texas City

Pamela Clanton · Family Health Care Center, 9300 E. F. Emmett Lowry Expressway, Suite 138, Texas City, TX 77591 · 409-986-9592

William F. Harper · Family Health Care Center, 9300 E. F. Emmett Lowry Expressway, Suite 138, Texas City, TX 77591 · 409-986-9592

Tyler

Ben F. Bridges · 520 Douglas Boulevard, Tyler, TX 75702 · 903-510-8758

David R. Shafer · (Diabetes, General Geriatric Medicine) · University of Texas Health Center-Tyler · University of Texas Health Center-Tyler, US Highway 271 and State Highway 155, P.O. Box 2003, Tyler, TX 75710-2003 · 903-877-7911

Waco

Gary K. Barbin · Waco Internal Medicine, 2800 Lyle Avenue, Waco, TX 76708 817-756-7091

J. Bond Browder · Providence Health Center · 405 Londonderry Drive, Suite 110, Waco, TX 76712 · 817-751-4949

Murray M. Colgin · Providence Health Center · 405 Londonderry Drive, Suite 201, Waco, TX 76712 · 817-751-4949

James L. Copeland, Jr. · Waco Internal Medicine, 2800 Lyle Avenue, Waco, TX 76708 · 817-756-7091

Roger W. Cowart · Providence Medical Clinic, 301 Richland West Circle, Waco, TX 76712 · 817-751-4955

Cathy A. Hurley · Providence Medical Clinic, 301 Richland West Circle, Waco, TX 76712 · 817-776-8333

Roxann M. Samples · Providence Health Center · Providence Medical Clinic, 301 Richland West Circle, Waco, TX 76712 · 817-776-8333

Darrell R. Slette · (General Gastroenterology) · Hillcrest Baptist Medical Center, Providence Health Center · 405 Londonderry Drive, Suite 201, Waco, TX 76712 817-751-4949

Arthur W. Sudan · Waco Internal Medicine, 2800 Lyle Avenue, Waco, TX 76708 817-756-7091

MEDICAL ONCOLOGY & HEMATOLOGY

Abilene

Victor J. Hirsch, Jr. · General Medical Oncology & Hematology · Texas Oncology, 1100 North 19th Street, Suite 1A, Abilene, TX 79601 · 915-672-4368

Amarillo

Sardar Karim Nawaz · General Medical Oncology & Hematology · 1901 Medical Park Drive, Suite 1049, Amarillo, TX 79106 · 806-355-9248

Mailan Patel · General Medical Oncology & Hematology · Don & Sybil Harrington Cancer Center, 1500 Wallace Boulevard, Amarillo, TX 79106 · 806-359-4673

Phillip O'Keefe Periman · (Multiple Myeloma, Prostate Cancer, Malignant Melanoma) · Don & Sybil Harrington Cancer Center · Don & Sybil Harrington Cancer Center, 1500 Wallace Boulevard, Amarillo, TX 79106-1745 · 806-359-4673

Narayana G. Pillai · (Lymphomas, Breast Cancer, Colon & Rectal Cancer) · High Plains Baptist Hospital, St. Anthony's Hospital, Amarillo Hospital District-Northwest Texas Hospital · 1901 Medi-Park, Suite 1010, Amarillo, TX 79106 · 806-358-8011

Brian T. Pruitt · General Medical Oncology & Hematology · Texas Tech University Health Sciences Center, Department of Medicine, 1400 Wallace Boulevard, Amarillo, TX 79106-1745 · 806-354-5486

Christopher O. Ruud · General Medical Oncology & Hematology (Lung Cancer, Gastrointestinal Cancer, Clotting Disorders) · High Plains Baptist Hospital, Amarillo Hospital District-Northwest Texas Hospital, St. Anthony's Hospital · Don & Sybil Harrington Cancer Center, 1500 Wallace Boulevard, Amarillo, TX 79106-1745 · 806-359-4673

Arlington

George Blumenschein · Breast Cancer · Arlington Cancer Center, Arlington Memorial Hospital, Columbia Medical Center of Arlington · 906 West Randol Mill Road, Arlington, TX 76012-6500 · 817-261-4906

Alfred DiStefano · General Medical Oncology & Hematology (Breast Cancer, Lung Cancer, Gastrointestinal Cancer) · Arlington Memorial Hospital, Columbia Medical Center of Arlington · Arlington Cancer Center, 906 West Randol Mill Road, Arlington, TX 76012 · 817-261-4906

Austin

John J. Costanzi · General Medical Oncology & Hematology (Solid Tumors, Lymphomas, Leukemia) · Seton Medical Center, Round Rock Hospital (Round Rock), Austin Diagnostic Medical Center, St. David's Healthcare Center, Brackenridge Hospital · Lone Star Oncology Consultants, 11044 Research Boulevard, Suite B-400, Austin, TX 78759 · 512-343-2103

Demetrius F. Loukas, Jr. · General Medical Oncology & Hematology (Breast Cancer, Lung Cancer, Lymphomas, Leukemia) · Seton Medical Center, St. David's Healthcare Center, Seton Northwest Hospital · Southwest Regional Cancer Center, 711 West 38th Street, Suite B-1, Austin, TX 78705 · 512-451-7387

John Franklin Sandbach · General Medical Oncology & Hematology (Breast Cancer) · Texas Oncology, 1600 West 38th Street, Suite 120, Austin, TX 78731 · 512-302-1771

Joseph D. Youman · General Medical Oncology & Hematology · Southwest Regional Cancer Center · Southwest Regional Cancer Center, 711 West 38th Street, Suite B-1, Austin, TX 78705 · 512-451-7387

Beaumont

Robert Rankin Birdwell · General Medical Oncology & Hematology · Mamie McFaddin Ward Cancer Center · 690 North 14th Street, Third Floor, Beaumont, TX 77702-1449 · 409-899-7180

Scott A. McKenney · General Medical Oncology & Hematology · Mamie McFaddin Ward Cancer Center, St. Elizabeth Hospital, Beaumont Regional Medical Center · Mamie McFaddin Ward Cancer Center, 690 North 14th Street, Third Floor, Beaumont, TX 77702-1449 · 409-899-7180

Jay R. Schachner · General Medical Oncology & Hematology (Leukemia, Lymphoma) · Mamie McFaddin Ward Cancer Center, St. Elizabeth Hospital · Mamie McFaddin Ward Cancer Center, 690 North 14th Street, Third Floor, Beaumont, TX 77702-1449 · 409-899-7180

Chris Trout · General Medical Oncology & Hematology · Mamie McFaddin Ward Cancer Center · Mamie McFaddin Ward Cancer Center, 690 North 14th Street, Third Floor, Beaumont, TX 77702-1449 · 409-899-7180

Corpus Christi

Kirby G. Barker, Jr. · General Medical Oncology & Hematology · Corpus Christi Cancer Center, 1625 Rodd Field Road, Corpus Christi, TX 78412 · 512-993-3456

Samuel Murphy · General Medical Oncology & Hematology · Corpus Christi Cancer Center, 1625 Rodd Field Road, Corpus Christi, TX 78412 · 512-993-3456

Albert J. Wood · General Medical Oncology & Hematology · Bay Area Medical Center, Spohn Hospital, Memorial Medical Center, Doctors Regional Medical Center · Corpus Christi Cancer Center, 1625 Rodd Field Road, Corpus Christi, TX 78412 · 512-993-3456

Dallas

Robert H. Collins, Jr. · Bone Marrow Transplantation (Immunotherapy, Cancer Biotherapy, Leukemia) · Baylor University Medical Center · Collins Building, Fifth Floor, 3535 Worth Street, Dallas, TX 75246 · 214-820-2619

Barry Cooper · General Medical Oncology & Hematology (Disorders of Bleeding, Thrombosis, Leukemia, Lymphomas) · Baylor University Medical Center · Baylor University Medical Center, Collins Building, Suite 200, 3535 Worth Street, Dallas, TX 75246 · 214-820-8347

Eugene Phillip Frenkel · General Medical Oncology & Hematology (Malignant Lymphomas, Breast Cancer, Prostate Cancer) · Zale Lipshy University Hospital, Parkland Memorial Hospital · University of Texas-Southwestern Medical Center at Dallas, 5323 Harry Hines Boulevard, Dallas, TX 75235 · 214-648-2647

Stephen E. Jones · Breast Cancer (Oncology only) · Charles A. Sammons Cancer Center · Charles A. Sammons Cancer Center, 3535 Worth Street, Suite 300, Dallas, TX 75246-2039 · 214-820-8309

Robert G. Mennel · General Medical Oncology & Hematology · Texas Oncology, 3535 Worth Street, Dallas, TX 75246 · 214-824-4901

John Dorrance Minna · Lung Cancer (Family Cancer Genetics) · Nancy B. & Jake L. Hamon Center for Therapeutic Oncology Research, Zale Lipshy University Hospital · University of Texas-Southwestern Medical Center at Dallas, Nancy B. & Jake L. Hamon Center for Therapeutic Oncology Research, 5323 Harry Hines Boulevard, Dallas, TX 75235-8593 · 214-648-4900

Douglas Wayne Orr · General Medical Oncology & Hematology · Baylor University Medical Center · Texas Oncology, 3535 Worth Street, Suite 230, Dallas, TX 75246 · 214-820-8672

Steven Paulson · Gastrointestinal Cancer · Baylor University Medical Center · Texas Oncology, 3535 Worth Street, Dallas, TX 75246 · 214-820-8672

Marvin Jules Stone · Myeloma (Lymphomas, Immunology) · Baylor University Medical Center · Baylor University Medical Center, 3500 Gaston Avenue, Dallas, TX 75246 · 214-820-3445

James F. Strauss · General Medical Oncology & Hematology (Disorders of Bleeding, Thrombosis) · Presbyterian Hospital of Dallas · 8230 Walnut Hill Lane, Suite 320, Dallas, TX 75231 · 214-739-4175

El Paso

Fred N. Ekery · General Medical Oncology & Hematology · Texas Oncology, 2800 North Stanton Street, El Paso, TX 79902-2509 · 915-545-2506

Raul M. Portillo · General Medical Oncology & Hematology · Providence Memorial Hospital · Texas Oncology, 2800 North Stanton Street, El Paso, TX 79902-2509 · 915-545-2506

Fort Worth

John L. E. Nugent · General Medical Oncology & Hematology · Hematology-Oncology Associates, 601 West Terrell Avenue, Fort Worth, TX 76104 · 817-338-4333

Michael Barry Ross · General Medical Oncology & Hematology · Oncology-Hematology Consultants, 1325 Pennsylvania Avenue, Suite 100, Fort Worth, TX 76104 · 817-336-5522

Galveston

Suzanne McClure · General Medical Oncology & Hematology (AIDS-Related Malignancies, Gastrointestinal Cancer) · University of Texas Medical Branch Hospitals, Columbia Mainland Center Hospital (Texas City) · University of Texas Medical Branch, Department of Hematology/Oncology, 301 University Boulevard, Room 4.164, Galveston, TX 77555-0565 · 409-772-1164

Houston

James Lewis Abbruzzese · Gastrointestinal Cancer (Pancreatic Cancer) · University of Texas-M. D. Anderson Cancer Center · University of Texas-M. D. Anderson Cancer Center, 1515 Holcombe Boulevard, Houston, TX 77030-4009 · 713-792-7770

Jaffer A. Ajani · Gastrointestinal Cancer · University of Texas-M. D. Anderson Cancer Center · University of Texas-M. D. Anderson Cancer Center, 1515 Holcombe Boulevard, Box 78, Houston, TX 77030 · 713-792-2828

Raymond Alexanian · Myeloma · University of Texas-M. D. Anderson Cancer Center · University of Texas-M. D. Anderson Cancer Center, 1515 Holcombe Boulevard, Box One, Houston, TX 77030 · 713-792-2850

Robert C. Bast, Jr. · Immunotherapy, Cancer Biotherapy, Gynecologic Cancer, Breast Cancer (Immunodiagnosis, Ovarian Cancer) · University of Texas-M. D. Anderson Cancer Center · University of Texas-M. D. Anderson Cancer Center, 1515 Holcombe Boulevard, Box 92, Houston, TX 77030 · 713-792-7770

Robert S. Benjamin · General Medical Oncology & Hematology (Melanomas, Sarcomas) · University of Texas-M. D. Anderson Cancer Center · University of Texas-M. D. Anderson Cancer Center, 1515 Holcombe Boulevard, Box 77, Houston, TX 77030 · 713-792-3626

Aman U. Buzdar · Breast Cancer · University of Texas-M. D. Anderson Cancer Center · University of Texas-M. D. Anderson Cancer Center, 1515 Holcombe Boulevard, Box 56, Houston, TX 77030 · 713-792-2817

Fernando Cabanillas · Lymphomas · University of Texas-M. D. Anderson Cancer Center · University of Texas-M. D. Anderson Cancer Center, 1515 Holcombe Boulevard, Box 68, Houston, TX 77030 · 713-792-2860

Luis T. Campos · General Medical Oncology & Hematology · 920 Frostwood Drive, Suite 780, Houston, TX 77024 · 713-827-9525

Richard Eugene Champlin · Leukemia, Bone Marrow Transplantation, Lymphomas, Breast Cancer (Leukemia) · University of Texas-M. D. Anderson Cancer Center · University of Texas-M. D. Anderson Cancer Center, 1515 Holcombe Boulevard, Box 65, Houston, TX 77030 · 713-792-3618

Elihu Harris Estey · Leukemia (Acute Leukemia) · University of Texas-M. D. Anderson Cancer Center · University of Texas-M. D. Anderson Cancer Center, Department of Hematology, Leukemia Section, 1515 Holcombe Boulevard, Box 61, Houston, TX 77030 · 713-792-7544

Emil J. Freireich · Leukemia (Therapy of Hematological Malignancies, Supportive Therapy for Bone Marrow Failure, General Medical Oncology & Hematology) University of Texas-M. D. Anderson Cancer Center · University of Texas-M. D. Anderson Cancer Center, 1515 Holcombe Boulevard, Box 55, Houston, TX 77030 713-792-2660

Bonnie S. Glisson · Lung Cancer (Head & Neck Cancer) · University of Texas-M. D. Anderson Cancer Center · University of Texas-M. D. Anderson Cancer Center, 1515 Holcombe Boulevard, Box 80, Houston, TX 77030 · 713-792-6363

Frankie N. Holmes · Breast Cancer · University of Texas-M. D. Anderson Cancer Center · University of Texas-M. D. Anderson Cancer Center, 1515 Holcombe Boulevard, Box 56, Houston, TX 77030 · 713-792-2817

Waun Ki Hong · Head & Neck Cancer, Lung Cancer (Cancer Chemoprevention, Retinoid Research) · University of Texas-M. D. Anderson Cancer Center · University of Texas-M. D. Anderson Cancer Center, 1515 Holcombe Boulevard, Box 80, Houston, TX 77030 · 713-792-6363

Gabriel N. Hortobagyi · Breast Cancer · University of Texas-M. D. Anderson Cancer Center, 1515 Holcombe Boulevard, Box 56, Houston, TX 77030 · 713-792-2817

Hagop M. Kantarjian · Leukemia (Chronic Leukemia) · University of Texas-M. D. Anderson Cancer Center, 1515 Holcombe Boulevard, Box 61, Houston, TX 77030 · 713-792-7026

John J. Kavanagh, Jr. · Gynecologic Cancer (Cervical Cancer, Ovarian Cancer) · University of Texas-M. D. Anderson Cancer Center · University of Texas-M. D. Anderson Cancer Center, 1515 Holcombe Boulevard, Box 39, Houston, TX 77030 713-792-7959

Michael J. Keating · Leukemia (Chronic Lymphocytic Leukemia) · University of Texas-M. D. Anderson Cancer Center, 1515 Holcombe Boulevard, Box 38, Houston, TX 77030 · 713-792-2933

Razelle Kurzrock · Immunotherapy, Cancer Biotherapy (Leukemia) · University of Texas-M. D. Anderson Cancer Center · University of Texas-M. D. Anderson Cancer Center, Department of Bioimmunotherapy, 1515 Holcombe Boulevard, Box 302, Houston, TX 77030-4009 · 713-794-1226

Jin Soo Lee · Lung Cancer (Thoracic Oncology, Malignant Thymoma, Chemoprevention) · University of Texas-M. D. Anderson Cancer Center · University of Texas-M. D. Anderson Cancer Center, 1515 Holcombe Boulevard, Box 80, Houston, TX 77030 · 713-792-6363

Sewa Singh Legha · General Medical Oncology & Hematology (Melanomas, Sarcomas, Breast Cancer) · University of Texas-M. D. Anderson Cancer Center · University of Texas-M. D. Anderson Cancer Center, 1515 Holcombe Boulevard, Box 77, Houston, TX 77030 · 713-792-2921

Scott M. Lippman · General Medical Oncology & Hematology · University of Texas-M. D. Anderson Cancer Center · University of Texas-M. D. Anderson Cancer Center, 1515 Holcombe Boulevard, Box 80, Houston, TX 77030 · 713-792-6363

Christopher J. Logothetis · Genito-Urinary Cancer · University of Texas-M. D. Anderson Cancer Center · University of Texas-M. D. Anderson Cancer Center, 1515 Holcombe Boulevard, Box 13, Houston, TX 77030 · 713-792-2830

Janet E. Macheledt · General Medical Oncology & Hematology · Memorial Hospital-Memorial City, Department of Medical Oncology & Hematology, 920 Frostwood Drive, Suite 640, Houston, TX 77024 · 713-827-8525

Peter McLaughlin · Lymphomas (Immunotherapy, Cancer Biotherapy) · University of Texas-M. D. Anderson Cancer Center · University of Texas-M. D. Anderson Cancer Center, 1515 Holcombe Boulevard, Box 68, Houston, TX 77030 713-792-2860

Joel Moake · Disorders of Bleeding, Thrombosis · Methodist Hospital · Methodist Hospital, 6565 Fannin Street, Mail Stop 902, Houston, TX 77030 · 713-790-2156

Susan O'Brien · Leukemia (Chronic Lymphocytic Leukemia) · University of Texas-M. D. Anderson Cancer Center · University of Texas-M. D. Anderson Cancer Center, Department of Hematology, 1515 Holcombe Boulevard, Box 61, Houston, TX 77030 · 713-792-7543

Richard Pazdur · Clinical Pharmacology (New Drug Development, Pancreatic Cancer, Colon & Rectal Cancer, Gastrointestinal Cancer) · University of Texas-M. D. Anderson Cancer Center · University of Texas-M. D. Anderson Cancer Center, 1515 Holcombe Boulevard, Box 92, Houston, TX 77030-4095 · 713-792-3634

Martin Newman Raber · Clinical Pharmacology (Clinical Trials, Unknown Primary Tumors) · University of Texas-M. D. Anderson Cancer Center · University of Texas-M. D. Anderson Cancer Center, 1515 Holcombe Boulevard, Box 318, Houston, TX 77030 · 713-792-7765

Moshe Talpaz · Immunotherapy, Cancer Biotherapy · University of Texas-M. D. Anderson Cancer Center · University of Texas-M. D. Anderson Cancer Center, 1515 Holcombe Boulevard, Box 302, Houston, TX 77030-4009 · 713-792-3522

W. K. Alfred Yung · Neuro-Oncology (Brain Tumors) · University of Texas-M. D. Anderson Cancer Center · University of Texas-M. D. Anderson Cancer Center, 1515 Holcombe Boulevard, Box 100, Houston, TX 77030 · 713-794-1285

Lubbock

Everardo Cobos · Bone Marrow Transplantation (Disorders of Bleeding, Thrombosis) · University Medical Center · Texas Tech University Health Sciences Center, Department of Internal Medicine, Division of Hematology & Medical Oncology, 3601 Fourth Street, Lubbock, TX 79430 · 806-743-3155

Rodolpho E. Martinez · General Medical Oncology & Hematology · 3702 Twentieth Street, Suite B, Lubbock, TX 79410 · 806-793-6654

H. Grant Taylor · General Medical Oncology & Hematology · 3506 Twenty-First Street, Suite 303, Lubbock, TX 79410 · 806-788-8105

McAllen

Joseph P. Litam · General Medical Oncology & Hematology · McAllen Medical Center Cancer Institute, 1800 South Fifth Street, Suite B, McAllen, TX 78503 · 210-687-1115

Nacogdoches

Gerard J. Ventura · General Medical Oncology & Hematology · University of Texas-M. D. Anderson Cancer Center (Houston) · 4848 Northeast Stallings Drive, Suite 207, Nacogdoches, TX 75961 · 409-569-0050

San Angelo

Fazlur Rahman · General Medical Oncology & Hematology (Breast Cancer, Lymphomas) · Columbia Medical Center of San Angelo · West Texas Medical Associates, 3555 Knickerbocker Road, San Angelo, TX 76904 · 915-949-9555

San Antonio

David H. Boldt · General Medical Oncology & Hematology (Hematology, Leukemia, Lymphoma, Bone Marrow Transplantation) · University Hospital-South Texas Medical Center, Cancer Therapy & Research Center · University of Texas Health Science Center at San Antonio, Department of Medicine, Division of Medical Hematology, 7703 Floyd Curl Drive, San Antonio, TX 78284-7884 · 210-567-4848

Howard A. Burris III · Clinical Pharmacology (Investigational Trials on New Drugs) · Brooke Army Medical Center (Fort Sam Houston), University Hospital-South Texas Medical Center · Grossman Cancer Center, 7979 Wurzbach Boulevard, San Antonio, TX 78229 · 210-616-5961

Natalie Scott Callander · Bone Marrow Transplantation (Coagulation Disorders, Disorders of Bleeding, Thrombosis) · University Hospital-South Texas Medical Center, Methodist Healthcare System · University of Texas Health Science Center at San Antonio, Department of Medicine, Division of Medical Hematology, 7703 Floyd Curl Drive, San Antonio, TX 78284-7884 · 210-567-4848

Charles A. Coltman, Jr. · Lymphomas (Hodgkin's Disease, Non-Hodgkin's Lymphoma) · The Cancer Therapy and Research Center · The Cancer Therapy & Research Center, 8122 Datapoint Drive, Suite 600, San Antonio, TX 78229 · 210-616-5580

Richard M. Elledge · Breast Cancer · University Hospital-South Texas Medical Center, St. Luke's Baptist Hospital, Audie L. Murphy Memorial Veterans Hospital · University of Texas Health Science Center at San Antonio, Department of Medicine, Division of Medical Oncology, 7703 Floyd Curl Drive, San Antonio, TX 78284-7884 · 210-567-4777

Cesar Ovidio Freytes · Bone Marrow Transplantation (Myeloma, Lymphomas) · Audie L. Murphy Memorial Veterans Hospital, University Hospital-South Texas Medical Center · University of Texas Health Science Center at San Antonio, Department of Medicine, Division of Hematology, 7703 Floyd Curl Drive, San Antonio, TX 78284-7884 · 210-617-5268

Steven Paul Kalter · General Medical Oncology & Hematology · Southwest Texas Methodist Hospital, St. Luke's Baptist Hospital, Santa Rosa Northwest Hospital · South Texas Oncology & Hematology Associates, 4450 Medical Drive, San Antonio, TX 78229 · 210-614-3307

Charles Frederick Le Maistre · Bone Marrow Transplantation · Southwest Texas Methodist Hospital · South Texas Cancer Institute, 7700 Floyd Curl Drive, San Antonio, TX 78229 · 210-593-3801

Jose Antonio Lopez · (General Medical Oncology, Breast Cancer, Lung Cancer) Northeast Baptist Hospital, Hill Country Memorial Hospital (Fredericksburg), Sid Peterson Memorial Hospital (Kerrville), Baptist Medical Center · 215 East Quincy Street, Suite 310, San Antonio, TX 78215 · 210-224-6531

Roger M. Lyons · Disorders of Bleeding, Thrombosis (AIDS, Cancer & Infections, General Medical Oncology & Hematology, Immunotherapy, Cancer Biotherapy, Leukemia, Lymphomas, Myeloma, Hematopathology) · Southwest Texas Methodist Hospital, San Antonio Community Hospital, Santa Rosa Northwest Hospital, St. Luke's Baptist Hospital · Hematology & Oncology Associates of South Texas, Methodist Plaza, Suite 233, 4499 Medical Drive, San Antonio, TX 78229 · 210-614-0463

C. Kent Osborne · Breast Cancer · University Hospital-South Texas Medical Center, The Cancer Therapy & Research Center · University of Texas Health Science Center at San Antonio, Department of Medicine, Division of Medical Oncology, 7703 Floyd Curl Drive, Room 5.210S, San Antonio, TX 78284-7884 · 210-567-4777

Victorio Rodriguez · General Medical Oncology & Hematology (Oncology) · 7390 Barlite Boulevard, Suite 306, San Antonio, TX 78224 · 210-923-7129

Mace Lawrence Rothenberg · Gynecologic Cancer (Gastrointestinal Cancer, Investigative New Drugs) · University Hospital-South Texas Medical Center, Audie L. Murphy Memorial Veterans Hospital, St. Luke's Baptist Hospital · University of Texas Health Science Center at San Antonio, Department of Medicine, Divi-

sion of Medical Oncology, 7703 Floyd Curl Drive, San Antonio, TX 78284-7884
210-567-4777

Lon Shelby Smith · General Medical Oncology & Hematology (Oncology) ·
South Texas Oncology, 7979 Wurzbach Road, Suite 230, San Antonio, TX 78229
210-614-3307

Daniel D. Von Hoff · Clinical Pharmacology, General Medical Oncology & He-
matology (New Drug Development) · The Cancer Therapy and Research Center
The Cancer Therapy & Research Center, 8122 Datapoint Drive, Suite 700, San
Antonio, TX 78229 · 210-616-5864

Geoffrey Roger Weiss · Gastrointestinal Cancer (Medical Oncology only, Genito-
Urinary Cancer, Investigational New Drugs, Biotherapy) · University Hospital-
South Texas Medical Center, Audie L. Murphy Memorial Veterans Hospital, St.
Luke's Baptist Hospital · University of Texas Health Science Center at San An-
tonio, Department of Medicine, Division of Medical Oncology, 7703 Floyd Curl
Drive, San Antonio, TX 78284-7884 · 210-617-5186

Temple

Arthur A. Trowbridge · Disorders of Bleeding, Thrombosis · Scott & White
Memorial Hospital & Clinic · Scott & White Memorial Hospital, 2401 South 31st
Street, Clinic 1A, Temple, TX 76508-0001 · 817-724-5918

Tyler

Gary E. Gross · General Medical Oncology & Hematology · East Texas Medical
Center, East Texas Medical Center-Athens (Athens), Trinity Mother Frances
Health Care Center · Tyler Hematology-Oncology, 619 South Fleishel Avenue,
Suite 309, Tyler, TX 75701 · 903-592-6152

Gary T. Kimmel · General Medical Oncology & Hematology · Tyler Cancer
Center, 910 East Houston Street, Suite 100, Tyler, TX 75702 · 903-592-6114

Arielle Shebay Lee · General Medical Oncology & Hematology · East Texas
Medical Center, Trinity Mother Frances Health Care Center, Nan Travis Memo-
rial Hospital (Jacksonville) · Tyler Hematology-Oncology, 619 South Fleishel
Avenue, Suite 309, Tyler, TX 75701 · 903-592-6152

Waco

Robert Anderson · General Medical Oncology & Hematology · Waco Medical Group, 2911 Herring Avenue, Suite 209, Waco, TX 76708-3240 · 817-755-4460

Lawrence Carroll Canning · General Medical Oncology & Hematology · Waco Medical Group, 2911 Herring Avenue, Waco, TX 76708-3240 · 817-755-4460

Webster

Roger William Rodgers · General Medical Oncology & Hematology · Clear Lake Regional Medical Center, University of Texas-M. D. Anderson Cancer Center (Houston), St. John Hospital (Nassau Bay) · 450 Blossom, Suite E, Webster, TX 77598 · 713-332-7608

Wichita Falls

Brian K. Ulrich · General Medical Oncology & Hematology · 501 Midwestern Parkway East, Wichita Falls, TX 76302 · 817-766-8875

NEPHROLOGY

Abilene

James D. Webster · General Nephrology · Abilene Area Dialysis Center, 1802 Pine Street, Abilene, TX 79601-2430 · 915-672-3243

Amarillo

Miguel A. Rios · General Nephrology · Amarillo Dialysis Center, 5920 Amarillo Boulevard, West, Amarillo, TX 79106-4148 · 806-353-9181

Carlos H. Santillan · General Nephrology · St. Anthony's Hospital · Amarillo Dialysis Center, 5920 Amarillo Boulevard, West, Amarillo, TX 79106 · 806-353-9181

Austin

Gerald A. Beathard · General Nephrology · Austin Diagnostic Medical Center, 12221 MoPac Expressway North, P.O. Box 85075, Austin, TX 78708-5075 · 512-901-4010

James Dawson Lindley · General Nephrology · Brackenridge Hospital, Seton Medical Center · Austin Diagnostic Medical Center, 12221 MoPac Expressway North, P.O. Box 85075, Austin, TX 78708-5075 · 512-901-4010

Peter L. Miller · General Nephrology (Dialysis, Glomerular Diseases, Kidney Transplantation) · Austin Diagnostic Medical Center, Brackenridge Hospital, Seton Medical Center, St. David's Healthcare Center · Austin Diagnostic Clinic, Department of Nephrology, 12221 MoPac Expressway North, Austin, TX 78758 512-901-4010

Jack W. Moncrief · Dialysis (Peritoneal Dialysis, Telemedicine, Peritoneal & Vascular Access, General Nephrology, Kidney Transplantation) · Austin Diagnostic Clinic, Brackenridge Hospital · Austin Diagnostic Medical Center, 12221 MoPac Expressway North, P.O. Box 85075, Austin, TX 78708-5075 · 512-901-4010

Paul Charles Nader · General Nephrology · Austin Diagnostic Medical Center, 12221 MoPac Expressway North, P.O. Box 85075, Austin, TX 78708-5075 · 512-901-4010

Byron Russell Welch · Kidney Transplantation (Vascular Access for Dialysis, General Nephrology) · Austin Diagnostic Medical Center, Brackenridge Hospital, St. David's Healthcare Center, South Austin Medical Center · Austin Diagnostic Medical Center, 12221 MoPac Expressway North, P.O. Box 85075, Austin, TX 78708-5075 · 512-901-4010

Beaumont

Raymond Derderian · General Nephrology · St. Elizabeth Hospital · Beaumont Nephrology, 3282 College Street, Beaumont, TX 77701-4610 · 409-832-4309

Jose Lozano-Mendez · General Nephrology · St. Elizabeth Hospital · Beaumont Nephrology, 3282 College Street, Beaumont, TX 77701-4610 · 409-832-4309

Corpus Christi

Janis L. Birchall · General Nephrology · Bay Area Kidney Disease Physicians, 1102 Santa Fe Street, Corpus Christi, TX 78404-3155 · 512-882-9278

Jack L. Cortese · General Nephrology · 1521 South Staples Street, Suite 401, Corpus Christi, TX 78404 · 512-887-8451

Clyde E. Rutherford III · General Nephrology · Bay Area Kidney Disease Physicians, 1102 Santa Fe Street, Corpus Christi, TX 78404 · 512-882-9278

William L. Shaffer · General Nephrology · Kidney Specialists of South Texas, 1521 South Staples Street, Suite 401, Corpus Christi, TX 78404 · 512-887-8451

Dallas

Robert J. Alpern · General Nephrology (Fluid & Electrolyte Abnormalities, Kidney Disease) · Zale Lipshy University Hospital, Parkland Memorial Hospital University of Texas-Southwestern Medical Center at Dallas, 5323 Harry Hines Boulevard, Dallas, TX 75235-8856 · 214-648-2754

Karl Robert Brinker · Kidney Transplantation · Methodist Medical Center · Dallas Nephrology Associates, 1150 North Bishop, Dallas, TX 75208 · 214-942-7900

Michael Emmett · General Nephrology (Renal Physiology, Acid-Base Disorders, Metabolic Bone Disease) · Baylor University Medical Center · Dallas Nephrology Associates, 3601 Swiss Avenue, Dallas, TX 75204 · 214-821-3939

Thomas A. Gonwa · Kidney Transplantation (Transplant Medicine, Liver Transplantation, Critical Care Medicine) · Baylor University Medical Center, Baylor Transplant Services · Dallas Nephrology Associates, 3601 Swiss Avenue, Dallas, TX 75204 · 214-827-7717

Judson Mark Hunt · General Nephrology (Transplantation Medicine) · Presbyterian Hospital of Dallas, Medical City Dallas Hospital · Dallas Nephrology Associates, 8230 Walnut Hill Lane, Suite 508, Dallas, TX 75231 · 214-373-6176

Robert Kunau · General Nephrology · Medical City Dallas Hospital · Dallas Nephrology Associates, 7777 Forest Lane, Suite B-245, Dallas, TX 75230 · 214-661-8464

Martin Louis Mai · General Nephrology (Kidney Transplantation, Critical Care Medicine) · Baylor University Medical Center · Baylor University Medical Center, 3600 Gaston Avenue, Dallas, TX 75246 · 214-827-7717

Larry B. Melton · Kidney Transplantation (General Nephrology) · Baylor University Medical Center · Dallas Nephrology Associates, 3601 Swiss Avenue, Dallas, TX 75204 · 214-827-7717

Steven Eric Rinner · General Nephrology · Presbyterian Hospital of Dallas · Dallas Nephrology, 8230 Walnut Hill Lane, Suite 508, Dallas, TX 75231 · 214-373-6176

Ruben L. Velez · General Nephrology · Methodist Medical Center · Dallas Nephrology Associates, 1150 North Bishop Court, Dallas, TX 75208 · 214-942-7900

Pedro J. Vergne-Marini · Kidney Transplantation (Pancreas Transplantation, Heart Transplantation, General Nephrology, Dialysis, Glomerular Disease) · Methodist Medical Center · Dallas Nephrology Associates, 6010 Forest Park Road, Suite 100, Dallas, TX 75235 · 214-358-2300

El Paso

Melvin Fox · (Peritoneal Dialysis, Diabetes, Hypertension) · Providence Memorial Hospital, Sierra Medical Center · 720 Arizona Avenue, El Paso, TX 79902-4402 · 915-544-2898

Fort Worth

James Patrick Brennan · General Nephrology · Harris Methodist-Fort Worth · Dialysis Associates, 950 West Magnolia Avenue, Fort Worth, TX 76104 · 817-336-5060

N. Kermit Olson · General Nephrology · John Peter Smith Hospital · Tarrant County Nephrology Center, 1408 St. Louis Street, Fort Worth, TX 76104 · 817-921-5191

Galveston

Richard W. Carson · General Nephrology (Glomerular Diseases, Kidney Transplantation) · University of Texas Medical Branch Hospitals · University of Texas Medical Branch, Division of Nephrology, John Sealy Annex, Room 4.200, 301 University Boulevard, Galveston, TX 77555-0562 · 409-772-8616

August Ray Remmers, Jr. · General Nephrology · University of Texas Medical Branch, 4.200 JSA Building, 301 University Boulevard, Galveston, TX 77555-0562 · 409-772-1811

Robert L. Safirstein · General Nephrology · University of Texas Medical Branch, Division of Nephrology, 301 University Boulevard, Galveston, TX 77555-0562 · 409-772-1811

Houston

Horacio Jose Adrogue · General Nephrology · VA Medical Center · Baylor College of Medicine, One Baylor Plaza, Houston, TX 77030 · 713-794-7244

Camilo Gustavo Barcenas · General Nephrology · St. Luke's Episcopal Hospital · 9197 Winkler Drive, Building D, Houston, TX 77017 · 713-947-9507

Charles Kenneth Crumb · General Nephrology · 7777 Southwest Freeway, Suite 736, Houston, TX 77074 · 713-270-4545

Thomas Durward DuBose, Jr. · (Acute and Chronic Renal Failure, Kidney Transplantation, Complicated Hypertension) · Hermann Hospital, University of Texas-M. D. Anderson Cancer Center, Lyndon B. Johnson General Hospital · University of Texas Medical School at Houston, 6431 Fannin Street, Room MSB 4.136, Houston, TX 77030 · 713-792-5425

Garabed Eknoyan · General Nephrology (Dialysis, Acute Renal Failure, Glomerulonephritis) · Ben Taub General Hospital, Methodist Hospital · Baylor College of Medicine, One Baylor Plaza, Houston, TX 77030 · 713-798-4748

Juan J. Olivero · General Nephrology (Dialysis, Glomerular Diseases, Kidney Disease) · Methodist Hospital · 6560 Fannin Street, Suite 1426, Houston, TX 77030 · 713-790-4615

Wadi N. Suki · General Nephrology, Hypertension, Kidney Transplantation, Dialysis (Hemodialysis, Peritoneal Dialysis) · Methodist Hospital · Baylor College of Medicine, 6550 Fannin Street, Suite 1273, Houston, TX 77030 · 713-790-3275

Lubbock

Neil A. Kurtzman · Kidney Disease (Electrolyte & Acid-Base Disorders) · University Medical Center · Texas Tech University Health Sciences Center, Department of Internal Medicine, 3601 Fourth Street, Lubbock, TX 79430 · 806-743-3155

William D. Myers · General Nephrology · Lubbock Methodist Hospital · South Plains Kidney Disease Center, 1607 West Loop 289, Lubbock, TX 79416 · 806-799-2991

Sandra Sabatini · General Nephrology (Dialysis, Kidney Transplantation) · University Medical Center · Texas Tech University Health Sciences Center, Division of Nephrology, 3601 Fourth Street, Lubbock, TX 79430 · 806-743-2520

Donald E. Wesson · (Renal Disease, Hypertension, Acid-Base Disorders) · University Medical Center · Texas Tech University Health Sciences Center, Division of Nephrology, 3601 Fourth Street, Lubbock, TX 79430 · 806-743-3155

Clarence J. Wheeler III · General Nephrology · Lubbock Methodist Hospital · Kidney & Blood Pressure Clinic, 4110 Twenty-Second Place, Suite 200, Lubbock, TX 79410 · 806-793-8447

Midland

Larry D. Oliver · (General Internal Medicine, Hypertension, Critical Care Medicine) · Memorial Hospital & Medical Center, Medical Center Hospital (Odessa) Midland-Odessa Medical Group—Nephrology, 10313 West County Road 117, P.O. Box 60250, Midland, TX 79711-0250 · 915-561-9328

San Antonio

Hanna Emile Abboud · General Nephrology · University Hospital-South Texas Medical Center · University of Texas Health Science Center at San Antonio, Department of Medicine, Division of Nephrology, 7703 Floyd Curl Drive, San Antonio, TX 78284-7882 · 210-567-4700

Gordon L. Bilbrey · Kidney Transplantation · San Antonio Community Hospital Renal Associates, 7434 Louis Pasteur Drive, Suite 120, San Antonio, TX 78229 · 210-614-1515

Carl Joseph Blond · General Nephrology · San Antonio Kidney Disease Center, 1222 McCullough Avenue, San Antonio, TX 78212 · 210-228-0743

Cleve Brantley Collins · General Nephrology · Renal Associates, 215 East Quincy Street, Suite 610, San Antonio, TX 78215 · 210-226-2001

Marvin Forland · General Nephrology (Glomerular Diseases, Kidney Disease, Urinary Tract Infection) · University Hospital-South Texas Medical Center, Audie L. Murphy Memorial Veterans Hospital · University of Texas Health Science

Center at San Antonio, Department of Medicine, Division of Nephrology, 7703 Floyd Curl Drive, San Antonio, TX 78284-7882 · 210-567-4431

Terrence Alan Fried · General Nephrology (Acute Kidney Failure, Dialysis, Glomerulonephritis) · Baptist Medical Center, Metropolitan Hospital, Santa Rosa Health Care · San Antonio Kidney Disease Center, 1222 McCullough Avenue, San Antonio, TX 78217 · 210-228-0743

Ronald Wayne Hamner · General Nephrology · Renal Associates, 215 East Quincy Street, Suite 610, San Antonio, TX 78215 · 210-226-2001

Denise Hart · General Nephrology · San Antonio Kidney Disease Center, 1222 McCullough Avenue, San Antonio, TX 78212 · 210-228-0743

Claudia E. Hura · General Nephrology (Glomerular Diseases, Kidney Transplantation) · Southwest Texas Methodist Hospital, San Antonio Community Hospital, University Hospital-South Texas Medical Center · San Antonio Kidney Disease Center, 7540 Louis Pasteur Drive, Suite 100, San Antonio, TX 78229 · 210-692-7228

Balakuntalam S. Kasinath · Glomerular Diseases (Diabetic Kidney Disease, Lupus Nephritis, General Nephrology) · University Hospital-South Texas Medical Center, Audie L. Murphy Memorial Veterans Hospital · University of Texas Health Science Center at San Antonio, Department of Medicine, Division of Nephrology, 7703 Floyd Curl Drive, San Antonio, TX 78284-7882 · 210-567-4707

Paraic Joseph Mulgrew · Kidney Transplantation · Metropolitan Hospital · Renal Associates, 7434 Louis Pasteur Drive, Suite 120, San Antonio, TX 78229 · 210-614-1515

David Mark Player · Kidney Transplantation (Body Composition Management, Immunologic Disease, General Nephrology, Dialysis) · San Antonio Community Hospital, Southwest Texas Methodist Hospital, St. Luke's Baptist Hospital · Health by Design, 9150 Huebner Road, Suite 160, San Antonio, TX 78240 · 210-558-3467

Henry John Reineck · General Nephrology · Southwest Texas Methodist Hospital · San Antonio Kidney Disease Center, 7540 Louis Pasteur Drive, Suite 100, San Antonio, TX 78229 · 210-692-7228

Steven Gerald Rosenblatt · General Nephrology · San Antonio Kidney Disease Center · San Antonio Kidney Disease Center, 7540 Louis Pasteur Drive, Suite 100, San Antonio, TX 78229 · 210-692-7228

Peter Smolens · General Nephrology · University Hospital-South Texas Medical Center, Baptist Medical Center · Northeast Kidney Disease Center, 2391 Northeast Loop 410, Suite 406, San Antonio, TX 78217 · 210-654-7326

Robert E. Stevens · General Nephrology (General Internal Medicine) · Nix Health Care System · San Antonio Medical Associates, 703 Nix Professional Building, San Antonio, TX 78205-2522 · 210-224-4811

Temple

Allan E. Nickel · General Nephrology (Dialysis, Glomerular Diseases) · Scott & White Memorial Hospital · Scott & White Memorial Hospital, Department of Nephrology, 2401 South 31st Street, Temple, TX 76508-0001 · 817-724-3666

Texarkana

C. Jackson Smith · General Nephrology (General Internal Medicine) · Collom & Carney Clinic, 4800 Texas Boulevard, Texarkana, TX 75503 · 903-792-7151

Tyler

James Russell Cotton, Jr. · General Nephrology · Tyler Nephrology Associates, 807 East First Street, Tyler, TX 75701 · 903-595-5486

Thomas Andrew Lowery · General Nephrology · Tyler Nephrology Associates, 807 East First Street, Tyler, TX 75701 · 903-595-5486

Waco

Richard Lee Gibney · General Nephrology · Kidney Disease Center, 3420 Pine Avenue, Waco, TX 76708-3130 · 817-752-5503

Woody Jene Reese · General Nephrology · Kidney Disease Center, 3420 Pine Avenue, Waco, TX 76708-3130 · 817-752-5503

NEUROLOGICAL SURGERY

Amarillo

Jeffrey D. Cone · General Neurological Surgery · Amarillo Hospital District-Northwest Texas Hospital · 320 South Polk Street, Suite 400, Amarillo, TX 79101 806-373-3177

Wayne S. Paullus, Jr. · (Cerebral Surgery, Pain Management) · High Plains Baptist Hospital, Amarillo Hospital District-Northwest Texas Hospital, Columbia Panhandle Surgical Hospital, St. Anthony's Hospital · Southwest Neuroscience Institute, 320 South Polk Street, Suite 500, Amarillo, TX 7910 · 806-373-8928

Austin

Michael Dorsen · Pediatric Neurological Surgery (General Neurological Surgery, Spinal Surgery) · Seton Medical Center · 2905 San Gabriel Street, Suite 310, Austin, TX 78705 · 512-474-8765

Gordon White · General Neurological Surgery · 4200 Marathon Boulevard, Suite 340, Austin, TX 78756 · 512-467-8596

Beaumont

Mark J. Kubala · General Neurological Surgery (Spinal Surgery) · St. Elizabeth Hospital · Southeast Texas Neurosurgery Associates, 2965 Harrison Street, Suite 111, Beaumont, TX 77702-1148 · 409-898-7800

Carl E. Shrontz · General Neurological Surgery · Southeast Texas Neurosurgery Associates, 2965 Harrison Street, Suite 111, Beaumont, TX 77702-1148 · 409-898-7800

Dallas

Derek A. Bruce · Pediatric Neurological Surgery (Trauma, Head Injury, Brain Tumors, Seizures) · Medical City Dallas Hospital · Medical City Dallas Hospital, Building C, Suite 737, 7777 Forest Lane, Dallas, TX 75230-2594 · 214-788-6640

Cole A. Giller · General Neurological Surgery (Surgery for Parkinson's Disease and Movement Disorders, Surgery for Epilepsy and Pain, Transcranial Doppler Ultrasound) · University of Texas-Southwestern Medical Center at Dallas, 5323 Harry Hines Boulevard, Dallas, TX 75235-8855 · 214-648-3373

Richard Henry Jackson · General Neurological Surgery · St. Paul Medical Center Dallas Neurosurgical Association, 8230 Walnut Hill Lane, Suite 610, Dallas, TX 75231 · 214-369-7596

Bruce E. Mickey · Epilepsy (Tumor Surgery) · Zale Lipshy University Hospital, Parkland Memorial Hospital · University of Texas-Southwestern Medical Center at Dallas, 5323 Harry Hines Boulevard, Dallas, TX 75235-8855 · 214-648-2369

Howard W. Morgan, Jr. · General Neurological Surgery (Spinal Surgery) · Zale Lipshy University Hospital, Parkland Memorial Hospital · University of Texas-Southwestern Medical Center at Dallas, 5323 Harry Hines Boulevard, Room CS5104C, Dallas, TX 75235-8855 · 214-648-8530

Duke S. Samson · Vascular Neurological Surgery (Cerebrovascular Surgery) · Zale Lipshy University Hospital, Parkland Memorial Hospital, VA Medical Center, Children's Medical Center of Dallas · University of Texas-Southwestern Medical Center at Dallas, 5323 Harry Hines Boulevard, Dallas, TX 75235-8855 · 214-648-3529

Bennie B. Scott · General Neurological Surgery · Baylor University Medical Center · Baylor University Medical Center, 3600 Gaston Avenue, Suite 605, Dallas, TX 75246 · 214-826-7060

Kenneth N. Shapiro · Pediatric Neurological Surgery (Tumor Surgery, Vascular Neurological Surgery, Craniofacial Surgery) · Children's Medical Center of Dallas, Medical City Dallas Hospital · Children's Medical Center of Dallas, Department of Neurological Surgery, 1935 Motor Street, Dallas, TX 75235 · 214-640-6660

Frederick H. Sklar · Pediatric Neurological Surgery (Pediatric Brain and Spinal Tumors, Congenital Malformations of the Brain and Spine, Pediatric Vascular Neurological Surgery) · Children's Medical Center of Dallas, Medical City Dallas Hospital · Children's Medical Center of Dallas, Center for Pediatric Neurosurgery, 1935 Motor Street, Dallas, TX 75235 · 214-640-6660

Dale Swift · Pediatric Neurological Surgery (Spinal Surgery, Stereotactic Radiosurgery, Trauma, Pediatric Tumor Surgery) · Children's Medical Center of Dallas · Children's Medical Center of Dallas, 1935 Motor Street, Dallas, TX 75235 214-640-6660

Richard L. Weiner · General Neurological Surgery (Stereotactic Radiosurgery, Spinal Surgery) · Presbyterian Hospital of Dallas, Doctors Hospital of Dallas, Presbyterian Hospital of Plano (Plano), Lake Pointe Medical Center (Rowlett), Baylor Medical Center-Garland (Garland) · Southwest Neurosurgical Associates, 8220 Walnut Hill Lane, Suite 308, Dallas, TX 75231-4413 · 214-363-8524

El Paso

Charles Shih-Cheng Chang · General Neurological Surgery · MRS Neurosurgery Group, 1600 Medical Center Drive, Suite 400, El Paso, TX 79902-5008 · 915-544-0544

Mitch Smeagel · General Neurological Surgery · MRS Neurosurgery Group, 1600 Medical Center Drive, Suite 400, El Paso, TX 79902-5008 · 915-544-0544

Fort Worth

Philip C. Bechtel · General Neurological Surgery · Harris Methodist-Fort Worth Southwest Neurological Surgery, 800 Eighth Avenue, Suite 220, Fort Worth, TX 76104-2710 · 817-336-1300

George F. Cravens · General Neurological Surgery · Center for Neurological Disorders, 1319 Summit Avenue, Suite 200, Fort Worth, TX 76102-4423 · 817-336-0551

Jack E. McCallum · General Neurological Surgery (Pediatric Neurological Surgery) · Harris Methodist-Fort Worth, Cook Children's Medical Center · Southwest Neurological Surgery, 800 Eighth Avenue, Suite 220, Fort Worth, TX 76104-2710 817-336-1300

Galveston

Jefferson W. Chen · General Neurological Surgery (Vascular Neurological Surgery, Tumor Surgery, Trauma) · University of Texas Medical Branch Hospitals · University of Texas Medical Branch, Department of Surgery, Division of Neurosurgery, 301 University Boulevard, Galveston, TX 77555-0517 · 409-772-6321

William W. Maggio · General Neurological Surgery · University of Texas Medical Branch, Department of Surgery, Division of Neurosurgery, 301 University Boulevard, Galveston, TX 77555-0517 · 409-772-8972

Haring J. Nauta · General Neurological Surgery · University of Texas Medical Branch, Department of Surgery, Division of Neurosurgery, 301 University Boulevard, Galveston, TX 77555-0517 · 409-772-1500

Daryl E. Warder · Pediatric Neurological Surgery (General Neurological Surgery) University of Texas Medical Branch Hospitals · University of Texas Medical Branch, Department of Surgery, Division of Neurosurgery, 301 University Boulevard, Galveston, TX 77555-0517 · 409-747-0738

Harlingen

F. Michael Fennegan · General Neurological Surgery (Spinal Surgery, Vascular & Tumor Brain Surgery) · Valley Baptist Medical Center · Neurosurgical Associates, 1725 Ed Carey Drive, Harlingen, TX 78550 · 210-423-0020

Houston

Lee V. Ansell · Spinal Surgery · Hermann Hospital, Memorial Hospital-Southwest Texas Center for Neurosurgery, 7777 Southwest Freeway, Suite 610, Houston, TX 77074 · 713-988-5677

David Stuart Baskin · Spinal Surgery (Pituitary Surgery, Intracranial Vascular Surgery, Spinal Microsurgery) · Methodist Hospital, St. Luke's Episcopal Hospital, Ben Taub General Hospital, VA Medical Center · Baylor College of Medicine, Department of Neurological Surgery, 6560 Fannin Street, Suite 944, Houston, TX 77030-2706 · 713-798-4696

Guy L. Clifton · General Neurological Surgery (Epilepsy Surgery) · Hermann Hospital · University of Texas Medical School at Houston, 6431 Fannin Street, Room 7.148, Houston, TX 77030 · 713-704-6445

Robert C. Dauser · Pediatric Neurological Surgery · Texas Children's Hospital Texas Children's Hospital, 6621 Fannin Street, Mail Code 3-3435, Houston, TX 77030-2399 · 713-770-3950

Franco DeMonte · Tumor Surgery (Skull-Base Surgery) · University of Texas-M. D. Anderson Cancer Center · University of Texas-M. D. Anderson Cancer Center, 1515 Holcombe Boulevard, Box 64, Houston, TX 77030 · 713-792-2400

Bruce L. Ehni · General Neurological Surgery · Methodist Hospital · Neurosurgical Group of Houston, 6560 Fannin Street, Suite 1250, Houston, TX 77030 · 713-797-0703

Robert G. Grossman · Epilepsy Surgery (Parkinson's Disease Surgery, Brain Tumors) · Methodist Hospital · Baylor College of Medicine, Department of Neurological Surgery, 6560 Fannin Street, Suite 944, Houston, TX 77030-2706 · 713-798-4696

Richard L. Harper · General Neurological Surgery (Spinal Surgery, Brain Tumors, Aneurysms, Hemifacial Spasms) · Methodist Hospital · 6560 Fannin Street, Suite 1250, Houston, TX 77030 · 713-797-0703

Samuel J. Hassenbusch · General Neurological Surgery (Pain) · University of Texas-M. D. Anderson Cancer Center · University of Texas-M. D. Anderson Cancer Center, Department of Neurosurgery, 1515 Holcombe Boulevard, Box 64, Houston, TX 77030 · 713-792-2400

John P. Laurent · Pediatric Neurological Surgery · Texas Children's Hospital · Texas Children's Hospital, Clinical Care Center, Suite 950, 6621 Fannin Street, Mail Code 3-3435, Houston, TX 77030-2303 · 713-770-3950

James E. Rose · General Neurological Surgery · Methodist Hospital · Baylor College of Medicine, Department of Neurological Surgery, 6560 Fannin Street, Suite 944, Houston, TX 77030-2706 · 713-798-4696

Raymond Sawaya · Tumor Surgery · University of Texas-M. D. Anderson Cancer Center · University of Texas-M. D. Anderson Cancer Center, 1515 Holcombe Boulevard, Box 64, Houston, TX 77030 · 713-792-2400

Lubbock

Richard E. George · Pediatric Neurological Surgery (Tumor Surgery) · Lubbock Methodist Hospital · Methodist Neurosurgical Associates, 3506 Twenty-First Street, Suite 400, Lubbock, TX 79410 · 806-792-7246

Ross R. Sedler · General Neurological Surgery · St. Mary of the Plains Hospital, Lubbock Methodist Hospital · Neurosurgery Associates, 3502 Ninth Street, Suite 240, Lubbock, TX 79415 · 806-792-4719

Midland

George Y. Lohmann, Jr. · (Spinal Surgery, Vascular Surgery, Pediatrics) · Memorial Hospital & Medical Center, Westwood Medical Center · 2205 West Tennessee Avenue, Midland, TX 79701 · 915-570-8880

William L. McGavran III · General Neurological Surgery (Tumors, Spinal Surgery, Trauma) · Memorial Hospital & Medical Center, Westwood Medical Center 2000 West Ohio Street, Suite H, Midland, TX 79701 · 915-682-4307

San Antonio

Sarah Gaskill · Pediatric Neurological Surgery · Women's & Children's Hospital, Santa Rosa Children's Hospital · 4499 Medical Drive, Suite 397, San Antonio, TX 78229 · 210-615-1218

Thomas Allen Kingman · General Neurological Surgery · Southwest Texas Methodist Hospital · 4410 Medical Drive, Suite 600, San Antonio, TX 78229 · 210-615-5200

Arthur E. Marlin · Pediatric Neurological Surgery · Southwest Texas Methodist Hospital, Santa Rosa Children's Hospital, Women's & Children's Hospital · 4499 Medical Drive, Suite 397, San Antonio, TX 78229 · 210-615-1218

Warren F. Neeley · General Neurological Surgery · Southwest Texas Methodist Hospital · 4410 Medical Drive, Suite 600, San Antonio, TX 78229 · 210-615-5200

Robert A. Partain III · General Neurological Surgery (Spinal Surgery, Cranial Nerve Surgery) · Southwest Texas Methodist Hospital · Neurosurgical Associates of San Antonio, Texas Neurosciences Institute Building, Suite 610, 4410 Medical Drive, San Antonio, TX 78229-3798 · 210-614-2453

Jim Lewis Story · Vascular Neurological Surgery (Cerebrovascular Surgery, Epilepsy & Movement Disorder Surgery, General Neurosurgery) · Santa Rosa Health Care, University Hospital-South Texas Medical Center · Santa Rosa Professional Pavilion, Suite 1240, 315 North San Saba, San Antonio, TX 78207 · 210-567-5625; 210-354-0877

Karl W. Swann · General Neurological Surgery · Southwest Texas Methodist Hospital, St. Luke's Baptist Hospital, San Antonio Community Hospital, Northeast Baptist Hospital, Santa Rosa Northwest Hospital · Neurosurgical Associates of San Antonio, Texas Neurosciences Institute Building, Suite 610, 4410 Medical Drive, San Antonio, TX 78229-3798 · 210-614-2453

Arnold Vardaman · General Neurological Surgery · 4410 Medical Drive, Suite 600, San Antonio, TX 78229 · 210-615-5200

Texarkana

George L. Bohmfalk · General Neurological Surgery (Trigeminal Neuralgia, Meningioma Surgery) · Wadley Regional Medical Center, St. Michael Health Care Center · 1001 Main Street, Texarkana, TX 75501 · 903-794-4196

Tyler

Ronald J. Donalson · General Neurological Surgery · East Texas Medical Center, Trinity Mother Frances Health Care Center · 700 Olympic Circle, Tyler, TX 75701 · 903-595-2441

Waco

Arthur F. Evans · General Neurological Surgery · Hillcrest Baptist Medical Center · 3115 Pine Avenue, Suite 803, Waco, TX 76708 · 817-753-2444

Robert H. Saxton · General Neurological Surgery · Hillcrest Baptist Medical Center · 3115 Pine Avenue, Suite 803, Waco, TX 76708 · 817-753-2444

Wichita Falls

John D. Reeves · General Neurological Surgery (Peripheral Nerve Surgery, Spinal Surgery) · Bethania Regional Health Care Center, Wichita General Hospital · 1004 Brook Street, Wichita Falls, TX 76301 · 817-723-0815

NEUROLOGY

Abilene

Paul C. Harris · General Neurology · Hendrick Medical Center, Abilene Regional Medical Center · Abilene Diagnostic, 1150 North 18th Street, Suite 200, Abilene, TX 79601 · 915-670-6488

Amarillo

Haydee Rohaidy · General Neurology · 1500 Coulter Drive, Suite Six, Amarillo, TX 79106 · 806-352-2742

Arlington

Kevin E. Conner · General Neurology (Neuromuscular Disease, Headache) · Columbia Medical Center of Arlington, Arlington Memorial Hospital · 3150 Matlock Road, Suite 405, Arlington, TX 76015 · 817-784-0316

Ganana Tesfa · General Neurology (Headache, Epilepsy) · Arlington Memorial Hospital, Columbia Medical Center of Arlington · Neurology Associates of Arlington, 1001 North Waldrop Street, Suite 816, Arlington, TX 76012 · 817-795-5566

Austin

Thomas A. Hill · General Neurology · Austin Diagnostic Medical Center, 12221 MoPac Expressway North, P.O. Box 85075, Austin, TX 78708-5075 · 512-459-1111

Harold Skaggs, Jr. · (Headaches, Electromyography—Evaluation of Neuropathy, Radiculopathy) · Seton Medical Center · 3705 Medical Parkway, Suite 540, Austin, TX 78705 · 512-458-6656

Jerry Ray Tindel · General Neurology (Neuromuscular Disease) · Austin Diagnostic Medical Center, 12221 MoPac Expressway North, P.O. Box 85075, Austin, TX 78708-5075 · 512-459-1111

Beaumont

Clifford J. Fraim · General Neurology · Neurological Associates of Southeast Texas, 3140 Medical Center Drive, Beaumont, TX 77701-4642 · 409-833-2212

Todd A. Maraist · General Neurology · 3560 Delaware Street, Suite 1201, Beaumont, TX 77706 · 409-899-9100

Clyde C. Meyers, Jr. · General Neurology · Neurological Associates of Southeast Texas, 3140 Medical Center Drive, Beaumont, TX 77701-4642 · 409-833-2212

Corpus Christi

Juan E. Bahamon-Dussan · General Neurology · Corpus Christi Neurology, 3301 South Alameda Street, Suite 501, Corpus Christi, TX 78411 · 512-853-0867

Ernesto H. Guido · General Neurology · Neurological Clinic, 3006 South Alameda Street, Corpus Christi, TX 78404 · 512-883-1731

Alexander R. Lim · General Neurology (Epilepsy, Movement Disorders) · Spohn Hospital, Spohn Hospital South, Memorial Medical Center, Bay Area Medical Center, Doctors Regional Medical Center · Neurological Clinic, 3006 South Alameda Street, Corpus Christi, TX 78404-2601 · 512-883-1731

Blake Bernard O'Lavin · General Neurology · Spohn Hospital · Neurological Clinic, 3006 South Alameda Street, Corpus Christi, TX 78404-2601 · 512-883-1731

Dallas

Richard J. Barohn · Neuromuscular Disease (Electromyography) · Zale Lipshy University Hospital, Parkland Memorial Hospital · University of Texas-Southwestern Medical Center at Dallas, 5323 Harry Hines Boulevard, Dallas, TX 75235-8897 · 214-648-6419

Wilson Werber Bryan · Neuromuscular Disease (Electromyography) · Zale Lipshy University Hospital, Parkland Memorial Hospital · University of Texas-Southwestern Medical Center at Dallas, 5323 Harry Hines Boulevard, Dallas, TX 75235-8897 · 214-648-6419

Richard B. Dewey, Jr. · Movement Disorders (Parkinson's Disease) · Zale Lipshy University Hospital, Parkland Memorial Hospital · University of Texas-Southwestern Medical Center at Dallas, Department of Neurology, 5323 Harry Hines Boulevard, Dallas, TX 75235-8897 · 214-648-7964

Ralph G. Greenlee, Jr. · Strokes (Electromyography) · Zale Lipshy University Hospital, Parkland Memorial Hospital · University of Texas-Southwestern Medical Center at Dallas, Department of Neurology, 5323 Harry Hines Boulevard, Dallas, TX 75235-7200 · 214-648-9574

Richard Charles Hinton · General Neurology (Stroke) · Presbyterian Hospital of Dallas · 8210 Walnut Hill Lane, Suite 915, Dallas, TX 75231-4407 · 214-750-9977

Robert F. LeRoy · Epilepsy · Medical City Dallas Hospital · The Neurological Clinic of Texas, Building B, Suite 410, 7777 Forest Lane, Dallas, TX 75230 · 214-661-7684

Alan William Martin · General Neurology · Baylor University Medical Center · Dallas Neurological Clinic, 712 North Washington Avenue, Suite 100, Dallas, TX 75246 · 214-827-3610

Allan Leslie Naarden · Movement Disorders (Tourette Syndrome, Alzheimer's & Related Disorders, Muscle Disease, Electromyography, General Neurology) · Medical City Dallas Hospital · Medical City Dallas Hospital, Neurological Clinic of Texas, Building B, Suite 410, 7777 Forest Lane, Dallas, TX 75230 · 214-661-7684

Richard Ralph North · Epilepsy · Medical City Dallas Hospital · Medical City Dallas Hospital, Neurological Clinic of Texas, Building B, Suite 410, 7777 Forest Lane, Dallas, TX 75230 · 214-661-7684

Roger N. Rosenberg · Neurogenetics (Degenerative Diseases, Alzheimer's Disease, General Neurology, Neuropsychiatry) · Parkland Memorial Hospital, Zale

Lipshy University Hospital · University of Texas-Southwestern Medical Center at Dallas, 5323 Harry Hines Boulevard, Dallas, TX 75235-9036 · 214-648-3239

S. Clifford Schold, Jr. · Neuro-Oncology (Brain Tumors) · Parkland Memorial Hospital, Zale Lipshy University Hospital · University of Texas-Southwestern Medical Center at Dallas, Department of Neurology, 5323 Harry Hines Boulevard, Room F2.318, Dallas, TX 75235-9036 · 214-648-2564

R. Malcolm Stewart · General Neurology (Movement Disorders, Degenerative Diseases) · Presbyterian Hospital of Dallas · Neurology Specialists of Dallas, 9400 North Central Expressway, Suite 1100, Dallas, TX 75231 · 214-265-5600

Kathy A. Toler · General Neurology · 10 Medical Parkway, Suite 103, Dallas, TX 75234 · 214-620-9048

Hal Unwin · (Critical Care Medicine, Stroke) · Zale Lipshy University Hospital, Parkland Memorial Hospital · 5323 Harry Hines Boulevard, Dallas, TX 75235-8897 · 214-648-3256

Paul C. Van Ness · Epilepsy (Clinical Neurophysiology, Epilepsy Surgery) · University of Texas-Southwestern Medical Center at Dallas, 5323 Harry Hines Boulevard, Dallas, TX 75235-9036 · 214-648-9356

El Paso

Albert C. Cuetter · General Neurology (Epilepsy, Electrodiagnostic Studies—Electromyogram, Electroencephalogram) · Thomason Hospital · Texas Tech University Health Sciences Center, Department of Neurology, 4800 Alberta Avenue, El Paso, TX 79905 · 915-545-6703

Martin Heitzman · General Neurology · 1250 East Cliff Drive, Suite 5C, El Paso, TX 79902-4847 · 915-533-5925

Fort Worth

Stephen P. Busby · General Neurology · 750 Eighth Avenue, Suite 430, Fort Worth, TX 76104-2500 · 817-870-2711

Lincoln F. Chin · General Neurology · 1350 South Main Street, Suite 4500, Fort Worth, TX 76104 · 817-336-1181

William R. Gulledge · General Neurology · 1307 Eighth Avenue, Suite 408, Fort Worth, TX 76104 · 817-921-4191

Shirley A. Molenich · General Neurology (Epilepsy, Headache) · Plaza Medical Center · Fort Worth Neurology Consultants, Saint Joseph's Professional Building, Suite 1400, 1350 South Main Street, Fort Worth, TX 76104 · 817-336-3968

Galveston

John R. Calverley · General Neurology · University of Texas Medical Branch Hospitals · University of Texas Medical Branch, Department of Neurology, 301 University Boulevard, Room E-39, Galveston, TX 77555-0539 · 409-772-2646

Karen A. Rasmusson · General Neurology · University of Texas Medical Branch Hospitals · University of Texas Medical Branch, Department of Neurology, 301 University Boulevard, Galveston, TX 77555-1354 · 409-772-7372

Harlingen

Thomas J. Brown · General Neurology (Electromyography, Headache, Movement Disorders) · Valley Baptist Medical Center · Valley Diagnostic Clinic, 2200 Haine Drive, Harlingen, TX 78550-8599 · 210-421-5173

Houston

Jack Nathaniel Alpert · General Neurology · St. Luke's Episcopal Hospital · 6624 Fannin Street, Suite 1550, Houston, TX 77030 · 713-795-4785

Stanley H. Appel · Degenerative Diseases, Neuromuscular Disease (Neurodegenerative Disease [Amyotrophic Lateral Sclerosis, Parkinson's Disease, Alzheimer's Disease]) · Methodist Hospital · Baylor College of Medicine, 6501 Fannin Street, Room NB-302, Houston, TX 77030 · 713-798-4072

Ronald DeVere · General Neurology (Memory Loss, Dementia) · Memorial Hospital-Southwest, Columbia Fort Bend Medical Center (Missouri City) · Houston Neurological Associates, 8200 Wednesbury Lane, Suite 111, Houston, TX 77074 713-777-4122

Rachelle S. Doody · General Neurology (Alzheimer's Disease, Behavioral Neurology, Degenerative Diseases) · Methodist Hospital · Baylor College of Medicine, Department of Neurology, Alzheimer's Disease Center, 6550 Fannin Street, Suite 1801, Houston, TX 77030 · 713-798-7416

Randolph W. Evans · General Neurology (Headache, Trauma) · St. Luke's Episcopal Hospital, Methodist Hospital, Park Plaza Hospital · 1200 Binz Street, Suite 1370, Houston, TX 77004 · 713-528-0725

Robert W. Fayle · General Neurology (Stroke, Sleep Disorders) · Hermann Hospital · Diagnostic Clinic of Houston, 6448 Fannin Street, Houston, TX 77030-1511 · 713-797-9191

James A. Ferrendelli · Epilepsy · Hermann Hospital · University of Texas Medical School at Houston, Department of Neurology, 6431 Fannin Street, Room 7.044, Houston, TX 77030 · 713-792-5777

James C. Grotta · Strokes · Hermann Hospital · Hermann Professional Building, Suite 520, 6410 Fannin Street, Houston, TX 77030 · 713-704-0780; 713-792-5777

Yadollah Harati · Neuromuscular Disease · Baylor College of Medicine, 6550 Fannin Street, Suite 1801, Houston, TX 77030 · 713-798-7411

Ernesto Infante · General Neurology (Neuromuscular Disease) · Diagnostic Center Hospital · Diagnostic Clinic of Houston, 6448 Fannin Street, Houston, TX 77030 · 713-797-9191

Kurt A. Jaeckle · Neuro-Oncology (Primary Brain Tumors, Para Neoplastic Disease) · University of Texas-M. D. Anderson Cancer Center · University of Texas-M. D. Anderson Cancer Center, 1515 Holcombe Boulevard, Box 100, Houston, TX 77030 · 713-794-1286

Joseph Jankovic · Movement Disorders · Methodist Hospital · Baylor College of Medicine, Department of Neurology, 6550 Fannin Street, Suite 1801, Houston, TX 77030-3498 · 713-798-5998

James M. Killian · General Neurology (Neuromuscular Disease, Stroke) · Methodist Hospital · Baylor College of Medicine, Department of Neurology, 6501 Fannin Street, Suite 302, Houston, TX 77030 · 713-798-7422

Victor Alan Levin · Neuro-Oncology (Brain and Spinal Tumors) · University of Texas-M. D. Anderson Cancer Center · University of Texas-M. D. Anderson Cancer Center, 1515 Holcombe Boulevard, Box 100, Houston, TX 77030 · 713-792-2573

Raymond A. Martin · General Neurology (Neuromuscular Disease, Stroke, Epilepsy) · Memorial Hospital-Southwest · Houston Neurological Associates, 8200 Wednesbury Lane, Suite 111, Houston, TX 77074 · 713-777-4122

Ninan T. Mathew · Headache (Migraine Pharmacotherapy, Clinical Research in Headache) · Methodist Hospital, Park Plaza Hospital, St. Luke's Episcopal Hospital, Hermann Hospital · Houston Headache Clinic, 1213 Hermann Drive, Suite 350, Houston, TX 77004 · 713-528-1916

Richard Payne · Neuro-Oncology (Pain Syndromes) · University of Texas-M. D. Anderson Cancer Center · University of Texas-M. D. Anderson Cancer Center, Department of Neuro-Oncology, 1515 Holcombe Boulevard, Box Eight, Houston, TX 77030 · 713-792-2824

Martin R. Steiner · General Neurology · Houston Neurological Associates, 8200 Wednesbury Lane, Suite 111, Houston, TX 77074 · 713-777-4122

Francine Joanna Vriesendorp · Neuromuscular Disease (Nerve Disorders, Electromyography) · Hermann Hospital · University of Texas Medical School at Houston, Department of Neurology, 6431 Fannin Street, Room 7.044, P.O. Box 20708, Houston, TX 77225 · 713-792-5777

L. James Willmore, Jr. · Epilepsy · Hermann Hospital · University of Texas Medical School at Houston, 6431 Fannin Street, Room 7.044, Houston, TX 77030 713-704-0780

Jerry S. Wolinsky · Infectious & Demyelinating Diseases (Neurovirology, Multiple Sclerosis, Infectious Diseases) · Hermann Hospital · University of Texas Medical School at Houston, 6431 Fannin Street, Room 7.044, Houston, TX 77030 713-792-5777

Frank M. Yatsu · Strokes (Dementia, Parkinson's Disease, Geriatric Neurology, Movement Disorders) · Hermann Hospital · University of Texas Medical School at Houston, 6431 Fannin Street, Room 7.044, Houston, TX 77030 · 713-792-5777

W. K. Alfred Yung · Neuro-Oncology (Brain Tumors) · University of Texas-M. D. Anderson Cancer Center · University of Texas-M. D. Anderson Cancer Center, 1515 Holcombe Boulevard, Box 100, Houston, TX 77030 · 713-794-1285

Lackland Air Force Base

Anthony Arnold Amato · Neuromuscular Disease · Wilford Hall Medical Center Wilford Hall Medical Center, 2200 Bergquist Drive, Suite One, Lackland Air Force Base, TX 78236-5300 · 210-670-4102

Thomas Duginsky · Epilepsy · Wilford Hall Medical Center · Wilford Hall Medical Center, 2200 Bergquist Drive, Suite One, Lackland Air Force Base, TX 78236 210-670-4102

April Lynn McVey · Neuromuscular Disease · Wilford Hall Medical Center · Wilford Hall Medical Center, 59 MDW/PSMN, 2200 Bergquist Drive, Suite One, Lackland Air Force Base, TX 78236-5300 · 210-670-7671

Michael L. Rosenberg · Neuro-Ophthalmology · Wilford Hall Medical Center · Wilford Hall Medical Center, Department of Neurology, 2200 Bergquist Drive, Suite One, Lackland Air Force Base, TX 78236-5300 · 210-670-7671

Lubbock

Richard W. Homan · Epilepsy (Clinical Neurophysiology, Behavioral Neurology) University Medical Center · Texas Tech University Health Sciences Center, 3601 Fourth Street, Lubbock, TX 79430 · 806-743-3111; 806-743-2391

Midland

Lawrence F. Buxton · General Neurology · 2201 West Tennessee Avenue, Midland, TX 79701-5953 · 915-570-1024

George H.D. Cirkovic · General Neurology · Westwood Medical Center · West Texas Neurology, 2114 West Michigan Street, Midland, TX 79701 · 915-686-7803

John W. Foster, Jr. · General Neurology · Memorial Hospital & Medical Center 2201 West Tennessee Avenue, Midland, TX 79701 · 915-687-0700

Plano

Paul W. Hurd · General Neurology · Clinical Neurology Associates, 4100 West 15th Street, Suite 100, Plano, TX 75093 · 214-596-2616

Jacob N. Wolfman · General Neurology · Clinical Neurology Associates, 4100 West 15th Street, Suite 100, Plano, TX 75075 · 214-596-2616

San Antonio

Walter F. Buell · General Neurology · San Antonio Community Hospital, Southwest Texas Methodist Hospital · The Neurology Clinic of San Antonio, 8042 Wurzbach Road, Suite 640, San Antonio, TX 78229 · 210-614-3959

John E. Carter · Neuro-Ophthalmology · University Hospital-South Texas Medical Center · University Eye Consultants, 4502 Medical Drive, San Antonio, TX 78229 · 210-567-1945

B. Peyton Delaney · General Neurology · Southwest Texas Methodist Hospital · 4499 Medical Drive, Suite 122, San Antonio, TX 78229 · 210-616-0665

Robert G. Hart · Strokes · Audie L. Murphy Memorial Veterans Hospital · University of Texas Health Science Center at San Antonio, Department of Medicine, Division of Neurology, 7703 Floyd Curl Drive, San Antonio, TX 78284-7883 · 210-617-5161

Carlayne Elizabeth Jackson · Neuromuscular Disease (Amyotrophic Lateral Sclerosis, Muscular Dystrophy, Peripheral Neuropathy, Electromyography) · University Hospital-South Texas Medical Center · University of Texas Health Science Center at San Antonio, Department of Medicine, Division of Neurology, 7703 Floyd Curl Drive, San Antonio, TX 78284-7883 · 210-567-4615

Bruce Ryan LeForce · Epilepsy (Electromyography, General Neurology) · St. Luke's Baptist Hospital, Southwest Texas Methodist Hospital, Santa Rosa Health Care, San Antonio Community Hospital · 2829 Babcock Road, Suite 407, San Antonio, TX 78229 · 210-616-0828

Douglas W. Marshall · General Neurology · 2829 Babcock Road, Suite 407, San Antonio, TX 78229 · 210-616-0828

Michael D. Merren · General Neurology · The Neurology Clinic of San Antonio, 8042 Wurzbach Road, Suite 640, San Antonio, TX 78229 · 210-614-3959

Pamela Z. New · Neuro-Oncology (Brain Tumors, Parkinson's Disease, General Internal Medicine) · University Hospital-South Texas Medical Center, St. Luke's Baptist Hospital, Audie L. Murphy Memorial Veterans Hospital · University of Texas Health Science Center at San Antonio, Department of Medicine, Division of Neurology, 7703 Floyd Curl Drive, San Antonio, TX 78284-7883 · 210-617-5161

David G. Sherman · Strokes · University Hospital-South Texas Medical Center University of Texas Health Science Center at San Antonio, Department of Medicine, Division of Neurology, 7703 Floyd Curl Drive, San Antonio, TX 78284-7883 · 210-617-5161

Temple

Alan B. Follender · General Neurology · Scott & White Memorial Hospital & Clinic · Scott & White Memorial Hospital, Division of Neurology, 2401 South 31st Street, Temple, TX 76508-0001 · 817-724-4170

Kyle H. Smith · Neuro-Ophthalmology · Scott & White Memorial Hospital · Scott & White Memorial Hospital, Department of Ophthalmology, 2401 South 31st Street, Temple, TX 76508-0001 · 817-724-4248

Tyler

Preston E. Harrison, Jr. · General Neurology · East Texas Medical Center · 910 East Houston Street, Suite 250, Tyler, TX 75702 · 903-597-3787

Richard F. Ulrich · General Neurology · East Texas Medical Center, Trinity Mother Frances Health Care Center, University of Texas Health Center-Tyler · 910 East Houston Street, Suite 250, Tyler, TX 75701-2025 · 903-597-3787

NEUROLOGY, CHILD

Austin

Dilip J. Karnik · (Attention Deficit Hyperactivity Disorder, Cerebral Palsy, Epilepsy) · Brackenridge Hospital, Healthsouth Rehabilitation Hospital of Austin, Seton Neonatal Center · Austin Neurology Clinic, 711 West 38th Street, Suite F-1, Austin, TX 78705 · 512-458-6121

Jeffrey Stuart Kerr · General Child Neurology · Children's Hospital of Austin · Austin Diagnostic Medical Center, 12221 MoPac Expressway North, P.O. Box 85075, Austin, TX 78708-5075 · 512-901-4011

Dallas

Mauricio R. Delgado-Ayala · General Child Neurology · Texas Scottish Rite Hospital for Children · Texas Scottish Rite Hospital for Children, Department of Neurology, 2222 Welborn Street, Dallas, TX 75219-3924 · 214-559-7479

Roy D. Elterman · Epilepsy (Neuro-Oncology, Infantile Spasms) · Medical City Dallas Hospital · Dallas Pediatric Neurology Associates, North Central Plaza, Building III, Suite 580, 12801 North Central Expressway, Dallas, TX 75243 · 214-991-2202

Susan Theresa Iannacone · Neuromuscular Disease · Texas Scottish Rite Hospital for Children · Texas Scottish Rite Hospital for Children, Department of Neurology, 2222 Welborn Street, Dallas, TX 75219-3924 · 214-559-7475

Steven LeRoy Linder · General Child Neurology (Headaches in Children) · Children's Medical Center of Dallas, Medical City Dallas Hospital · Dallas Pediatric Neurology Associates, North Central Plaza, Building III, Suite 580, 12801 North Central Expressway, Dallas, TX 75243-1708 · 214-991-2202

Van Strickland Miller · General Child Neurology (Neonatal Neurology) · Children's Medical Center of Dallas · University of Texas-Southwestern Medical Center at Dallas, Division of Pediatric Neurology, 5323 Harry Hines Boulevard, Dallas, TX 75235-9129 · 214-648-9732

David Bruce Owen · General Child Neurology (Epilepsy in Children, Learning Problems in Children) · Children's Medical Center of Dallas, Medical City Dallas Hospital · Dallas Pediatric Neurology Associates, North Central Plaza, Building III, Suite 580, 12801 North Central Expressway, Dallas, TX 75243-1708 · 214-991-2202

Anthony Richard Riela · Epilepsy · Children's Medical Center of Dallas · University of Texas-Southwestern Medical Center at Dallas, 5323 Harry Hines Boulevard, Dallas, TX 75235-9129 · 214-648-9735

Ewell S. Roach · General Child Neurology (Genetic Disorders Affecting the Brain, Stroke/Vascular Disorders in Children, Brain Tumors in Children) · Texas Scottish Rite Hospital for Children, Children's Medical Center of Dallas, Pediatric Center for Restorative Care · University of Texas-Southwestern Medical Center at Dallas, Department of Neurology, 5323 Harry Hines Boulevard, Dallas, TX 75235-9036 · 214-640-2751

David Bartow Sperry · General Child Neurology (Child Development, Epilepsy) Presbyterian Hospital of Dallas, Children's Medical Center of Dallas, Medical City Dallas Hospital, Medical Center of Plano (Plano) · 12801 North Central Expressway, Suite 580, Dallas, TX 75243 · 214-991-2202

El Paso

Johanan Levine · General Child Neurology (Epilepsy, Neuromuscular Disease) · 10400 Vista del Sol, Suite 104, El Paso, TX 79925-7923 · 915-593-3172

Robert Craig Woody · General Child Neurology · 125 West Hague Road, Suite 310, El Paso, TX 79902 · 915-577-9191

Fort Worth

Howard M. Kelfer · General Child Neurology (Child Development, Epilepsy) · Cook Children's Medical Center · Cook Children's Physicians Group, Department of Neurology, 709 West Leuda Street, Fort Worth, TX 76104-3115 · 817-335-3258

Samuel Mark Laney · General Child Neurology · Cook Children's Medical Center · Cook Children's Physicians Group, Department of Neurology, 709 West Leuda Street, Fort Worth, TX 76104-3115 · 817-335-3258

Warren Alan Marks · General Child Neurology · Cook Children's Medical Center · Cook Children's Physicians Group, Department of Neurology, 709 West Leuda Street, Fort Worth, TX 76104-3115 · 817-335-3258

Bryan Douglas Ryals · General Child Neurology (Epilepsy, Child Development) Cook Children's Medical Center · Cook Children's Physicians Group, Department of Neurology, 709 West Leuda Street, Fort Worth, TX 76104-3115 · 817-335-3258

Galveston

Jay D. Cook · General Child Neurology (Neuromuscular Disease) · University of Texas Medical Branch Hospitals · University of Texas Medical Branch, Department of Neurology, Division of Pediatric Neurology, 301 University Boulevard, Galveston, TX 77555-0342 · 409-772-0201

Houston

Ian J. Butler · General Child Neurology, Movement Disorders (Tourette's Syndrome, General Child Neurology, Neuromuscular Disease) · Hermann Hospital, University of Texas-M. D. Anderson Cancer Center, Shriners Hospitals for Crippled Children · University of Texas Medical School at Houston, 6431 Fannin Street, Room 7.044, Houston, TX 77030 · 713-792-5777 x35

Marvin A. Fishman · General Child Neurology · Texas Children's Hospital · Texas Children's Hospital, Pediatric Neurology, 6621 Fannin Street, Mail Code 3-3311, Houston, TX 77030 · 713-770-3964

Daniel G. Glaze · General Child Neurology (Sleep Disorders, Epilepsy) · Methodist Hospital, Texas Children's Hospital, Blue Bird Circle Clinic for Pediatric Neurology · Methodist Hospital, Blue Bird Circle Clinic for Pediatric Neurology, 6501 Fannin Street, Room NB-100, Houston, TX 77030 · 713-790-5046

Eli M. Mizrahi · Epilepsy (Neonatal Neurology, Clinical Neurophysiology [Electroencephalography, EEG/Video Monitoring]) · Methodist Hospital, Texas Children's Hospital, St. Luke's Episcopal Hospital, Ben Taub General Hospital · Baylor College of Medicine, Department of Neurology, Section of Neurophysiology, 6565 Fannin Street, Room M-587, Houston, TX 77030-3411 · 713-790-3109

Barry R. Tharp · Epilepsy · Methodist Hospital · Methodist Hospital, Blue Bird Circle Clinic for Pediatric Neurology, 6501 Fannin Street, Room NB-100, Houston, TX 77030 · 713-790-5046

James W. Wheless · Epilepsy · Hermann Hospital, Hermann Children's Hospital University of Texas Medical School at Houston, Department of Neurology, 6431 Fannin Street, Room 7.044, Houston, TX 77030 · 713-792-5777

Robert S. Zeller · General Child Neurology · Texas Children's Hospital · Child Neurology, 7400 Fannin Street, Suite 760, Houston, TX 77054-1920 · 713-795-5588

Huda Zoghbi · (Neurogenetics, Inherited Ataxias, Rett Syndrome, Aicardi Syndrome) · Texas Children's Hospital · Baylor College of Medicine, One Baylor Plaza, Houston, TX 77030 · 713-798-6558

Lubbock

Daniel L. Hurst · General Child Neurology · University Medical Center · Texas Tech University Health Sciences Center, Department of Neurology, 3601 Fourth Street, Room 4A126, Lubbock, TX 79430 · 806-743-2391

San Antonio

Wilfred Castro · General Child Neurology · Southwest Texas Methodist Hospital 4410 Medical Drive, Suite 400, San Antonio, TX 78229-3710 · 210-615-1401

Charles F. Dreyer · General Child Neurology (Epilepsy) · University Hospital-South Texas Medical Center, Santa Rosa Children's Hospital · University of Texas Health Science Center at San Antonio, Department of Pediatric Neurology, 7703 Floyd Curl Drive, San Antonio, TX 78284-7814 · 210-567-5275

Charles Thomas Gay · General Child Neurology · University Hospital-South Texas Medical Center · University of Texas Health Science Center at San Antonio, Department of Pediatric Neurology, 7703 Floyd Curl Drive, San Antonio, TX 78284-7883 · 210-567-5275

Sheldon G. Gross · General Child Neurology · Southwest Texas Methodist Hospital · Southwest Neurology, 4499 Medical Drive, Suite 396, San Antonio, TX 78229 · 210-614-3737

Jorge A. Saravia · General Child Neurology · 2829 Babcock Road, Suite 436, San Antonio, TX 78229 · 210-614-3657

John Raymond Seals · General Child Neurology (Epilepsy, Movement Disorders) · Southwest Texas Methodist Hospital, Women's & Children's Hospital, Santa Rosa Children's Hospital · 4410 Medical Drive, Suite 400, San Antonio, TX 78229-3710 · 210-615-2222

Jerry Jack Tomasovic · General Child Neurology · Southwest Texas Methodist Hospital · 4410 Medical Drive, Suite 400, San Antonio, TX 78229-3710 · 210-615-2333

Temple

Ricardo Calvo · General Child Neurology · Scott & White Memorial Hospital · Scott & White Memorial Hospital, Division of Pediatric Neurology, 2401 South 31st Street, Temple, TX 76508-0001 · 817-724-3409

E. Darrell Crisp · General Child Neurology · Scott & White Memorial Hospital & Clinic · Scott & White Memorial Hospital, Division of Pediatric Neurology, 2401 South 31st Street, Temple, TX 76508-0001 · 817-724-3409

Tyler

Jerry J. Bettinger · General Child Neurology · 935 South Baxter Avenue, Suite 105, Tyler, TX 75701 · 903-593-2022

Lloyd F. Mercer, Jr. · General Child Neurology · 514 South Beckham Avenue, Tyler, TX 75702 · 903-595-3414

NUCLEAR MEDICINE

Amarillo

Bill F. Byrd · General Nuclear Medicine · 7008 Smoketree Drive, P.O. Box 3160, Amarillo, TX 79116-3160 · 806-359-8102

Austin

Joseph Anthony Volpe · (Nuclear Cardiology, Nuclear Endocrinology, Nuclear Medicine of the Bones) · Austin Diagnostic Medical Center · Austin Diagnostic Medical Center, 12221 MoPac Expressway North, P.O. Box 85075, Austin, TX 78708-5075 · 512-901-1305

Beaumont

Henry O. Williams · General Nuclear Medicine · St. Elizabeth Hospital · Cancer Treatment Center, 690 North 14th Street, Beaumont, TX 77702 · 409-899-7181

Dallas

Frederick J. Bonte · Brain, General Nuclear Medicine (Thyroid Disease) · Parkland Memorial Hospital, Zale Lipshy University Hospital · University of Texas-Southwestern Medical Center at Dallas, Nuclear Medicine Center, 5323 Harry Hines Boulevard, Dallas, TX 75235-9061 · 214-648-2025

Landis K. Griffeth · General Nuclear Medicine (Oncology, Positron Emission Tomography) · Baylor University Medical Center, 3500 Gaston Avenue, Dallas, TX 75246 · 214-820-4057

William C. Harvey · General Nuclear Medicine · Presbyterian Hospital of Dallas Presbyterian Hospital of Dallas, 8200 Walnut Hill Lane, Dallas, TX 75231 · 214-345-2556

Robert W. Parkey · General Nuclear Medicine (Nuclear Cardiology, Nuclear Radiology) · Parkland Memorial Hospital, Zale Lipshy University Hospital, Children's Medical Center of Dallas, St. Paul Medical Center, Baylor University Medical Center, VA Medical Center · University of Texas-Southwestern Medical Center at Dallas, Department of Radiology, 5323 Harry Hines Boulevard, Dallas, TX 75235-8896 · 214-648-8016

Fort Sam Houston

Scott C. Williams · General Nuclear Medicine · Brooke Army Medical Center · Brooke Army Medical Center, Department of Nuclear Medicine, 1950 Stanley Road, Fort Sam Houston, TX 78234 · 210-916-9314

Fort Worth

H. Daniel Fawcett · General Nuclear Medicine · Harris Methodist-Fort Worth, Department of Radiology, 1401 Pennsylvania Avenue, Fort Worth, TX 76104 · 817-882-3550

Galveston

Martin L. Nusynowitz · General Nuclear Medicine (Thyroidology, Nuclear Cardiology) · University of Texas Medical Branch Hospitals · University of Texas Medical Branch, 301 University Boulevard, Room 207B, Route G-93, Galveston, TX 77555-0793 · 409-772-2921

Houston

Ralph J. Gorten · General Nuclear Medicine (Nuclear Cardiology) · Kelsey-Seybold Clinic · 6624 Fannin Street, Suite 2000, Houston, TX 77030 · 713-791-8738

Milton J. Guiberteau · General Nuclear Medicine (Nuclear Cardiology, Oncology) · St. Joseph Hospital · St. Joseph Radiology Associates, 3465 West Alabama Street, P.O. Box 27705, Houston, TX 77227 · 713-757-7467

Thomas Powell Haynie III · General Nuclear Medicine, Oncology · University of Texas-M. D. Anderson Cancer Center, Ben Taub General Hospital · The Levit Radiologic-Pathologic Institute, 1515 Holcombe Boulevard, Mail Code 208, Houston, TX 77030 · 713-792-3007

Satish G. Jhingran · General Nuclear Medicine · Methodist Hospital · Methodist Hospital, 6565 Fannin Street, Suite MBI-68, Houston, TX 77030 · 713-790-2282

E. Edmund Kim · General Nuclear Medicine, Oncology (Positron Emission Tomography [PET], Magnetic Resonance Imaging, Nuclear Radiology) · University of Texas-M. D. Anderson Cancer Center · University of Texas-M. D. Anderson Cancer Center, Department of Nuclear Medicine, 1515 Holcombe Boulevard, Box 59, Houston, TX 77030 · 713-794-1052

Lamk M. Lamki · Oncology (Brain, Total Quality Management, Nuclear Radiology, General Nuclear Medicine) · Hermann Hospital, Lyndon B. Johnson General Hospital · University of Texas Medical School at Houston, 6431 Fannin Street, Room MSB 2.132, Houston, TX 77030 · 713-704-1788

Warren Hamilton Moore · General Nuclear Medicine (Nuclear Cardiology, Pediatric Nuclear Medicine) · St. Luke's Episcopal Hospital, Texas Children's Hospital, Ben Taub General Hospital, VA Medical Center, Texas Heart Institute St. Luke's Episcopal Hospital/Texas Children's Hospital, Department of Nuclear Medicine, 6720 Bertner Avenue, Mail Code 3-261, Houston, TX 77030 · 713-791-3126

Donald A. Podoloff · Oncology, General Nuclear Medicine (Radioisotopic Therapy) · University of Texas-M. D. Anderson Cancer Center · University of Texas-M. D. Anderson Cancer Center, Department of Nuclear Medicine, 1515 Holcombe Boulevard, Box 83, Houston, TX 77030 · 713-792-6535

Lackland Air Force Base

Angelita Ramos-Gabatin · General Nuclear Medicine (Endocrine, Thyroid) · Wilford Hall Medical Center · Wilford Hall Medical Center, Nuclear Medicine Service/SGHRI, 2200 Bergquist Drive, Lackland Air Force Base, TX 78236-5300 210-670-5290

San Antonio

Ralph Blumhardt · General Nuclear Medicine (Nuclear Cardiology, Thyroidology) · University Hospital-South Texas Medical Center · University of Texas Health Science Center at San Antonio, Department of Radiology, Division of Nuclear Medicine, 7703 Floyd Curl Drive, San Antonio, TX 78284-7800 · 210-567-5600

Gerald W. Growcock · General Nuclear Medicine · Radiology Associates of San Antonio, 343 West Houston Street, Suite 209, San Antonio, TX 78205 · 210-222-2255

John C. Lasher · Nuclear Cardiology · University Hospital-South Texas Medical Center · University of Texas Health Science Center at San Antonio, Department of Radiology, Division of Nuclear Medicine, 7703 Floyd Curl Drive, San Antonio, TX 78284-7800 · 210-567-5600

William Thomas Phillips · General Nuclear Medicine (Infection Imaging, Gastric Emptying) · University Hospital-South Texas Medical Center · University of Texas Health Science Center at San Antonio, Department of Radiology, Division of Nuclear Medicine, 7703 Floyd Curl Drive, San Antonio, TX 78284-7800 · 210-567-5550

Fred Whitcomb Riley, Jr. · General Nuclear Medicine · St. Luke's Baptist Hospital, Southwest Texas Methodist Hospital, Women's & Children's Hospital South Texas Radiology Group, 7950 Floyd Curl Drive, Suite SL1-21, P.O. Box 29407, San Antonio, TX 78229-0407 · 210-616-7796

Temple

William R. Carpentier · General Nuclear Medicine · Scott & White Memorial Hospital · Scott & White Memorial Hospital, Department of Nuclear Medicine, 2401 South 31st Street, Temple, TX 76508-0001 · 817-724-2745

OBSTETRICS & GYNECOLOGY

Amarillo

Brian J. Eades · General Obstetrics & Gynecology · 1901 Medical Park Plaza, Suite 200, Amarillo, TX 79106-2107 · 806-358-5121

Robert C. Henderson · General Obstetrics & Gynecology · High Plains Baptist Hospital · 1911 Port Lane, Amarillo, TX 79106 · 806-359-5468

Thomas J. Hickman III · General Obstetrics & Gynecology · Amarillo Hospital District-Northwest Texas Hospital · 301 Amarillo Boulevard, West, Suite 208, Amarillo, TX 79107 · 806-345-2100

Todd H. Overton · (Gynecology, Gynecologic Surgery, Abnormal Uterine Bleeding, Gynecologic Ovarian, Uterine & Cervix Cancer and Pre-Cancer, Preventive Medicine) · St. Anthony's Hospital, High Plains Baptist Hospital, Columbia Panhandle Surgical Hospital · Saint Anthony's Professional Office Building, Suite 201, 301 Amarillo Boulevard, West, Amarillo, TX 79107 · 806-345-2188

Bobby Alan Rimer · (Gynecology) · Amarillo Hospital District-Northwest Texas Hospital · Texas Tech University Health Sciences Center, Department of Obstetrics & Gynecology, 1400 Wallace Boulevard, Amarillo, TX 79106-1745 · 806-354-5500 x231

Michael D. Williams · General Obstetrics & Gynecology · High Plains Baptist Hospital · 1911 Port Lane, Amarillo, TX 79106-2430 · 806-352-5234

Austin

Charles E. L. Brown · Maternal & Fetal Medicine · Seton Medical Center, Brackenridge Hospital, St. David's Healthcare Center · Central Texas Perinatal Associates, 4201 Marathon Boulevard, Suite 303, Austin, TX 78756 · 512-459-1131

Mark Allen Crozier · Gynecologic Cancer · St. David's Healthcare Center, Seton Medical Center, Brackenridge Hospital · Southwest Regional Cancer Center, 711 West 38th Street, Suite B-1, Austin, TX 78705 · 512-451-7387

Byron G. Darby · (Ultrasonography) · Seton Medical Center · Central Texas Perinatal Associates, 4201 Marathon Boulevard, Suite 303, Austin, TX 78756 · 512-459-1131

Joseph L. Des Rosiers · (Gynecology) · 1301 West 38th Street, Suite 403, Austin, TX 78705 · 512-454-5188

Noble W. Doss, Jr. · General Obstetrics & Gynecology · St. David's Healthcare Center · 4201 Marathon Boulevard, Suite 301, Austin, TX 78756 · 512-451-7991

Jo Bess Hammer · General Obstetrics & Gynecology · St. David's Healthcare Center · 805 East 32nd Street, Austin, TX 78705 · 512-477-1954

Donna Schroeder Hurley · General Obstetrics & Gynecology · Women Partners in Health, 1305 West 34th Street, Suite 308, Austin, TX 78705 · 512-458-6138

Terrence A. Kuhlmann · General Obstetrics & Gynecology · St. David's Healthcare Center · Gynics Associates, 1007 East 41st Street, Austin, TX 78751 · 512-451-3131

Douglas K. McIntyre · General Obstetrics & Gynecology · 4201 Marathon Boulevard, Suite 201, Austin, TX 78756 · 512-454-6765

Patrick D. Nunnelly · General Obstetrics & Gynecology · Seton Medical Center 1301 West 38th Street, Suite 403, Austin, TX 78705 · 512-454-5188

Kaylen Mark Silverberg · Reproductive Endocrinology · Austin Diagnostic Medical Center, Seton Medical Center, St. David's Healthcare Center, Brackenridge Hospital · 3705 Medical Parkway, Suite 230, Austin, TX 78705-1022 · 512-451-0149

Ellen Blair Smith · Gynecologic Cancer · Seton Medical Center, St. David's Healthcare Center, Seton Northwest Hospital · Southwest Regional Cancer Center, 711 West 38th Street, Suite B-1, Austin, TX 78705 · 512-451-7387

Karen Grace Swenson · General Obstetrics & Gynecology · Seton Medical Center · Women Partners in Health, 1305 West 34th Street, Suite 308, Austin, TX 78705 · 512-459-8082

Margaret M. Thompson · General Obstetrics & Gynecology · 3705 Medical Parkway, Suite 260, Austin, TX 78705 · 512-451-7436

Thomas C. Vaughn · Reproductive Endocrinology (Infertility) · Seton Medical Center, St. David's Healthcare Center, Austin Diagnostic Medical Center · 3705 Medical Parkway, Suite 230, Austin, TX 78705 · 512-451-0149

Diana Gay Weihs · General Obstetrics & Gynecology · Seton Medical Center · Women Partners in Health, 1305 West 34th Street, Suite 308, Austin, TX 78705 512-459-8082

Robert H. Wernecke · (Gynecology) · 1301 West 38th Street, Suite 403, Austin, TX 78705 · 512-454-5188

Christopher J. Wilson · General Obstetrics & Gynecology · Seton Medical Center, St. David's Healthcare Center · Gynics Associates, 1007 East 41st Street, Austin, TX 78751 · 512-451-3131

Beaumont

Brent W. Bost · General Obstetrics & Gynecology (Infertility) · St. Elizabeth Hospital, Beaumont Surgical Center · Southeast Texas Ob-Gyn Associates, 3030 North Street, Suite 310, Beaumont, TX 77702 · 409-899-1499

James F. Kirby · (Gynecology) · Southeast Texas Ob-Gyn Associates, 3030 North Street, Suite 310, Beaumont, TX 77702 · 409-899-5880

Doreen L. Mowers · General Obstetrics & Gynecology · 2965 Harrison Street, Suite 320, Beaumont, TX 77702-1150 · 409-899-1360

Pamela A. St. Amand · General Obstetrics & Gynecology · 2965 Harrison Street, Suite 320, Beaumont, TX 77702-1150 · 409-899-1360

College Station

Randy W. Smith · General Obstetrics & Gynecology · 1602 Rock Prairie Road, Suite 230, College Station, TX 77845 · 409-693-0737

Corpus Christi

William H. Barth · General Obstetrics & Gynecology · OB-GYN Associates, 5920 Saratoga Boulevard, Suite 200, Corpus Christi, TX 78414 · 512-994-5454

C. Dale Eubank, Jr. · General Obstetrics & Gynecology · Spohn Hospital · 7121 South Padre Island Drive, Suite 200, Corpus Christi, TX 78412 · 512-993-6000

Billy N. Griffin · General Obstetrics & Gynecology (Perimenopause/Menopause, Osteoporosis) · Doctors Regional Medical Center, Spohn Hospital, Bay Area Medical Center · OB-GYN Associates, 5920 Saratoga Boulevard, Suite 200, Corpus Christi, TX 78414-4105 · 512-994-5454

Terry R. Groff · General Obstetrics & Gynecology · Doctors Regional Medical Center · Corpus Christi Women's Clinic, 3240 Fort Worth Street, Suite 100, Corpus Christi, TX 78411 · 512-851-5000

Robert E. Mastin · General Obstetrics & Gynecology · Spohn Hospital · Corpus Christi Women's Clinic, 3240 Fort Worth Street, Suite 100, Corpus Christi, TX 78411 · 512-851-5000

Bernhardt F. Rothschild · General Obstetrics & Gynecology · Coastal Bend Women's Center, 7121 South Padre Island Drive, Suite 200, Corpus Christi, TX 78412 · 512-993-6000

Dallas

Karen D. Bradshaw · Reproductive Endocrinology (Infertility, Menopause, Pediatric & Adolescent Gynecology) · Zale Lipshy University Hospital, Children's Medical Center of Dallas, St. Paul Medical Center, Parkland Memorial Hospital University of Texas-Southwestern Medical Center at Dallas, Department of Obstetrics & Gynecology, 5323 Harry Hines Boulevard, Dallas, TX 75235-9032 · 214-648-3791

Bruce R. Carr · Reproductive Endocrinology (Reproductive Surgery, Menopause) Zale Lipshy University Hospital, Parkland Memorial Hospital, St. Paul Medical Center · University of Texas-Southwestern Medical Center at Dallas, Department of Obstetrics & Gynecology, 5323 Harry Hines Boulevard, Dallas, TX 75235-9032 214-648-4747

Susan M. Cox · Infectious Disease, Maternal & Fetal Medicine · Parkland Memorial Hospital · University of Texas-Southwestern Medical Center at Dallas, Department of Obstetrics & Gynecology, 5323 Harry Hines Boulevard, Dallas, TX 75235-9032 · 214-648-4770

F. Gary Cunningham · Maternal & Fetal Medicine · Parkland Memorial Hospital University of Texas-Southwestern Medical Center at Dallas, Department of Obstetrics & Gynecology, 5323 Harry Hines Boulevard, Dallas, TX 75235-9032 · 214-648-3639

Norman F. Gant, Jr. · Maternal & Fetal Medicine (Hypertension in Pregnancy, High Risk Pregnancy) · Parkland Memorial Hospital · 5323 Harry Hines Boulevard, Dallas, TX 75235 · 214-871-1619

Larry C. Gilstrap III · Maternal & Fetal Medicine · Parkland Memorial Hospital, St. Paul Medical Center · University of Texas-Southwestern Medical Center at Dallas, Department of Obstetrics & Gynecology, 5323 Harry Hines Boulevard, Dallas, TX 75235-9032 · 214-648-2646

David L. Hemsell · Infectious Disease · University of Texas-Southwestern Medical Center at Dallas, Department of Obstetrics & Gynecology, 5323 Harry Hines Boulevard, Dallas, TX 75235-9032 · 214-648-3019

Kenneth J. Leveno · Maternal & Fetal Medicine · Parkland Memorial Hospital · University of Texas-Southwestern Medical Center at Dallas, 5323 Harry Hines Boulevard, Dallas, TX 75235-9032 · 214-648-3793

James Donald Madden · Reproductive Endocrinology · Presbyterian Hospital of Dallas · 8160 Walnut Hill Lane, Suite 320, Dallas, TX 75231-4355 · 214-363-6322

Carolyn M. Matthews · Gynecologic Cancer · Baylor University Medical Center Texas Oncology, 3320 Live Oak Street, Dallas, TX 75204 · 214-820-8672

C. Allen Stringer, Jr. · Gynecologic Cancer · Baylor University Medical Center · Texas Oncology, 3535 Worth Street, Second Floor, Dallas, TX 75246 · 214-824-4901

William Kemp Strother III · General Obstetrics & Gynecology (Reproductive Surgery, Laparoscopic Surgery, Genital Dermatological Disease, Gynecologic Cancer, Infectious Disease, Pediatric & Adolescent Gynecology) · Baylor University Medical Center · 1311 North Washington Street, Dallas, TX 75204 · 214-824-2563

Denison

Darius Roderick Maggi · General Obstetrics & Gynecology · 900 North Armstrong Avenue, Denison, TX 75020-2230 · 903-463-5416

El Paso

Kellie Flood-Shaffer · General Obstetrics & Gynecology (Maternal & Fetal Medicine, Cultural Obstetrics & Gynecology) · Thomason Hospital, Providence Memorial Hospital, Columbia Medical Center-East · Texas Tech University Health Sciences Center, Department of Obstetrics & Gynecology, 4800 Alberta Avenue, El Paso, TX 79905 · 915-545-6710

Frederick E. Harlass · Maternal & Fetal Medicine · Thomason Hospital, Columbia Medical Center-East, Columbia Medical Center-West, Providence Memorial Hospital · Texas Tech University Health Sciences Center, Department of Obstetrics & Gynecology, 4800 Alberta Avenue, El Paso, TX 79920-5001 · 915-545-6710

Linda S. Lacy · General Obstetrics & Gynecology · 1600 Medical Center Drive, Suite 307, El Paso, TX 79902 · 915-541-1144

Joseph Sakakini, Jr. · Maternal & Fetal Medicine · Thomason Hospital · Texas Tech University Health Sciences Center, Department of Obstetrics & Gynecology, 4800 Alberta Avenue, El Paso, TX 79905-2700 · 915-545-6710

Fort Worth

Kevin J. Doody · Reproductive Endocrinology (Infertility, Reproductive Surgery, In Vitro Fertilization) · Center for Assisted Reproduction, 1325 Pennsylvania Avenue, Suite 440, Fort Worth, TX 76104 · 817-878-5360

Kenneth C. Hancock · Gynecologic Cancer · Harris Methodist-Fort Worth, All Saints Episcopal Hospital-Fort Worth · Texas Oncology, 918 Eighth Avenue, Fort Worth, TX 76104 · 817-332-7394

D. Alan Johns · General Obstetrics & Gynecology · Harris Methodist-Fort Worth Texas Health Care, 1325 Pennsylvania Avenue, Suite 750, Fort Worth, TX 76104 817-332-7733

Mark C. Maberry · Maternal & Fetal Medicine · Texas Maternal Fetal Medicine, 1325 Pennsylvania Avenue, Suite 690, Fort Worth, TX 76104 · 817-878-5298

Bannie L. Tabor · Maternal & Fetal Medicine · John Peter Smith Hospital · Texas Maternal Fetal Medicine, 1325 Pennsylvania Avenue, Suite 690, Fort Worth, TX 76104 · 817-878-5298

Galveston

Garland D. Anderson · Maternal & Fetal Medicine (Perinatology) · University of Texas Medical Branch Hospitals · University of Texas Medical Branch, Department of Obstetrics & Gynecology, 301 University Boulevard, Galveston, TX 77555-0587 · 409-772-1572

Gary D. V. Hankins · Maternal & Fetal Medicine (Infectious Disease, Critical Care Obstetrics) · University of Texas Medical Branch Hospitals · University of Texas Medical Branch, Department of Obstetrics & Gynecology, 301 University Boulevard, Room 3.400 Old John Sealy, Galveston, TX 77555-0587 · 409-772-1957

Gayle Olson · Maternal & Fetal Medicine · University of Texas Medical Branch Hospitals, John Sealy Hospital · University of Texas Medical Branch, Department of Obstetrics & Gynecology, 301 University Boulevard, Room 3.400 Old John Sealy, Galveston, TX 77555-0587 · 409-747-4905

Harlingen

William L. Spilker · General Obstetrics & Gynecology (Reproductive Surgery) · Valley Baptist Medical Center · Women's Medical Associates, 1713 Treasure Hills Boulevard, Suite 1D, Harlingen, TX 78550-8321 · 210-425-8545

Houston

Karolina Adam · Maternal & Fetal Medicine · St. Luke's Episcopal Hospital, Methodist Hospital · Houston Perinatal Associates, 7400 Fannin Street, Suite 700, Houston, TX 77054 · 713-791-9700

Robert L. Andres · Maternal & Fetal Medicine (Substance Abuse, Autoimmune Disease, Addicted Pregnant Women) · Hermann Hospital · University of Texas Medical School at Houston, Department of Obstetrics, Gynecology & Reproductive Sciences, 6431 Fannin Street, Room 3.204, Houston, TX 77030 · 713-792-5360

Isam Y. A. Balat · General Obstetrics & Gynecology (Endometriosis, Infertility) Park Plaza Hospital, Hermann Hospital, The Woman's Hospital of Texas · 1200 Binz Street, Suite 1100, Houston, TX 77004 · 713-522-3333

Michael A. Belfort · Maternal & Fetal Medicine (Pre-Eclampsia, Pregnancy-Induced Hypertension, Obstetric Anesthesia, Critical Care Medicine) · St. Luke's Episcopal Hospital, Methodist Hospital, Ben Taub General Hospital · Baylor College of Medicine, Department of Obstetrics & Gynecology, 6550 Fannin Street, Suite 901, Houston, TX 77030 · 713-793-3570

Jorge D. Blanco · Maternal & Fetal Medicine · 908 Town & Country Boulevard, Suite 120, Houston, TX 77020 · 713-984-7509

Dale Brown, Jr. · Genital Dermatological Disease (Vulvar Disease) · St. Luke's Episcopal Hospital, Methodist Hospital · 6624 Fannin Street, Suite 2180, Houston, TX 77030 · 713-797-1144

Thomas W. Burke · Gynecologic Cancer · University of Texas-M. D. Anderson Cancer Center · University of Texas-M. D. Anderson Cancer Center, Department of Gynecologic Oncology, 1515 Holcombe Boulevard, Box 67, Houston, TX 77030 · 713-792-2770

John E. Buster · Reproductive Endocrinology (Infertility, Reproductive Surgery, Menopause) · Methodist Hospital, Texas Children's Hospital, St. Luke's Episcopal Hospital · Baylor College of Medicine, Department of Obstetrics & Gynecology, 6550 Fannin Street, Suite 801, Houston, TX 77030 · 713-798-8399

Jan Byrne · Maternal & Fetal Medicine · Baylor College of Medicine, Department of Perinatal Medicine, 6550 Fannin Street, Suite 901, Houston, TX 77030 713-798-7500

Robert J. Carpenter, Jr. · Maternal & Fetal Medicine (Genetics) · St. Luke's Episcopal Hospital · 6624 Fannin Street, Suite 2720, Houston, TX 77030 · 713-795-4600

Sandra A. Carson · Reproductive Endocrinology · Methodist Hospital · Baylor College of Medicine, Department of Reproductive Endocrinology and Infertility, 6550 Fannin Street, Suite 801, Houston, TX 77030 · 713-798-8484

Peter R. Casson · Reproductive Endocrinology (Infertility, Reproductive Surgery) · Methodist Hospital, Ben Taub General Hospital, St. Luke's Episcopal Hospital · Baylor College of Medicine, Department of Reproductive Endocrinology and Infertility, 6550 Fannin Street, Suite 801, Houston, TX 77030 · 713-798-7580

Robert K. Creasy · Maternal & Fetal Medicine · Hermann Hospital · University of Texas Medical School at Houston, 6431 Fannin Street, Room 3.286, Houston, TX 77030 · 713-792-5362

Mohamed Yusoff Dawood · Reproductive Endocrinology (Reproductive Surgery, General Obstetrics & Gynecology) · Hermann Hospital, St. Joseph Hospital, Lyndon B. Johnson General Hospital · University of Texas Medical School at Houston, Department of Obstetrics, Gynecology & Reproductive Sciences, 6431 Fannin Street, Room 3.204, Houston, TX 77030 · 713-792-5360

Randall Clifford Dunn · Reproductive Endocrinology (Infertility, Reproductive Surgery, In Vitro Fertilization) · St. Luke's Episcopal Hospital, The Woman's Hospital of Texas, Methodist Hospital · Obstetrical & Gynecological Associates, 7550 Fannin Street, Suite 104, Houston, TX 77030 · 713-797-9123 x5280

Creighton L. Edwards · Gynecologic Cancer · University of Texas-M. D. Anderson Cancer Center · University of Texas-M. D. Anderson Cancer Center, Department of Gynecology, 1515 Holcombe Boulevard, Box 67, Houston, TX 77030-4095 · 713-792-2980

Sherman Elias · Genetics (Reproductive Genetics) · Methodist Hospital, St. Luke's Episcopal Hospital, Ben Taub General Hospital · Baylor College of Medicine, Department of Obstetrics & Gynecology, 6550 Fannin Street, Suite 701-A, Houston, TX 77030 · 713-798-4717

Arthur Monroe Faris, Jr. · (Gynecology) · 4818 San Jacinto Street, Houston, TX 77004 · 713-527-0153

Robert Ray Franklin · Reproductive Surgery · The Woman's Hospital of Texas Obstetrical & Gynecological Associates, 7550 Fannin Street, Suite 200, Houston, TX 77054 · 713-797-9123 x5390

Geri-Lynn Fromm · Gynecologic Cancer · The Woman's Hospital of Texas · 7400 Fannin Street, Suite 1180, Houston, TX 77054 · 713-796-1957

David M. Gershenson · Gynecologic Cancer · University of Texas-M. D. Anderson Cancer Center · University of Texas-M. D. Anderson Cancer Center, Department of Gynecologic Oncology, 1515 Holcombe Boulevard, Box 67, Houston, TX 77030 · 713-745-2565

Mark J. Gottesman · General Obstetrics & Gynecology (Reproductive Surgery, Pelviscopy) · Methodist Hospital · 7515 South Main Street, Suite 300, Houston, TX 77030-4519 · 713-797-0060

Hunter A. Hammill · Infectious Disease · Baylor College of Medicine, Department of Obstetrics & Gynecology, 6550 Fannin Street, Suite 701, Houston, TX 77030-2719 · 713-798-4065

Eric J. Haufrect · General Obstetrics & Gynecology · 6560 Fannin Street, Suite 1402, Houston, TX 77030 · 713-797-9666

Lynn P. Hoffman · General Obstetrics & Gynecology · Methodist Hospital · 6550 Fannin Street, Suite 2221, Houston, TX 77030 · 713-790-9133

Alan Leslie Kaplan · Gynecologic Cancer (Gynecologic Surgery) · Methodist Hospital, St. Luke's Episcopal Hospital · Baylor College of Medicine, Department of Obstetrics & Gynecology, 6550 Fannin Street, Suite 701, Houston, TX 77030-3411 · 713-798-7675

Allan R. Katz · General Obstetrics & Gynecology · Hermann Hospital, Harris County Hospital District · University of Texas Medical School at Houston, Department of Obstetrics & Gynecology, 6431 Fannin Street, Room 3.270, Houston, TX 77030 · 713-792-5360

Raymond H. Kaufman · Genital Dermatological Disease (Vulvar Disease, Gynecologic Pathology) · Methodist Hospital, St. Luke's Episcopal Hospital · Baylor College of Medicine, Department of Obstetrics & Gynecology, 6550 Fannin Street, Suite 701, Houston, TX 77030-2719 · 713-798-3189

Dirk Kiebach · Gynecologic Cancer · Methodist Hospital · Baylor College of Medicine, 6560 Fannin Street, Suite 740, Houston, TX 77030 · 713-798-7500

Brian Kirshon · Maternal & Fetal Medicine (High-Risk Obstetrics, Fetal Anomalies, Prenatal Diagnosis) · The Woman's Hospital of Texas, St. Luke's Episcopal Hospital, Methodist Hospital · Houston Perinatal Associates, 7400 Fannin Street, Suite 700, Houston, TX 77054 · 713-791-9700

Samuel W. Law II · General Obstetrics & Gynecology · St. Luke's Episcopal Hospital, Methodist Hospital · 6550 Fannin Street, Suite 1402, Houston, TX 77030 · 713-797-9666

Leroy J. Leeds · General Obstetrics & Gynecology · The Woman's Hospital of Texas · Obstetrical & Gynecological Associates, 7550 Fannin Street, Suite 107, Houston, TX 77054 · 713-797-9123 x5480

Maurice N. Leibman · General Obstetrics & Gynecology (Infertility) · Memorial Hospital-Southwest · Memorial Hospital-Southwest, 7500 Beechnut Street, Suite 366, Houston, TX 77074 · 713-270-0527

Maurizio Maccato · Infectious Disease · Houston Perinatal Associates, 7400 Fannin Street, Suite 700, Houston, TX 77054 · 713-791-9700

L. Russell Malinak · Reproductive Endocrinology, Reproductive Surgery (Endometriosis) · Methodist Hospital, St. Luke's Episcopal Hospital · Baylor College of Medicine, Department of Obstetrics & Gynecology, 6550 Fannin Street, Suite 801, Houston, TX 77030 · 713-798-5095

Harold J. Miller · General Obstetrics & Gynecology (Pelvic Reconstruction) · Methodist Hospital, St. Luke's Episcopal Hospital · Baylor College of Medicine,

Department of Obstetrics & Gynecology, 6550 Fannin Street, Suite 901, Houston, TX 77030 · 713-798-8987

Michele Follen Mitchell · Gynecologic Cancer · University of Texas-M. D. Anderson Cancer Center · University of Texas-M. D. Anderson Cancer Center, Department of Gynecologic Oncology, 1515 Holcombe Boulevard, Box 67, Houston, TX 77030-4009 · 713-792-2770

Kenneth Joseph Moise, Jr. · Maternal & Fetal Medicine · St. Luke's Episcopal Hospital · Baylor College of Medicine, Department of Obstetrics & Gynecology, One Baylor Plaza, Houston, TX 77030 · 713-793-3539

Alan G. Moore · General Obstetrics & Gynecology · Center for Women's Health, 17030 Nanes Drive, Suite 111, Houston, TX 77090 · 713-440-7462

Edward R. Newton · General Obstetrics & Gynecology · University of Texas Medical School at Houston, 6410 Fannin Street, Suite 350, Houston, TX 77030 · 713-794-5131

Ferdinand J. Plavidal · General Obstetrics & Gynecology · The Woman's Hospital of Texas, St. Luke's Episcopal Hospital, Methodist Hospital · 7580 Fannin Street, Suite 335, Houston, TX 77054 · 713-795-5450 x3001

Susan F. Pokorny · Pediatric & Adolescent Gynecology · Texas Children's Hospital · Kelsey Seybold Clinic, Department of Obstetrics & Gynecology, 7800 Fannin Street, Suite 300, Houston, TX 77054 · 713-795-5444

Alex A. Reiter · Maternal & Fetal Medicine (Critical Care Medicine, Genetics) · Methodist Hospital, St. Luke's Episcopal Hospital, The Woman's Hospital of Texas · Houston Perinatal Associates, 7400 Fannin Street, Suite 700, Houston, TX 77054 · 713-791-9700

Geoffrey Schnider · General Obstetrics & Gynecology (Reproductive Surgery, Minimally Invasive Laparoscopic Surgery) · The Woman's Hospital of Texas · 7580 Fannin Street, Suite 310, Houston, TX 77054 · 713-797-9701

Terry Lee Simon · General Obstetrics & Gynecology (Laparoscopy, Pelviscopy, Dysplasia) · Methodist Hospital, St. Luke's Episcopal Hospital · 7515 South Main Street, Suite 340, Houston, TX 77030 · 713-797-9209

Joe Leigh Simpson · Genetics (Reproductive Genetics, Prenatal Genetic Diagnosis, Disorders of Sexual Differentiation) · Methodist Hospital, St. Luke's Episcopal Hospital, Ben Taub General Hospital · Baylor College of Medicine, Department of Obstetrics & Gynecology, 6550 Fannin Street, Suite 729-A, Houston, TX 77030 · 713-798-8052

Douglas A. Thibodeaux · General Obstetrics & Gynecology · West Oaks Obstetrics & Gynecology, 12121 Richmond Avenue, Suite 315, Houston, TX 77082 · 713-589-0156

Peter K. Thompson · (Urogynecology) · The Woman's Hospital of Texas · Obstetrical & Gynecological Associates, 7550 Fannin Street, Houston, TX 77054 · 713-512-7000

Rachel A. Thompson · General Obstetrics & Gynecology · The Woman's Hospital of Texas · Obstetrical & Gynecological Associates, 7550 Fannin Street, Houston, TX 77054 · 713-797-9123

Cecilia T. Valdes · Reproductive Endocrinology (Infertility, Reproductive Surgery, In Vitro Fertilization) · The Woman's Hospital of Texas · Obstetrical & Gynecological Associates, 7550 Fannin Street, Suite 104, Houston, TX 77054 · 713-797-9123 x5280

Mary L. Van Sickle · General Obstetrics & Gynecology (Menopausal Issues for Women, Adolescent Gynecology) · St. Luke's Episcopal Hospital, Methodist Hospital, Memorial Hospital-Southwest, The Woman's Hospital of Texas · Baylor College of Medicine, 6550 Fannin Street, Suite 843A, Houston, TX 77030 · 713-798-7500

J. Taylor Wharton · Gynecologic Cancer · University of Texas-M. D. Anderson Cancer Center · University of Texas-M. D. Anderson Cancer Center, Department of Gynecologic Oncology, 1515 Holcombe Boulevard, Box 67, Houston, TX 77030 · 713-792-8628

Isabelle A. Wilkins · Maternal & Fetal Medicine · St. Luke's Episcopal Hospital, Methodist Hospital · Baylor College of Medicine, Department of Obstetrics & Gynecology, Smith Tower, Suite 901, 6550 Fannin Street, Houston, TX 77030 · 713-798-5072

Ronald L. Young · Reproductive Endocrinology (Critical Care Medicine, General Obstetrics & Gynecology, Maternal & Fetal Medicine, Reproductive Surgery) · Methodist Hospital, St. Luke's Episcopal Hospital, The Woman's Hospital of Texas, Texas Children's Hospital · Baylor College of Medicine, Department of Obstetrics & Gynecology, 6550 Fannin Street, Suite 901, Houston, TX 77030-2719 · 713-798-7648

David E. Zepeda · General Obstetrics & Gynecology (Advanced Operative Laparoscopy and Hysterectomy, Major Pelvic Surgery) · Methodist Hospital, St. Luke's Episcopal Hospital · Baylor College of Medicine, 6550 Fannin Street, Suite 901, Houston, TX 77030-4519 · 713-798-8956

Huntsville

Billy J. Atkins · General Obstetrics & Gynecology · Huntsville Memorial Hospital Women and Children's Clinic, 2135 I-45, Suite A, Huntsville, TX 77340 · 409-295-6436

Lubbock

Melin Cañez · (Reproductive Endocrinology, Reproductive Surgery, Infertility) · University Medical Center · Texas Tech University Health Sciences Center, Department of Reproductive Endocrinology & Infertility, 3601 Fourth Street, Lubbock, TX 79430 · 806-743-1200

Robert Haskell Messer · (Gynecology, Endocrinology, Reproductive Surgery) · University Medical Center · Texas Tech University Health Sciences Center, Department of Obstetrics & Gynecology, 3601 Fourth Street, Lubbock, TX 79430 · 806-743-2295

Mikal Janelle Odom-Dorsett · Reproductive Endocrinology (Infertility, In Vitro Fertilization) · Lubbock Methodist Hospital, St. Mary of the Plains Hospital, University Medical Center · 3506 Twenty-First Street, Suite 605, Lubbock, TX 79410 · 806-788-1212

Selman I. Welt · General Obstetrics & Gynecology (Pediatric & Adolescent Gynecology, Maternal & Fetal Medicine, Obstetrical & Gynecological Ultrasound) · University Medical Center, St. Mary of the Plains Hospital · University Medical Center, Department of Obstetrics & Gynecology, 602 Indiana Avenue, Lubbock, TX 79415 · 806-743-2356

McAllen

Daniel A. Chester · General Obstetrics & Gynecology · Landrum & Chester OBGYN Associates, 222 East Ridge Road, Suite 216, McAllen, TX 78503 · 210-686-6588

Wayne B. Wilson · General Obstetrics & Gynecology · Rio Grande Regional Hospital, McAllen Medical Center · Landrum & Chester OBGYN Associates, 222 East Ridge Road, Suite 216, McAllen, TX 78503 · 210-686-6588

Midland

Gary D. Madden · General Obstetrics & Gynecology · Midland Odessa Medical Group, 2009 West Wall Street, Midland, TX 79701 · 915-682-7341

San Angelo

O. Sterling Gillis III · General Obstetrics & Gynecology · West Texas Medical Associates, 3555 Knickerbocker Road, San Angelo, TX 76904 · 915-949-9555

Leslie D. Mueller · General Obstetrics & Gynecology · West Texas Medical Associates, 3555 Knickerbocker Road, San Angelo, TX 76904 · 915-949-9555

San Antonio

Bruce Donald Akright · General Obstetrics & Gynecology · Northeast Baptist Hospital · 8500 Village Drive, Suite 101, San Antonio, TX 78217 · 210-653-5501

Joe Childress · General Obstetrics & Gynecology · 8601 Village Drive, Suite 118, San Antonio, TX 78217 · 210-654-6371

Bryan Matthew Cox · General Obstetrics & Gynecology · 4499 Medical Drive, Suite 370, San Antonio, TX 78229 · 210-614-1707

Christine de la Garza · General Obstetrics & Gynecology · Southwest Texas Methodist Hospital, Women's & Children's Hospital · 4499 Medical Drive, Suite 274, San Antonio, TX 78229 · 210-692-9500

Mark Gerard Doherty · Gynecologic Cancer (Premalignant Disease, Chemotherapy, Genital Dermatological Disease, General Gynecology) · Southwest Texas Methodist Hospital, Methodist Healthcare System, Santa Rosa Health Care, Baptist Memorial Healthcare System · South Texas Medical Plaza, 7922 Ewing Halsell Drive, Suite 220, San Antonio, TX 78229-3725 · 210-614-9548

S. Ender Dolen · General Obstetrics & Gynecology (Urogynecology) · Methodist Healthcare System, Women's & Children's Hospital, St. Luke's Baptist Hospital, Santa Rosa Northwest Hospital · 7922 Ewing Halsell Drive, Suite 320, San Antonio, TX 78229 · 210-692-0831

Lillian Beth Engelsgjerd · General Obstetrics & Gynecology (Gynecology) · 4499 Medical Drive, Suite 275, San Antonio, TX 78229 · 210-616-0676

Bruce Fine · Gynecologic Cancer · University of Texas Health Science Center at San Antonio, Department of Obstetrics & Gynecology, 7703 Floyd Curl Drive, San Antonio, TX 78284-7836 · 210-567-6248

Michael D. Garcia · General Obstetrics & Gynecology · Baptist Medical Center, Metropolitan Hospital, Santa Rosa Health Care · South Texas Obstetrics & Gynecology Associates, 215 East Quincy Street, Suite 505, San Antonio, TX 78215 210-225-5930

Michelle A. Harden · General Obstetrics & Gynecology · Methodist Healthcare System, St. Luke's Baptist Hospital · 4499 Medical Drive, Suite 274, San Antonio, TX 78229 · 210-692-9500

Brian Harle · General Obstetrics & Gynecology · 4499 Medical Drive, Suite 218, San Antonio, TX 78229 · 210-692-9422

Heidi Rebecca Heck · General Obstetrics & Gynecology · Southwest Texas Methodist Hospital, Women & Children's Hospital · 4499 Medical Drive, Suite 251, San Antonio, TX 78229 · 210-614-1404

Parke Joseph Hedges · General Obstetrics & Gynecology · 4499 Medical Drive, Suite 280, San Antonio, TX 78229 · 210-614-3556

Charles R. Honore · General Obstetrics & Gynecology · Southwest Texas Methodist Hospital · Oak Hills Medical Building, Suite 902, 7711 Louis Pasteur Drive, San Antonio, TX 78229-3465 · 210-614-0457

Robert W. Huff · Maternal & Fetal Medicine (Prenatal Diagnosis, Genetics) · University Hospital-South Texas Medical Center · University of Texas Health Science Center at San Antonio, Department of Obstetrics & Gynecology, 7703 Floyd Curl Drive, San Antonio, TX 78284-7836 · 210-567-4999

Roberta Lynn Krueger · General Obstetrics & Gynecology · Women's & Children's Hospital, Southwest Texas Methodist Hospital · 7922 Ewing Halsell Drive, Suite 310, San Antonio, TX 78229 · 210-692-9230

Richard Mark Lackritz · Reproductive Endocrinology · Metropolitan Hospital · Metropolitan OB-Gyn Associates, 4499 Medical Drive, Suite 230, San Antonio, TX 78229 · 210-615-0866

Oded Langer · Maternal & Fetal Medicine (Diabetes) · University Hospital-South Texas Medical Center · University of Texas Health Science Center at San Antonio, Department of Obstetrics & Gynecology, 7703 Floyd Curl Drive, San Antonio, TX 78284-7836 · 210-567-5000

Joseph E. Martin · General Obstetrics & Gynecology (Fertility) · Southwest Texas Methodist Hospital · Fertility Center of San Antonio, 4499 Medical Drive, Suite 360, San Antonio, TX 78229 · 210-692-0577

Freddy M. Massey · Gynecologic Cancer · South Texas Medical Plaza, 7922 Ewing Halsell Drive, Suite 220, San Antonio, TX 78229-3725 · 210-614-9548

Mohammad Hossein Saidi · General Obstetrics & Gynecology · Northeast Baptist Hospital · Northeast Obstetrics & Gynecology, 8500 Village Drive, Suite 101, San Antonio, TX 78217 · 210-653-5501

Robert S. Schenken · Reproductive Endocrinology (Infertility, Endometriosis) · University Hospital-South Texas Medical Center, Women's & Children's Hospital, St. Luke's Baptist Hospital · South Texas Women's Health Center, 8122 Datapoint Drive, Suite 1300, San Antonio, TX 78229-3264 · 210-567-4930

Robert E. Schorlemer · General Obstetrics & Gynecology · 4499 Medical Drive, Suite 178, San Antonio, TX 78229 · 210-614-9400

Patrick M. Tolar · General Obstetrics & Gynecology · 4499 Medical Drive, Suite 178, San Antonio, TX 78229 · 210-614-3510

Thierry G. Vancaillie · Reproductive Surgery (Laparoscopic Surgery) · 4499 Medical Drive, Suite 289, San Antonio, TX 78229 · 210-616-0711

Marilyn Jean Vanover · General Obstetrics & Gynecology · Northeast Baptist Hospital · 1777 Northeast Loop 410, Suite 200, San Antonio, TX 78217 · 210-826-2494

Allan James White · Gynecologic Cancer · Southwest Texas Methodist Hospital 7711 Louis Pasteur Drive, Suite 503, San Antonio, TX 78229 · 210-616-0603

Carol E. Wratten · General Obstetrics & Gynecology · 1777 Northeast Loop 410, Suite 200, San Antonio, TX 78217 · 210-826-2494

Temple

Steven R. Allen · Maternal & Fetal Medicine · Scott & White Memorial Hospital Scott & White Memorial Hospital, Department of Obstetrics & Gynecology, 2401 South 31st Street, Temple, TX 76508-0001 · 817-724-2589

Dudley P. Baker · Gynecologic Cancer · Scott & White Memorial Hospital & Clinic · Scott & White Memorial Hospital, Texas A&M University Health Science Center, Department of Obstetrics & Gynecology, 2401 South 31st Street, Temple, TX 76508-0001 · 817-724-2576

Charles V. Capen · Gynecologic Cancer · Scott & White Memorial Hospital, Department of Obstetrics & Gynecology, 2401 South 31st Street, Temple, TX 76508-0001 · 817-724-2576

Alfred B. Knight · Maternal & Fetal Medicine (Prenatal Diagnosis, High Risk Pregnancy, Genetics) · Scott & White Memorial Hospital · Scott & White Memorial Hospital, Department of Obstetrics & Gynecology, 2401 South 31st Street, Temple, TX 76508-0001 · 817-724-2589

Jose F. Pliego · Reproductive Endocrinology (Reproductive Surgery) · Scott & White Memorial Hospital & Clinic · Scott & White Memorial Hospital, Texas A&M University Health Science Center, Department of Obstetrics & Gynecology, 2401 South 31st Street, Temple, TX 76508-0001 · 817-724-2738

Bob L. Shull · Reproductive Surgery (Pelvic Reconstructive Surgery, Urogynecology) · Scott & White Memorial Hospital · Scott & White Memorial Hospital, Department of Obstetrics & Gynecology, 2401 South 31st Street, Temple, TX 76508-0001 · 817-724-2677

Patricia J. Sulak · General Obstetrics & Gynecology (Hormone Replacement Therapy, Contraception) · Scott & White Memorial Hospital · Scott & White Memorial Hospital, Department of Obstetrics & Gynecology, 2401 South 31st Street, Temple, TX 76508-0001 · 817-724-4034

Thomas J. Wincek · Reproductive Endocrinology · Scott & White Memorial Hospital, Department of Obstetrics & Gynecology, 2401 South 31st Street, Temple, TX 76508-0001 · 817-724-2738

Texarkana

Jack H. McCubbin · General Obstetrics & Gynecology · Collom & Carney, 4800 Texas Boulevard, Texarkana, TX 75503 · 903-792-7151

Victoria

Stephen Schneberger · General Obstetrics & Gynecology (Gynecologic Urology, Hysteroscopy) · Victoria Regional Medical Center, Detar Hospital, Citizens Medical Center · 115 Medical Drive, Suite 202, Victoria, TX 77904 · 512-572-0464

Waco

Robert W. Grayson · General Obstetrics & Gynecology · Hillcrest Baptist Medical Center · Hillcrest OB-GYN Associates, 3115 Pine Avenue, Suite 708, Waco, TX 76708-3201 · 817-753-3190

Donald K. Lewis · General Obstetrics & Gynecology · Hillcrest Baptist Medical Center · Hillcrest OB-GYN Associates, 3115 Pine Avenue, Suite 708, Waco, TX 76708-3201 · 817-753-3190

Wilbur G. Murff · General Obstetrics & Gynecology · Hillcrest Baptist Medical Center · 3115 Pine Avenue, Suite 1001, Waco, TX 76708 · 817-752-9221

Dianne W. Sawyer · General Obstetrics & Gynecology · 3115 Pine Avenue, Suite 903, Waco, TX 76708-3201 · 817-753-5858

OPHTHALMOLOGY

Amarillo

Robert E. Gerald · General Ophthalmology · High Plains Baptist Hospital · 7308 Fleming Avenue, Amarillo, TX 79106 · 806-359-7603

Paul M. Munden · Glaucoma · 3501 Soncy Road, Suite 100, Amarillo, TX 79121 806-355-7021

J. Avery Rush · (Anterior Segment—Cataract & Refractive) · High Plains Baptist Hospital, Amarillo Hospital District-Northwest Texas Hospital · 7308 Fleming Avenue, Amarillo, TX 79106 · 806-353-0125

Coleman Taylor · General Ophthalmology · High Plains Baptist Hospital · 15 Medical Drive, Amarillo, TX 79106 · 806-355-9811

Bruce L. Weinberger · General Ophthalmology · High Plains Baptist Hospital · 700 Quail Creek Drive, Amarillo, TX 79124 · 806-353-6691

Austin

Peter H. Broberg · General Ophthalmology · South Austin Medical Center · 4207 James Casey Street, Suite 306, Austin, TX 78745-3362 · 512-447-6096

M. Coleman Driver, Jr. · Vitreo-Retinal Surgery · Seton Medical Center, St. David's Healthcare Center, HealthSouth Surgical Hospital, Brackenridge Hospital · Austin Retina Associates, 801 West 38th Street, Austin, TX 78705-1106 · 512-451-0103

Thomas T. Henderson · General Ophthalmology (Anterior Segment—Cataract & Refractive, Optics & Refraction) · HealthSouth Surgical Hospital, Seton Medical Center, Brackenridge Hospital, St. David's Healthcare Center, South Austin Medical Center · Eye Clinic of Austin, 3410 Far West Boulevard, Suite 140, Austin, TX 78731 · 512-794-9984

Ernest E. Howerton · General Ophthalmology · Howerton Eye Center, 2610 Interstate 35 South, Austin, TX 78704 · 512-443-9715

Oscar Branche Jackson, Jr. · Pediatric Ophthalmology · Seton Medical Center · 3509 Lawton Avenue, Austin, TX 78731 · 512-451-0234

Lyle D. Koen · Vitreo-Retinal Surgery (Uveitis) · Seton Medical Center · Austin Retina Associates, 801 West 38th Street, Austin, TX 78705-1106 · 512-451-0103

Jose A. Martinez · (Retinal Disease, Uveitis, Vitreo-Retinal Surgery) · Seton Medical Center, St. David's Healthcare Center, Brackenridge Hospital · Austin Retina Associates, 801 West 38th Street, Austin, TX 78705-1106 · 512-451-0103

John McCrary · Neuro-Ophthalmology · Austin Retina Associates, 801 West 38th Street, Austin, TX 78705-1106 · 512-451-0103

James D. McNabb · General Ophthalmology · Cataract & Eye Center, 1101 West 40th Street, Austin, TX 78756 · 512-467-7744

Russell W. Neuhaus · Oculoplastic & Orbital Surgery · Seton Medical Center, St. David's Healthcare Center, Brackenridge Hospital · 3705 Medical Parkway, Suite 370, Austin, TX 78705 · 512-458-2141

Robert L. Rock · General Ophthalmology (Anterior Segment—Cataract & Refractive Surgery) · St. David's Healthcare Center · 5011 Burnet Road, Austin, TX 78756-2611 · 512-454-8744

Gary R. Rylander · General Ophthalmology (Anterior Segment—Cataract & Refractive, Corneal Diseases & Transplantation) · Seton Medical Center · 5011 Burnet Road, Austin, TX 78756 · 512-454-8744

H. Grady Rylander III · General Ophthalmology · 5011 Burnet Road, Austin, TX 78756 · 512-454-8744

George C. Thorne · General Ophthalmology · 5011 Burnet Road, Austin, TX 78756 · 512-454-8744

Sue Ellen Young · General Ophthalmology (Anterior Segment—Cataract & Refractive, Glaucoma, Neuro-Ophthalmology, Ophthalmic Plastic Surgery) · Brackenridge Hospital · 1313 Red River Street, Suite 206, Austin, TX 78701 · 512-472-4011

Beaumont

Graham D. Avery · Vitreo-Retinal Surgery · Retina Consultant of Beaumont, 810 Hospital Drive, Suite 350, Beaumont, TX 77701 · 409-832-8883

Mark K. Harmon · General Ophthalmology (Glaucoma, Anterior Segment—Cataract & Refractive) · Levacy & Harmon Eye Center, 3345 Plaza 10 Drive, Suite B, Beaumont, TX 77707-2508 · 409-833-0444

Jerry Spruce Lehmann · General Ophthalmology (Anterior Segment—Cataract & Refractive) · Surgery Center of Southeast Texas, St. Elizabeth Hospital, Baptist Hospital Beaumont, Beaumont Regional Medical Center · Beaumont Eye Associates, 3129 College Street, Beaumont, TX 77701-4649 · 409-838-3725

Richard A. Levacy · Corneal Diseases & Transplantation (Anterior Segment—Cataract & Refractive, General Ophthalmology) · Beaumont Surgical Center, Southeast Texas Surgical Center, St. Elizabeth Hospital, Baptist Hospital Beaumont, Beaumont Regional Medical Center · Levacy & Harmon Eye Center, 3345 Plaza 10 Drive, Suite B, Beaumont, TX 77707-2508 · 409-833-0444

Big Spring

John R. Fish · Anterior Segment—Cataract & Refractive · Scenic Mountain Medical Center · Fish Ophthalmology Clinic, 207 East Seventh Street, Big Spring, TX 79720-2706 · 915-267-3649

Bryan

Mark B. Lindsay · General Ophthalmology · Columbia Medical Center (College Station) · 2725 East 29th Street, Bryan, TX 77802 · 409-776-2020

William H. Marr · General Ophthalmology · Marr Eye Center, 2801 East 29th Street, Suite 101, Bryan, TX 77802-2602 · 409-776-7564

College Station

Paul Wutrich · General Ophthalmology · Scott & White Clinic, Department of Ophthalmology, 1600 University Drive, East, College Station, TX 77840 · 817-691-3200

Corpus Christi

Paul K. Ayars, Jr. · General Ophthalmology · Spohn Hospital · 1521 South Staples Street, Suite 202, Corpus Christi, TX 78404-3122 · 512-882-2651

Charles Harvey Campbell · Vitreo-Retinal Surgery · Spohn Hospital, Driscoll Children's Hospital, Bay Area Medical Center, Columbia Valley Regional Hospital (Brownsville), McAllen Medical Center (McAllen) · South Texas Retina Consultants, 5540 Saratoga Boulevard, Corpus Christi, TX 78413-2953 · 512-993-8510

William C. Newberry · General Ophthalmology · Spohn Hospital · Eye Associates of Corpus Christi, 3301 South Alameda Street, Suite 403, Corpus Christi, TX 78411-1871 · 512-853-7319

R. Michael Nisbet · Vitreo-Retinal Surgery (Retinal Diseases) · Memorial Medical Center · 3301 South Alameda Street, Suite 307, Corpus Christi, TX 78411-1829 · 512-853-2226

Dallas

Rajiv Anand · Vitreo-Retinal Surgery (Ocular Oncology, Retinal Diseases, Uveitis) · Presbyterian Hospital of Dallas, Medical City Dallas Hospital · Texas Retina Associates, 7150 Greenville Avenue, Suite 400, Dallas, TX 75231 · 214-692-6941

Charles R. Barnett · Neuro-Ophthalmology (Ocular Motility) · Medical City Dallas Hospital · Dallas Diagnostic Association, Building C, Suite 300, 7777 Forest Lane, Dallas, TX 75230 · 214-991-6000

George R. Beauchamp · Pediatric Ophthalmology (Strabismus) · Children's Medical Center of Dallas, Presbyterian Hospital of Dallas, Baylor University Medical Center · Pediatric Ophthalmology, 8201 Preston Road, Suite 140A, Lock Box 23, Dallas, TX 75225 · 214-369-6434

Walter E. Beebe · Corneal Diseases & Transplantation (Anterior Segment—Cataract & Refractive) · Presbyterian Hospital of Dallas · Cornea Associates of Texas, 7150 Greenville Avenue, Suite 600, Dallas, TX 75231-5165 · 214-692-0146

Priscilla M. Berry · Pediatric Ophthalmology (Strabismus, Amblyopia) · Children's Medical Center of Dallas, Presbyterian Hospital of Dallas, Medical City Dallas Hospital, Baylor University Medical Center, Texas Scottish Rite Hospital for Children · Pediatric Ophthalmology, 8201 Preston Road, Suite 140A, Dallas, TX 75225 · 214-369-6434

William Larkin Berry · General Ophthalmology (Glaucoma, Cataracts) · Baylor University Medical Center · Texas Eye Care Associates, Barnett Tower, Suite 609, 3600 Gaston Avenue, Dallas, TX 75246 · 214-826-8201

Bradley Bowman · Corneal Diseases & Transplantation (Anterior Segment— Cataract & Refractive, Radial Keratotomy, Photorefractive Keratectomy) · Presbyterian Hospital of Dallas, Baylor University Medical Center, Arlington Memorial Hospital (Arlington), Medical City Dallas Hospital · Cornea Associates of Texas, Greenville Medical Tower, Suite 600, 7150 Greenville Avenue, Dallas, TX 75231-5165 · 214-692-0146

Robert Wayne Bowman · Corneal Diseases & Transplantation · University of Texas-Southwestern Medical Center at Dallas, 5323 Harry Hines Boulevard, Dallas, TX 75235-9057 · 214-648-3847

Peter Robert Bringewald · Neuro-Ophthalmology · Medical City Dallas Hospital, Presbyterian Hospital of Dallas · Neurological Clinic, Building B, Suite 410, 7777 Forest Lane, Dallas, TX 75230 · 214-661-7684

Donald P. Brotherman · General Ophthalmology · 10 Medical Parkway, Suite 102, Dallas, TX 75234-7838 · 214-328-3597

John E. Eisenlohr · General Ophthalmology (Anterior Segment—Cataract & Refractive, Glaucoma, Optics & Refraction) · Mary Shiels Hospital · 2811 Lemmon Avenue, East, Dallas, TX 75204-2860 · 214-521-5620

Ronald L. Fellman · Glaucoma · Presbyterian Hospital of Dallas, Baylor University Medical Center · Glaucoma Associates of Texas, 7150 Greenville Avenue, Suite 300, Dallas, TX 75231-5165 · 214-360-0000

Gary Edd Fish · Uveitis, Medical Retinal Diseases (Macular Diseases) · Presbyterian Hospital of Dallas · Texas Retina Associates, 7150 Greenville Avenue, Suite 400, Dallas, TX 75231 · 214-692-6941

Dwain G. Fuller · Ocular Oncology (Vitreo-Retinal Surgery, Retinal Diseases) · Presbyterian Hospital of Dallas · Texas Retina Associates, 7150 Greenville Avenue, Suite 400, Dallas, TX 75231 · 214-692-6941

Lawrence O. Gahagan · Anterior Segment—Cataract & Refractive (Cataract only) · Presbyterian Hospital of Dallas · 6120 Sherry Lane, Dallas, TX 75225 · 214-361-1232

Henry Gelender · Corneal Diseases & Transplantation (Anterior Segment—Cataract & Refractive) · Presbyterian Hospital of Dallas, Medical City Dallas Hospital · Cornea Associates of Texas, Greenville Medical Tower, Suite 600, 7150 Greenville Avenue, Dallas, TX 75231-5165 · 214-692-0146

John Norris Harrington · Oculoplastic & Orbital Surgery (Ophthalmic Plastic & Reconstructive Surgery, Lacrimal Surgery) · Baylor University Medical Center, Mary Shiels Hospital, Presbyterian Hospital of Dallas · Texas Ophthalmic, Plastic, Reconstructive & Orbital Surgery Associates, 2731 Lemmon Avenue East, Suite 304, Dallas, TX 75204 · 214-522-7733

William L. Hutton · Vitreo-Retinal Surgery, Medical Retinal Diseases (Uveitis) · Presbyterian Hospital of Dallas · Texas Retina Associates, 7150 Greenville Avenue, Suite 400, Dallas, TX 75231-5165 · 214-692-6941

Bradley F. Jost · Medical Retinal Diseases, Vitreo-Retinal Surgery · Presbyterian Hospital of Dallas, Baylor University Medical Center · Texas Retina Associates, 7150 Greenville Avenue, Suite 400, Dallas, TX 75231 · 214-692-6941

James P. McCulley · Corneal Diseases & Transplantation (Anterior Segment—Cataract & Refractive, General Ophthalmology) · Parkland Memorial Hospital, Zale Lipshy University Hospital · University of Texas-Southwestern Medical Center at Dallas, 5323 Harry Hines Boulevard, Dallas, TX 75235-9057 · 214-648-3407

David W. Meltzer · General Ophthalmology (Anterior Segment—Cataract & Refractive, Optics & Refraction) · Presbyterian Hospital of Dallas · 8210 Walnut Hill Lane, Suite 109, Dallas, TX 75231-4418 · 214-368-2020

James H. Merritt · Oculoplastic & Orbital Surgery (Reconstructive Surgery) · Presbyterian Hospital of Dallas, Baylor University Medical Center, Medical City Dallas Hospital, Children's Medical Center of Dallas, Presbyterian Hospital of Plano (Plano) · 8230 Walnut Hill Lane, Suite 518, Dallas, TX 75231 · 214-369-0555

Susannah Soon-Chun Park · Vitreo-Retinal Surgery · University of Texas-Southwestern Medical Center at Dallas, 5323 Harry Hines Boulevard, Dallas, TX 75235-9057 · 214-648-3838

Craig D. Smith · General Ophthalmology (Contact Lenses, Anterior Segment—Cataract & Refractive [Laser]) · Medical City Dallas Hospital · Four Forest Plaza, 12222 Merit Drive, Suite 400, Dallas, TX 75251-2229 · 214-233-6237

William B. Snyder · Vitreo-Retinal Surgery (Retinal Diseases, Uveitis) · Presbyterian Hospital of Dallas, Baylor University Medical Center, St. Paul Medical Center, Medical City Dallas Hospital · Texas Retina Associates, 7150 Greenville Avenue, Suite 400, Dallas, TX 75231-5165 · 214-692-6941

Rand (William Bertrand) Spencer · Vitreo-Retinal Surgery (Retinopathy of Prematurity, Diabetic Retinopathy, Medical Retinal Diseases) · Baylor University Medical Center, Presbyterian Hospital of Dallas · Baylor University Medical Center, 3600 Gaston Avenue, Suite 1055, Dallas, TX 75246 · 214-821-4540

David R. Stager · Pediatric Ophthalmology (Adult Strabismus) · Children's Medical Center of Dallas, Presbyterian Hospital of Dallas, Baylor University Medical Center, Medical City Dallas Hospital, St. Paul Medical Center · Pediatric Ophthalmology, 8201 Preston Road, Suite 140-A, Dallas, TX 75225-5906 · 214-369-6434

Richard J. Starita · Glaucoma · Presbyterian Hospital of Dallas, Medical City Dallas Hospital, Baylor University Medical Center · Glaucoma Associates of Texas, 7150 Greenville Avenue, Suite 300, Dallas, TX 75231-5165 · 214-360-0000

Bruce C. Taylor · Vitreo-Retinal Surgery, Medical Retinal Diseases · 2811 Lemmon Avenue, East, Suite 402, Dallas, TX 75204 · 214-521-1153

Robert Mayo Tenery, Jr. · General Ophthalmology (Corneal Disease & Transplantation, Anterior Segment—Cataract & Refractive) · Medical City Dallas Hospital · Eye Associates, 7777 Forest Lane, Suite 333, Dallas, TX 75230-2502 · 214-233-3488

Robert Eugene Torti · Medical Retinal Diseases, Vitreo-Retinal Surgery (Diabetic Retinopathy) · Methodist Medical Center of Dallas, RHD Memorial Medical Center, St. Paul Medical Center · 1330 North Beckley Avenue, Suite 103, Dallas, TX 75203 · 214-620-0270

David Robert Weakley · Pediatric Ophthalmology · Children's Medical Center of Dallas, Zale Lipshy University Hospital, St. Paul Medical Center · University of Texas-Southwestern Medical Center at Dallas, 5323 Harry Hines Boulevard, Dallas, TX 75235-8895 · 214-648-3837

Steven Eugene Wilson · Corneal Diseases & Transplantation · University of Texas-Southwestern Medical Center at Dallas, 5323 Harry Hines Boulevard, Dallas, TX 75235-9057 · 214-648-2427

Richard Lee Winslow · Vitreo-Retinal Surgery, Medical Retinal Diseases (Uveitis) · Mary Shiels Hospital, Baylor University Medical Center · 2811 Lemmon Avenue, East, Suite 402, Dallas, TX 75204 · 214-521-1153

Carol F. Zimmerman · Neuro-Ophthalmology · Zale Lipshy University Hospital, Parkland Memorial Hospital, Children's Medical Center of Dallas · University of Texas-Southwestern Medical Center at Dallas, Department of Ophthalmology, 5323 Harry Hines Boulevard, Dallas, TX 75235 · 214-648-2427

El Paso

David S. Doka · Pediatric Ophthalmology · 10201 Gateway Boulevard West, Suite 140, El Paso, TX 79925-7647 · 915-591-4441

Roy A. Levit · (Vitreo-Retinal Diseases & Surgery, Uveitis) · Sierra Medical Center, Columbia Medical Center-West, Columbia Medical Center-East · Southwest Retina Consultants, 1700 Curie Drive, Suite 3800, El Paso, TX 79902 · 915-532-3912

Fort Worth

Lee Stewart Anderson · Vitreo-Retinal Surgery · Retina Consultants, 1350 South Main Street, Suite 3200, Fort Worth, TX 76104-7605 · 817-332-1782

Ronald L. Antinone · Pediatric Ophthalmology · 901 Travis Street, Fort Worth, TX 76104 · 817-338-0322

Clifton H. Beasley, Jr. · Vitreo-Retinal Surgery · Harris Methodist-Fort Worth · Retina Consultants, 1350 South Main Street, Suite 3200, Fort Worth, TX 76104-7605 · 817-332-1782

Daniel Edward Bruhl · Anterior Segment—Cataract & Refractive (Cataract only) The Fort Worth Surgery Center, Plaza Medical Center · Ophthalmology Associates, 1201 Summit Avenue, Fort Worth, TX 76102-4514 · 817-332-2020

Frederick Thomason Feaster · Corneal Diseases & Transplantation · All Saints Episcopal Hospital-Fort Worth · Ophthalmology Associates, 1201 Summit Avenue, Fort Worth, TX 76104-4514 · 817-335-5435

Stephen M. Goode · Glaucoma · Plaza Medical Center · 1350 South Main Street, Suite 1600, Fort Worth, TX 76104-7605 · 817-332-4005

Judson Paul Smith III · (Comprehensive Ophthalmology, Cataract, Intraocular Lens, Glaucoma) · Plaza Day Surgery Center · 1350 South Main Street, Suite 3100, Fort Worth, TX 76104-7605 · 817-338-4081

Galveston

Allan H. Fradkin · General Ophthalmology · The Eye Clinic of Texas, 2302 Avenue P, Galveston, TX 77550 · 409-765-6324

Daniel H. Gold · Medical Retinal Diseases (Anterior Segment—Cataract & Refractive, General Ophthalmology) · Mainland Center Hospital (Texas City), Clear Lake Regional Medical Center (Webster), University of Texas Medical Branch Hospitals · The Eye Clinic of Texas, 2302 Avenue P, Galveston, TX 77550 · 409-765-6324

Bernard A. Milstein · General Ophthalmology (Anterior Segment—Cataract & Refractive, Glaucoma) · Mainland Center Hospital (Texas City), Clear Lake Regional Medical Center (Webster), University of Texas Medical Branch Hospitals · The Eye Clinic of Texas, 2302 Avenue P, Galveston, TX 77550 · 409-765-6324

Katherine Ochsner · Glaucoma (General Ophthalmology) · University of Texas Medical Branch Hospitals · University of Texas Medical Branch, Department of Ophthalmology, 301 University Boulevard, Galveston, TX 77555-0521 · 409-772-8102

Rosa A. Tang · Neuro-Ophthalmology (Ocular Oncology) · Hermann Hospital (Houston), University of Texas-M. D. Anderson Cancer Center (Houston), St. Luke's Episcopal Hospital (Houston), Lyndon B. Johnson General Hospital (Houston), John Sealy Hospital, St. Mary Hospital (Port Arthur) · 700 University Boulevard, Galveston, TX 77555-1041 · 713-942-8624

Harlingen

Donald C. Meadows · General Ophthalmology · Valley Baptist Medical Center · Valley Eye Center, 2001 Ed Carey Drive, Harlingen, TX 78550-8257 · 210-423-2100

Houston

Michael A. Bloome · Medical Retinal Diseases (Diabetic Retinopathy, Macular Degeneration, Hereditary Retinal Diseases) · Gramercy Surgery Center, Hermann Hospital, Diagnostic Center Hospital, St. Joseph Hospital · Houston Eye Associates, 2855 Gramercy Street, Houston, TX 77025 · 713-668-6828

Milton Boniuk · General Ophthalmology (Ocular Oncology, Oculoplastic & Orbital Surgery) · Methodist Hospital, St. Luke's Episcopal Hospital · Baylor College of Medicine, Department of Ophthalmology, 6560 Fannin Street, Suite 902, Houston, TX 77030 · 713-798-5955

Jared M. Emery · Anterior Segment—Cataract & Refractive · Methodist Hospital Baylor College of Medicine, Cullen Eye Institute, Room NC-200, 6501 Fannin Street, Houston, TX 77030 · 713-798-5941

John D. Goosey · Anterior Segment—Cataract & Refractive, Corneal Diseases & Transplantation · Hermann Hospital · Houston Eye Associates, 2855 Gramercy Street, Houston, TX 77025 · 713-668-6828

Ronald L. Gross · Glaucoma · Methodist Hospital · Baylor College of Medicine, Cullen Eye Institute, Room NC-200, 6501 Fannin Street, Houston, TX 77030 · 713-798-4538

Jack T. Holladay · Optics & Refraction, Anterior Segment—Cataract & Refractive · Hermann Hospital, Park Plaza Hospital, St. Joseph Hospital, Gramercy Outpatient Surgery Center, Laser Eye Institute of Texas · Houston Eye Associates, 2855 Gramercy Street, Houston, TX 77025-1635 · 713-668-6828

Dan B. Jones · Corneal Diseases & Transplantation (Infectious Diseases) · Methodist Hospital · Baylor College of Medicine, Cullen Eye Institute, Room NC-200, 6501 Fannin Street, Houston, TX 77030 · 713-798-5951

Douglas D. Koch · Anterior Segment—Cataract & Refractive, Corneal Diseases & Transplantation · Methodist Hospital · Baylor College of Medicine, Cullen Eye Institute, Room NC-200, 6501 Fannin Street, Houston, TX 77030 · 713-798-6443

H. Michael Lambert · Vitreo-Retinal Surgery (Retinal Detachment, Macular and Submacular Surgery, Pediatric Surgery) · Methodist Hospital, St. Luke's Episcopal Hospital, Texas Children's Hospital, Ben Taub General Hospital, Victoria Regional Medical Center (Victoria), The Institute for Rehabilitation and Research Baylor College of Medicine, Cullen Eye Institute, Room NC-200, 6501 Fannin Street, Houston, TX 77030 · 713-798-6100

Jeffrey D. Lanier · Corneal Diseases & Transplantation · Hermann Hospital · Houston Eye Associates, 2855 Gramercy Street, Houston, TX 77025-1635 · 713-668-6828

Andrew G. Lee · Neuro-Ophthalmology · Methodist Hospital, St. Luke's Episcopal Hospital, Texas Children's Hospital · Baylor College of Medicine, Cullen Eye Institute, Room NC-200, 6501 Fannin Street, Houston, TX 77030 · 713-798-6100

Richard Alan Lewis · Ophthalmic Genetics, Medical Retinal Diseases (Uveitis, Diagnostic Testing) · Texas Children's Hospital, Methodist Hospital · Baylor College of Medicine, Cullen Eye Institute, Room NC-206, One Baylor Plaza, Houston, TX 77030 · 713-798-3030

Malcolm L. Mazow · Pediatric Ophthalmology (Strabismus) · Hermann Hospital, Texas Children's Hospital, Park Plaza Hospital · Houston Eye Associates, 2855 Gramercy Street, Houston, TX 77025-1635 · 713-668-6828

Robert A. Moura · Vitreo-Retinal Surgery · St. Luke's Episcopal Hospital, Methodist Hospital, VA Medical Center · McPherson Associates, Scurlock Tower, Suite 2200, 6560 Fannin Street, Houston, TX 77030 · 713-797-1903

James R. Patrinely · Oculoplastic & Orbital Surgery (Ocular Oncology, Facial Aesthetic Surgery) · University of Texas-M. D. Anderson Cancer Center, Methodist Hospital, St. Luke's Episcopal Hospital, Texas Children's Hospital, Cullen Eye Institute · Baylor College of Medicine, Cullen Eye Institute/Alkek Eye Clinic, 6550 Fannin Street, Suite 1501, Houston, TX 77030 · 713-786-6100

Richard S. Ruiz · Ocular Oncology (General Ophthalmology, Retinal Diseases) · Hermann Hospital · Hermann Eye Center, 6411 Fannin Street, Houston, TX 77030 · 713-704-1777

Paul M. Scott · General Ophthalmology · Memorial Hospital-Southwest, St. Luke's Episcopal Hospital · 7500 Beechnut Street, Suite 256, Houston, TX 77074 713-988-0121

Hayne J. Sheffield · General Ophthalmology · 530 Wells Fargo, Suite 117, Houston, TX 77090 · 713-444-1677

Gerald M. Sheldon · General Ophthalmology · Rosewood Medical Center · Rosewood Eye Clinic, 9034 Westheimer Street, Suite 106, Houston, TX 77063 · 713-789-3937

Paul G. Steinkuller · Pediatric Ophthalmology · Texas Children's Hospital · Texas Children's Hospital, 6621 Fannin Street, Mail Code 3-2700, Houston, TX 77030 · 713-770-3230

Rosa A. Tang · Neuro-Ophthalmology (Ocular Oncology) · Hermann Hospital, University of Texas-M. D. Anderson Cancer Center, St. Luke's Episcopal Hospital, Lyndon B. Johnson General Hospital, John Sealy Hospital, St. Mary Hospital (Port Arthur) · 1315 Calhoun Street, Suite 1205, Houston, TX 77002 · 713-942-8624

Gunter K. von Noorden · Pediatric Ophthalmology (Strabismus) · Texas Children's Hospital · Texas Children's Hospital, Department of Ophthalmology, 6621 Fannin Street, Mail Code 3-2700, Houston, TX 77030-0269 · 713-770-3230

Kirk R. Wilhelmus · Corneal Diseases & Transplantation (Ocular Microbiology, External Eye Diseases) · Cullen Eye Institute, Methodist Hospital · Baylor College of Medicine, Cullen Eye Institute, Room NC-200, 6501 Fannin Street, Houston, TX 77030 · 713-798-6100

Robert Benson Wilkins · Oculoplastic & Orbital Surgery · Hermann Hospital, Diagnostic Center Hospital, St. Luke's Episcopal Hospital · Houston Eye Associates, 2855 Gramercy Street, Houston, TX 77025-1635 · 713-668-6828

Jacksonville

Scott J. Sands · General Ophthalmology · Ophthalmology Associates, 928 Bolton Street, Jacksonville, TX 75766 · 903-586-0521

Longview

Michael B. Guillory · General Ophthalmology (Anterior Segment—Cataract & Refractive) · Longview Regional Hospital, Good Shepherd Medical Center · 3209 North Fourth Street, Suite 100, Longview, TX 75605 · 903-757-4662

Lubbock

Sandra M. Brown · Pediatric Ophthalmology · University Medical Center · Texas Tech University Health Sciences Center, Division of Ophthalmology & Visual Sciences, Sixth and Flynt Street, Lubbock, TX 79408 · 806-743-2020

Curt Cockings · Pediatric Ophthalmology · Lubbock Methodist Hospital, St. Mary of the Plains Hospital, St. Mary's SurgiCenter · 3606 Twenty-First Street, Suite 209, Lubbock, TX 79410 · 806-796-1551

David W. Lamberts · Corneal Diseases & Transplantation · 4003 Twenty-Second Street, Lubbock, TX 79410 · 806-792-3400

David L. McCartney · Corneal Diseases & Transplantation (Anterior Segment—Cataract & Refractive, Optics & Refraction) · University Medical Center, Lubbock Methodist Hospital, St. Mary of the Plains Hospital, St. Mary's SurgiCenter Texas Tech University Health Sciences Center, Thompson Hall, 3601 Fourth Street, Lubbock, TX 79430 · 806-743-2020

Jose Morales · Glaucoma · University Medical Center · Texas Tech University Health Sciences Center, Division of Ophthalmology & Visual Sciences, 3601 Fourth Street, Lubbock, TX 79430 · 806-743-2020

Donald F. Naegle · Medical Retinal Diseases, Vitreo-Retinal Surgery · 4020 Twenty-First Street, Suite Two, Lubbock, TX 79410 · 806-793-8733

Michel Shami · Medical Retinal Diseases, Vitreo-Retinal Surgery · University Medical Center, St. Mary of the Plains Hospital · Texas Tech University Health Sciences Center, Division of Ophthalmology & Visual Sciences, 3601 Fourth Street, Lubbock, TX 79430 · 806-743-2020

Midland

Ronald W. Ingram · General Ophthalmology · Eye Center of West Texas, 3001 West Illinois Avenue, Midland, TX 79701 · 915-694-0999

Patrick K. Riggs · General Ophthalmology · Riggs Eye Center, 4534 Sinclair Avenue, Midland, TX 79707-6454 · 915-682-0088

New Braunfels

David Mott Way · General Ophthalmology · McKenna Memorial Hospital · 457 Landa Street, Suite A, New Braunfels, TX 78130 · 210-625-2335

Odessa

John H. Sheets · Anterior Segment—Cataract & Refractive · Medical Center Hospital · Eyes of Texas Clinic & Surgery Center, 155 South East Loop 338, Suite 100, Odessa, TX 79762-9745 · 915-367-7241

Alan D. Smith · Anterior Segment—Cataract & Refractive · Medical Center Hospital · Eyes of Texas Clinic & Surgery Center, 155 South East Loop 338, Suite 100, Odessa, TX 79762-9745 · 915-367-7241

Thomas C. Turner · General Ophthalmology · Medical Center Hospital · Turner Eye Clinic, 419 West Fourth Street, Suite 812, Odessa, TX 79761-5063 · 915-580-0246

San Angelo

John L. Barnes · Anterior Segment—Cataract & Refractive · 319 West Harris Street, San Angelo, TX 76903 · 915-658-8595

Kenton H. Fish · General Ophthalmology · Shannon Medical Center · Shannon Clinic, Department of Ophthalmology, 120 East Beauregard Avenue, San Angelo, TX 76903 · 915-658-1511

Douglas J. Kappelmann · General Ophthalmology (Anterior Segment—Cataract & Refractive, Glaucoma) · Angelo Community Hospital · West Texas Medical Associates, 3555 Knickerbocker Road, San Angelo, TX 76904 · 915-949-9555

San Antonio

Gilberto Aguirre · General Ophthalmology · Santa Rosa Health Care · 315 North San Saba, Suite 970, San Antonio, TX 78207 · 210-225-6705

Harrison N. Bowes · Glaucoma · Baptist Medical Center · 730 North Main Avenue, Suite 424, San Antonio, TX 78205 · 210-223-4273

Sheldon P. Braverman · General Ophthalmology (Vitreo-Retinal Surgery, Anterior Segment—Cataract & Refractive, Pediatric Ophthalmology) · Baptist Medical Center · Eye Consultants of San Antonio, 1100 North Main Avenue, San Antonio, TX 78212 · 210-222-2154

Daniel Gist Duke · General Ophthalmology (Anterior Segment—Cataract & Refractive) · Northeast Baptist Hospital · 8601 Village Drive, Suite 212, San Antonio, TX 78217 · 210-656-3533

Michael Ference III · Corneal Diseases & Transplantation (Glaucoma, Anterior Segment—Cataract & Refractive) · Santa Rosa Northwest Hospital, St. Luke's Baptist Hospital, Methodist Healthcare System, San Antonio Community Hospital · Santa Rosa Northwest Tower II, Suite 345, 2833 Babcock Road, San Antonio, TX 78229 · 210-614-3600

Kristin Story Held · General Ophthalmology (Glaucoma, Anterior Segment—Cataract & Refractive) · North Central Baptist Hospital · 540 Madison Oak Drive, Suite 450, San Antonio, TX 78258 · 210-490-6759

Donald Hollsten · Oculoplastic & Orbital Surgery · St. Luke's Baptist Hospital, Southwest Texas Methodist Hospital, Women's & Children's Hospital · Medical Center Tower I, Suite 505, 7950 Floyd Curl Drive, San Antonio, TX 78229 · 210-616-0739

Jean Edwards Holt · General Ophthalmology · 540 Madison Oak Drive, Suite 450, San Antonio, TX 78258 · 210-490-6759

Jane B. L. Hughes · General Ophthalmology (Anterior Segment—Cataract & Refractive) · St. Luke's Baptist Hospital, Southwest Texas Methodist Hospital · Opthalmology/Ophthalmic Surgery, Medical Center Tower II, Suite 1020, 7940 Floyd Curl Drive, San Antonio, TX 78229 · 210-614-5566

David M. Hunter · General Ophthalmology (Vitreo-Retinal Diseases, Photorefractive Keratectomy) · Nix Health Care System · Ophthalmology Associates, 414 Navarro Street, Suite 400, San Antonio, TX 78205 · 210-223-5561

Lina Mohamad Marouf · Vitreo-Retinal Surgery · 7940 Floyd Curl Drive, Suite 820, San Antonio, TX 78229 · 210-615-8413

Calvin E. Mein · Vitreo-Retinal Surgery (Pediatric, Adult) · Southwest Texas Methodist Hospital, St. Luke's Baptist Hospital · 4499 Medical Drive, Suite 166, San Antonio, TX 78229 · 210-615-1311

James L. Mims III · Pediatric Ophthalmology · 311 Camden Street, Suite 511, San Antonio, TX 78215 · 210-225-0084

John V. Mumma · Pediatric Ophthalmology · San Antonio Community Hospital 8038 Wurzbach Road, Suite 520, San Antonio, TX 78229 · 210-615-8474

Patrick S. O'Connor · General Ophthalmology (Neuro-Ophthalmology) · Southeast Baptist Hospital · 4242 East Southcross Boulevard, Suite 10, San Antonio, TX 78222 · 210-337-1910

Kenneth L. Piest · Oculoplastic & Orbital Surgery (Pediatric, Adult, Ocular Oncology, Ophthalmic Genetics) · North Central Baptist Hospital, Santa Rosa Health Care, Southwest Texas Methodist Hospital, Northeast Methodist Hospital, San Antonio Community Hospital, Women's & Children's Hospital, Metropolitan Hospital, South Texas Ambulatory Surgery Hospital, University Health System · Stone Oak Medical Building, Suite 450, 540 Madison Oak Drive, San Antonio, TX 78258 · 210-494-8859

Robert H. Poirier · Anterior Segment—Cataract & Refractive, Corneal Diseases & Transplantation · Southwest Texas Methodist Hospital · South Texas Family Eye Center, 7810 Louis Pasteur Drive, San Antonio, TX 78229 · 210-692-0218

Edward Raymond Rashid · General Ophthalmology (Corneal Diseases & Transplantation, Anterior Segment—Cataract & Refractive) · 54030 Fredericksburg Road, Suite 100, San Antonio, TX 78229 · 210-340-1212

Robert san Martin · General Ophthalmology · 315 North San Saba, San Antonio, TX 78207 · 210-225-3937

David G. Shulman · General Ophthalmology · St. Luke's Baptist Hospital · 999 East Basse Road, Suite 116, San Antonio, TX 78209 · 210-821-6901

Robert Charles Snip · Corneal Diseases & Transplantation (Glaucoma, Anterior Segment—Cataract & Refractive) · San Antonio Community Hospital, St. Luke's Baptist Hospital, Methodist Healthcare System, Santa Rosa Northwest Hospital, San Antonio Surgery Center · 2833 Babcock Road, Suite 345, San Antonio, TX 78229 · 210-614-3600

James William Speights · Vitreo-Retinal Surgery · St. Luke's Baptist Hospital, San Antonio Community Hospital, Santa Rosa Health Care, Methodist Healthcare System · 7940 Floyd Curl Drive, Suite 820, San Antonio, TX 78229 · 210-615-8413

William E. Sponsel · Glaucoma · University Hospital-South Texas Medical Center · University of Texas Health Science Center at San Antonio, Department of Ophthalmology, 7703 Floyd Curl Drive, San Antonio, TX 78284-6230 · 210-567-8414

Arlo C. Terry · Corneal Diseases & Transplantation · Nix Health Care System · Ophthalmology Associates, 414 Navarro Street, Suite 400, San Antonio, TX 78205 210-223-5561

Stuart A. Terry · Glaucoma (Anterior Segment—Cataract & Refractive) · Baptist Medical Center · Advanced Family Eye Center, 215 East Quincy Street, Suite 200, San Antonio, TX 78215-2030 · 210-226-5191

Elmer Yuchen Tu · Corneal Diseases & Transplantation (Anterior Segment—Cataract & Refractive) · University of Texas Health Science Center at San Antonio, Department of Ophthalmology, 7703 Floyd Curl Drive, San Antonio, TX 78284-6230 · 210-567-8401

Wichard A. J. van Heuven · Medical Retinal Diseases, Vitreo-Retinal Surgery · University Hospital-South Texas Medical Center, Audie L. Murphy Memorial Veterans Hospital, Santa Rosa Northwest Hospital · University of Texas Health Science Center at San Antonio, Department of Ophthalmology, 7703 Floyd Curl Drive, San Antonio, TX 78284-6230 · 210-567-8400

Martha A. Walton · General Ophthalmology · North Central Baptist Hospital, South Texas Ambulatory Surgery Hospital, St. Luke's Baptist Hospital · Diagnostic Clinic of San Antonio, 4647 Medical Drive, San Antonio, TX 78229 · 210-615-1300

William D. Willerson, Jr. · Vitreo-Retinal Surgery (Vitreo-Retinal Diseases, General Ophthalmology, Diabetes Mellitus) · Baptist Medical Center, Southwest Texas Methodist Hospital, San Antonio Community Hospital, Santa Rosa Health Care · 303 East Quincy Street, Suite 100, San Antonio, TX 78215 · 210-271-7648

Temple

Glen O. Brindley · General Ophthalmology (Glaucoma, Oculoplastic & Orbital Surgery) · Scott & White Memorial Hospital, Department of Ophthalmology, 2401 South 31st Street, Temple, TX 76508-0001 · 817-724-2394

Richard D. Cunningham · General Ophthalmology (Optics & Refraction, Neuro-Ophthalmology) · Scott & White Memorial Hospital · Scott & White Memorial Hospital, Department of Ophthalmology, 2401 South 31st Street, Temple, TX 76508-0001 · 817-724-2287

R. Douglas Davis · General Ophthalmology (Retinal Diseases) · Scott & White Memorial Hospital · Scott & White Memorial Hospital, Department of Ophthalmology, 2401 South 31st Street, Temple, TX 76508-0001 · 817-724-5541

J. Paul Dieckert · (Vitreo-Retinal Surgery) · Scott & White Memorial Hospital · Scott & White Memorial Hospital, Division of Ophthalmology, 2401 South 31st Street, Temple, TX 76508-0001 · 817-724-5050

Tyler

Jerry A. Parrish · General Ophthalmology (Anterior Segment—Cataract & Refractive) · Medical Center Hospital, Trinity Mother Frances Health Care Center 1133 Medical Drive, Tyler, TX 75701 · 903-593-2523

Ronald J. Pinkenburg · General Ophthalmology (Anterior Segment—Cataract & Refractive) · Trinity Mother Frances Health Care Center, East Texas Medical Center · Tyler Eye Associates, 820 South Baxter Avenue, Tyler, TX 75701 · 903-593-2461

Jon T. Schreiber · General Ophthalmology (Anterior Segment—Cataract & Refractive, Radial Keratotomy Surgery) · Trinity Mother Frances Health Care Center, East Texas Medical Center · 618 South Broadway, Tyler, TX 75701 · 903-595-4468

Ali Vagefi · Vitreo-Retinal Surgery · Trinity Mother Frances Health Care Center, East Texas Medical Center · Tyler Retina Consultants, 1519 East Front Street, Tyler, TX 75702 · 903-597-4644

Waco

James V. Campbell · Vitreo-Retinal Surgery · 3500 Hillcrest Drive, Suite 2A, Waco, TX 76708 · 817-753-7007

John Liu · General Ophthalmology · Waco Eye Associates, 3500 Hillcrest Drive, Suite Six, Waco, TX 76708 · 817-756-4457

Herman J. Quinius · General Ophthalmology (Anterior Segment—Cataract & Refractive) · Hillcrest Baptist Medical Center, Providence Health Center · Central Texas Eye Clinic, 3115 Pine Avenue, Suite 202, Waco, TX 76708 · 817-752-8328

Russell E. Swann · General Ophthalmology (Anterior Segment—Cataract & Refractive) · Providence Health Center, Hillcrest Baptist Medical Center, West Community Hospital (West), Goodall-Witcher Hospital (Clifton) · 405 Londonderry Drive, Suite 301, Waco, TX 76712-7918 · 817-751-4994

Wichita Falls

Jeffrey V. Harrington · General Ophthalmology · 1508 Brook Avenue, Wichita Falls, TX 76301 · 817-761-2317

Phillip W. Kelly · General Ophthalmology (Anterior Segment—Cataract & Refractive, Glaucoma) · Bethania Regional Health Care Center, Wichita General Hospital, Texoma Outpatient Surgery Center · North Texas Ophthalmology Associates, 1704 Eleventh Street, Wichita Falls, TX 76301-5020 · 817-723-1274

Marylin H. White · General Ophthalmology · Bethania Regional Health Care Center · North Texas Ophthalmology Associates, 1704 Eleventh Street, Wichita Falls, TX 76301-5020 · 817-723-1274

ORTHOPAEDIC SURGERY

Amarillo

Bill S. Barnhill · Sports Medicine/Arthroscopy (Knee Surgery, Shoulder Surgery) · Columbia Panhandle Surgical Hospital, St. Anthony's Hospital · Panhandle Sports Medicine Institute, 7000 West Ninth Street, Amarillo, TX 79106 · 806-359-1800

Howard L. Berg · General Orthopaedic Surgery · High Plains Baptist Hospital · 13 Medical Drive, Amarillo, TX 79106-4151 · 806-358-4531

Andrew F. Brooker · Trauma, Reconstructive Surgery · 13 Medical Drive, Amarillo, TX 79106 · 806-355-6552

Richard F. McKay · General Orthopaedic Surgery (Hip Surgery, Knee Surgery) · St. Anthony's Hospital, High Plains Baptist Hospital · Eight Medical Drive, Amarillo, TX 79106-4136 · 806-353-3529

Earl C. Smith, Jr. · General Orthopaedic Surgery · 320 South Polk Street, Suite 300, Amarillo, TX 79101 · 806-376-5511

Bobby Loyd Stafford · General Orthopaedic Surgery · St. Anthony's Hospital · Eight Medical Drive, Amarillo, TX 79106-4151 · 806-355-9887

Austin

Christopher S. Chenault · General Orthopaedic Surgery · Austin Bone & Joint Clinic, 1015 East 32nd Street, Suite 101, Austin, TX 78705-2700 · 512-477-6341

Donald Robert Davis · General Orthopaedic Surgery · The Orthopaedic Group, 630 West 34th Street, Suite 302, Austin, TX 78705-1203 · 512-459-3228

John A. Genung · General Orthopaedic Surgery · The Orthopaedic Group, 630 West 34th Street, Suite 302, Austin, TX 78705-1203 · 512-459-3228

Charles Bruce Malone III · General Orthopaedic Surgery (Reconstructive Surgery, Trauma) · Seton Medical Center, Brackenridge Hospital, St. David's Healthcare Center · Austin Bone & Joint Clinic, 1015 East 32nd Street, Suite 101, Austin, TX 78705-2700 · 512-477-6341

John Charles Pearce · General Orthopaedic Surgery (Sports Medicine/Arthroscopy, Joint Replacement, Foot & Ankle Surgery, Hip Surgery, Knee Surgery, Reconstructive Surgery, Shoulder Surgery, Trauma) · St. David's Healthcare Center, Seton Medical Center, Brackenridge Hospital · Austin Bone & Joint Clinic, 1015 East 32nd Street, Suite 101, Austin, TX 78705-2700 · 512-477-6341

Stephen Moe Pearce · General Orthopaedic Surgery · St. David's Healthcare Center · Austin Bone & Joint Clinic, 1015 East 32nd Street, Suite 101, Austin, TX 78705-2700 · 512-477-6341

Eugene Paul Schoch III · General Orthopaedic Surgery · Texas Bone & Joint, 711 West 38th Street, Suite E-4, Austin, TX 78705 · 512-452-9584

William Peyton Taylor · Spinal Surgery · Seton Medical Center · Central Texas Spine Institute, 6818 Austin Center Boulevard, Suite 200, Austin, TX 78731 · 512-795-2225

Archie Kent Whittemore · General Orthopaedic Surgery · Seton Medical Center The Orthopaedic Group, 630 West 34th Street, Suite 302, Austin, TX 78705 · 512-459-3228

Beaumont

Jerry D. Clark · General Orthopaedic Surgery (Total Joint Replacement & Revisions) · St. Elizabeth Hospital · Beaumont Bone & Joint Clinic, 3650 Laurel Street, Beaumont, TX 77707-2216 · 409-838-0346

Charles C. Domingues · Foot & Ankle Surgery · Beaumont Bone & Joint Clinic, 3650 Laurel Street, Beaumont, TX 77702-1841 · 409-838-0346

Marshall W. Hayes · Sports Medicine/Arthroscopy (Total Joint Replacement, General Orthopaedic Surgery) · St. Elizabeth Hospital · Beaumont Bone & Joint Clinic, 3650 Laurel Street, Beaumont, TX 77702-1841 · 409-838-0346

Henry A. Reid · Sports Medicine/Arthroscopy (Knee Surgery) · 3129 College Street, Suite 200, Beaumont, TX 77701-4649 · 409-835-5537

Thomas M. Smith · Sports Medicine/Arthroscopy · St. Elizabeth Hospital · Beaumont Bone & Joint Clinic, 3650 Laurel Street, Beaumont, TX 77707-2216 · 409-838-0346

Elizabeth A. Szalay · Pediatric Orthopaedic Surgery (Scoliosis, Congenital Musculoskeletal Abnormalities) · St. Elizabeth Hospital, Baptist Hospital Beaumont · Beaumont Bone & Joint Clinic, 3650 Laurel Street, Beaumont, TX 77707-2216 · 409-838-0346

David D. Teuscher · Sports Medicine/Arthroscopy (Reconstructive Surgery) · St. Elizabeth Hospital, Baptist Hospital Beaumont, Beaumont Surgical Center, Beaumont Regional Medical Center · Beaumont Bone & Joint Clinic, 3650 Laurel Street, Beaumont, TX 77702-1841 · 409-838-0346

Corpus Christi

Charles Clark, Jr. · Knee Surgery · Orthopaedic Surgeons and Sports Medicine, 1333 Third Street, Suite 200, Corpus Christi, TX 78404 · 512-883-2000

James R. Dinn · General Orthopaedic Surgery (Sports Medicine/Arthroscopy) · Spohn Hospital, Doctors Regional Medical Center, Driscoll Children's Hospital · Orthopaedic Surgeons and Sports Medicine, 1333 Third Street, Suite 200, Corpus Christi, TX 78404 · 512-883-2000

Michael M. Heckman · Sports Medicine/Arthroscopy (Knee Surgery, Shoulder Surgery) · Orthopaedic Surgeons and Sports Medicine, 1333 Third Street, Suite 200, Corpus Christi, TX 78404 · 512-883-2000

Christopher H. Isensee · General Orthopaedic Surgery · 3302 South Alameda Street, Corpus Christi, TX 78411-1826 · 512-854-6231

Dallas

John G. Birch · Pediatric Orthopaedic Surgery · Texas Scottish Rite Hospital for Children · Texas Scottish Rite Hospital for Children, Department of Orthopaedics, 2222 Welborn Street, Dallas, TX 75219 · 214-559-7557

James W. Brodsky · Foot & Ankle Surgery · Orthopedic Associates of Dallas, 411 North Washington Avenue, Suite 7000, Dallas, TX 75246-1777 · 214-823-7090

Robert W. Bucholz · Trauma (Reconstructive Hip & Knee Surgery, Biomaterials in Orthopaedic Surgery) · Parkland Memorial Hospital, Zale Lipshy University Hospital, Children's Medical Center of Dallas, VA Medical Center, Healthsouth Dallas Rehabilitation Institute, Texas Scottish Rite Hospital for Children · University of Texas-Southwestern Medical Center at Dallas, Department of Orthopaedic Surgery, 5323 Harry Hines Boulevard, Dallas, TX 75235-8883 · 214-648-3871

Wayne Z. Burkhead, Jr. · Shoulder Surgery (Elbow Surgery, Sports Medicine/Arthroscopy) · Baylor University Medical Center, Mary Shiels Hospital, Presbyterian Hospital of Dallas · W. B. Carrell Memorial Clinic, 2909 Lemmon Avenue, Dallas, TX 75204 · 214-220-2468

Daniel E. Cooper · Sports Medicine/Arthroscopy, Foot & Ankle Surgery (Knee Surgery, Shoulder Surgery) · Baylor University Medical Center, Mary Shiels Hospital, Presbyterian Hospital of Dallas · W. B. Carrell Memorial Clinic, 2909 Lemmon Avenue, Dallas, TX 75204-2385 · 214-220-2468

Phillip E. Hansen · Shoulder Surgery (Hand Surgery) · Orthopaedic Associates of Dallas, 411 North Washington Avenue, Suite 7000, Dallas, TX 75246 · 214-823-7090

John A. Herring · Pediatric Orthopaedic Surgery (Spinal Surgery) · Texas Scottish Rite Hospital for Children · Texas Scottish Rite Hospital for Children, Department of Orthopaedics, 2222 Welborn Street, Dallas, TX 75219-3993 · 214-559-7556

Robert W. Jackson · Sports Medicine/Arthroscopy (Knee Surgery) · Baylor University Medical Center · Baylor University Medical Center, 3500 Gaston Avenue, Dallas, TX 75246 · 214-820-3434

Richard Edward Jones III · Reconstructive Surgery (Total Joint Replacement, Hip Surgery, Knee Surgery, Shoulder Surgery) · St. Paul Medical Center · Southwest Orthopaedic Institute, 5920 Forest Park Road, Suite 600, Dallas, TX 75235 214-350-7500

Roby Dan Mize · Trauma (Severe Fractures, Pediatric Orthopaedic Surgery, Sports Medicine/Arthroscopy) · Presbyterian Hospital of Dallas · Texas Orthopaedics Associates, 8210 Walnut Hill Lane, Suite 416, Dallas, TX 75231 · 214-750-1207

James B. Montgomery · Sports Medicine/Arthroscopy (Knee Surgery) · St. Paul Medical Center · Southwest Orthopaedic Institute, 5920 Forest Park Road, Suite 600, Dallas, TX 75235-6411 · 214-350-7500

Paul Conrad Peters, Jr. · Reconstructive Surgery (Hip Surgery, Knee Surgery) · Presbyterian Hospital of Dallas, Baylor University Medical Center · W. B. Carrell Memorial Clinic, 2909 Lemmon Avenue, Dallas, TX 75204-2385 · 214-220-2468

Charles Marshall Reinert · Trauma (Pelvic Fractures, Acetabular Fractures, Complex Extremity Fractures, Trauma Reconstruction) · Parkland Memorial Hospital, Zale Lipshy University Hospital, Children's Medical Center of Dallas · University of Texas-Southwestern Medical Center at Dallas, Department of Orthopaedic Surgery, 5323 Harry Hines Boulevard, Dallas, TX 75235-8883 · 214-648-6771

B. Stephens Richards III · Pediatric Orthopaedic Surgery · Texas Scottish Rite Hospital for Children · Texas Scottish Rite Hospital for Children, Department of Orthopaedics, 2222 Welborn Street, Dallas, TX 75219-3924 · 214-559-7561

Timothy G. Schacherer · Trauma (Upper Extremity, Hand Surgery, Soft Tissue Reconstruction) · Parkland Memorial Hospital, Zale Lipshy University Hospital, Children's Medical Center of Dallas · University of Texas-Southwestern Medical Center at Dallas, Department of Orthopaedic Surgery, 5323 Harry Hines Boulevard, Dallas, TX 75235-8883 · 214-648-8739

Robert R. Scheinberg · General Orthopaedic Surgery (Sports Medicine/Arthroscopy, Knee Surgery, Shoulder Surgery) · Presbyterian Hospital of Dallas, Presbyterian Hospital of Plano (Plano), Medical Arts Hospital of Dallas, Doctors Hospital of Dallas, Baylor-Richardson Medical Center (Richardson) · Texas Orthopaedics Associates, 8210 Walnut Hill Lane, Suite 416, Dallas, TX 75231 · 214-750-1207

Richard D. Schubert · General Orthopaedic Surgery (Total Joint Replacement) · Baylor University Medical Center · W. B. Carrell Memorial Clinic, 2909 Lemmon Avenue, Dallas, TX 75204-2385 · 214-220-2468

Robert D. Vandermeer · Sports Medicine/Arthroscopy · Baylor University Medical Center, Mary Shiels Hospital · W. B. Carrell Memorial Clinic, 2909 Lemmon Avenue, Dallas, TX 75204-2385 · 214-220-2468

Robert G. Viere · Spinal Surgery (Spinal Cord Injury, Diseases of the Cervical Spine, Spinal Deformity) · Zale Lipshy University Hospital, VA Medical Center University of Texas-Southwestern Medical Center at Dallas, Department of Orthopaedic Surgery, 5323 Harry Hines Boulevard, Dallas, TX 75235-8883 · 214-648-3065

El Paso

Thomas J. Scully · General Orthopaedic Surgery · William Beaumont Army Medical Center, 5005 North Piedras Street, El Paso, TX 79920-5001 · 915-569-2316; 915-569-1834

Fort Worth

George N. Armstrong, Jr. · General Orthopaedic Surgery · 556 Eighth Avenue, Fort Worth, TX 76104-2010 · 817-336-6222

Ajai Cadambi · Hip Surgery, Knee Surgery · Texas Hip & Knee Center, 750 Eighth Avenue, Suite 300, Fort Worth, TX 76104-2500 · 817-877-3432

John Conway · Sports Medicine/Arthroscopy · Harris Methodist-Fort Worth · Orthopaedic Specialty Associates, 1325 Pennsylvania Avenue, Suite 890, Fort Worth, TX 76104 · 817-878-5300

Harry Anderson Dollahite · General Orthopaedic Surgery · Harris Methodist-Fort Worth, All Saints Episcopal Hospital-Fort Worth · 1201 Eighth Avenue, Suite A, Fort Worth, TX 76104-4104 · 817-332-3869

Gary L. Douglas · Pediatric Orthopaedic Surgery (Spinal Surgery) · Cook Children's Medical Center · Cook Children's Medical Center, Department of Pediatric Orthopaedic Surgery, 801 Seventh Avenue, Fort Worth, TX 76104-2796 · 817-885-4405

Hinton H. Hamilton III · Pediatric Orthopaedic Surgery · Cook Children's Orthopaedic Services, 1430 West Humbolt Street, Fort Worth, TX 76104 · 817-336-2664

Robert W. Hunnicutt · General Orthopaedic Surgery · 5701 Bryant Irvin Road, South, Suite 101, Fort Worth, TX 76132 · 817-346-4116

Larry D. Messer · Pediatric Orthopaedic Surgery · Cook Children's Orthopaedics, 1430 West Humbolt Street, Fort Worth, TX 76104-2712 · 817-332-4818

John A. Richards · (Adult Hip Surgery, Adult Knee Surgery, Sports Medicine/Arthroscopy) · All Saints Episcopal Hospital, Harris Methodist-Fort Worth, Harris Methodist-Southwest, Plaza Medical Center · 556 Eighth Avenue, Fort Worth, TX 76104-2010 · 817-336-6222

James William Roach · Pediatric Orthopaedic Surgery (Scoliosis Surgery, Spinal Surgery) · Cook Children's Medical Center · Cook Children's Medical Center, 801 Seventh Avenue, Fort Worth, TX 76104-2796 · 817-885-4405

Robert H. Schmidt · Hip Surgery, Knee Surgery · Texas Hip & Knee Center, 750 Eighth Avenue, Suite 300, Fort Worth, TX 76104-2500 · 817-877-3432

Keith C. Watson · Shoulder Surgery (Elbow Surgery) · Harris Methodist-Fort Worth, Tarrant County Hospital, All Saints Episcopal Hospital-Fort Worth, Plaza Medical Center · Orthopaedic Specialty Associates, 1325 Pennsylvania Avenue, Suite 890, Fort Worth, TX 76104-2145 · 817-878-5300

Galveston

Jason H. Calhoun · General Orthopaedic Surgery (Foot & Ankle Surgery, Osteomyelitis, Musculoskeletal Infections) · University of Texas Medical Branch Hospitals · University of Texas Medical Branch, Department of Orthopaedics and Rehabilitation, 301 University Boulevard, Galveston, TX 77555-0792 · 409-772-2565

Houston

Donald E. Baxter · Foot & Ankle Surgery (Runners' Injuries) · Methodist Hospital, Memorial Hospital-Southwest · 2500 Fondren Street, Suite 350, Houston, TX 77063 · 713-782-4532

James R. Bocell, Jr. · Knee Surgery · 6560 Fannin Street, Suite 400, Houston, TX 77030 · 713-790-2954

William J. Bryan · Sports Medicine/Arthroscopy (Total Joint Replacement, Hip Surgery, Knee Surgery, Shoulder Disorders) · Methodist Hospital · Baylor College of Medicine, Department of Orthopaedic Surgery, 6560 Fannin Street, Suite 400, Houston, TX 77030 · 713-790-2951

Thomas O. Clanton · Sports Medicine/Arthroscopy (Knee Surgery, Foot & Ankle Surgery) · Hermann Hospital, Diagnostic Center Hospital, Columbia Medical Center · 2500 Fondren Street, Suite 350, Houston, TX 77063 · 713-782-4532; 713-791-9088

Jesse H. Dickson · Spinal Surgery (Scoliosis) · Methodist Hospital, Texas Children's Hospital, St. Luke's Episcopal Hospital · Baylor College of Medicine, Department of Orthopaedic Surgery, 6550 Fannin Street, Suite 2501, Houston, TX 77030 · 713-790-2791

Richard H. Eppright · General Orthopaedic Surgery (Total Joint Arthroplasty, Acetabular Dysplasia, Dial Osteotomy) · Methodist Hospital, Texas Children's Hospital · 6550 Fannin Street, Suite 2201, Houston, TX 77030 · 713-790-6425

Wendell Dwight Erwin · Pediatric Orthopaedic Surgery (Scoliosis) · Texas Children's Hospital, Methodist Hospital, St. Luke's Episcopal Hospital · Texas Children's Hospital, 6621 Fannin Street, Suite 200, Mail Code 3-2295, Houston, TX 77030 · 713-770-3110

Stephen Ivor Esses · Spinal Surgery · Methodist Hospital · Baylor College of Medicine, Department of Orthopaedic Surgery, 6550 Fannin Street, Suite 2501, Houston, TX 77030 · 713-790-3709

Gary M. Gartsman · Shoulder Surgery · Texas Orthopaedic Hospital, St. Luke's Episcopal Hospital, Methodist Hospital · Fondren Orthopaedic Group, 7401 South Main Street, Houston, TX 77030 · 713-799-2300

Michael H. Heggeness · Spinal Surgery · Methodist Hospital, St. Luke's Episcopal Hospital, Texas Children's Hospital · Baylor College of Medicine, 6560 Fannin Street, Suite 1900, Houston, TX 77030 · 713-790-6410

Richard J. Kearns · General Orthopaedic Surgery (Joint Replacements, Orthopaedic Oncology, Hip Surgery, Knee Surgery, Tumor Surgery) · Methodist Hospital · Fondren Orthopaedic Group, 7401 South Main Street, Houston, TX 77030 713-799-2300

Glenn C. Landon · (Joint Replacement, Orthopaedic Infections, Hip Surgery, Knee Surgery, Reconstructive Surgery) · St. Luke's Episcopal Hospital, Methodist Hospital · Kelsey-Seybold Clinic, 6624 Fannin Street, 18th Floor, Houston, TX 77030 · 713-791-8700

Ronald W. Lindsey · Trauma, Spinal Surgery (Spine, Pelvic, Limb) · Baylor College of Medicine, Department of Orthopaedic Surgery, 6550 Fannin Street, Suite 2625, Houston, TX 77030 · 713-790-4818

Kenneth Bradford Mathis · General Orthopaedic Surgery (Joint Replacement, Hip Surgery, Knee Surgery) · Methodist Hospital, Memorial Hospital-Southeast · Memorial Hospital-Southeast, 11914 Astoria Boulevard, Suite 670, Houston, TX 77089 · 713-484-4800

James Bruce Moseley, Jr. · Sports Medicine/Arthroscopy · Methodist Hospital · Baylor College of Medicine, Department of Orthopaedic Surgery, 6560 Fannin Street, Suite 400, Houston, TX 77030 · 713-790-3851

John A. Murray · Tumor Surgery · University of Texas-M. D. Anderson Cancer Center · University of Texas-M. D. Anderson Cancer Center, Department of Surgical Oncology, 1515 Holcombe Boulevard, Box 106, Houston, TX 77030 · 713-792-8828

Jeffrey D. Reuben · General Orthopaedic Surgery (Lower Extremity) · Orthopaedic Consultants of Houston, 6410 Fannin Street, Suite 1100, Houston, TX 77030 · 713-704-2580

Hugh S. Tullos · Hip Surgery (Total Joint Surgery of Hip, Knee, and Shoulder) · Methodist Hospital · Baylor College of Medicine, Department of Orthopaedic Surgery, 6550 Fannin Street, Suite 2625, Houston, TX 77030 · 713-790-3112

Lubbock

Eugene Jean Dabezies · Trauma (Hand Surgery, Arthritis) · University Medical Center · Texas Tech University Health Sciences Center, 3601 Fourth Street, Room 1A113, Lubbock, TX 79430 · 806-743-2465

Mark Scioli · Foot & Ankle Surgery (Spine Reconstruction, Total Joint Reconstruction) · St. Mary of the Plains Hospital, Lubbock Methodist Hospital, University Medical Center · Center for Orthopaedic Surgery, 4102 Twenty-Fourth Street, Suite 300, Lubbock, TX 79410 · 806-797-4985

Peter Stasikelis · Pediatric Orthopaedic Surgery · University Medical Center, Lubbock Methodist Hospital, St. Mary of the Plains Hospital · Texas Tech University Health Sciences Center, Department of Orthopaedic Surgery, 3601 Fourth Street, Lubbock, TX 79430 · 806-743-3038

Midland

Thurston E. Dean · General Orthopaedic Surgery · 509 North Garfield Street, Midland, TX 79701 · 915-682-0433

Donald W. Floyd · General Orthopaedic Surgery · Southwest Orthopaedics, 4304 Andrews Highway, Midland, TX 79703 · 915-520-3050

David J. Power · General Orthopaedic Surgery · Southwest Orthopaedics, 4304 Andrews Highway, Midland, TX 79703 · 915-520-3020

Plano

Roger Hill Emerson, Jr. · Reconstructive Surgery (Hip Surgery, Knee Surgery) · Presbyterian Hospital of Plano · Texas Center for Joint Replacement, 6300 West Parker Road, Suite 220, Plano, TX 75093 · 214-608-8868

William C. Head · Reconstructive Surgery (Hip Surgery, Knee Surgery) · Presbyterian Hospital of Dallas (Dallas) · Texas Center for Joint Replacement, 6300 West Parker Road, Suite 220, Plano, TX 75093 · 214-608-8868

Stephen Howard Hochschuler · Spinal Surgery (Failed Lumbar Surgery, Sports & the Spine, Rehabilitation of the Spine) · Medical Center of Plano, Presbyterian Hospital of Plano · Texas Back Institute, 6300 West Parker Road, Plano, TX 75093-7916 · 214-608-5000

Ralph F. Rashbaum · Spinal Surgery (Spinal Disorders, Management of Chronic Spinal Pain States with Spinal Cord Stimulation & Spine Administered Narcotics) · Presbyterian Hospital of Plano · Texas Back Institute, 6300 West Parker Road, Plano, TX 75093 · 214-608-5000

San Antonio

Robert M. Campbell, Jr. · Pediatric Orthopaedic Surgery (Complex Chest Wall/ Spinal Deformities in Infants and Children) · Santa Rosa Children's Hospital, University Hospital-South Texas Medical Center · University of Texas Health Science Center at San Antonio, Department of Orthopaedics, 7703 Floyd Curl Drive, San Antonio, TX 78284-7774 · 210-567-5125

Ralph John Curtis, Jr. · Shoulder Surgery · Nix Health Care System, Southwest Texas Methodist Hospital, San Antonio Community Hospital, St. Luke's Baptist Hospital, Santa Rosa Northwest Hospital · Orthopaedic Surgery Associates of San Antonio, 9150 Huebner Road, Suite 250A, San Antonio, TX 78240-1501 · 210-561-7100

Jesse C. Delee · Sports Medicine/Arthroscopy (Reconstructive, Total Joint Replacement) · South Texas Ambulatory Surgery Hospital, Nix Health Care System, Southwest Texas Methodist Hospital, Baptist Medical Center, Santa Rosa Northwest Hospital · Orthopaedic Surgery Associates of San Antonio, 9150 Huebner Road, Suite 250A, San Antonio, TX 78240 · 210-561-7100

John Allan Evans · General Orthopaedic Surgery (Total Joint Replacement) · Orthopaedic Surgery Associates of San Antonio, 9150 Huebner Road, Suite 250A, San Antonio, TX 78240 · 210-561-7100

Mayo J. Galindo, Jr. · Foot & Ankle Surgery · Southwest Texas Methodist Hospital · 9150 Huebner Road, Suite 200, San Antonio, TX 78240 · 210-561-7060

Brad B. Hall · General Orthopaedic Surgery (Spine) · St. Luke's Baptist Hospital South Texas Orthopaedics & Spinal Surgery Associates, 9150 Huebner Road, Suite 350, San Antonio, TX 78240 · 210-561-7234

James Donald Heckman · Foot & Ankle Surgery · University Hospital-South Texas Medical Center · University of Texas Health Science Center at San Antonio, Department of Orthopaedics, 7703 Floyd Curl Drive, San Antonio, TX 78284-7774 · 210-567-5125

Peter F. Holmes · Sports Medicine/Arthroscopy · Metropolitan Hospital · Orthopaedic Surgery Associates of San Antonio, 9150 Huebner Road, Suite 250A, San Antonio, TX 78240 · 210-561-7100

Jay D. Mabrey · General Orthopaedic Surgery (Hip Surgery, Knee Surgery, Total Joint Replacement) · University Hospital-South Texas Medical Center · University of Texas Health Science Center at San Antonio, Department of Orthopaedics, 7703 Floyd Curl Drive, San Antonio, TX 78284-7774 · 210-567-6290

Peter L. J. McGanity · Trauma · University Hospital-South Texas Medical Center University of Texas Health Science Center at San Antonio, Department of Orthopaedics, 7703 Floyd Curl Drive, San Antonio, TX 78284-7774 · 210-567-5125

Charles A. Rockwood, Jr. · Reconstructive Surgery, Shoulder Surgery · University Hospital-South Texas Medical Center · University of Texas Health Science Center at San Antonio, Department of Orthopaedics, 7703 Floyd Curl Drive, San Antonio, TX 78284-7774 · 210-567-5125

Albert Earnest Sanders · Spinal Surgery (Scoliosis) · Nix Health Care System · 1431 Nix Professional Building, 414 Navarro Street, San Antonio, TX 78205 · 210-271-7767

James O. Sanders · Pediatric Orthopaedic Surgery · Pediatric Orthopaedic Associates of San Antonio, Medical Center Tower II, Suite 630, 7940 Floyd Curl Drive, San Antonio, TX 78229 · 210-692-1613

Robert Cumming Schenck, Jr. · Sports Medicine/Arthroscopy · University of Texas Health Science Center at San Antonio, Department of Orthopaedics, 7703 Floyd Curl Drive, San Antonio, TX 78284-7774 · 210-567-6447

David Richard Schmidt · Sports Medicine/Arthroscopy (Knee Surgery, General Orthopaedic Surgery) · St. Luke's Baptist Hospital, Southwest Texas Methodist Hospital, San Antonio Community Hospital, South Texas Ambulatory Surgery Hospital · Orthopaedic Surgery Associates of San Antonio, 9150 Huebner Road, Suite 250A, San Antonio, TX 78240 · 210-561-7100

Earl Austin Stanley · Pediatric Orthopaedic Surgery (Spinal Surgery) · Santa Rosa Children's Hospital · Pediatric Orthopaedic Associates of San Antonio, 343 West Houston Street, Suite 303, San Antonio, TX 78205 · 210-692-1613

John S. Toohey · Spinal Surgery · University Hospital-South Texas Medical Center, Baptist Memorial Healthcare System, Santa Rosa Health Care · University of Texas Health Science Center at San Antonio, Department of Orthopaedics, 7703 Floyd Curl Drive, San Antonio, TX 78284-7774 · 210-567-4997

Lorence Wain Trick · General Orthopaedic Surgery (Total Joint Replacement, Revision Joint Replacement) · Metropolitan Hospital, Nix Health Care System, Southwest Texas Methodist Hospital · 414 Navarro Street, Suite 1128, San Antonio, TX 78205 · 210-351-6500

Jeffrey R. Warmann · Pediatric Orthopaedic Surgery (Spinal Surgery, Hip Surgery, Foot Surgery) · Santa Rosa Children's Hospital, Southwest Texas Methodist Hospital/Children's Hospital · Pediatric Orthopaedic Associates of San Antonio, 7940 Floyd Curl Drive, Suite 630, San Antonio, TX 78229 · 210-692-1613

Kaye Evan Wilkins · Pediatric Orthopaedic Surgery · Pediatric Orthopaedic Associates of San Antonio, 343 West Houston Street, Suite 303, San Antonio, TX 78205-2103 · 210-692-1613

Ronald Paul Williams · Tumor Surgery (Orthopaedic Oncology) · University Hospital-South Texas Medical Center, Audie L. Murphy Memorial Veterans Hospital, St. Luke's Baptist Hospital, Santa Rosa Health Care · University of Texas Health Science Center at San Antonio, Department of Orthopaedics, 7703 Floyd Curl Drive, San Antonio, TX 78284-7774 · 210-567-6446

Michael A. Wirth · Shoulder Surgery (Total Joint Replacement) · University Hospital-South Texas Medical Center · University of Texas Health Science Center at San Antonio, Department of Orthopaedics, 7703 Floyd Curl Drive, San Antonio, TX 78284-7774 · 210-567-5125

Temple

George W. Brindley · General Orthopaedic Surgery · Scott & White Memorial Hospital · Scott & White Memorial Hospital, Department of Orthopaedic Surgery, 2401 South 31st Street, Temple, TX 76508-0001 · 817-724-2422

Hanes H. Brindley, Jr. · Pediatric Orthopaedic Surgery · Scott & White Memorial Hospital · Scott & White Memorial Hospital, Department of Orthopaedic Surgery, 2401 South 31st Street, Temple, TX 76508-0001 · 817-724-2749

Tyler

William E. Schreiber · General Orthopaedic Surgery · Azalea Orthopaedic and Sports Medicine Clinic, 700 Olympic Plaza, Suite 700, Tyler, TX 75701 · 903-595-1049

John F. Walker · General Orthopaedic Surgery · Azalea Orthopaedic and Sports Medicine Clinic, 700 Olympic Plaza, Suite 700, Tyler, TX 75701 · 903-595-3464

Waco

Jerry A. Benham · General Orthopaedic Surgery · Providence Health Center · Waco Orthopaedic Clinic, 2200 North 25th Street, Waco, TX 76708 · 817-752-9638

Ray W. Covington · General Orthopaedic Surgery · Hillcrest Baptist Medical Center · Waco Bone & Joint Clinic, 3500 Hillcrest Drive, Waco, TX 76708 · 817-754-0375

John K. Ethridge · General Orthopaedic Surgery · Providence Health Center · Waco Orthopaedic Clinic, 2200 North 25th Street, Waco, TX 76708-3318 · 817-752-9638

David W. Sudbrink · General Orthopaedic Surgery · Hillcrest Baptist Medical Center · Waco Bone & Joint Clinic, 3500 Hillcrest Drive, Waco, TX 76708 · 817-754-0375

OTOLARYNGOLOGY

Amarillo

Gary W. Bryan · General Otolaryngology · High Plains Baptist Hospital · 7305-B Wallace Boulevard, Amarillo, TX 79106-1806 · 806-355-8948

Michael D. Guttenplan · General Otolaryngology · High Plains Baptist Hospital, Amarillo Hospital District-Northwest Texas Hospital · Amarillo Ear, Nose & Throat, 3501 Soncy Road, Suite 106, Amarillo, TX 79121 · 806-355-5625

Martin L. Schneider · General Otolaryngology · St. Anthony's Hospital · 5311 West Ninth Street, Suite 104, Amarillo, TX 79106 · 806-358-4327

Geoffrey L. Wright · General Otolaryngology · Amarillo Hospital District-Northwest Texas Hospital · Amarillo Ear, Nose & Throat, 3501 Soncy Road, Suite 106, Amarillo, TX 79121 · 806-355-5625

Austin

George Paul Burns · General Otolaryngology · Austin Ear, Nose & Throat Clinic, 3705 Medical Parkway, Suite 320, Austin, TX 78705 · 512-454-0392

Christopher Paul Dehan · General Otolaryngology (Sinus & Nasal Surgery, Head & Neck Surgery) · Seton Medical Center, St. David's Healthcare Center, Brackenridge Hospital · Austin Ear, Nose & Throat Clinic, 3705 Medical Parkway, Suite 320, Austin, TX 78705 · 512-454-0392

Steven Trey Fyfe · General Otolaryngology (Head & Neck Surgery) · Seton Medical Center, Children's Hospital of Austin · Austin Ear, Nose & Throat Clinic, 3705 Medical Parkway, Suite 320, Austin, TX 78705 · 512-454-0392

Arthur Boyd Morgan · General Otolaryngology · 1111 West 34th Street, Suite 100, Austin, TX 78705 · 512-459-8783

John Howard Nowlin · Pediatric Otolaryngology · Children's Hospital of Austin 711 West 38th Street, Suite C-8, Austin, TX 78705-1126 · 512-452-0231

Drew Grant Sawyer · Pediatric Otolaryngology · Seton Medical Center, Children's Hospital of Austin · 711 West 38th Street, Suite C-8, Austin, TX 78705-1126 · 512-452-0231

John W. Youngblood, Jr. · General Otolaryngology · Seton Medical Center · Austin Ear Clinic, 711 West 38th Street, Suite C-1, Austin, TX 78705-1126 · 512-454-0341

Beaumont

Ray Fontenot, Jr. · General Otolaryngology (Allergy, Sinus & Nasal Surgery) · St. Elizabeth Hospital · Southeast Texas Ear, Nose & Throat, 3030 North Street, Suite 520, Beaumont, TX 77702 · 409-892-6401

Carl C. Jordan · General Otolaryngology · St. Elizabeth Hospital · Southeast Texas Ear, Nose & Throat, 3030 North Street, Suite 520, Beaumont, TX 77702 409-892-6401

Thomas J. Killian · General Otolaryngology · St. Elizabeth Hospital · Southeast Texas Ear, Nose & Throat, 3030 North Street, Suite 520, Beaumont, TX 77702 409-892-6401

Harold S. Parks, Jr. · General Otolaryngology (Head & Neck Cancer Surgery, Sinus & Nasal Surgery, Laryngology, Otology, Pediatric Otolaryngology) · St. Elizabeth Hospital, Baptist Hospital Beaumont, Beaumont Regional Medical Center · Southeast Texas Ear, Nose & Throat, 3030 North Street, Suite 520, Beaumont, TX 77702 · 409-892-6401

Corpus Christi

George H. Fisher · General Otolaryngology · Ear, Nose & Throat Associates, 3318 South Alameda Street, Corpus Christi, TX 78411-1868 · 512-854-7000

Michael L. Mintz · General Otolaryngology · Ear, Nose & Throat Associates, 3318 South Alameda Street, Corpus Christi, TX 78411-1868 · 512-854-7000

James M. Motes, Jr. · General Otolaryngology · Ear, Nose & Throat Associates, 3318 South Alameda Street, Corpus Christi, TX 78411-1868 · 512-854-7000

Robert D. Oshman · General Otolaryngology · Ear, Nose & Throat Associates, 3318 South Alameda Street, Corpus Christi, TX 78411-1868 · 512-854-7000

Alan I. Zane · General Otolaryngology · Ear, Nose & Throat Associates, 3318 South Alameda Street, Corpus Christi, TX 78411-1868 · 512-854-7000

Dallas

Orval E. Brown · Pediatric Otolaryngology (Choanal Atresia, Extensive Skull Base and Neck Cystic Hygroma, Laryngeal Reconstruction) · Children's Medical Center of Dallas · University of Texas-Southwestern Medical Center at Dallas, Department of Otolaryngology, 5323 Harry Hines Boulevard, Dallas, TX 75235-9035 · 214-648-3103

Henry M. Carder · General Otolaryngology (Otology, Pediatric Otolaryngology, Sinus & Nasal Surgery) · Children's Medical Center of Dallas, Presbyterian Hospital of Dallas · 8315 Walnut Hill Lane, Suite 135, Dallas, TX 75231-4211 · 214-369-8121

Marvin C. Culbertson, Jr · Pediatric Otolaryngology (Otology) · Children's Medical Center of Dallas, St. Paul Medical Center, Parkland Memorial Hospital University of Texas-Southwestern Medical Center at Dallas, Department of Otolaryngology, 5323 Harry Hines Boulevard, Dallas, TX 75235-9060 · 214-368-1316

Joseph Lee Leach, Jr. · General Otolaryngology (Facial Plastic Surgery, Sinus & Nasal Surgery) · Zale Lipshy University Hospital, St. Paul Medical Center, Parkland Memorial Hospital, Children's Medical Center of Dallas · University of Texas-Southwestern Medical Center at Dallas, 5323 Harry Hines Boulevard, Dallas, TX 75235-9035 · 214-648-3071

Richard L. Mabry · General Otolaryngology (Allergy of the Nose & Sinuses, Sinus & Nasal Surgery) · Zale Lipshy University Hospital · University of Texas-Southwestern Medical Center at Dallas, Department of Otolaryngology, 5323 Harry Hines Boulevard, Dallas, TX 75235-9035 · 214-648-2243; 214-648-3071

William L. Meyerhoff · Otology/Neurotology (Otology) · Zale Lipshy University Hospital · University of Texas-Southwestern Medical Center at Dallas, Department of Otolaryngology, 5323 Harry Hines Boulevard, Dallas, TX 75235-9035 · 214-648-2432

Fred D. Owens · Otology (Otology/Neurotology, Skull-Base Surgery) · Baylor University Medical Center · Baylor University Medical Center, 3600 Gaston Avenue, Suite 1103, Dallas, TX 75246 · 214-742-2194

Peter S. Roland · Otology (Otology/Neurotology, Skull-Base Surgery) · Zale Lipshy University Hospital, St. Paul Medical Center, Children's Medical Center of Dallas, Parkland Memorial Hospital · University of Texas-Southwestern Medical Center at Dallas, Department of Otolaryngology, 5323 Harry Hines Boulevard, Dallas, TX 75235-9035 · 214-648-3102

John Morrow Truelson · Head & Neck Surgery (Microvascular Reconstruction, Sleep Apnea, Sinus Surgery) · Zale Lipshy University Hospital, Parkland Memorial Hospital, VA Medical Center, St. Paul Medical Center · University of Texas-Southwestern Medical Center at Dallas, Department of Otolaryngology, 5323 Harry Hines Boulevard, Mail Code 9035, Dallas, TX 75235-9035 · 214-648-3071

El Paso

Jorge J. Arango · General Otolaryngology (Head & Neck Cancer, Sinus & Nasal Surgery, Facial Surgery, Otology, Maxillofacial Surgery, Reconstructive Nasal Surgery) · Columbia Medical Center-West, Columbia Medical Center-East, Providence Memorial Hospital, Sierra Medical Center · El Paso Ear, Nose & Throat Associates, 5959 Gateway Boulevard West, Suite 160, El Paso, TX 79925-3331 · 915-779-5866

Richard A. D. Morton, Jr. · General Otolaryngology · Sierra Medical Center · 1733 Curie Drive, Suite 100, El Paso, TX 79902-2907 · 915-533-5461

Mark J. Wegleitner · General Otolaryngology (Diagnostic Otology, Head & Neck Cancer, Sinus & Nasal Surgery) · Providence Memorial Hospital, Sierra Medical Center, Columbia Medical Center-West, Columbia Medical Center-East · El Paso Ear, Nose & Throat Associates, 5959 Gateway Boulevard West, Suite 160, El Paso, TX 79925-3331 · 915-779-5866

Euless

John R. Marchbanks · General Otolaryngology · Midcity Ear, Nose, Throat and Facial Plastic Surgery, 451 Westpark Way, Suite Seven, Euless, TX 76040-3994 · 817-540-3121

John C. Ponder · General Otolaryngology · Harris Methodist HEB (Bedford) · Midcity Ear, Nose, Throat and Facial Plastic Surgery, 451 Westpark Way, Suite One, Euless, TX 76040 · 817-540-3121

Charles H. Railsback · General Otolaryngology · 451 Westpark Way, Suite One, Euless, TX 76040 · 817-540-3121

Fort Worth

Philip Fowler Anthony · Otology · 901 Hemphill Street, Fort Worth, TX 76104-3111 · 817-332-4060

Robert J. Burkett · General Otolaryngology · 800 Eighth Avenue, Suite 618, Fort Worth, TX 76104 · 817-335-6336

J. Mark Palmer · General Otolaryngology (Pediatric, Adult, Head & Neck Surgery, Laryngology, Sinus & Nasal Surgery) · Cook Children's Medical Center, All Saints Episcopal Hospital-Fort Worth, Plaza Medical Center, Harris Methodist-Fort Worth · 800 Eighth Avenue, Suite 426, Fort Worth, TX 76104 · 817-334-0686

Howard L. Shaffer · General Otolaryngology (Endoscopic Sinus Surgery, Facial Plastic Surgery, Head & Neck Surgery, Pediatric Otolaryngology, Sinus & Nasal Surgery) · Harris Methodist-Southwest, Cook Children's Medical Center, Plaza Medical Center, All Saints Hospital-Cityview, Surgery Center · 6100 Harris Parkway, Suite 350, Fort Worth, TX 76132 · 817-346-5350

Leslie C. Strange III · General Otolaryngology · 800 Eighth Avenue, Suite 326, Fort Worth, TX 76104 · 817-870-2611

Galveston

Byron J. Bailey · Laryngology, Head & Neck Surgery (Laryngeal Cancer, Laryngeal Reconstruction) · University of Texas Medical Branch Hospitals · University of Texas Medical Branch, Department of Otolaryngology, 301 University Boulevard, Galveston, TX 77555-0521 · 409-772-2704

Karen H. Calhoun · General Otolaryngology (Head & Neck Cancer, Facial Plastic & Reconstructive Surgery) · University of Texas Medical Branch Hospitals · University of Texas Medical Branch, Department of Otolaryngology, 301 University Boulevard, Galveston, TX 77555-0521 · 409-772-2705

Ronald W. Deskin · Pediatric Otolaryngology (Neonatal & Infant Airway) · University of Texas Medical Branch Hospitals · University of Texas Medical Branch, Department of Otolaryngology, 301 University Boulevard, Galveston, TX 77555-0521 · 409-772-2703

Christopher H. Rassekh · Head & Neck Surgery (Sinus & Nasal Surgery, Skull-Base Surgery) · University of Texas Medical Branch Hospitals · University of Texas Medical Branch, Department of Otolaryngology, 301 University Boulevard, Galveston, TX 77555-0521 · 409-772-4688

Jeffrey T. Vrabec · Otology/Neurotology (Skull-Base Surgery) · University of Texas Medical Branch Hospitals · University of Texas Medical Branch, Department of Otolaryngology, 301 University Boulevard, Galveston, TX 77555-0521 · 409-772-4688

Houston

Bobby R. Alford · Otology/Neurotology (Head & Neck Surgery) · Methodist Hospital · Baylor College of Medicine, One Baylor Plaza, Room NA-102, Houston, TX 77030 · 713-798-5906

Newton J. Coker · Otology/Neurotology · Methodist Hospital · Baylor College of Medicine, One Baylor Plaza, Room SM-1727, Houston, TX 77030 · 713-798-5900

J. Rayner Dickey · General Otolaryngology · 9034 Westheimer Street, Suite 103, Houston, TX 77063 · 713-781-9660

Donald Thomas Donovan · Head & Neck Surgery (Head & Neck Tumors, Laryngeal Disorders, Sinus & Nasal Surgery) · Methodist Hospital, St. Luke's Episcopal Hospital, Texas Children's Hospital · Baylor College of Medicine, 6550 Fannin Street, Suite 1701, Houston, TX 77030-2717 · 713-798-5900

Newton Oran Duncan III · Pediatric Otolaryngology · Texas Children's Hospital Texas Children's Hospital, Pediatric Otolaryngology, 1102 Bates Street, Suite 340, Houston, TX 77030 · 713-770-3267

Ellen M. Friedman · Pediatric Otolaryngology (Congenital Airway Problems, Congenital Malformations of the Head & Neck) · Texas Children's Hospital · Texas Children's Hospital, 6621 Fannin Street, Suite 340, Houston, TX 77030 · 713-770-3268

Helmuth Goepfert · Head & Neck Surgery, Skull-Base Surgery (Head & Neck Cancer) · University of Texas-M. D. Anderson Cancer Center · University of Texas-M. D. Anderson Cancer Center, 1515 Holcombe Boulevard, Box 69, Houston, TX 77030-4095 · 713-792-6925

Melton Jay Horwitz · Otology/Neurotology (Neurotology) · Diagnostic Center Hospital, St. Luke's Episcopal Hospital, St. Joseph Hospital, Methodist Hospital, Texas Children's Hospital, Park Plaza Hospital · Medical Center Ear, Nose and Throat Associates, 6624 Fannin Street, Suite 1500, Houston, TX 77030 · 713-795-0111

Herman A. Jenkins · Otology/Neurotology, Skull-Base Surgery (General Otolaryngology) · Methodist Hospital · Baylor College of Medicine, Smith Tower, Suite 1701, 6550 Fannin Street, Houston, TX 77030 · 713-798-5900

Jimmy W. C. Lee · General Otolaryngology · Cypress Fairbanks Medical Center Cypress Fairbanks Ear, Nose & Throat, 11301 Fallbrook Drive, Suite 310, Houston, TX 77065 · 713-890-6155

H. Edward Maddox III · Otology/Neurotology (Cochlear Implants) · Memorial Hospital-Southwest · Houston Ear, Nose & Throat Clinic, 7777 Southwest Freeway, Suite 820, Houston, TX 77074 · 713-776-2211

S. Harold Reuter · General Otolaryngology · St. Luke's Episcopal Hospital, Methodist Hospital, Hermann Hospital, Texas Children's Hospital, Park Plaza Hospital · 6550 Fannin Street, Suite 2001, Houston, TX 77030 · 713-796-2001

Charles M. Stiernberg · Head & Neck Surgery (General Otolaryngology, Laryngology) · Hermann Hospital, West Houston Medical Center, Lyndon B. Johnson General Hospital · 7400 Fannin Street, Suite 900, Houston, TX 77054 · 713-792-4752; 713-265-4300

Marcelle Sulek · Pediatric Otolaryngology (Chronic Sinusitis) · Texas Children's Hospital, Methodist Hospital · Texas Children's Hospital, 1102 Bates Street, Suite 340, Houston, TX 77030 · 713-770-3250

Samuel Coleman Weber · General Otolaryngology (Adult & Pediatric, Thyroid, Head & Neck Surgery, Otology, Sinus & Nasal Surgery) · St. Luke's Episcopal Hospital, Methodist Hospital, Texas Children's Hospital · St. Luke's Medical Towers, Suite 1480, 6624 Fannin Street, Houston, TX 77030 · 713-795-5343

Irving

Natalie A. Roberge · General Otolaryngology · Irving Healthcare System, Baylor Medical Center-Grapevine (Grapevine), Children's Medical Center of Dallas (Dallas) · The Medical and Surgical Clinic of Irving, 2023 West Park Drive, Irving, TX 75061 · 214-253-2500

Frank William Theilen · General Otolaryngology · Irving Healthcare System, St. Paul's Medical Center (Dallas), Children's Medical Center of Dallas (Dallas), American Transitional Care-Dallas/Fort Worth · 2001 North MacArthur Boulevard, Suite 205, Irving, TX 75061 · 214-254-0640

Kingwood

Thomas J. Clegg · General Otolaryngology · Houston Ear, Nose & Throat, 1414 Green Oak Terrace Court, Kingwood, TX 77339 · 713-358-2314

Lubbock

Thomas Frederick Neal · General Otolaryngology · 3621 Twenty-Second Street, Suite 400, Lubbock, TX 79410 · 806-792-5331

Robert C. Wang · General Otolaryngology · University Medical Center · Texas Tech University Health Sciences Center, 3502 Ninth Street, Suite 410, Lubbock, TX 79415 · 806-743-1350

Midland

Roberta M. S. Case · General Otolaryngology · Memorial Hospital & Medical Center, Westwood Medical Center · 2010 West Ohio Street, Midland, TX 79701-5946 · 915-687-1981

Roger M. Traxel · General Otolaryngology (Otology, Sinus & Nasal Surgery) · Memorial Hospital & Medical Center, Westwood Medical Center, Surgicare · 2012 West Ohio Street, Midland, TX 79701-5946 · 915-683-1856

San Angelo

Leslie Kay Williamson · General Otolaryngology · Shannon Clinic, Department of Otolaryngology, 120 East Beauregard Avenue, San Angelo, TX 76903 · 915-658-1511

San Antonio

James H. Atkins, Jr. · General Otolaryngology (Sinus & Nasal Surgery, Pediatric Otolaryngology) · Southwest Texas Methodist Hospital, St. Luke's Baptist Hospital, San Antonio Community Hospital · 7940 Floyd Curl Drive, Suite 400, San Antonio, TX 78229 · 210-616-0096

Juan Alfredo Bonilla · Pediatric Otolaryngology · Women's & Children's Hospital, Santa Rosa Children's Hospital · Pediatric Ear, Nose & Throat Institute, 8122 Datapoint Drive, Suite 1050, San Antonio, TX 78229 · 210-614-0171

Anita King Bowes · Pediatric Otolaryngology (Pediatric Bronchoesophagology) · Women's & Children's Hospital · Pediatric Ear, Nose & Throat Institute, 8122 Datapoint Drive, Suite 1050, San Antonio, TX 78229 · 210-615-0293

Kevin Brian Browne · Sinus & Nasal Surgery · Affiliated Head & Neck Surgeons, 4499 Medical Drive, Suite 330, San Antonio, TX 78229-3712 · 210-615-8177

Robert A. Dobie · Otology/Neurotology · University Hospital-South Texas Medical Center · University of Texas Health Science Center at San Antonio, Department of Otolaryngology-Head & Neck Surgery, 7703 Floyd Curl Drive, San Antonio, TX 78284-7777 · 210-567-5655

Mark William Hatch · General Otolaryngology · Southwest Texas Methodist Hospital · South Texas Ear, Nose & Throat, 2727 Babcock Road, Suite A, San Antonio, TX 78229 · 210-692-7668

George Richard Holt · Head & Neck Surgery (Laryngology, Facial Plastic Surgery) · North Central Baptist Hospital, University Hospital-South Texas Medical Center · 540 Madison Oak Drive, Suite 450, San Antonio, TX 78258 · 210-490-6371

Wesley W. O. Krueger · Otology/Neurotology (Ear and Related Skull-Base Structures) · Southwest Texas Methodist Hospital · Texas Neurosciences Institute, 4410 Medical Drive, Suite 340, San Antonio, TX 78229 · 210-615-3695

Susan Marenda · Otology/Neurotology · Southwest Texas Methodist Hospital, St. Luke's Baptist Hospital, Women's & Children's Hospital · Texas Neurosciences Institute, Ear Medical Group, 4410 Medical Drive, Suite 550, San Antonio, TX 78229 · 210-614-6070

Roderick Donald Moe, Jr. · Pediatric Otolaryngology · Pediatric Ear, Nose & Throat Institute, 8122 Datapoint Drive, Suite 1050, San Antonio, TX 78229 · 210-614-0171

Richard Kurt Newman · General Otolaryngology (Head & Neck Surgery, Skull-Base Surgery) · Southwest Texas Methodist Hospital, St. Luke's Baptist Hospital 4499 Medical Drive, Suite 330, San Antonio, TX 78229 · 210-615-8177

James Edward Olsson · Otology/Neurotology (Otology, Skull-Base Surgery) · Southwest Texas Methodist Hospital · Texas Neurosciences Institute, 4410 Medical Drive, Suite 550, San Antonio, TX 78229 · 210-614-6070

Randal Allen Otto · Head & Neck Surgery (Head & Neck Cancer, Sinus Disease) University Hospital-South Texas Medical Center · University of Texas Health Science Center at San Antonio, Department of Otolaryngology-Head & Neck Surgery, 7703 Floyd Curl Drive, San Antonio, TX 78284-7777 · 210-567-5669

Gilbert M. Ruiz · General Otolaryngology · Santa Rosa Health Care · 315 North San Saba, Suite 1195, San Antonio, TX 78207 · 210-225-3136

Stephen J. Talley · General Otolaryngology (Sinus & Nasal Surgery) · Northeast Baptist Hospital · San Antonio Head & Neck Surgical Associates, 8711 Village Drive, Suite 200, San Antonio, TX 78217 · 210-590-2597

Temple

Lewis R. Hutchinson · Pediatric Otolaryngology · Scott & White Memorial Hospital · Scott & White Memorial Hospital, Department of Otolaryngology, 2401 South 31st Street, Temple, TX 76508-0001 · 817-724-2996

Tyler

Steuart L. Heaton · General Otolaryngology · 700 South Fleishel Avenue, Tyler, TX 75701 · 903-592-5601

James D. Toney · General Otolaryngology · Tyler ENT, 417 South Saunders Street, Tyler, TX 75702 · 903-533-1491

Waco

Mace L. Brindley · General Otolaryngology · Hillcrest Baptist Medical Center, Providence Health Center · Waco Otolaryngology, 3115 Pine Avenue, Suite 408, Waco, TX 76708-3201 · 817-753-0351

Ronald L. Johnson · General Otolaryngology · Providence Health Center, Hillcrest Baptist Medical Center · Waco Otolaryngology, 3115 Pine Avenue, Suite 408, Waco, TX 76708-3201 · 817-753-0351

John M. Reid III · General Otolaryngology · Providence Health Center, Hillcrest Baptist Medical Center · Waco Otolaryngology, 3115 Pine Avenue, Suite 408, Waco, TX 76708-3201 · 817-753-0351

Wichita Falls

Donald L. Bomer · General Otolaryngology · Head & Neck Surgical Associates, 1622 Eleventh Street, Wichita Falls, TX 76301-4309 · 817-322-6953

Cameron D. Godfrey · General Otolaryngology · Bethania Regional Health Care Center · 501 Midwestern Parkway East, Wichita Falls, TX 76302 · 817-766-8772

Barry B. Prestridge · General Otolaryngology · Head & Neck Surgical Associates, 1622 Eleventh Street, Wichita Falls, TX 76301-4309 · 817-322-6953

Earl F. Singleton · General Otolaryngology · Head & Neck Surgical Associates, 1622 Eleventh Street, Wichita Falls, TX 76301-4309 · 817-322-6953

PATHOLOGY

Amarillo

James M. Goforth · General Pathology · 200 Northwest Seventh Street, Amarillo, TX 79107 · 806-378-6111

James E. Hamous · General Pathology · 3423 Danbury Drive, Amarillo, TX 79109 · 806-378-6111

Arlington

Dudley D. Jones · General Pathology (Anatomic & Clinical Pathology, Dermatopathology, Liver Pathology, Surgical Pathology) · Arlington Memorial Hospital · Arlington Pathology Association, 908 Wright Street, Arlington, TX 76012 · 817-460-4366

Austin

Phillip C. Collins · General Pathology (Surgical Pathology, Transfusion Medicine) · Brackenridge Hospital, South Austin Medical Center, Austin Diagnostic Medical Center · Brackenridge Hospital, Department of Pathology, 601 East 15th Street, Austin, TX 78701-1930 · 512-480-1516

Bruce A. Hurt · (Dermatopathology, Medical Microbiology) · Seton Medical Center · Clinical Pathology Laboratories, 8613 Cross Park Drive, Austin, TX 78754 · 512-323-1183

Stephen Jurco · General Pathology (Surgical Pathology, Clinical Chemistry) · St. David's Healthcare Center, Seton Medical Center · Clinical Pathology Laboratories, 8613 Cross Park Drive, Austin, TX 78754 · 512-339-1275

Margaret B. Listrom · (Cytopathology) · Clinical Pathology Laboratories, 8613 Cross Park Drive, Austin, TX 78754 · 512-323-1183

Alan T. Moore · Hematopathology · Clinical Pathology Laboratories, 8613 Cross Park Drive, Austin, TX 78754 · 512-339-1275

Robert Dean Niemeyer · General Pathology · Seton Medical Center · Clinical Pathology Laboratories, 8613 Cross Park Drive, Austin, TX 78754 · 512-339-1275

Max M. Wells · (Dermatopathology, Medical Microbiology) · Seton Medical Center · Clinical Pathology Laboratories, 8613 Cross Park Drive, Austin, TX 78754 · 512-323-1183

Sheryl Diane Zeisman · Hematopathology · Clinical Pathology Laboratories, 8613 Cross Park Drive, Austin, TX 78754 · 512-339-1275

Beaumont

Larry E. Kane · General Pathology · Diagnostic Pathology Associates, 3155 Stagg Drive, Suite 316, Beaumont, TX 77701-4506 · 409-838-6456

Michael L. Kessler · General Pathology · Baptist Hospital Beaumont · Diagnostic Pathology Associates, 3155 Stagg Drive, Suite 316, Beaumont, TX 77701-4506 · 409-838-6456

Corpus Christi

Joe A. Lewis · General Pathology · Spohn Hospital · Pathology Associates, 600 Elizabeth Street, Corpus Christi, TX 78404 · 512-881-3924

James D. Mullins · General Pathology · Spohn Hospital, Department of Pathology, 600 Elizabeth Street, P.O. Box 3666, Corpus Christi, TX 78404 · 512-881-3925

Dallas

Jorge Albores-Saavedra · General Pathology (Surgical Pathology) · University of Texas-Southwestern Medical Center at Dallas, Department of Pathology, 5323 Harry Hines Boulevard, Dallas, TX 75235-9072 · 214-590-8328

Raheela Ashfaq · General Pathology (Fine Needle Aspiration Biopsy, Automated Gyn-Cytology, New Technologies in Cytology) · Parkland Hospital, Department of Cytology, 5201 Harry Hines Boulevard, Dallas, TX 75235 · 214-590-8743

Jeffrey J. Barnard · General Pathology (Forensic) · Southwestern Institute of Forensic Sciences, 5230 Medical Center Drive, Dallas, TX 75235-0728 · 214-920-5913

Dennis K. Burns · Neuropathology · Parkland Memorial Hospital · University of Texas-Southwestern Medical Center at Dallas, H Building, Second Floor, Room 130, 5323 Harry Hines Boulevard, Dallas, TX 75235-9072 · 214-648-6867

Clay J. Cockerell · Dermatopathology (Clinical Dermatology, Cutaneous Lymphomas, HIV Infection, AIDS, Melanoma, Clinicopathologic Correlation) · Zale Lipshy University Hospital, Parkland Memorial Hospital, Methodist Medical Center, Baylor University Medical Center, Presbyterian Hospital of Dallas, St. Paul Medical Center · Freeman-Cockerell Dermatopathology Laboratories, 2330 Butler Street, Suite 115, Dallas, TX 75235-9930 · 214-638-2222

Peter A. Dysert · General Pathology · Baylor University Medical Center · Baylor University Medical Center, 3500 Gaston Avenue, Dallas, TX 75246-2017 · 214-820-3303

Robert G. Freeman · Dermatopathology (General Pathology, Surgical Pathology) Parkland Memorial Hospital · Freeman-Cockerell Dermatopathology Laboratories, 2330 Butler Street, Suite 115, Dallas, TX 75235-9930 · 214-638-2222

Jose Alberto Hernandez · Hematopathology · Parkland Memorial Hospital · University of Texas-Southwestern Medical Center at Dallas, Department of Pathology, 5323 Harry Hines Boulevard, Dallas, TX 75235-9072 · 214-590-8125

Edwin P. Jenevein, Jr. · General Pathology (Surgical Pathology) · St. Paul Medical Center · St. Paul Medical Center, 5909 Harry Hines Boulevard, Dallas, TX 75235-6285 · 214-879-3888

Harold S. Kaplan · General Pathology (Transfusion Medicine) · University of Texas-Southwestern Medical Center at Dallas, Department of Pathology, 5323 Harry Hines Boulevard, Dallas, TX 75235-9072 · 214-648-7885

Joseph H. Keffer · (Clinical Pathology, Thyroid Function, Myocardial Markers of Injury, Laboratory Utilization and Point-of-Care Testing) · Zale Lipshy University Hospital, Parkland Memorial Hospital · University of Texas-Southwestern Medical Center at Dallas, 5323 Harry Hines Boulevard, Dallas, TX 75235-9072 · 214-648-7887

Edward L. Lee · General Pathology (Gastrointestinal) · VA Medical Center · VA Medical Center, 4500 South Lancaster Road, Dallas, TX 75216 · 214-376-5451

Robert W. McKenna · Hematopathology · Parkland Memorial Hospital, Children's Medical Center of Dallas, Zale Lipshy University Hospital · University of Texas-Southwestern Medical Center at Dallas, Department of Pathology, 5323 Harry Hines Boulevard, Dallas, TX 75235-9072 · 214-648-4004

William V. Miller · General Pathology (Blood Banking/Transfusion Medicine, Bone Marrow Transplantation) · BloodCare Dallas, 9000 Harry Hines Boulevard, Dallas, TX 75235-1730 · 214-351-8561

Nancy R. Schneider · General Pathology (Cytogenetics) · Parkland Memorial Hospital · University of Texas-Southwestern Medical Center at Dallas, Department of Pathology, Division of Cytogenetics, 5323 Harry Hines Boulevard, Dallas, TX 75235-9072 · 214-648-3357

Paul M. Southern · General Pathology (Clinical Microbiology, Parasitology) · Parkland Memorial Hospital · University of Texas-Southwestern Medical Center at Dallas, Department of Pathology, 5323 Harry Hines Boulevard, Dallas, TX 75235-9072 · 214-648-3587

Wayne E. Taylor · General Pathology (Surgical Pathology) · Medical City Dallas Hospital · Department of Pathology, 7777 Forest Lane, Dallas, TX 75230 · 214-661-7285

Glenn Weldon Tillery · General Pathology · Baylor University Medical Center · Baylor University Medical Center, 3500 Gaston Avenue, Dallas, TX 75246-2017 214-820-3023

Milan F. Vuitch · Surgical Pathology (Cytopathology) · Parkland Memorial Hospital, Zale Lipshy University Hospital · University of Texas-Southwestern Medical Center at Dallas, 5323 Harry Hines Boulevard, Dallas, TX 75235-9072 · 214-590-8690

Arthur G. Weinberg · Pediatric Pathology · Children's Medical Center of Dallas Children's Medical Center of Dallas, Department of Pathology, 1935 Motor Street, Dallas, TX 75235-7794 · 214-640-2324

Charles L. White III · Neuropathology · Parkland Memorial Hospital, Zale-Lipshy University Hospital · University of Texas-Southwestern Medical Center at Dallas, Department of Pathology, Division of Neuropathology, 5323 Harry Hines Boulevard, Dallas, TX 75235-9072 · 214-648-2148

El Paso

Darius A. Boman · Surgical Pathology · Thomason Hospital · Texas Tech University Health Sciences Center, Department of Pathology, 4800 Alberta Avenue, El Paso, TX 79905 · 915-545-6775

Jodie Lawrence · General Pathology · Sierra Hospital, 1625 Medical Center Drive, El Paso, TX 79902 · 915-544-5323

William G. McGee · Surgical Pathology · Corning Clinical Laboratories, 16 Concord Street, El Paso, TX 79936 · 915-775-2622

Fort Worth

Bryan L. Bartlett · General Pathology · All Saints Episcopal Hospital-Fort Worth All Saints Episcopal Hospital-Fort Worth, Department of Pathology, 1400 Eighth Avenue, Fort Worth, TX 76104-4192 · 817-926-2544

Robert W. Collison · General Pathology · Plaza Medical Center · Plaza Medical Center, 900 Eighth Avenue, Fort Worth, TX 76104 · 817-336-2100

LaDon W. Homer · General Pathology · Huguley Memorial Medical Center · 11803 South Freeway, Suite 210, Fort Worth, TX 76115 · 817-293-4304

Margie B. Peschel · General Pathology (Transfusion Medicine) · Carter Blood Center, 1263 West Rosedale Street, Fort Worth, TX 76194-2801 · 817-335-4935

Stephen M. Russell · General Pathology (Clinical Pathology) · Harris Methodist-Fort Worth · Harris Methodist-Fort Worth, Department of Pathology and Laboratory Medicine, 1401 Pennsylvania Avenue, Fort Worth, TX 76104-2122 · 817-878-5622

Galveston

Daniel F. Cowan · Surgical Pathology (Breast Pathology) · University of Texas Medical Branch, Surgical Pathology, 301 University Boulevard, Galveston, TX 77555-0588 · 409-772-7220

David H. Walker · General Pathology (Infectious Diseases) · University of Texas Medical Branch, Department of Pathology, 301 University Boulevard, Galveston, TX 77555-0609 · 409-772-3989

Houston

Alberto G. Ayala · Surgical Pathology (Urologic Pathology, Soft Tissue Pathology, Bone & Joint Pathology, Breast Pathology, General Pathology, Urologic Pathology) · University of Texas-M. D. Anderson Cancer Center · University of Texas-M. D. Anderson Cancer Center, 1515 Holcombe Boulevard, Box 85, Houston, TX 77030 · 713-792-3151

John G. Batsakis · Surgical Pathology, ENT Pathology · University of Texas-M. D. Anderson Cancer Center · University of Texas-M. D. Anderson Cancer Center, Department of Pathology, 1515 Holcombe Boulevard, Box 85, Houston, TX 77030-4009 · 713-792-3100

Arthur W. Bracey · General Pathology (Clinical Pathology, Transfusion Medicine) · St. Luke's Episcopal Hospital · St. Luke's Episcopal Hospital, Department of Pathology, 6720 Bertner Avenue, Room P125T, Houston, TX 77030 · 713-791-3274

Richard W. Brown · Surgical Pathology · Methodist Hospital, Department of Pathology, 6565 Fannin Street, Mail Stop 205, Houston, TX 77030 · 713-790-2419

Janet M. Bruner · Neuropathology (Brain Tumors) · University of Texas-M. D. Anderson Cancer Center · University of Texas-M. D. Anderson Cancer Center, Department of Pathology, 1515 Holcombe Boulevard, Box 85, Houston, TX 77030-4009 · 713-792-7935

Louis Maximilian Buja · General Pathology (Anatomic Pathology, Cardiovascular Disease) · Hermann Hospital · University of Texas Medical School at Houston, 6431 Fannin Street, Room G.010, Houston, TX 77030 · 713-792-5000

Philip T. Cagle · General Pathology (Pulmonary) · Baylor College of Medicine, Department of Pathology, One Baylor Plaza, Houston, TX 77030 · 713-790-5219

Harry Launius Evans · Surgical Pathology (Soft Tissue, Dermatopathology) · University of Texas-M. D. Anderson Cancer Center · University of Texas-M. D. Anderson Cancer Center, 1515 Holcombe Boulevard, Box 85, Houston, TX 77030-4009 · 713-792-3152

Tina V. Fanning · General Pathology (Cytopathology) · University of Texas-M. D. Anderson Cancer Center · University of Texas-M. D. Anderson Cancer Center, Department of Pathology, 1515 Holcombe Boulevard, Box 53, Houston, TX 77030-4009 · 713-794-5625

Milton J. Finegold · Pediatric Pathology (Liver Pathology, Pediatric Gastroenterology) · Texas Children's Hospital · Texas Children's Hospital, 6621 Fannin Street, Mail Code 1-2261, Houston, TX 77030 · 713-770-1856

Ramon L. Font · General Pathology (Ophthalmic Pathology) · Baylor School of Medicine, Department of Pathology, 6501 Fannin Street, Room NC-200, Houston, TX 77030 · 713-798-4644

Armand B. Glassman · General Pathology (Clinical Pathology, Blood Banking/Transfusion Medicine, Genetics, General Nuclear Medicine, Hematopathology) · University of Texas-M. D. Anderson Cancer Center · University of Texas-M. D. Anderson Cancer Center, 1515 Holcombe Boulevard, Box 73, Houston, TX 77030 713-792-6311

Richard J. Hausner · Surgical Pathology · Cypress Fairbanks Medical Center · Cypress Fairbanks Medical Center, Department of Pathology, 10655 Steepletop Drive, Houston, TX 77065 · 713-897-3165

Ruth L. Katz · General Pathology (Cytopathology) · University of Texas-M. D. Anderson Cancer Center · University of Texas-M. D. Anderson Cancer Center, 1515 Holcombe Boulevard, Box 53, Houston, TX 77030-4009 · 713-794-5625

Joel B. Kirkpatrick · Neuropathology · Methodist Hospital · Baylor College of Medicine, Department of Pathology, One Baylor Plaza, Houston, TX 77030 · 713-790-2370

Juan Lechago · General Pathology (Surgical Pathology, Gastrointestinal and Liver Pathology, Endocrine Pathology) · The Methodist Hospital, Department of Pathology, 6565 Fannin Street, Mail Stop 205, Houston, TX 77030 · 713-793-1189

Benjamin Lichtiger · General Pathology (Transfusion Medicine) · University of Texas-M. D. Anderson Cancer Center · University of Texas-M. D. Anderson Cancer Center, 1515 Holcombe Boulevard, Box Seven, Houston, TX 77030 · 713-792-2644

Michael W. Lieberman · General Pathology (Molecular Pathology) · Methodist Hospital · Baylor College of Medicine, Department of Pathology, One Baylor Plaza, Houston, TX 77030 · 713-798-3859

Mario A. Luna · Surgical Pathology (Head & Neck Cancer, Surgical Pathology of Opportunistic Infections, Surgical Pathology of Cancer Chemotherapy-Induced Pathology) · University of Texas-M. D. Anderson Cancer Center · University of Texas-M. D. Anderson Cancer Center, 1515 Holcombe Boulevard, Box Seven, Houston, TX 77030-4009 · 713-792-3138

Bruce Makay · Surgical Pathology (Pulmonary, Electron Microscopy) · University of Texas-M. D. Anderson Cancer Center · University of Texas-M. D. Anderson Cancer Center, Department of Pathology, 1515 Holcombe Boulevard, Box 085, Houston, TX 77030-4009 · 713-792-3310

Hugh A. McAllister, Jr. · General Pathology (Cardiovascular Pathology) · St. Luke's Episcopal Hospital, Texas Heart Institute · St. Luke's Episcopal Hospital, 6720 Bertner Avenue, P.O. Box 20269, Houston, TX 77030-2699 · 713-791-4685

John D. Milam · General Pathology (Transfusion Medicine) · Lyndon B. Johnson General Hospital · Lyndon B. Johnson General Hospital, Pathology Department, 5656 Kelley Street, Third Floor, Houston, TX 77026 · 713-636-5266

Dina R. Mody · Surgical Pathology (Cytopathology, Obstetric & Gynecologic Pathology, Skeletal Pathology) · Methodist Hospital · Baylor College of Medicine, Department of Pathology, One Baylor Plaza, Houston, TX 77030-3498 · 713-790-2370

Nelson G. Ordonez · Surgical Pathology (Immunocytochemistry, Renal Pathology, Immunohistochemistry, Electron Microscopy, Cytopathology) · University of Texas-M. D. Anderson Cancer Center · University of Texas-M. D. Anderson

Cancer Center, 1515 Holcombe Boulevard, Box 85, Houston, TX 77030-4009 · 713-792-3167

William C. Pugh · Hematopathology (Molecular Pathology, Immunobiology) · University of Texas-M. D. Anderson Cancer Center · University of Texas-M. D. Anderson Cancer Center, Department of Pathology, 1515 Holcombe Boulevard, Box 85, Houston, TX 77030-4009 · 713-794-5501; 713-794-5446

Ibrahim Ramzy · General Pathology (Cytopathology, Fine Needle Aspiration, Gynecologic Pathology) · Methodist Hospital · Baylor College of Medicine, Department of Pathology, One Baylor Plaza, Houston, TX 77030 · 713-790-4508

Jay Y. Ro · Surgical Pathology (Prostate, Lung, Soft Tissue) · University of Texas-M. D. Anderson Cancer Center · University of Texas-M. D. Anderson Cancer Center, Department of Pathology, 1515 Holcombe Boulevard, Box 85, Houston, TX 77030-4009 · 713-792-8134

Harvey Rosenberg · Pediatric Pathology · University of Texas Medical School at Houston, Department of Pathology, 6431 Fannin Street, Room MSB 2.137, Houston, TX 77030 · 713-792-3020

Mary R. Schwartz · Surgical Pathology (Cytopathology, Dermatopathology) · Methodist Hospital · Methodist Hospital, Department of Laboratory Medicine, 6565 Fannin Street, Mail Stop 205, Houston, TX 77030 · 713-790-2370

Elvio G. Silva · Gynecologic Pathology (Surgical Pathology) · University of Texas-M. D. Anderson Cancer Center · University of Texas-M. D. Anderson Cancer Center, Department of Pathology, 1515 Holcombe Boulevard, Box 85, Houston, TX 77030-4009 · 713-792-3108

Nour Sneige · Breast Pathology (Cytopathology, Fine Needle Aspiration Cytology, Surgical Pathology [Breast]) · University of Texas-M. D. Anderson Cancer Center · University of Texas-M. D. Anderson Cancer Center, Department of Pathology, 1515 Holcombe Boulevard, Box 53, Houston, TX 77030-4009 · 713-794-5625

Harlan J. Spjut · Surgical Pathology (Orthopaedic Pathology) · Methodist Hospital · Baylor College of Medicine, Department of Pathology, One Baylor Plaza, Room 286-A, Houston, TX 77030 · 713-798-4661

Margaret O. Uthman · Hematopathology · Hermann Hospital · University of Texas Medical School at Houston, Department of Pathology, 6431 Fannin Street, Houston, TX 77030 · 713-792-8303

Thomas M. Wheeler · Surgical Pathology (Prostate, Urologic, Cytopathology, Thyroid Disease) · Methodist Hospital · Baylor College of Medicine, Department of Pathology, One Baylor Plaza, Houston, TX 77030-2707 · 713-790-2681

David H. Yawn · General Pathology (Transfusion Medicine) · Methodist Hospital Baylor College of Medicine, Department of Pathology, One Baylor Plaza, Houston, TX 77030 · 713-790-2434

Lackland Air Force Base

Kevin M. McCabe · Surgical Pathology (Cytopathology) · Wilford Hall Medical Center · Wilford Hall Medical Center, Department of Pathology/PSLA, 2200 Bergquist Drive, Suite One, Lackland Air Force Base, TX 78236-5300 · 210-670-7313

Lubbock

Dale M. Dunn · (Transfusion Medicine, Histo-Compatability Testing) · University Medical Center · Texas Tech University Health Sciences Center, Department of Pathology, 3601 Fourth Street, Room 1A96, Lubbock, TX 79430 · 806-743-2172

Viviane Mamlok · Pediatric Pathology · University Medical Center · Texas Tech University Health Sciences Center, Department of Pathology, 3601 Fourth Street, Lubbock, TX 79430 · 806-743-2155

McAllen

Domingo H. Useda · General Pathology · Rio Grande Regional Hospital, Department of Pathology, 101 East Ridge Road, McAllen, TX 78503 · 210-632-6405

Midland

Terry R. Burns · General Pathology · Memorial Hospital & Medical Center, Department of Pathology, 2200 West Illinois Street, Midland, TX 79701 · 915-685-1631

Sherri Gillham · General Pathology · Memorial Hospital & Medical Center, Department of Pathology, 2200 West Illinois Street, Midland, TX 79701 · 915-685-1631

Christopher L. Hall · General Pathology · Memorial Hospital & Medical Center Memorial Hospital & Medical Center, Department of Pathology, 2200 West Illinois Street, Midland, TX 79701 · 915-685-1631

Odessa

Krishnakumari Challapalli · General Pathology · 500 Adams Avenue, Suite 600, Odessa, TX 79761 · 915-337-8441

San Antonio

Oscar D. Abbott · General Pathology · Severance & Associates, 750 East Mulberry, Suite 325, San Antonio, TX 78212 · 210-271-9363

Craig D. Allred · Breast Pathology (Immunopathology, Surgical Pathology) · University Hospital-South Texas Medical Center · University of Texas Health Science Center at San Antonio, Department of Pathology, 7703 Floyd Curl Drive, San Antonio, TX 78284-7750 · 210-567-4091

Peter M. Banks · Hematopathology · University Hospital-South Texas Medical Center, Audie L. Murphy Memorial Veterans Hospital · University of Texas Health Science Center at San Antonio, Department of Pathology, 7703 Floyd Curl Drive, San Antonio, TX 78284-7750 · 210-567-4034

George Abcar Bannayan · Surgical Pathology (Renal) · San Antonio Community Hospital · San Antonio Community Hospital, Department of Pathology, 8026 Floyd Curl Drive, San Antonio, TX 78229 · 210-692-8150

Kathy Cagan-Hallett · Neuropathology · Audie L. Murphy Memorial Veterans Hospital · Audie L. Murphy Memorial Veterans Hospital, 7400 Merton Minter Boulevard, Mail Code 67113, San Antonio, TX 78284-5700 · 210-617-5300 x4350

Charlotte Nanette Clare · Hematopathology (Cytogenetics, Peripheral Blood & Bone Marrow) · Audie L. Murphy Memorial Veterans Hospital · University of Texas Health Science Center at San Antonio, Department of Pathology, 7703 Floyd Curl Drive, San Antonio, TX 78284-7750 · 210-567-4067

Fiona E. Craig · Hematopathology (Flow Cytometry) · University Hospital-South Texas Medical Center, Audie L. Murphy Memorial Veterans Hospital · University of Texas Health Science Center at San Antonio, Department of Pathology, 7703 Floyd Curl Drive, San Antonio, TX 78284-7750 · 210-567-4125

Everett M. Donowho, Jr. · Surgical Pathology · Southwest Texas Methodist Hospital · Southwest Texas Methodist Hospital, Department of Pathology, 7700 Floyd Curl Drive, San Antonio, TX 78229-3902 · 210-692-4745

Randall C. Harper · Surgical Pathology (Cytopathology, General Pathology) · St. Luke's Baptist Hospital · 7940 Floyd Curl Drive, Suite 220, San Antonio, TX 78229 · 210-614-0045

David N. Henkes · (Fine Needle Aspiration, Cytopathology, Clinical Pathology, General Surgical Pathology) · Santa Rosa Northwest Hospital · Santa Rosa Northwest Hospital, Department of Pathology, 2827 Babcock Road, San Antonio, TX 78229 · 210-705-6463

William W. Hinchey · Surgical Pathology · Baptist Medical Center · Baptist Medical Center, Department of Pathology, 111 Dallas Street, San Antonio, TX 78205-1230 · 210-222-8431

Thomas F. Kardos · Surgical Pathology (Cytopathology, Fine Needle Aspiration) · Baptist Medical Center · Baptist Medical Center, Department of Pathology, 111 Dallas Street, San Antonio, TX 78205-1230 · 210-271-3035

Paula Larson · Surgical Pathology (Cytopathology, Fine Needle Aspiration) · Southwest Texas Methodist Hospital · Southwest Texas Methodist Hospital, Department of Pathology, 7700 Floyd Curl Drive, San Antonio, TX 78229 · 210-692-4850

Jacqueline H. Longbotham · Hematopathology, Surgical Pathology · Baptist Medical Center · Baptist Medical Center, Department of Pathology, 111 Dallas Street, San Antonio, TX 78205-1201 · 210-302-2405

Donald R. Pulitzer · Dermatopathology · University of Texas Health Science Center at San Antonio, Department of Pathology, 7703 Floyd Curl Drive, San Antonio, TX 78284-7750 · 210-567-4085

Cliff M. Richmond · General Pathology (Surgical Pathology, Cytogenetics) · Santa Rosa Northwest Hospital · Santa Rosa Northwest Hospital, Department of Pathology, 2827 Babcock Road, San Antonio, TX 78229 · 210-616-6300

Valerie René Rone · Surgical Pathology (Cytopathology) · Severance & Associates, 750 East Mulberry Avenue, Suite 325, San Antonio, TX 78212 · 210-271-9363

Victor A. Saldivar · Pediatric Pathology (General Pathology, Breast Pathology) · Santa Rosa Health Care · Santa Rosa Health Care, Department of Pathology, 519 West Houston Street, San Antonio, TX 78207-3108 · 210-228-2311

Joyce G. Schwartz · General Pathology (Clinical Chemistry) · University Hospital-South Texas Medical Center · University of Texas Health Science Center at San Antonio, Department of Pathology, 7703 Floyd Curl Drive, San Antonio, TX 78284-7750 · 210-567-4072

Cathy J. Spadaccini · Hematopathology (Transfusion Medicine, Coagulation) · Baptist Medical Center · Baptist Medical Center, Department of Pathology, 111 Dallas Street, San Antonio, TX 78205-1230 · 210-222-8431

Philip T. Valente · General Pathology (Cytopathology, Surgical Pathology, Gynecologic Pathology) · University Hospital-South Texas Medical Center · University of Texas Health Science Center at San Antonio, Department of Pathology, 7703 Floyd Curl Drive, San Antonio, TX 78284-7750 · 210-567-4134

Temple

Robert F. Peterson · General Pathology · Scott & White Memorial Hospital · Scott & White Memorial Hospital, Department of Pathology, 2401 South 31st Street, Temple, TX 76508-0001 · 817-724-3691

Tyler

Marian F. Fagan · Hematopathology · University of Texas Health Center-Tyler University of Texas Health Center-Tyler, Department of Pathology, US Highway 271 and State Highway 155, P.O. Box 2003, Tyler, TX 75710-2003 · 903-877-7884

Brent R. Harris · General Pathology · Pathology Associates, 901 Turtle Creek, Tyler, TX 75701 · 903-593-0481

LeRoy R. Hieger · General Pathology (Pulmonary) · University of Texas Health Center-Tyler · University of Texas Health Center-Tyler, Department of Pathology, US Highway 271 and State Highway 155, P.O. Box 2003, Tyler, TX 75710-2003 · 903-877-7880

Waco

Simon Milford Bunn, Jr. · General Pathology · Hillcrest Baptist Medical Center Hillcrest Baptist Medical Center, Department of Pathology, 3000 Herring Avenue, Waco, TX 76708 · 817-756-8011

Ronald E. Henderson, Jr. · General Pathology · Providence Health Center · Medical Laboratory Services of Waco, 3115 Pine Street, Suite 108, Waco, TX 76708 · 817-752-9621

David M. McTaggart · General Pathology · Providence Health Center · Medical Laboratory Services of Waco, 3115 Pine Street, Suite 108, Waco, TX 76708 · 817-752-9621

Douglas B. Michaels · General Pathology (Anatomic & Clinical Pathology) · Providence Health Center · Waco Clinical Pathology Laboratory, 2112 Washington Avenue, Waco, TX 76701 · 817-753-2406

Edwin B. Morrison · General Pathology (Blood Banking, Surgical Pathology) · Hillcrest Baptist Medical Center · Medical Laboratory Services of Waco, 3115 Pine Street, Suite 108, Waco, TX 76708 · 817-752-9621

Wichita Falls

Susan M. Strate · (Surgical Pathology) · Wichita General Hospital · North Texas Medical Lab, 1600 Eighth Street, Wichita Falls, TX 76301 · 817-761-8340

PEDIATRICS

Amarillo

Rolf W. O. Habersang · Pediatric Critical Care (Children with Special Health Care Needs) · Amarillo Hospital District-Northwest Texas Hospital · Healthcare Professional Associates, 1600 Coulter Drive, Suite F-600, Amarillo, TX 79106 · 806-358-2192

Mubariz Naqvi · Neonatal-Perinatal Medicine · Amarillo Hospital District-Northwest Texas Hospital · Texas Tech University Health Sciences Center, Department of Pediatrics, 1400 Wallace Boulevard, Amarillo, TX 79106 · 806-354-5525

Austin

David Lee Anglin · Pediatric Critical Care · Children's Hospital of Austin · Children's Hospital of Austin, 601 East 15th Street, Austin, TX 78701-1996 · 512-480-1987

David R. Breed · Neonatal-Perinatal Medicine · St. David's Healthcare Center · Capital Neonatology Associates, 900 East 30th Street, Suite 305, Austin, TX 78705 · 512-476-0895

James S. Creswell · Neonatal-Perinatal Medicine · Seton Medical Center · Seton Medical Center, Department of Neonatal Medicine, 1201 West 38th Street, Austin, TX 78705 · 512-323-1000

Betty J. Edmond · Pediatric Infectious Disease · Children's Hospital of Austin · 4007 James Casey Street, Suite D-250, Austin, TX 78745-1182 · 512-448-4544

James Patrick Finnigan · Pediatric Cardiology · Brackenridge Hospital · Children's Cardiology Associates, 1313 Red River Street, Suite 112, Austin, TX 78701 512-472-6066

William Harold Hyde · Neonatal-Perinatal Medicine · Seton Medical Center · Seton Medical Center, Department of Neonatal Medicine, 1201 West 38th Street, Austin, TX 78705-1006 · 512-323-1000

Sharon Kay Lockhart · Pediatric Hematology-Oncology · Children's Hospital of Austin · The Park at Children's Hospital, 601 East 15th Street, Box 48, Austin, TX 78701 · 512-480-1480

Stuart A. Rowe · Pediatric Cardiology · Children's Hospital of Austin, Brackenridge Hospital · Children's Cardiology Associates, 1313 Red River Street, Suite 112, Austin, TX 78701 · 512-454-1110

John Todd Scharnberg, Jr. · Neonatal-Perinatal Medicine · Seton Medical Center · Seton Medical Center, Department of Neonatal Medicine, 1201 West 38th Street, Austin, TX 78705-1006 · 512-323-1000

James C. Sharp, Jr. · Pediatric Hematology-Oncology · Children's Hospital of Austin, Brackenridge Hospital · The Park at Children's Hospital, 601 East 15th Street, Box 48, Austin, TX 78701 · 512-480-1480

George L. Sharpe · Neonatal-Perinatal Medicine · Brackenridge Hospital, Seton Medical Center · Brackenridge Hospital, 601 East 15th Street, Room 2.202, Austin, TX 78701-1996 · 512-476-6461

David E. Wermer · Neonatal-Perinatal Medicine · Seton Medical Center · Seton Medical Center, Department of Neonatal Medicine, 1201 West 38th Street, Austin, TX 78705-1006 · 512-323-1000

Beaumont

Aiyanadar Bharathi · Neonatal-Perinatal Medicine · St. Elizabeth Hospital · St. Elizabeth Hospital, Department of Neonatology, 2830 Calder Avenue, Beaumont, TX 77702 · 409-899-7892

Krishna Devaru Bhat · Pediatric Pulmonology, Pediatric Critical Care (Asthma, Cystic Fibrosis, Lung Infections) · 2627 Laurel Street, Beaumont, TX 77702-2204 409-835-5382

Vijay S. Kusnoor · Pediatric Cardiology · St. Elizabeth Hospital · Southeast Texas Cardiology, 2693 North Street, Beaumont, TX 77702 · 409-832-8862

William Jerome Reed · Abused Children (Attention Deficit Hyperactive Disorder and Its Spectrum) · St. Elizabeth Hospital, Baptist Hospital Beaumont, Beaumont Regional Medical Center · 2900 North Street, Suite 408, Beaumont, TX 77702-1542 · 409-892-8362

Brownsville

Ruth Ann F. Plotkin · Pediatric Endocrinology · Brownsville Medical Center · 1064 East Los Ebanos, Brownsville, TX 78520 · 210-541-5383

Corpus Christi

Cathryn B. Howarth · Pediatric Hematology-Oncology · Driscoll Children's Hospital · Driscoll Children's Hospital, Department of Pediatric Hematology-Oncology, 3533 South Alameda Street, Corpus Christi, TX 78411-1721 · 512-850-5311

Raymond C. Lewandowski · (Genetics) · Driscoll Children's Hospital · Center for Genetic Services, 7121 South Padre Island Drive, Suite 202, Corpus Christi, TX 78412 · 512-985-6600

Judith K. Mullins · Pediatric Hematology-Oncology · Driscoll Children's Hospital Driscoll Children's Hospital, 3533 South Alameda Street, Corpus Christi, TX 78411-1721 · 512-850-5311

Donald Paul Pinkel · Pediatric Hematology-Oncology (Pediatric Leukemia) · Driscoll Children's Hospital · Driscoll Children's Hospital, 3533 South Alameda Street, Corpus Christi, TX 78411 · 512-850-5311

Donnie P. Wilson · Pediatric Endocrinology · Driscoll Children's Hospital · Driscoll Children's Hospital, Department of Endocrinology, 3533 South Alameda Street, Corpus Christi, TX 78411 · 512-850-5444

Dallas

Steven Roy Alexander · Pediatric Nephrology (Dialysis, Kidney Transplantation, General Clinical Pediatric Nephrology) · Children's Medical Center of Dallas · University of Texas-Southwestern Medical Center at Dallas, 5323 Harry Hines Boulevard, Dallas, TX 75235-9063 · 214-648-3438; 214-640-2980

John Milton Andersen · Pediatric Gastroenterology (Esophageal Disease, Inflammatory Bowel Disease, Liver Disease) · Children's Medical Center of Dallas Children's Medical Center of Dallas, Center for Pediatric Gastroenterology, 1935 Motor Street, Dallas, TX 75235-7794 · 214-640-8000

Michel G. Baum · Pediatric Nephrology · Children's Medical Center of Dallas · University of Texas-Southwestern Medical Center at Dallas, 5323 Harry Hines Boulevard, Dallas, TX 75235-9063 · 214-648-3438

Sarah Blumenschein · Pediatric Cardiology (Preventive Cardiology in Children, Hypercholesterolemia in Children & their Families, Congenital Heart Disease) · Children's Medical Center, 1935 Motor Street, Dallas, TX 75235 · 214-640-2333

George R. Buchanan · Pediatric Hematology-Oncology (Pediatric Leukemia, Sickle Cell Disease, Hemophilia) · Children's Medical Center of Dallas · University of Texas-Southwestern Medical Center at Dallas, 5323 Harry Hines Boulevard, Dallas, TX 75235-9063 · 214-648-8594

Bryan A. Dickson · Pediatric Endocrinology (Diabetes, Growth Disorders, Disorders of Puberty) · Children's Medical Center of Dallas · University of Texas-Southwestern Medical Center at Dallas, 5323 Harry Hines Boulevard, Dallas, TX 75235-9063 · 214-640-5959

Duane L. Dowell · Adolescent & Young Adult Medicine · Children's Medical Center of Dallas, Parkland Memorial Hospital · 6303 Harry Hines Boulevard, Suite 101, Dallas, TX 75235-5228 · 214-640-0300

Chester Walter Fink · Pediatric Rheumatology (Classification & Genetics of Juvenile Arthritis, Vasculitis in Children, Systemic Lupus Erythematosus) · Children's Medical Center of Dallas, Texas Scottish Rite Hospital for Children · University of Texas-Southwestern Medical Center at Dallas, 5323 Harry Hines Boulevard, Dallas, TX 75235-9063 · 214-648-3388

David E. Fixler · Pediatric Cardiology · Children's Medical Center of Dallas · Children's Medical Center of Dallas, Department of Cardiology, 1935 Motor Street, Dallas, TX 75235 · 214-640-2333

Jose L. Gonzalez · Pediatric Endocrinology (Growth & Maturational Disorders in Children & Adolescents) · Children's Medical Center of Dallas · Children's Medical Center of Dallas, 6300 Harry Hines Boulevard, Suite 1200, Dallas, TX 75235-7794 · 214-640-5959

Barton A. Kamen · Pediatric Hematology-Oncology (Clinical Pharmacology, Experimental Chemotherapy) · Children's Medical Center of Dallas · University of Texas-Southwestern Medical Center at Dallas, 5323 Harry Hines Boulevard, Dallas, TX 75235-9063 · 214-648-3896

David J. Keljo · Pediatric Gastroenterology (Inflammatory Bowel Disease, Short Bowel Syndrome, Disorders of Elimination) · Children's Medical Center of Dallas · Children's Medical Center of Dallas, Center for Pediatric Gastroenterology, 1935 Motor Street, Dallas, TX 75235-7794 · 214-640-8000

Kathleen Ann Kennedy · Neonatal-Perinatal Medicine · St. Paul Medical Center, Parkland Memorial Hospital, Children's Medical Center of Dallas · University of Texas-Southwestern Medical Center at Dallas, Department of Pediatrics, Division of Neonatal-Perinatal Medicine, 5323 Harry Hines Boulevard, Dallas, TX 75235-9063 · 214-648-3753

Daniel L. Levin · Pediatric Critical Care · Children's Medical Center of Dallas · Children's Medical Center of Dallas, Pediatric Intensive Care, 1935 Motor Street, Dallas, TX 75235 · 214-640-2360

Lynn Mahony · Pediatric Cardiology (Marfan's Syndrome, Congenital Heart Disease, Cardiovascular Evaluation of Student Athletes) · Children's Medical Center of Dallas · Children's Medical Center of Dallas, Department of Cardiology, 1935 Motor Street, Dallas, TX 75235 · 214-640-2333

James F. Marks · Pediatric Endocrinology (Type I Diabetes Mellitus) · Children's Medical Center of Dallas · University of Texas-Southwestern Medical Center at Dallas, 5323 Harry Hines Boulevard, Dallas, TX 75235-9063 · 214-648-3501

George H. McCracken, Jr. · Pediatric Infectious Disease (Bacterial Meningitis, Pediatric Antibiotic Therapy, General Infectious Disease) · Children's Medical Center of Dallas, Parkland Memorial Hospital · University of Texas-Southwestern Medical Center at Dallas, 5323 Harry Hines Boulevard, Dallas, TX 75235-9063 · 214-648-3439

Charles E. Mize · Metabolic Diseases · Children's Medical Center of Dallas · University of Texas-Southwestern Medical Center at Dallas, Department of Pediatrics, 5323 Harry Hines Boulevard, Dallas, TX 75235-9063 · 214-648-3382

Trudy V. Murphy · Pediatric Infectious Disease · Children's Medical Center of Dallas, Parkland Memorial Hospital · University of Texas-Southwestern Medical Center at Dallas, 5323 Harry Hines Boulevard, Dallas, TX 75235-9063 · 214-648-3720

John D. Nelson · Pediatric Infectious Disease (Antibiotic Pharmacology, General Infectious Disease) · Parkland Memorial Hospital, Children's Medical Center of Dallas · University of Texas-Southwestern Medical Center at Dallas, 5323 Harry Hines Boulevard, Dallas, TX 75235-9063 · 214-648-3391

Edgar A. Newfeld · Pediatric Cardiology (Congenital Heart Disease, Acquired Heart Disease in Children) · 8230 Walnut Hill Lane, Suite 800, Dallas, TX 75231 214-363-0000

Perry D. Nisen · Pediatric Hematology-Oncology · Children's Medical Center of Dallas · University of Texas-Southwestern Medical Center at Dallas, 5323 Harry Hines Boulevard, Dallas, TX 75235-9063 · 214-648-3896

Jeffrey M. Perlman · Neonatal-Perinatal Medicine (Prevention of Conditions that Presdispose to Cerebral Palsy, eg Intraventricular Hemorrhage, Hypoxic Ischemic Brain Injury, Delivery Room Resuscitation, Neurologic Complications of In Utero Drug Exposure) · Children's Medical Center of Dallas, Parkland Memorial Hospital, St. Paul Medical Center · University of Texas-Southwestern Medical Center at Dallas, 5323 Harry Hines Boulevard, Dallas, TX 75235-9063 · 214-648-3903

Marilynn G. Punaro · Pediatric Rheumatology · Texas Scottish Rite Hospital for Children · Scottish Rite Hospital, 2222 Welborn Street, Dallas, TX 75219-3924 · 214-521-3168

Albert Haine Quan · Pediatric Nephrology · University of Texas-Southwestern Medical Center at Dallas, Department of Pediatrics, 5323 Harry Hines Boulevard, Dallas, TX 75235-9063 · 214-648-3438

Raymond P. Quigley · Pediatric Nephrology · Children's Medical Center of Dallas · University of Texas-Southwestern Medical Center at Dallas, Department of Pediatrics, 5323 Harry Hines Boulevard, Dallas, TX 75235-9063 · 214-648-3438

Charles R. Roe · Metabolic Diseases (Fatty Acid Oxidation) · Baylor University Medical Center · Baylor University Medical Center, Four Hoblitzelle Building, 3500 Gaston Avenue, Dallas, TX 75246-2017 · 214-820-4533

Charles Richard Rosenfeld · Neonatal-Perinatal Medicine (Diagnosis of Neonatal Infection—Neutrophil Values, Cardiovascular Adaptation in Fetus and Newborn, Mechanisms Maintaining Uteroplacental and Umbilical Blood Flows) · Parkland Memorial Hospital, Children's Medical Center of Dallas, St. Paul Medical Center · University of Texas-Southwestern Medical Center at Dallas, 5323 Harry Hines Boulevard, Dallas, TX 75235-9063 · 214-648-3903

Kathleen Rotondo · Pediatric Cardiology · Children's Medical Center of Dallas, Department of Cardiology, 1935 Motor Street, Dallas, TX 75235 · 214-640-2333

Pablo J. Sanchez · Pediatric Infectious Disease (Neonatal-Perinatal Medicine, Neonatal Infectious Diseases, Congenital Syphilis) · Children's Medical Center of Dallas, Parkland Memorial Hospital, St. Paul Medical Center · University of Texas-Southwestern Medical Center at Dallas, Department of Pediatrics, 5323 Harry Hines Boulevard, Dallas, TX 75235-9063 · 214-648-3753

Eric S. Sandler · Pediatric Hematology-Oncology (Pediatric Bone Marrow Transplantation) · Children's Medical Center of Dallas · University of Texas-Southwestern Medical Center at Dallas, Department of Pediatrics, 5323 Harry Hines Boulevard, Dallas, TX 75235-9063 · 214-640-2382

William Scott · Pediatric Cardiology (Arrhythmias, Syncope, Pacemakers) · Children's Medical Center of Dallas · University of Texas-Southwestern Medical Center at Dallas, Department of Pediatrics, 5323 Harry Hines Boulevard, Dallas, TX 75235 · 214-640-2333

Mouin G. Seikaly · Pediatric Nephrology (Hypertension, Rickets, General Nephrology) · Children's Medical Center of Dallas, Parkland Memorial Hospital, Texas Scottish Rite Hospital for Children · University of Texas-Southwestern Medical Center at Dallas, 5323 Harry Hines Boulevard, Dallas, TX 75235-9063 · 214-640-6005

Jane D. Siegel · Pediatric Infectious Disease (Hospital-Acquired Infections, Tuberculosis, Neonatal Bacterial Infections, Group B Strep) · Children's Medical Center of Dallas · University of Texas-Southwestern Medical Center at Dallas, 5323 Harry Hines Boulevard, Dallas, TX 75235-9063 · 214-648-3720

Robert H. Squires, Jr. · Pediatric Gastroenterology · Children's Medical Center of Dallas · Children's Medical Center of Dallas, Center for Pediatric Gastroenterology, 1935 Motor Street, Dallas, TX 75235 · 214-640-8000

Gail Elizabeth Tomlinson · Pediatric Hematology-Oncology (Pediatric Oncology [Solid Tumors], Genetic Testing for Cancer Predisposition) · Children's Medical Center of Dallas · University of Texas-Southwestern Medical Center at Dallas, Department of Pediatrics, 5323 Harry Hines Boulevard, Dallas, TX 75235 · 214-648-3896

Jon Edward Tyson · Neonatal-Perinatal Medicine · St. Paul Medical Center, Parkland Memorial Hospital · University of Texas-Southwestern Medical Center at Dallas, 5323 Harry Hines Boulevard, Dallas, TX 75235-9063 · 214-648-3753

Lewis J. Waber · Metabolic Diseases (Genetics) · University of Texas-Southwestern Medical Center at Dallas, 5323 Harry Hines Boulevard, Dallas, TX 75235-9063 · 214-648-8996

Ellen Weinstein · Pediatric Cardiology (Echocardiography) · Children's Medical Center of Dallas, Department of Cardiology, 1935 Motor Street, Dallas, TX 75235 214-640-2333

Perrin C. White · Pediatric Endocrinology (Diabetes) · Children's Medical Center of Dallas · University of Texas-Southwestern Medical Center at Dallas, Department of Pediatric Endocrinology, 5323 Harry Hines Boulevard, Dallas, TX 75235-9060 · 214-648-3501

Golder N. Wilson · Metabolic Diseases (Genetics, Congenital Anomalies) · Children's Medical Center of Dallas, Parkland Memorial Hospital · University of Texas-Southwestern Medical Center at Dallas, 5323 Harry Hines Boulevard, Dallas, TX 75235-9063 · 214-648-8996

Naomi J. Winick · Pediatric Hematology-Oncology (Leukemia, Lymphomas, Methotrexate/6-Mercaptopurine) · Children's Medical Center of Dallas · University of Texas-Southwestern Medical Center at Dallas, Department of Hematology-Oncology, Sixth Floor Clinic, 1935 Motor Street, Dallas, TX 75235 · 214-640-2382

Thomas Michael Zellers · Pediatric Cardiology · University of Texas-Southwestern Medical Center at Dallas, Department of Pediatrics, 5323 Harry Hines Boulevard, Dallas, TX 75235 · 214-640-2333

Robert Jeffrey Zwiener · Pediatric Gastroenterology (Pediatric Liver Disease, Pediatric Endoscopy, Pediatric Inflammatory Bowel Disease) · Children's Medical Center of Dallas · Children's Medical Center of Dallas, Center for Pediatric Gastroenterology, 1935 Motor Street, Dallas, TX 75235 · 214-640-8000

El Paso

Roberto Canales · Pediatric Hematology-Oncology · 1733 Curie Drive, Suite 103, El Paso, TX 79902 · 915-532-2985

Robert Christianson · Pediatric Endocrinology · Texas Tech University Health Sciences Center, Department of Pediatrics, 4800 Alberta Avenue, El Paso, TX 79905-2709 · 915-545-6785

Delia M. Gallo · Abused Children (Preventive Programs for Children, Parenting Skills Program) · Providence Memorial Hospital, Sierra Medical Center, Thomason Hospital · Texas Tech Outpatient Clinic, 424 Executive Center, Suite 101, El Paso, TX 79902 · 915-533-2471; 915-545-6785

Gilberto A. Handal · Pediatric Critical Care, Pediatric Infectious Disease · Thomason Hospital, Sierra Medical Center, Providence Memorial Hospital · Texas Tech University Health Sciences Center, Department of Pediatrics, 4800 Alberta Avenue, El Paso, TX 79905-2709 · 915-545-6785

Merle A. Ipson · Neonatal-Perinatal Medicine · Texas Tech University Health Sciences Center, Department of Pediatric Neonatology, 4800 Alberta Avenue, El Paso, TX 79905-2709 · 915-545-6785

Carlos Antonio Jesurun · Neonatal-Perinatal Medicine · Thomason Hospital · Texas Tech University Health Sciences Center, Department of Pediatrics, 4800 Alberta Avenue, El Paso, TX 79905-2700 · 915-545-6785

Garrett Stephen Levin · Neonatal-Perinatal Medicine · Texas Tech University Health Sciences Center, Department of Pediatrics, 4800 Alberta Avenue, El Paso, TX 79905 · 915-545-6785

Manuel Schydlower · Adolescent Medicine · Providence Memorial Hospital, Columbia Medical Center-West, Columbia Medical Center-East, Thomason Hospital · Texas Tech University Health Sciences Center, Department of Pediatrics, Adolescent Medicine Clinic, 4800 Alberta Avenue, El Paso, TX 79905 · 915-545-6785

Fort Sam Houston

Judith Ann O'Connor · Pediatric Gastroenterology · Brooke Army Medical Center · Brooke Army Medical Center, Department of Pediatrics, 1950 Stanley Road, Fort Sam Houston, TX 78234 · 210-916-9160

Terry Eugene Pick · Pediatric Hematology-Oncology · Brooke Army Medical Center · Brooke Army Medical Center, Department of Pediatrics, 1950 Stanley Road, Fort Sam Houston, TX 78234 · 210-916-9160

Fort Worth

William R. Allen · Pediatric Nephrology (Diabetes) · Cook Children's Medical Center · Cook Children's Medical Center, 801 Seventh Avenue, Fort Worth, TX 76104-2796 · 817-885-4260

James Hudson Allender · Pediatric Cardiology (Congenital Heart Disease, Cardiac Pacing in Children) · Cook Children's Medical Center · Pediatric Cardiology Associates, 1516 Cooper Street, Fort Worth, TX 76104 · 817-332-1085

William Paul Bowman · Pediatric Hematology-Oncology (Leukemia, Lymphomas) · Cook Children's Medical Center · Cook Children's Medical Center, Department of Hematology-Oncology, 801 Seventh Avenue, Fort Worth, TX 76104-2796 · 817-885-4006

Roberto Caballero · Pediatric Critical Care · Cook Children's Medical Center · Cook Children's Medical Center, 801 Seventh Avenue, Fort Worth, TX 76104-2796 · 817-885-4000

James Calvin Cunningham · Pediatric Pulmonology (Cystic Fibrosis) · Cook Children's Medical Center · Cook Children's Medical Center, 801 Seventh Avenue, Fort Worth, TX 76104-2796 · 817-885-4202

Nancy N. Dambro · Pediatric Pulmonology · Cook Children's Medical Center · Cook Children's Medical Center, Department of Pulmonary Medicine, 801 Seventh Avenue, Fort Worth, TX 76104-2796 · 817-885-4202

Maynard C. Dyson · Pediatric Pulmonology · Cook Children's Medical Center, Department of Pediatric Pulmonary Medicine, 801 Seventh Avenue, Fort Worth, TX 76104-2796 · 817-885-4202

Gretchen M. Eames · Pediatric Hematology-Oncology (Bone Marrow Transplantation, Late Effects of Cancer Therapy) · Cook Children's Medical Center · Cook Children's Medical Center, Department of Hematology-Oncology, 801 Seventh Avenue, Fort Worth, TX 76104-2796 · 817-885-4006

David Friedman · Pediatric Hematology-Oncology (Bone Marrow Transplantation, Medical Hematology) · Cook Children's Medical Center, Harris Methodist-Fort Worth · Cook Children's Medical Center, Department of Hematology-Oncology, 801 Seventh Avenue, Fort Worth, TX 76104-2796 · 817-885-4006

Timothy C. Griffin · Pediatric Hematology-Oncology · Cook Children's Medical Center · Cook Children's Medical Center, Department of Hematology-Oncology, 801 Seventh Avenue, Fort Worth, TX 76104-2796 · 817-885-4006

Sami K. Wassouf Hadeed · Pediatric Pulmonology · Cook Children's Medical Center · Cook Children's Medical Center, Department of Pulmonary Medicine, 801 Seventh Avenue, Fort Worth, TX 76104-2796 · 817-885-4202

Susan Lynn Hess · Pediatric Cardiology · Pediatric Cardiology Associates, 1516 Cooper Street, Fort Worth, TX 76104 · 817-332-1085

Lyn I. Hunt · Pediatric Gastroenterology · Pediatric Gastroenterology, 800 Seventh Avenue, Fort Worth, TX 76104 · 817-332-2233

Stephen Yuer-Mon Lai · Pediatric Cardiology · Pediatric Cardiology Associates, 1516 Cooper Street, Fort Worth, TX 76104 · 817-332-1085

Jan Leah Lamb · Abused Children · Cook Children's Medical Center · Cook Children's Medical Center, Department of Pediatrics, 801 Seventh Avenue, Fort Worth, TX 76104-2796 · 817-885-3960

Michael P. Morris · Pediatric Gastroenterology · Cook Children's Medical Center Pediatric Gastroenterology, 800 Seventh Avenue, Fort Worth, TX 76104 · 817-332-2233

Donald K. Murphey · Pediatric Infectious Disease · Cook Children's Medical Center · Cook Children's Medical Center, Department of Infectious Diseases, 801 Seventh Avenue, Fort Worth, TX 76104-2796 · 817-885-4312

Jeffrey C. Murray · Pediatric Hematology-Oncology · Cook Children's Medical Center · Cook Children's Medical Center, Department of Hematology-Oncology, 801 Seventh Avenue, Fort Worth, TX 76104-2796 · 817-885-4006

William B. Nelson · Pediatric Critical Care · Cook Children's Medical Center · Cook Children's Medical Center, Pediatric Intensive Care Unit, 801 Seventh Avenue, Fort Worth, TX 76104-2796 · 817-885-4205

Richard I. Readinger · Pediatric Cardiology · Pediatric Cardiology Associates, 1516 Cooper Street, Fort Worth, TX 76104 · 817-332-1085

Joann Marie Sanders · Pediatric Hematology-Oncology · Cook Children's Medical Center · Cook Children's Medical Center, Department of Hematology-Oncology, 801 Seventh Avenue, Fort Worth, TX 76104-2796 · 817-885-4006

Mark McGregor Shelton · Pediatric Infectious Disease · Cook Children's Medical Center · Cook Children's Medical Center, Department of Infectious Diseases, 801 Seventh Avenue, Fort Worth, TX 76104-2796 · 817-885-4312

Richard A. Sidebottom · Neonatal-Perinatal Medicine · Cook Children's Medical Center, Harris Methodist-Fort Worth · Cook Children's Medical Center, Department of Neonatology, 801 Seventh Avenue, Fort Worth, TX 76104-2796 · 817-885-4283

Michael Dale Stanley · Neonatal-Perinatal Medicine · Cook Children's Medical Center, Harris Methodist-Fort Worth · Harris Methodist-Fort Worth, 1301 Pennsylvania Avenue, Fort Worth, TX 76104 · 817-885-4382

Michael J. Stevener · Neonatal-Perinatal Medicine · Cook Children's Medical Center, Harris Methodist-Fort Worth · Cook Children's Medical Center, Department of Neonatology, 801 Seventh Avenue, Fort Worth, TX 76104-2796 · 817-885-4283

Galveston

Blanche P. Alter · Pediatric Hematology-Oncology (Hematology) · University of Texas Medical Branch Hospitals · University of Texas Medical Branch, Division of Pediatric Hematology-Oncology, 301 University Boulevard, Galveston, TX 77555-0361 · 409-772-2341

John S. Dallas · Pediatric Endocrinology · University of Texas Medical Branch, Department of Pediatric Endocrinology & Diabetes, 301 University Boulevard, Galveston, TX 77555-0363 · 409-772-3365

Steven C. Diven · Pediatric Nephrology · University of Texas Medical Branch Hospitals · University of Texas Medical Branch, Department of Pediatrics, Division of Pediatric Nephrology, 301 University Boulevard, Galveston, TX 77555-0373 · 409-772-2538

Joan R. Hebeler · Abused Children · University of Texas Medical Branch Hospitals · University of Texas Medical Branch, Department of Psychiatry, 3.258 Graves Building, 301 University Boulevard, Galveston, TX 77550 · 409-772-1066

Alok Kalia · Pediatric Nephrology · University of Texas Medical Branch Hospitals University of Texas Medical Branch, Division of Pediatric Nephrology, 301 University Boulevard, Galveston, TX 77555-0373 · 409-772-2538

Bruce Stone Keenan · Pediatric Endocrinology (Pediatric Diabetes) · University of Texas Medical Branch Hospitals · University of Texas Medical Branch, Division of Pediatric Endocrinology, 301 University Boulevard, Galveston, TX 77555-0363 · 409-772-3365

Susan E. Keeney · Neonatal-Perinatal Medicine · University of Texas Medical Branch Hospitals · University of Texas Medical Branch, Division of Neonatology, 301 University Boulevard, Galveston, TX 77555-0526 · 409-772-2815

Lillian H. Lockhart · Metabolic Diseases (Medical Genetics) · University of Texas Medical Branch, Department of Pediatrics, Division of Pediatric Genetics, 301 University Boulevard, Galveston, TX 77555-0359 · 409-772-3466

Michael H. Malloy · Neonatal-Perinatal Medicine · University of Texas Medical Branch, Division of Neonatology, 301 University Boulevard, Galveston, TX 77555-0526 · 409-772-2815

Pearay L. Ogra · Pediatric Infectious Disease (Vaccines, Mucosal Immunity) · Children's Hospital of University of Texas Medical Branch · Children's Hospital, Department of Pediatrics, 301 University Boulevard, Galveston, TX 77555-0351 · 409-772-1596

Janak A. Patel · Pediatric Infectious Disease · University of Texas Medical Branch Hospitals · University of Texas Medical Branch, Department of Pediatrics, Division of Pediatric Infectious Disease, 301 University Boulevard, Galveston, TX 77555-0371 · 409-772-2798

Carol Joan Richardson · Neonatal-Perinatal Medicine · University of Texas Medical Branch Hospitals · University of Texas Medical Branch, Department of Pediatrics, 301 University Boulevard, Galveston, TX 77555-0526 · 409-772-2815

David W. Sapire · Pediatric Cardiology (Congenital Heart Disease in Adults) · University of Texas Medical Branch Hospitals · University of Texas Medical Branch, Department of Pediatrics, Division of Pediatric Cardiology, 301 University Boulevard, Galveston, TX 77555-0367 · 409-772-2507

Karen E. Shattuck · Neonatal-Perinatal Medicine · University of Texas Medical Branch Hospitals · University of Texas Medical Branch, Department of Pediatrics, Division of Neonatology, 301 University Boulevard, Galveston, TX 77555-0526 · 409-772-2815

Luther B. Travis · Pediatric Nephrology (Diabetes, Renal Disease, Pediatric Metabolic Disease) · Children's Hospital of University of Texas Medical Branch · Children's Hospital of University of Texas Medical Branch, 301 University Boulevard, Room 2.330, Galveston, TX 77555-0373 · 409-772-2538

Houston

James Mervyn Adams · Neonatal-Perinatal Medicine · Texas Children's Hospital · Texas Children's Hospital, Department of Neonatal Medicine, 6621 Fannin Street, Mail Code 1-3460, Houston, TX 77030 · 713-770-1380

Joann L. Ater · Pediatric Hematology-Oncology (Neuro-Oncology, Pediatric Brain Tumor) · University of Texas-M. D. Anderson Cancer Center · University of Texas-M. D. Anderson Cancer Center, 1515 Holcombe Boulevard, Box 87, Houston, TX 77030 · 713-792-6665

Jane Troendle Atkins · Pediatric Infectious Disease (Congenital Syphillis, Congenital Cytomegalovirus Infections) · Hermann Hospital, Lyndon B. Johnson General Hospital · University of Texas Medical School at Houston, Department of Pediatrics, 6431 Fannin Street, Mail Code GSB1739, Houston, TX 77030 · 713-792-5330 x3114

Nancy A. Ayres · Pediatric Cardiology (Echocardiography) · Texas Children's Hospital · Texas Children's Hospital, Department of Cardiology, 6621 Fannin Street, Mail Code 2-2280, Houston, TX 77030 · 713-770-5600

Bruce Kenneth Bacot · Pediatric Pulmonology (General Pediatrics) · Texas Children's Hospital · Texas Children's Hospital, Department of Pulmonary Medicine, 6621 Fannin Street, Mail Code 3-2571, Houston, TX 77030 · 713-770-2575

Carol Jane Baker · Pediatric Infectious Disease · Texas Children's Hospital · Baylor College of Medicine, Department of Pediatrics, One Baylor Plaza, Room 307-E, Houston, TX 77030 · 713-798-4790

Arthur Louis Beaudet · Metabolic Diseases (General Pediatrics, Cystic Fibrosis, Urea Cycle Disorders, Genetics) · Texas Children's Hospital, Methodist Hospital, Harris County Hospital District, St. Joseph Hospital, The Woman's Hospital of Texas, St. Luke's Episcopal Hospital · Baylor College of Medicine, Department of Molecular & Human Genetics, One Baylor Plaza, Room T-619, Houston, TX 77030 · 713-798-4795

Thomas N. Belhorn · Pediatric Infectious Disease (Virology) · Hermann Hospital University of Texas Medical School at Houston, 6431 Fannin Street, Mail Code JFB 1.739, Houston, TX 77030 · 713-792-5330

John W. Belmont · Metabolic Diseases (Genetics) · Texas Children's Hospital · Baylor College of Medicine, Department of Molecular & Human Genetics, One Baylor Plaza, Room T-826, Houston, TX 77030 · 713-798-4634

Stacey L. Berg · Pediatric Hematology-Oncology · Texas Children's Hospital, 6621 Fannin Street, Mail Code 3-3320, Houston, TX 77030 · 713-770-4200

Dennis M. Bier · Pediatric Endocrinology (Growth Hormone, Metabolism, Nutrition) · Texas Children's Hospital, Harris County Hospital District · Children's Nutrition Research Center, 1100 Bates Street, Houston, TX 77030-2600 · 713-798-7022

Susan M. Blaney · Pediatric Hematology-Oncology (Pediatric Neuro-Oncology) · Texas Children's Cancer Center · Texas Children's Cancer Center, Department of Hematology-Oncology, 6621 Fannin Street, Mail Code 3-3320, Houston, TX 77030 · 713-770-4200

W. Archie Bleyer · Pediatric Hematology-Oncology (Neuro-Oncology, New Agent Trials, Pediatric Leukemia) · University of Texas-M. D. Anderson Cancer Center · University of Texas-M. D. Anderson Cancer Center, 1515 Holcombe Boulevard, Box 87, Houston, TX 77030 · 713-792-6603

Melvin A. Bonilla-Felix · Pediatric Nephrology (Renal Tubular Acidosis, Kidney Transplantation, Glomerular Diseases) · Hermann Children's Hospital, Lyndon B. Johnson General Hospital · University of Texas Medical School at Houston, Department of Pediatrics, Division of Pediatric Nephrology, 6431 Fannin Street, Room 3.124, Houston, TX 77030 · 713-792-5330

L. Eileen Doyle Brewer · Pediatric Nephrology (Dialysis, Kidney Transplantation) · Texas Children's Hospital · Texas Children's Hospital, 6621 Fannin Street, Mail Code 3-2482, Houston, TX 77030-2303 · 713-770-3800

John Timothy Bricker · Pediatric Cardiology (Exercise Physiology, Preventive Cardiology) · Texas Children's Hospital · Texas Children's Hospital, 6621 Fannin Street, Mail Code 2-2280, Houston, TX 77030 · 713-770-5600

Judith Rochelle Campbell · Pediatric Infectious Disease · Baylor School of Medicine, Department of Infectious Disease, One Baylor Plaza, Room 307E, Houston, TX 77030 · 713-798-4790

Mariam R. Chacko · Adolescent & Young Adult Medicine (Medical Evaluation of the Sexually Abused Child) · Texas Children's Hospital · Texas Children's Hospital, 1102 Bates Street, Mail Code 3-2305, P.O. Box 300630, Houston, TX 77230-0630 · 713-770-3440

Ka Wah Chan · Pediatric Hematology-Oncology (Bone Marrow Transplantation) University of Texas-M. D. Anderson Cancer Center · University of Texas-M. D. Anderson Cancer Center, Department of Pediatrics, 1515 Holcombe Boulevard, Box 87, Houston, TX 77030-4009 · 713-792-7751

Murali M. Chintagumpala · Pediatric Hematology-Oncology · Texas Children's Hospital · Texas Children's Hospital, 6621 Fannin Street, Mail Code 3-3320, Houston, TX 77030-2399 · 713-770-4200

Thomas G. Cleary · Pediatric Infectious Disease (Diarrhea, Daycare Infections) · University of Texas Medical School at Houston, 6431 Fannin Street, Mail Code JFB 1.739, Houston, TX 77030 · 713-792-5330 x3114

Timothy R. Cooper · Neonatal-Perinatal Medicine · Texas Children's Hospital, Ben Taub General Hospital, The Woman's Hospital of Texas, Methodist Hospital Texas Children's Hospital, Department of Neonatology, 6621 Fannin Street, Houston, TX 77030 · 713-770-1380

Kenneth C. Copeland · Pediatric Endocrinology (General Pediatrics, Growth, Diabetes) · Texas Children's Hospital · Texas Children's Hospital, Department of Pediatrics (Diabetes-Metabolism), 6621 Fannin Street, Mail Code 3-2351, Houston, TX 77030-2399 · 713-770-3780

Armando Gerardo Correa · Pediatric Infectious Disease (Tuberculosis) · Texas Children's Hospital · Texas Children's Hospital, 6621 Fannin Street, Mail Code 3-2371, Houston, TX 77030-2399 · 713-770-4330

William J. Craigen · Metabolic Diseases (Genetics) · Texas Children's Hospital Baylor College of Medicine, Department of Molecular & Human Genetics, One Baylor Plaza, Room S-911-A, Houston, TX 77030 · 713-798-8305

Sharon Sue Crandell · Neonatal-Perinatal Medicine · Hermann Hospital · University of Texas Medical School at Houston, 6431 Fannin Street, Room 3.244, Houston, TX 77030 · 713-792-5330 x8

Steven J. Culbert · Pediatric Hematology-Oncology · University of Texas-M. D. Anderson Cancer Center · University of Texas-M. D. Anderson Cancer Center, Department of Pediatrics, 1515 Holcombe Boulevard, Box 87, Houston, TX 77030 · 713-792-6634

Gail J. Demmler · Pediatric Infectious Disease (Virology, Cytomegalovirus, Chicken Pox) · Texas Children's Hospital · Texas Children's Hospital, 6621 Fannin Street, Mail Code 3-2371, Houston, TX 77030 · 713-770-4330

Susan Warren Denfield · Pediatric Cardiology (Transplantation, Cardiomyopathy, General Cardiology) · Texas Children's Hospital · Texas Children's Hospital, Department of Cardiology, 6621 Fannin Street, Mail Code 2-2280, Houston, TX 77030 · 713-770-5600

Susan E. Denson · Neonatal-Perinatal Medicine · Hermann Hospital · University of Texas Medical School, Department of Pediatrics, Division of Neonatology, 6431 Fannin Street, Room 3.256, Houston, TX 77030 · 713-792-5330

Marilyn Doyle · Pediatric Infectious Disease (HIV Infections, AIDS) · Hermann Hospital · University of Texas Medical School at Houston, Department of Pediatrics, 6410 Fannin Street, Suite 720, Houston, TX 77030 · 713-794-4044

Zoann Eckert Dreyer · Pediatric Hematology-Oncology (Late Effects of Childhood Cancer Therapy, Infant Acute Lymphoid Leukemia) · Texas Children's Hospital · Texas Children's Hospital, 6621 Fannin Street, Mail Code 3-3320, Houston, TX 77030 · 713-770-4207

Morven Spencer Edwards · Pediatric Infectious Disease · Texas Children's Hospital · Baylor College of Medicine, Department of Pediatrics, One Baylor Plaza, Room 307-E, Houston, TX 77030 · 713-798-4790

Janet A. Englund · Pediatric Infectious Disease · Baylor College of Medicine, Department of Microbiology & Immunology, One Baylor Plaza, Room 632-EA, Houston, TX 77030 · 713-798-4469

Khoulood F. Fakhoury · Pediatric Pulmonology (Asthma, Cystic Fibrosis, Bronchopulmonary Dysplasia) · Texas Children's Hospital · Texas Children's Hospital, Department of Pulmonary Medicine, 6621 Fannin Street, Mail Code 3-2571, Houston, TX 77030 · 713-770-3300

Leland L. Fan · Pediatric Pulmonology, Pediatric Critical Care (Interstitial Lung Disease) · Texas Children's Hospital · Texas Children's Hospital, 6621 Fannin Street, Mail Code 3-2571, Houston, TX 77030-2399 · 713-770-3300

Ralph D. Feigin · Pediatric Infectious Disease (Meningitis) · Texas Children's Hospital · Texas Children's Hospital, 6621 Fannin Street, Mail Code 1-3420, Houston, TX 77030-2303 · 713-798-4780

Timothy Francis Feltes · Pediatric Cardiology (Intensive Care, Echocardiography) · Texas Children's Hospital · Texas Children's Hospital, 6621 Fannin Street, Mail Code 2-2280, Houston, TX 77030 · 713-770-5640

George D. Ferry · Pediatric Gastroenterology (Inflammatory Bowel Disease) · Texas Children's Hospital · Texas Children's Hospital, 6621 Fannin Street, Mail Code 3-3391, Houston, TX 77030-2303 · 713-770-3600

Robert Cecil Franks · Pediatric Endocrinology · Lyndon B. Johnson General Hospital, Hermann Children's Hospital · University of Texas Medical School at Houston, 6431 Fannin Street, Room MSB 3.020, Houston, TX 77030 · 713-636-5845

Jose Garcia · Neonatal-Perinatal Medicine · Lyndon B. Johnson General Hospital · Lyndon B. Johnson General Hospital, Department of Pediatrics, Neonatal Division, 5656 Kelley Street, Houston, TX 77026 · 713-636-5846

Joseph Arthur Garcia-Prats · Neonatal-Perinatal Medicine · Ben Taub General Hospital, Texas Children's Hospital, The Woman's Hospital of Texas, Methodist Hospital · Ben Taub General Hospital, Third Floor, Room 3NT91002, 1502 Taub Loop, Houston, TX 77030 · 713-793-2000

Wallace Anselm Gleason, Jr. · Pediatric Gastroenterology (Hepatology, Nutrition) · Hermann Hospital · University of Texas Medical School at Houston, Department of Pediatrics, 6431 Fannin Street, Room 3.142, Houston, TX 77030 · 713-792-5330

W. Paul Glezen · Pediatric Infectious Disease (Influenza) · Harris County Hospital District · Baylor College of Medicine, Influenza Research Center, Department of Microbiology & Immunology, One Baylor Plaza, Houston, TX 77030 · 713-798-5249

Ronald G. Grifka · Pediatric Cardiology (Cardiac Catheterization, Pediatric Critical Care) · Texas Children's Hospital · Texas Children's Hospital, Department of Cardiology, 6621 Fannin Street, Mail Code 2-2280, Houston, TX 77030 · 713-770-5600

Alfred L. Guest · Neonatal-Perinatal Medicine · Texas Children's Hospital, Department of Neonatology, 6621 Fannin Street, Houston, TX 77030 · 713-770-1380

Charleta Guillory · Neonatal-Perinatal Medicine · Texas Children's Hospital, Department of Neonatology, 6621 Fannin Street, Houston, TX 77030 · 713-770-1380

Gunyon M. Harrison · Pediatric Pulmonology · Texas Children's Hospital · Texas Children's Hospital, Department of Pulmonary Medicine, 6621 Fannin Street, Mail Code 3-2571, Houston, TX 77030 · 713-770-3300

Gail E. Herman · Metabolic Diseases (Genetics) · Texas Children's Hospital · Baylor College of Medicine, Department of Molecular & Human Genetics, One Baylor Plaza, Room T-821, Houston, TX 77030 · 713-798-6526

Cynthia E. Herzog · Pediatric Hematology-Oncology · University of Texas-M. D. Anderson Cancer Center · University of Texas-M. D. Anderson Cancer Center, Department of Pediatrics, 1515 Holcombe Boulevard, Box 087, Houston, TX 77030 · 713-795-0157

Peter W. Hiatt · Pediatric Pulmonology · Texas Children's Hospital · Texas Children's Hospital, Department of Pulmonary Medicine, 6621 Fannin Street, Mail Code 3-2571, Houston, TX 77030 · 713-770-3300

Louis Leighton Hill · Pediatric Nephrology · Texas Children's Hospital · Baylor College of Medicine, One Baylor Plaza, Houston, TX 77030 · 713-798-4794

W. Keith Hoots · Pediatric Hematology-Oncology (Hemophilia, Coagulopathy Associated with Head Injury, Disorders of Bleeding, Thrombosis) · Hermann Hospital · The Gulf States Hemophilia Center, 6410 Fannin Street, Suite 416, Houston, TX 77030 · 713-704-1986

Marc E. Horowitz · Pediatric Hematology-Oncology (Pediatric Brain Tumors, Pediatric Solid Tumors, Informatics) · Texas Children's Hospital · Texas Children's Hospital, Hematology-Oncology Service, 6621 Fannin Street, Mail Code 3-3320, Houston, TX 77030 · 713-770-4200

Richard L. Hurwitz · Pediatric Hematology-Oncology · Texas Children's Hospital · Texas Children's Hospital, 6621 Fannin Street, Mail Code 3-3320, Houston, TX 77030 · 713-770-4200

Norman Jaffe · Pediatric Hematology-Oncology (Bone Sarcomas) · University of Texas-M. D. Anderson Cancer Center, 1515 Holcombe Boulevard, Box 87, Houston, TX 77030 · 713-792-6626

Larry S. Jefferson · Pediatric Critical Care · Texas Children's Hospital · Texas Children's Hospital, Critical Care & Surgical Facility, Suite 440, 6621 Fannin Street, Mail Code 2-3450, Houston, TX 77030-2399 · 713-770-6232

Karen E. Johnson · Neonatal-Perinatal Medicine · Texas Children's Hospital, Department of Neonatology, 6621 Fannin Street, Houston, TX 77030 · 713-770-1380

Sheldon Lee Kaplan · Pediatric Infectious Disease (Meningitis) · Texas Children's Hospital · Texas Children's Hospital, 6621 Fannin Street, Mail Code 3-2371, Houston, TX 77030-2303 · 713-770-4330

Julie P. Katkin · Pediatric Pulmonology · Texas Children's Hospital · Texas Children's Hospital, Department of Pulmonary Medicine, 6621 Fannin Street, Mail Code 3-2571, Houston, TX 77030 · 713-770-3300

John Lindsey Kirkland III · Pediatric Endocrinology (Growth & Development) · Texas Children's Hospital · Texas Children's Hospital, 6621 Fannin Street, Houston, TX 77030-2399 · 713-798-4793

Rebecca T. Kirkland · Pediatric Endocrinology · Texas Children's Hospital · Baylor College of Medicine, Department of Pediatrics, One Baylor Plaza, Houston, TX 77030 · 713-770-3442

Mark W. Kline · Pediatric Infectious Disease (Immunology, HIV Infections) · Texas Children's Hospital · Texas Children's Hospital, Department of Allergy/Immunology, 6621 Fannin Street, Suite A-380, Houston, TX 77030 · 713-770-1319

William John Klish · Pediatric Gastroenterology (Nutrition) · Texas Children's Hospital · Texas Children's Hospital, 6621 Fannin Street, Mail Code 3-3391, Houston, TX 77030-2303 · 713-770-3600

John Kuttesch · Pediatric Hematology-Oncology (Neuro-Oncology, Pediatric Brain Tumor, Trials of Investigational Drugs in Children with Recurrent Tumors) · University of Texas-M. D. Anderson Cancer Center · University of Texas-M. D. Anderson Cancer Center, Department of Pediatrics, 1515 Holcombe Boulevard, Box 087, Houston, TX 77030 · 713-792-6559

Donald Hopkins Mahoney, Jr. · Pediatric Hematology-Oncology · Texas Children's Hospital · Texas Children's Hospital, 6621 Fannin Street, Mail Code 3-3320, Houston, TX 77030 · 713-770-4200

Judith F. Margolin · Pediatric Hematology-Oncology · Texas Children's Hospital · Texas Children's Hospital, 6621 Fannin Street, Mail Code 3-3320, Houston, TX 77030 · 713-770-4583

Kenneth Louis McClain · Pediatric Hematology-Oncology (Lymphomas, Hematological Diseases) · Texas Children's Hospital · Texas Children's Hospital, 6621 Fannin Street, Mail Code 3-3320, Houston, TX 77030 · 713-770-4208

Alicia A. Moise · Neonatal-Perinatal Medicine · Texas Children's Hospital, Ben Taub General Hospital, The Woman's Hospital of Texas, Methodist Hospital · Texas Children's Hospital, Department of Neonatology, 6621 Fannin Street, Houston, TX 77030 · 713-770-1380

Robert H. Moore · Pediatric Pulmonology · Texas Children's Hospital · Texas Children's Hospital, 6621 Fannin Street, Mail Code 3-2571, Houston, TX 77030-2399 · 713-770-3300

Aamar B. Morad · Pediatric Hematology-Oncology · Texas Children's Hospital Texas Children's Hospital, 6621 Fannin Street, Mail Code 3-3320, Houston, TX 77030 · 713-770-4200

Charles Edward Mullins · Pediatric Cardiology (Therapeutic Catheterization) · Texas Children's Hospital · Texas Children's Hospital, 6621 Fannin Street, Mail Code 2-2531, Houston, TX 77030 · 713-770-5901

Barry Lee Myones · Pediatric Rheumatology (Lupus, Vasculitis, Antiphospholipid Syndrome, Immunodeficiency) · Texas Children's Hospital · Texas Children's Hospital, 6621 Fannin Street, Mail Code 3-2290, Houston, TX 77030 · 713-770-3830

Michael R. Nihill · Pediatric Cardiology (Interventional Catheterization, Pulmonary Hypertension, Health Informatics) · Texas Children's Hospital · Texas Children's Hospital, Department of Cardiology, 6621 Fannin Street, Mail Code 2-2280, Houston, TX 77030 · 713-770-5600

Hope Northrup · Metabolic Diseases (Medical Genetics) · Shriners Hospitals for Crippled Children, Lyndon B. Johnson General Hospital, Hermann Hospital · University of Texas Medical School at Houston, Department of Pediatrics, Division of Medical Genetics, 6431 Fannin Street, Room 3.144, Houston, TX 77030 713-792-5330 x3060

Angela Kent Ogden · Pediatric Hematology-Oncology · Texas Children's Hospital · Texas Children's Hospital, Department of Hematology-Oncology, 6621 Fannin Street, Mail Code 3-3320, Houston, TX 77030-2399 · 713-770-4200

Maria de Los Angeles Perez · Pediatric Rheumatology · Texas Children's Hospital · Texas Children's Hospital, Department of Rheumatology, 6621 Fannin Street, Mail Code 3-2290, Houston, TX 77030 · 713-770-3830

David G. Poplack · Pediatric Hematology-Oncology (Pediatric Leukemia) · Texas Children's Hospital · Texas Children's Hospital, 6621 Fannin Street, Mail Code 3-3320, Houston, TX 77030 · 713-770-4556

Ronald Jay Portman · Pediatric Nephrology (Hypertension, Transplantation, Chronobiology, Dialysis) · Hermann Children's Hospital, University of Texas-M. D. Anderson Cancer Center · University of Texas Medical School at Houston, 6431 Fannin Street, Room 3.124, Houston, TX 77030 · 713-792-5330 x3075

David R. Powell · Pediatric Nephrology (General Nephrology) · Texas Children's Hospital · Texas Children's Hospital, Section of Pediatric Nephrology, 6621 Fannin Street, Suite 800, Mail Code 3-2482, Houston, TX 77030 · 713-770-3800

Irma Ramirez · Pediatric Hematology-Oncology · University of Texas-M. D. Anderson Cancer Center · University of Texas-M. D. Anderson Cancer Center, Department of Pediatrics, 1515 Holcombe Boulevard, Box 87, Houston, TX 77030-4009 · 713-792-3497

Richard Beverly Raney, Jr. · Pediatric Hematology-Oncology (Pediatric Rhabdomyosarcoma, Langerhans Cell Histiocytosis, Malignant Germ Cell Tumors) · University of Texas-M. D. Anderson Cancer Center · University of Texas-M. D. Anderson Cancer Center, 1515 Holcombe Boulevard, Box 87, Houston, TX 77030-4095 · 713-792-6624

Barbara Sue Reid · Pediatric Gastroenterology · Texas Children's Hospital · Texas Children's Hospital, 6621 Fannin Street, Mail Code 3-3391, Houston, TX 77030 · 713-790-3636

William J. Riley · Pediatric Endocrinology (Diabetes) · Hermann Hospital · University of Texas Medical School at Houston, 6431 Fannin Street, Room 3.122, Houston, TX 77030 · 713-792-5330 x3082

W. Mark Roberts · Pediatric Hematology-Oncology · University of Texas-M. D. Anderson Cancer Center · University of Texas-M. D. Anderson Cancer Center, 1515 Holcombe Boulevard, Box 87, Houston, TX 77030-4009 · 713-745-1718

Dan K. Seilheimer · Pediatric Pulmonology (Asthma, Cystic Fibrosis) · Texas Children's Hospital · Texas Children's Hospital, Clinical Care Center, Suite 410, 6621 Fannin Street, Mail Code 3-2571, Houston, TX 77030-2399 · 713-770-3300

Stuart K. Shapira · Metabolic Diseases (Genetics) · Texas Children's Hospital · Texas Children's Hospital, Department of Genetics, 6621 Fannin Street, Mail Code 3-3370, Houston, TX 77030 · 713-770-4280

Robert Jay Shulman · Pediatric Gastroenterology (Nutrition) · Texas Children's Hospital · Texas Children's Hospital, 6621 Fannin Street, Mail Code 3-3391, Houston, TX 77030 · 713-770-3600

Marianna M. Sockrider · Pediatric Pulmonology · Texas Children's Hospital · Texas Children's Hospital, Department of Pulmonary Medicine, 6621 Fannin Street, Mail Code 3-2571, Houston, TX 77030 · 713-770-3300

John Wesley Sparks · Neonatal-Perinatal Medicine · Hermann Hospital · University of Texas Medical School at Houston, Department of Pediatrics, 6431 Fannin Street, Houston, TX 77030 · 713-792-5330 x1

Michael Emery Speer · Neonatal-Perinatal Medicine · Texas Children's Hospital, Methodist Hospital, St. Luke's Episcopal Hospital, The Woman's Hospital of Texas · Texas Children's Hospital, 6621 Fannin Street, Suite A.340, Houston, TX 77030 · 713-790-4593

Jeffrey R. Starke · Pediatric Infectious Disease (Tuberculosis, Infection Control) · Ben Taub General Hospital, Texas Children's Hospital · Texas Children's Hospital, 1102 Bates Street, Mail Code 3-2371, Houston, TX 77030 · 713-770-4330

Fernando Stein · Pediatric Critical Care · Texas Children's Hospital · Texas Children's Hospital, Critical Care & Surgical Facility, Suite 440, 6621 Fannin Street, Mail Code 2-3450, Houston, TX 77030-2399 · 713-770-6231

Charles P. Steuber · Pediatric Hematology-Oncology · Texas Children's Hospital · Texas Children's Hospital, 6621 Fannin Street, Mail Code 3-3320, Houston, TX 77030 · 713-770-4207

Douglas Strother · Pediatric Hematology-Oncology (Neuroblastoma, Pediatric Brain Tumors, General Pediatrics) · Texas Children's Hospital · Texas Children's Cancer Center, 6621 Fannin Street, Mail Code 3-3320, Houston, TX 77030 · 713-770-4200

Larry Taber · Pediatric Infectious Disease (Congenital Infections) · Texas Children's Hospital, Department of Infectious Disease, 6621 Fannin Street, Mail Code 3-2371, Houston, TX 77030 · 713-770-4330

David G. Tubergen · Pediatric Hematology-Oncology · University of Texas-M. D. Anderson Cancer Center · University of Texas-M. D. Anderson Cancer Center, 1515 Holcombe Boulevard, Box 87, Houston, TX 77030-4009 · 713-745-0886

Robert Wells Warren · Pediatric Rheumatology · Texas Children's Hospital · Texas Children's Hospital, 6621 Fannin Street, Mail Code 3-2290, Houston, TX 77030 · 713-770-3830

Mary Elizabeth Wearden · Neonatal-Perinatal Medicine · Baylor College of Medicine, Department of Pediatrics, One Baylor Plaza, Room 326-D, Houston, TX 77030 · 713-798-4675

Leonard Emil Weisman · Neonatal-Perinatal Medicine · Texas Children's Hospital, Ben Taub General Hospital, Methodist Hospital, St. Luke's Episcopal Hospital, The Woman's Hospital of Texas · Texas Children's Hospital, 6621 Fannin Street, Mail Code 1-3460, Houston, TX 77030 · 713-770-1380

Stephen E. Welty · Neonatal-Perinatal Medicine · Texas Children's Hospital, Department of Neonatology, 6621 Fannin Street, Houston, TX 77030 · 713-770-1380

Barbara Lynn West · (Asthma, Infant Apnea) · Texas Children's Hospital · Texas Children's Hospital, 6621 Fannin Street, Mail Code 3-2571, Houston, TX 77030 · 713-770-3300

Andrew P. Wilking · Pediatric Rheumatology · Texas Children's Hospital · Texas Children's Hospital, Department of Rheumatology, 6621 Fannin Street, Mail Code 3-2290, Houston, TX 77030 · 713-770-3830

Theodore Zipf · Pediatric Hematology-Oncology · University of Texas-M. D. Anderson Cancer Center · University of Texas-M. D. Anderson Cancer Center, 1515 Holcombe Boulevard, Houston, TX 77030-4009 · 713-792-4855

Lackland Air Force Base

David Peter Ascher · Pediatric Infectious Disease · Wilford Hall Medical Center · Wilford Hall Medical Center, 2200 Bergquist Drive, Suite One, Lackland Air Force Base, TX 78236-5300 · 210-670-7347

Sven Thomas Berg · Pediatric Hematology-Oncology · Wilford Hall Medical Center · Wilford Hall Medical Center, 2200 Bergquist Drive, Suite One, Lackland Air Force Base, TX 78236-5300 · 210-670-6642

Robert M. Haws · Pediatric Nephrology · Wilford Hall Medical Center · Wilford Hall Medical Center, 2200 Bergquist Drive, Suite One, Lackland Air Force Base, TX 78236-5300 · 210-670-7347

Michael Ryan Kuskie · Pediatric Infectious Disease · Wilford Hall Medical Center · Wilford Hall Medical Center, 2200 Bergquist Drive, Suite One, Lackland Air Force Base, TX 78236-5300 · 210-670-7347

Charles T. Morton · Developmental & Behavioral Pediatrics (Developmental Disabilities) · Wilford Hall Medical Center · Wilford Hall Medical Center, 2200 Bergquist Drive, Suite One, Lackland Air Force Base, TX 78236-5300 · 210-670-7844

Lubbock

Michael J. Bourgeois · Pediatric Endocrinology · University Medical Center, Lubbock Methodist Hospital · Texas Tech University Health Sciences Center, Department of Pediatrics, 3601 Fourth Street, Lubbock, TX 79430 · 806-743-2301

Edwin Aldo Contreras · Neonatal-Perinatal Medicine · Lubbock Methodist Hospital · Lubbock Methodist Hospital, Neonatal Intensive Care Unit, 3615 Nineteenth Street, Lubbock, TX 79410 · 806-793-4212

Rafael R. Garcia · Abused Children (General Pediatrics, Pediatric & Adolescent Gynecology) · University Medical Center, St. Mary of the Plains Hospital · Texas Tech University Health Sciences Center, CARE Center, Thompson Hall, Room C-108, Lubbock, TX 79430 · 806-743-2121

James V. Higgins · Pediatric Gastroenterology · University Medical Center Children's Hospital, Methodist Children's Hospital, St. Mary of the Plains Hospital · 3502 Ninth Street, Suite 380, Lubbock, TX 79415 · 806-762-8500

J. J. Lambert · Pediatric Critical Care · University Medical Center · University Medical Center, Department of Pediatrics, 602 Indiana Avenue, Lubbock, TX 79415 · 806-743-2330

Richard Michael Lampe · Pediatric Infectious Disease · University Medical Center · Texas Tech University Health Sciences Center, Department of Pediatrics, 3601 Fourth Street, Lubbock, TX 79430 · 806-743-3088

Milton James Law · Developmental & Behavioral Pediatrics · UMC Texas Tech Health Sciences Center · Texas Tech University Health Sciences Center, Department of Pediatrics, 3601 Fourth Street, Lubbock, TX 79430 · 806-743-2332

Marian Kathryn S. Myers · Neonatal-Perinatal Medicine · University Medical Center · University Medical Center, Department of Pediatrics, 602 Indiana Avenue, Lubbock, TX 79415-3364 · 806-743-2319

Terry L. Myers · (Genetics) · University Medical Center, Amarillo Hospital District-Northwest Texas Hospital (Amarillo) · Texas Tech University Health Sciences Center, Department of Pediatrics, 3601 Fourth Street, Lubbock, TX 79430-0001 · 806-743-2266

Melanie G. Oblender · Pediatric Hematology-Oncology (Pediatric Pain Control) Methodist Children's Hospital, University Medical Center · Methodist Hospital, Children's Hematology-Oncology Team, 3606 Twenty-First Street, Suite 106, Lubbock, TX 79410 · 806-793-6629

Joon M. Park · Pediatric Cardiology · University Medical Center · Texas Tech University Health Sciences Center, Department of Pediatrics, 3601 Fourth Street, Lubbock, TX 79430 · 806-743-2333

Fortunato Perez-Benavides · Neonatal-Perinatal Medicine · University Medical Center · University Medical Center, Department of Pediatrics, 602 Indiana Avenue, Lubbock, TX 79415-3364 · 806-743-2319

Doanh Phan · Neonatal-Perinatal Medicine (Perinatal Medicine) · Lubbock Methodist Hospital · St. Mary of the Plains Hospital, Neonatal Intensive Care Unit, 4000 Twenty-Fourth Street, Lubbock, TX 79410 · 806-796-6472

Antonio Santiago · Neonatal-Perinatal Medicine · Lubbock Methodist Hospital Lubbock Methodist Hospital, Neonatal Intensive Care Unit, 3615 Nineteenth Street, Lubbock, TX 79410 · 806-793-4212

Somkid Sridaromont · Pediatric Cardiology · Methodist Children's Hospital · 3606 Twenty-First Street, Suite 305, Lubbock, TX 79410 · 806-791-5930

Thelma Kwan Sutter · Neonatal-Perinatal Medicine · St. Mary of the Plains Hospital · St. Mary of the Plains Hospital, Neonatal Intensive Care Unit, 4000 Twenty-Fourth Street, Lubbock, TX 79410 · 806-796-6472

Surendra Kumar Varma · Pediatric Endocrinology (Diabetes, Growth, Thyroid) University Medical Center, Lubbock Methodist Hospital, St. Mary of the Plains Hospital, Highland Medical Center · Texas Tech University Health Sciences Center, Department of Pediatrics, 3601 Fourth Street, Lubbock, TX 79430 · 806-743-2301

Baluswamy Viswanathan · Pediatric Critical Care · Lubbock Methodist Hospital Methodist Children's Hospital, Department of Pediatrics, 3610 Twenty-First Street, Lubbock, TX 79410 · 806-784-5019

David C. Waagner · Pediatric Infectious Disease · University Medical Center · Texas Tech University Health Sciences Center, Department of Pediatrics, 3601 Fourth Street, Lubbock, TX 79430 · 806-743-2268

Catherine L. Watts · Neonatal-Perinatal Medicine · University Medical Center · University Medical Center, Department of Pediatrics, 602 Indiana Avenue, Lubbock, TX 79415-3364 · 806-743-2319

Midland

John D. Bray · Pediatric Pulmonology · 606-B North Kent Street, Midland, TX 79701 · 915-686-8658

San Antonio

Remedios Ching Agrawal · Neonatal-Perinatal Medicine · Santa Rosa Children's Hospital · South Texas Newborn Associates, 4115 Medical Drive, Suite 301, San Antonio, TX 78229 · 210-614-3472

Kenneth Bloom · Pediatric Cardiology · 4499 Medical Drive, Suite 272, San Antonio, TX 78229 · 210-614-3264

Howard A. Britton · Pediatric Hematology-Oncology · Santa Rosa Children's Hospital, University Hospital-South Texas Medical Center · Santa Rosa Children's Hospital, Children's Cancer Clinic, Eighth Floor, 519 West Houston Street, San Antonio, TX 78207-3108 · 210-704-2187

Dennis Allen Conrad · Pediatric Infectious Disease · Santa Rosa Children's Hospital, University Hospital-South Texas Medical Center · University of Texas Health Science Center at San Antonio, Department of Pediatrics, 7703 Floyd Curl Drive, San Antonio, TX 78284-7811 · 210-567-5309

Anthony J. Corbet · Neonatal-Perinatal Medicine (Prematurity, Respiratory Distress Syndrome) · Santa Rosa Children's Hospital · South Texas Newborn Associates, 4115 Medical Drive, Suite 301, San Antonio, TX 78229 · 210-614-3472

Mark Maxwell Danney · Pediatric Endocrinology · Santa Rosa Children's Hospital, University Hospital-South Texas Medical Center · University of Texas Health Science Center at San Antonio, Department of Pediatrics, Division of Endocrinology, 7703 Floyd Curl Drive, San Antonio, TX 78284-7806 · 210-704-3612

Terence I. Doran · Pediatric Infectious Disease · University of Texas Health Science Center at San Antonio, Department of Pediatrics, 7703 Floyd Curl Drive, San Antonio, TX 78284-7811 · 210-567-5301

Ihsan Elshihabi · Pediatric Nephrology · University of Texas Health Science Center at San Antonio, Department of Pediatric Nephrology, 7703 Floyd Curl Drive, San Antonio, TX 78284-7809 · 210-567-5279

Marilyn Barnard Escobedo · Neonatal-Perinatal Medicine · University Hospital-South Texas Medical Center · University of Texas Health Science Center at San Antonio, Department of Pediatrics, Division of Neonatology, 7703 Floyd Curl Drive, San Antonio, TX 78284-7812 · 210-567-5225

Clementina Funaro Geiser · Pediatric Hematology-Oncology (Solid Tumor, Leukemia, Histiocytosis in Children) · University Hospital-South Texas Medical Center, Santa Rosa Children's Hospital · University of Texas Health Science Center at San Antonio, Department of Pediatrics, Division of Hematology, Oncology & Immunology, 7703 Floyd Curl Drive, San Antonio, TX 78284-7810 · 210-567-5265

Alice Kim Gong · Neonatal-Perinatal Medicine · University Hospital-South Texas Medical Center, Baptist Memorial Healthcare System · University of Texas Health Science Center at San Antonio, Department of Pediatrics, Division of Neonatology, 7703 Floyd Curl Drive, San Antonio, TX 78284-7812 · 210-567-5227

Roni Grad · Pediatric Pulmonology · 4499 Medical Drive, Suite 255, San Antonio, TX 78229 · 210-614-3403

Guy Howard Grayson · Pediatric Hematology-Oncology (Bone Marrow Transplantation) · Southwest Texas Methodist Hospital · South Texas Cancer Institute, 7700 Floyd Curl Drive, San Antonio, TX 78229 · 210-593-3801

Humberto Arturo Hidalgo · Pediatric Pulmonology · University of Texas Health Science Center at San Antonio, Department of Pediatrics, Division of Pulmonology, 7703 Floyd Curl Drive, San Antonio, TX 78284 · 210-567-5320

J. Leonard Hilliard · Neonatal-Perinatal Medicine · Santa Rosa Children's Hospital · South Texas Newborn Associates, 4115 Medical Drive, Suite 301, San Antonio, TX 78229 · 210-614-3472

Eduardo Ibarguen · Pediatric Gastroenterology · 4499 Medical Drive, Suite 240, San Antonio, TX 78229 · 210-614-3100

Hal Brockbank Jenson · Pediatric Infectious Disease (Pediatric AIDS, Transplantation Infections, Herpes Virus Infections) · University Hospital-South Texas Medical Center, Santa Rosa Children's Hospital · University of Texas Health Science Center at San Antonio, Department of Pediatrics, 7703 Floyd Curl Drive, San Antonio, TX 78284-7811 · 210-567-5301

Chris P. Johnson · Developmental & Behavioral Pediatrics (Developmental Disabilities) · The Village of Hope—Center for Children with Developmental Disabilities, University Hospital-South Texas Medical Center · The Village of Hope—Center for Children with Developmental Disabilities, 703 South Zarzamora Street, San Antonio, TX 78207 · 210-433-9723

Javier R. Kane · Pediatric Hematology-Oncology (General Pediatrics) · University Hospital-South Texas Medical Center, Santa Rosa Children's Hospital · University of Texas Health Science Center at San Antonio, Department of Pediatric-Hematology/Oncology, 7703 Floyd Curl Drive, San Antonio, TX 78284-7810 · 210-567-5264

Celia I. Kaye · Metabolic Diseases (Genetics) · Santa Rosa Children's Hospital, University Hospital-South Texas Medical Center · University of Texas Health Science Center at San Antonio, Department of Pediatrics, 7703 Floyd Curl Drive, San Antonio, TX 78284-7809 · 210-567-5195

Nancy Denny Kellogg · Abused Children · University Hospital-South Texas Medical Center, Santa Rosa Children's Hospital · University of Texas Health Science Center at San Antonio, Department of Pediatrics, 7703 Floyd Curl Drive, San Antonio, TX 78284-7808 · 210-270-3971

Anne Marie Langewin · Pediatric Hematology-Oncology · Santa Rosa Children's Hospital · University of Texas Health Science Center at San Antonio, Department of Pediatrics, Division of Hematology, Oncology & Immunology, 7703 Floyd Curl Drive, San Antonio, TX 78284-7810 · 210-567-5265

Kenneth Hillard Lazarus · Pediatric Hematology-Oncology · Southwest Texas Methodist Hospital, Methodist Women's and Children's Hospital · 4499 Medical Drive, Suite 260, San Antonio, TX 78229-3712 · 210-616-0800

Charles Thomas Leach · Pediatric Infectious Disease · University Hospital-South Texas Medical Center, Santa Rosa Children's Hospital, Southwest Texas Methodist Hospital · University of Texas Health Science Center at San Antonio, Department of Pediatrics, 7703 Floyd Curl Drive, San Antonio, TX 78284-7811 · 210-567-5301

Nola R. Marx · Developmental & Behavioral Pediatrics (Children with Differences in Psychomotor Development) · 8042 Wurzbach Road, Suite 110, San Antonio, TX 78229 · 210-692-3439

Thomas Cullee Mayes · Pediatric Critical Care (Pediatric Transport) · University Hospital-South Texas Medical Center, Santa Rosa Children's Hospital · University of Texas Health Science Center at San Antonio, Department of Pediatrics, 7703 Floyd Curl Drive, San Antonio, TX 78284-7829 · 210-567-5314

Martha Ruth Morse · Pediatric Pulmonology (Asthma, Cystic Fibrosis, Lung Infections) · Southwest Texas Methodist Hospital · 4499 Medical Drive, Suite 255, San Antonio, TX 78229 · 210-614-3403

David C. Mullins · Neonatal-Perinatal Medicine · Santa Rosa Children's Hospital, Southwest Texas Methodist Hospital, Women's & Children's Hospital ·

South Texas Newborn Associates, 4115 Medical Drive, Suite 301, P.O. Box 29067, San Antonio, TX 78229 · 210-614-3472

Deborah Ann Neigut · Pediatric Gastroenterology · University Hospital-South Texas Medical Center, Santa Rosa Children's Hospital, Methodist Healthcare System, Women's & Children's Hospital · University of Texas Health Science Center at San Antonio, Department of Pediatrics, Division of Gastroenterology, 7703 Floyd Curl Drive, San Antonio, TX 78284-7703 · 210-567-5280

Carlos Nieto, Jr. · Neonatal-Perinatal Medicine · Santa Rosa Children's Hospital South Texas Newborn Associates, Oak on Bluff Creek Building, 4115 Medical Drive, Suite 301, San Antonio, TX 78229 · 210-614-3472

William John Norberg · Pediatric Critical Care (Pediatric Cardiology, Pediatric Transport Medicine) · Southwest Texas Methodist Hospital, University Hospital-South Texas Medical Center, Santa Rosa Children's Hospital · Southwest Texas Methodist Hospital, Pediatric Intensive Care Unit, 7700 Floyd Curl Drive, San Antonio, TX 78229 · 210-692-4483

Emil Ortiz · Neonatal-Perinatal Medicine · Southwest Texas Methodist Hospital South Texas Newborn Associates, 4115 Medical Drive, Suite 301, San Antonio, TX 78229 · 210-614-3472

Rajam S. Ramamurthy · Neonatal-Perinatal Medicine · University Hospital-South Texas Medical Center, Santa Rosa Children's Hospital, Baptist Memorial Healthcare System · University of Texas Health Science Center at San Antonio, Department of Pediatrics, Division of Neonatology, 7703 Floyd Curl Drive, San Antonio, TX 78284-7812 · 210-567-5228

James Henry Rogers, Jr. · Pediatric Cardiology · Santa Rosa Children's Hospital, University Hospital-South Texas Medical Center · The Children's Heart Network, 1901 Babcock Road, Suite 301, San Antonio, TX 78229 · 210-341-7722

Michael Joseph Romano · Pediatric Critical Care · Southwest Texas Methodist Hospital · Southwest Texas Methodist Hospital, Pediatric Intensive Care Unit, 7700 Floyd Curl Drive, San Antonio, TX 78229 · 210-692-4483

Robert F. Stratton · (Genetics) · 730 North Main Avenue, Suite 615, San Antonio, TX 78205 · 210-227-4363

Paul Jan Thomas · Pediatric Hematology-Oncology · Santa Rosa Children's Hospital · University of Texas Health Science Center at San Antonio, Department of Pediatrics, Division of Hematology, Oncology & Immunology, 7703 Floyd Curl Drive, San Antonio, TX 78284-7810 · 210-567-5265

Temple

E. Darrell Crisp · Metabolic Diseases · Scott & White Memorial Hospital & Clinic · Scott & White Memorial Hospital, Division of Pediatric Neurology, 2401 South 31st Street, Temple, TX 76508-0001 · 817-724-3409

James F. Daniel · Pediatric Gastroenterology · Scott & White Memorial Hospital Scott & White Memorial Hospital, Department of Pediatrics, 2401 South 31st Street, Temple, TX 76508-0001 · 817-724-2708

Lawrence S. Frankel · Pediatric Hematology-Oncology · Scott & White Memorial Hospital & Clinic · Scott & White Memorial Hospital, Department of Pediatrics, 2401 South 31st Street, Temple, TX 76508-0001 · 817-724-2111

Bess G. Gold · Pediatric Infectious Disease · Scott & White Memorial Hospital · Scott & White Memorial Hospital, Department of Pediatrics, 2401 South 31st Street, Temple, TX 76508-0001 · 817-724-2708

David Ray Hardy · Pediatric Critical Care · Scott & White Memorial Hospital & Clinic · Scott & White Memorial Hospital, Department of Pediatrics, 2401 South 31st Street, Temple, TX 76508-0001 · 817-724-1199

Linda J. Kirby-Keyser · Pediatric Nephrology · Scott & White Memorial Hospital Scott & White Memorial Hospital, Department of Pediatrics, 2401 South 31st Street, Temple, TX 76508-0001 · 817-724-2708

Joseph W. Kraft · Adolescent & Young Adult Medicine (Sports Medicine, General Pediatrics) · Scott & White Memorial Hospital · Scott & White Memorial Hospital, Department of Pediatrics, 2401 South 31st Street, Temple, TX 76508-0001 · 817-724-3109

David Roy Krauss · Neonatal-Perinatal Medicine · Scott & White Memorial Hospital & Clinic · Scott & White Memorial Hospital, Department of Neonatology, 2401 South 31st Street, Temple, TX 76508-0001 · 817-724-2310

Susan M. P. Nickel · Adolescent & Young Adult Medicine, Abused Children · Scott & White Memorial Hospital & Clinic · Scott & White Memorial Hospital, Department of Pediatrics, 2401 South 31st Street, Temple, TX 76508-0001 · 817-724-3109

Stephen W. Ponder · Pediatric Endocrinology · Scott & White Memorial Hospital Scott & White Memorial Hospital, Department of Pediatrics, 2401 South 31st Street, Temple, TX 76508-0001 · 817-724-2708

Lori Lou Wick · Pediatric Critical Care · Scott & White Memorial Hospital · Scott & White Memorial Hospital, Department of Pediatrics, 2401 South 31st Street, Temple, TX 76508-0001 · 817-724-1199

Tyler

Robert B. Klein · Pediatric Pulmonology · University of Texas Health Center-Tyler, US Highway 271 and State Highway 155, P.O. Box 2003, Tyler, TX 75710-2003 · 903-877-7039

PEDIATRICS (GENERAL)

Abilene

Stephen T. Faehnle · Hendrick Medical Center · Professional Association of Pediatrics, 1101 North 19th Street, Abilene, TX 79601-2314 · 915-677-2801

George D. Pope · Hendrick Medical Center · Professional Association of Pediatrics, 1101 North 19th Street, Abilene, TX 79601-2314 · 915-677-2801

Jimmy Lee Strong · Professional Association of Pediatrics, 1101 North 19th Street, Abilene, TX 79601-2314 · 915-677-2801

A. Gregory Tuegel · Hendrick Medical Center · Professional Association of Pediatrics, 1101 North 19th Street, Abilene, TX 79601-2314 · 915-677-2801

Austin

Leslie Franklin Aiello · (Infectious Disease, Cardiology) · Children's Hospital of Austin, Seton Medical Center · Pediatric Associates of Austin, 1500 West 38th Street, Suite 20, Austin, TX 78731 · 512-458-5323

Michael Bayer · Seton Medical Center, St. David's Healthcare Center, Children's Hospital of Austin · 711 West 38th Street, Suite C-2, Austin, TX 78705 · 512-458-6717

William David Caldwell · (Psychosocial Development and Disorders) · Seton Medical Center, Children's Hospital of Austin, St. David's Healthcare Center · 1500 West 38th Street, Suite 10, Austin, TX 78731 · 512-454-0406

Thomas Britton Dawson · 514 Medical Park Tower, 1301 West 38th Street, Austin, TX 78705 · 512-467-1600

David Earl Gamble · Children's Hospital of Austin · Pediatric Associates of Austin, 1500 West 38th Street, Suite 20, Austin, TX 78731 · 512-476-6424

Ellis Charles Gill · Brackenridge Hospital · Pediatric Associates of Austin, 1500 West 38th Street, Suite 20, Austin, TX 78731 · 512-458-5323

Stephen Randal Griggs · Pediatric Associates of Austin, 1500 West 38th Street, Suite 20, Austin, TX 78731 · 512-458-5323

Jack C. Kidd · Children's Hospital of Austin · 621 Radam Lane, Austin, TX 78745 512-443-4800

Maia Killian · 514 Medical Park Tower, 1301 West 38th Street, Austin, TX 78705 512-467-1600

Jack A. Louis · 711 West 38th Street, Suite C-2, Austin, TX 78705 · 512-458-6717

Beth W. Nauert · (Abused Children) · Children's Hospital of Austin, Brackenridge Hospital · 621 Radam Lane, Austin, TX 78745 · 512-443-4800

Jaime E. Ramirez · Seton Medical Center, Children's Hospital of Austin, St. David's Healthcare Center · 514 Medical Park Tower, 1301 West 38th Street, Austin, TX 78705 · 512-467-1600

Karen Williams Teel · Children's Hospital of Austin · 1305 West 34th Street, Suite 410, Austin, TX 78705 · 512-454-6616

Charlotte Ann Weaver · Children's Hospital of Austin · Westlake Children's Clinic, 4615 West Bee Cave Road, Austin, TX 78746 · 512-327-0562

John Richard Worrel · (Adolescent Medicine) · Children's Hospital of Austin · 1500 West 38th Street, Suite 46, Austin, TX 78731-6319 · 512-454-2080

Beaumont

Benfard Earl Hicks · St. Elizabeth Hospital · 3030 North Street, Suite 410, Beaumont, TX 77702-1542 · 409-899-1433

Uma Mahesh Kanojia · (Adolescent & Young Adult Medicine, General Pediatrics) · St. Elizabeth Hospital, Baptist Hospital Beaumont, Beaumont Regional Medical Center · 3455 Stagg Drive, Suite 101, Beaumont, TX 77701-4520 · 409-835-2082

William Jerome Reed · (Adolescent & Young Adult Medicine) · St. Elizabeth Hospital, Baptist Hospital Beaumont, Beaumont Regional Medical Center · 2900 North Street, Suite 408, Beaumont, TX 77702-1542 · 409-892-8362

Conroe

Richard T. Calvin · Conroe Pediatrics, 704 Longmire Road, Suite Eight, Conroe, TX 77304 · 409-756-8108

William L. Nix · Conroe Pediatrics, 9001 Interstate 45, Suite 500, Conroe, TX 77385 · 713-367-5100

Susan J. R. O'Neil · Memorial Hospital-The Woodlands (The Woodlands) · Conroe Pediatrics, 9001 Interstate 45, Suite 500, Conroe, TX 77385 · 713-367-5100

Corpus Christi

Peggy L. Wakefield · Children's Clinic, 3435 South Alameda Street, Corpus Christi, TX 78411-1728 · 512-855-7346

Dallas

Michael Edwin Brown · Children's Medical Center of Dallas, Presbyterian Hospital of Dallas · 8355 Walnut Hill Lane, Suite 200, Dallas, TX 75231 · 214-369-7661

Debra Lou Burns · Children's Medical Center of Dallas, Presbyterian Hospital of Dallas · 8315 Walnut Hill Lane, Suite 140, Dallas, TX 75231 · 214-750-8496

Duane L. Dowell · (Adolescents) · Children's Medical Center of Dallas, Parkland Memorial Hospital · 6303 Harry Hines Boulevard, Suite 101, Dallas, TX 75235-5228 · 214-640-0300

Molly Droge · Children's Medical Center of Dallas, Medical City Dallas Hospital 5525A Arapaho Road, Dallas, TX 75248 · 214-385-6450

Ross Leland Finkelman · Children's Medical Center of Dallas, Medical City Dallas Hospital, Presbyterian Hospital of Dallas · 8355 Walnut Hill Lane, Suite 200, Dallas, TX 75231-4200 · 214-369-7661

John Foster · Children's Medical Center of Dallas, Presbyterian Hospital of Dallas, Presbyterian Hospital of Plano (Plano), Medical City Dallas Hospital, Baylor University Medical Center, St. Paul Medical Center · 8355 Walnut Hill Lane, Suite 200, Dallas, TX 75231 · 214-369-7661

Charles Morris Ginsburg · (Pediatric Infectious Disease, Pediatric Emergency Medicine, Medical Toxicology, General Pediatrics) · Children's Medical Center of Dallas · University of Texas-Southwestern Medical Center at Dallas, 5323 Harry Hines Boulevard, Dallas, TX 75235-9063 · 214-648-3563

Jules Greif · Parkland Memorial Hospital, Children's Medical Center of Dallas · Bluitt Flowers Health Center, 303 Overton Road, Dallas, TX 75216 · 214-590-4340

Joseph Arthur Hanig · Children's Medical Center of Dallas · 8355 Walnut Hill Lane, Suite 105, Dallas, TX 75231 · 214-368-3659

James Patrick Hieber · Clinic of Pediatric Associates, 8355 Walnut Hill Lane, Suite 105, Dallas, TX 75231 · 214-368-3659

Hugh Leslie Moore II · (Pediatric Nephrology, General Infectious Disease, General Pediatrics) · Children's Medical Center of Dallas · Clinical Pediatric Associates, 8355 Walnut Hill Lane, Suite 105, Dallas, TX 75231 · 214-368-3659

Daniel Dean Nale · Children's Medical Center of Dallas · 9304 Forest Lane, Suite 150, Dallas, TX 75243-8953 · 214-343-9696

Joseph Paul Peterman · 8222 Douglas Avenue, Dallas, TX 75225 · 214-987-0777

Claude Brockman Prestidge · (Pediatric Pulmonology, Cystic Fibrosis, Asthma, General Pediatrics) · Children's Medical Center of Dallas, Presbyterian Hospital of Dallas, Baylor University Medical Center, St. Paul Medical Center · 8355 Walnut Hill Lane, Suite 200, Dallas, TX 75231 · 214-369-7661

Wilfred Leroy Raine · Children's Medical Center of Dallas, Medical City Dallas Hospital, St. Paul Medical Center · 7310 South Westmoreland Road, Dallas, TX 75237 · 214-296-6666

Janet E. Squires · (Infectious Disease, AIDS, Abused Children) · Children's Medical Center of Dallas · Children's Medical Center of Dallas, 1935 Motor Street, Dallas, TX 75235-7794 · 214-640-2329

Joel B. Steinberg · (Pediatric Sleep Disorders, Pediatric Obesity & Nutrition Problems, General Pediatrics) · Children's Medical Center of Dallas · Children's Medical Center of Dallas, 1935 Motor Street, Dallas, TX 75235-7794 · 214-640-2730

El Paso

Arturo Casillas · 1501 North Mesa Avenue, Suite 2A, El Paso, TX 79902 · 915-577-0444

Jagdish Patel · 10501 Vista del Sol, Building I, Suite 100, El Paso, TX 79925 · 915-593-5444

Euless

Albert L. Blakes · 350 Westpark Way, Suite 112, Euless, TX 76040 · 817-379-6933

Sharon Rae · 350 Westpark Way, Suite 112, Euless, TX 76040 · 817-379-6933

Fort Worth

John Howard Dalton · Cook Children's Medical Center, Harris Methodist-Fort Worth · 6862 Grapevine Highway, Fort Worth, TX 76180-8818 · 817-284-2714

Walter Halpenny · Cook Children's Medical Center · Health Partners Pediatrics, 851 West Terrell Avenue, Fort Worth, TX 76104 · 817-335-1104

Deborah Susan Hucaby · 6100 Harris Parkway, Suite 235, Fort Worth, TX 76132 · 817-346-5444

Alan Kent Lassiter · Cook Children's Medical Center · Cook Children's Medical Center, Department of Pediatrics, 801 Seventh Avenue, Fort Worth, TX 76104-2796 · 817-885-1475

James E. Louis · 1050 Fifth Avenue, Suite F, Fort Worth, TX 76104 · 817-336-2757

Ray N. Rhodes, Jr. · Cook Children's Medical Center · Health Partners Pediatrics, 851 West Terrell Avenue, Fort Worth, TX 76104 · 817-335-1104

John M. Richardson · 1129 Sixth Avenue, Fort Worth, TX 76104 · 817-336-4896

Tom Rogers, Jr. · Harris Methodist-Fort Worth · Cook Children's Primary Care Services, 3200 Riverfront Drive, Suite 103, Fort Worth, TX 76107 · 817-336-3800

Galveston

Rima Chamseddine · (Behavioral Pediatrics, Pediatric Endocrinology) · University of Texas Medical Branch Hospitals · Gulf Coast Medical Group, Pediatric Division, 200 University Boulevard, Suite 604, Galveston, TX 77550 · 409-762-9667

David P. McCormick · University of Texas Medical Branch, Department of Pediatrics, 301 University Boulevard, Galveston, TX 77555-0319 · 409-772-6283

Ralph W. Noble III · St. Mary's Hospital · Pediatric Associates, 624 Rosenberg Street, Galveston, TX 77550-1706 · 409-763-0311

Mary J. Owen · University of Texas Medical Branch, Department of Pediatrics, 301 University Boulevard, Galveston, TX 77555-0319 · 409-772-3536

Ben G. Raimer · Pediatric Associates, 301 University Boulevard, Suite 1019, Galveston, TX 77555-0814 · 409-763-0311

Sally Sue Robinson · University of Texas Medical Branch Hospitals · Gulf Coast Medical Group, Pediatric Division, 200 University Boulevard, Suite 604, Galveston, TX 77550 · 409-762-9667

Leigh R. Smith · University of Texas Medical Branch, Department of Pediatrics, Division of Ambulatory Pediatrics, 301 University Boulevard, Galveston, TX 77555-0319 · 409-772-2357

Harlingen

Roland J. Dominguez · Harlingen Pediatrics & Associates, 2226 Haine Drive, Harlingen, TX 78550 · 210-425-8761

Houston

James Eblen Allison III · Texas Children's Hospital · 5620 Greenbriar Street, Suite 104, Houston, TX 77005 · 713-524-9009

Dennis Richard Boardman · Texas Children's Hospital · 4110 Bellaire Boulevard, Suite 210, Houston, TX 77025 · 713-666-1953

Stephen C. Bolline · 4110 Bellaire Boulevard, Suite 210, Houston, TX 77025 · 713-666-1953

Debra Mucasey Bootin · 1200 Binz Street, Suite 530, Houston, TX 77004 · 713-630-0660

Robert Allen Boyd · Texas Children's Hospital, Hermann Hospital · Houston Pediatric Associates, 4110 Bellaire Boulevard, Suite 210, Houston, TX 77025-1099 713-666-1953

Nancy Byrd · 7400 Fannin Street, Suite 880, Houston, TX 77054 · 713-790-0320

John Wilhite Caudill, Jr. · Texas Children's Hospital, Methodist Hospital, Park Plaza Hospital, St. Luke's Episcopal Hospital · 1630 Fountain View Road, Houston, TX 77057 · 713-782-4830

Kenneth E. Cohen · Town & Country Pediatric Association, 909 Frostwood Drive, Suite 126, Houston, TX 77024 · 713-461-6414

David Michael Cotlar · Texas Children's Hospital · 7777 Southwest Freeway, Suite 946, Houston, TX 77074 · 713-776-3045

Philip R. Dreessen · Pediatric Medical Group, 4101 Greenbriar Street, Suite 100, Houston, TX 77098 · 713-526-6443

Jan Edwin Drutz · Texas Children's Hospital · Texas Children's Hospital, Department of Pediatrics, 1102 Bates Street, Mail Code 3-2305, Houston, TX 77030 · 713-770-3441

Leon David Freedman · Texas Children's Hospital · Town & Country Pediatric Association, 909 Frostwood Drive, Suite 126, Houston, TX 77024 · 713-461-6414

Susan E. Gardner · 17030 Nanes Drive, Suite 105, Houston, TX 77090-2504 · 713-440-4150

Mario Garza · Cypress Fairbanks Medical Center · Steeple Chase Pediatric Center, 11037 FM 1960 West, Suite B-2, Houston, TX 77065-3600 · 713-469-2838

Clyde H. Gilless · (Learning Dysfunction, Attention Problems, Behavioral Problems) · Houston Northwest Medical Center, Cypress Fairbanks Medical Center, Hermann Hospital · FM 1960 Pediatric Center, 17070 Red Oak Drive, Suite 101, Houston, TX 77090 · 713-440-1950

Neal J. Grossman · 12121 Richmond Avenue, Suite 124, Houston, TX 77082 · 713-589-9700

Sheryl Ann Hausinger · Ben Taub General Hospital · 9055 Katy Freeway, Suite 420, Houston, TX 77024 · 713-464-0560

Paul S. Herman · Cypress Fairbanks Medical Center · Steeple Chase Pediatric Center, 11037 FM 1960 West, Suite B-2, Houston, TX 77065-3600 · 713-467-2838

Frank Douglass Hill III · Texas Children's Hospital · Pediatric Medical Group, 4101 Greenbriar Street, Suite 100, Houston, TX 77098-5244 · 713-526-6443

Harold S. Joachim · Memorial Hospital-Northwest · Northwest Pediatrics, 1820 West 43rd Street, Houston, TX 77018 · 713-681-9263

Arnold G. Kagan · Texas Children's Hospital · 12929 Gulf Freeway, Suite 200, Houston, TX 77034 · 713-484-9332

Abbas A. Kapasi · 17030 Nanes Drive, Suite 105, Houston, TX 77090 · 713-440-4150

Ian A. Kavin · Memorial Pediatric Association, 902 Frostwood Drive, Suite 227, Houston, TX 77024 · 713-467-4434

Michael S. Kessler · (Birth Defects, Child Abuse, Sickle Cell Disease, Diagnostic Puzzles) · Texas Children's Hospital, St. Luke's Episcopal Hospital, Methodist Hospital, The Woman's Hospital of Texas, Hermann Hospital · Pediatric Consultants of Houston, 1160 Scurlock Tower, 6560 Fannin Street, Houston, TX 77030 · 713-797-9700

R. Peter Killinger · 1630 Fountain View Road, Houston, TX 77057 · 713-782-4830

Allen H. Kline · 3838 Hillcroft Street, Houston, TX 77057 · 713-782-2770

Michael F. Knapick · Houston Northwest Medical Center · FM 1960 Pediatric Center, 11301 Fallbrook Drive, Suite 200, Houston, TX 77065 · 713-890-6514

Campbell Montgomery Lange · Texas Children's Hospital · 1630 Fountain View Road, Houston, TX 77057 · 713-782-4830

Marilyn J. B. Lemos · Texas Children's Hospital, St. Luke's Episcopal Hospital, The Woman's Hospital of Texas · Kelsey-Seybold Clinic, 1111 Augusta Drive, Houston, TX 77057 · 713-780-1661

John Mallory Long · Texas Children's Hospital, The Woman's Hospital of Texas, St. Luke's Episcopal Hospital, Methodist Hospital, Hermann Hospital, Park Plaza Hospital · Pediatric Medical Group, 4101 Greenbriar Street, Suite 100, Houston, TX 77098-5244 · 713-526-6443

Jerry W. Moye · FM 1960 Pediatric Center, 17070 Red Oak Drive, Suite 101, Houston, TX 77090 · 713-440-1950

Virginia A. Moyer · (Newborn Medicine) · Lyndon B. Johnson General Hospital Lyndon B. Johnson General Hospital, 5656 Kelley Street, Houston, TX 77026 · 713-636-4540

Abel Paredes · 902 Frostwood Drive, Suite 108, Houston, TX 77024 · 713-932-6261

Margaret Lee Payne · Texas Children's Hospital · 7505 South Main Street, Suite 300, Houston, TX 77030 · 713-791-9902

Norris S. Payne · Texas Children's Hospital · 7505 South Main Street, Suite 300, Houston, TX 77030 · 713-791-9902

Alfred Jon Phillips · Texas Children's Hospital, Memorial Hospital-Memorial City · Town & Country Pediatric Association, 909 Frostwood Drive, Suite 126, Houston, TX 77024 · 713-461-6414

Ciro Jorge Porras · Texas Children's Hospital · Parkview Clinic, 5724 Chimney Rock Road, Houston, TX 77081 · 713-663-6186

Jesse D. Ragan, Jr. · 1630 Fountain View Road, Houston, TX 77057 · 713-782-4830

George E. S. Reynolds III · 17150 El Camino Real, Houston, TX 77058 · 713-488-6347

Patti M. Savrick · 1200 Binz Street, Suite 530, Houston, TX 77004 · 713-630-0660

Don Minchen Schaffer · Texas Children's Hospital · 1200 Binz Street, Suite 530, Houston, TX 77004 · 713-630-0660

Rhonda G. Smith · Texas Children's Hospital · Pediatric Medical Group, 4101 Greenbriar Street, Suite 100, Houston, TX 77098 · 713-526-6443

Stanley W. Spinner · (Pediatric Allergy, Pediatric Asthma, General Pediatrics) · Memorial Hospital-Memorial City · Town & Country Pediatric Association, 909 Frostwood Drive, Suite 126, Houston, TX 77024 · 713-461-6414

Barbara J. Taylor-Cox · West Houston Pediatrics, 12121 Richmond Avenue, Suite 204, Houston, TX 77082 · 713-496-7093

Richard Michael Thaller · (General Pediatrics, Well Child & Adolescent Care) · Texas Children's Hospital · 9055 Katy Freeway, Suite 420, Houston, TX 77024 713-464-0560

M. Everett Truitt · 12700 North Featherwood Drive, Suite 200, Houston, TX 77034 · 713-481-8984

James A. Twining · 17150 El Camino Real, Houston, TX 77058 · 713-488-6347

Richard M. Vadala · 17030 Nanes Drive, Suite 105, Houston, TX 77090 · 713-440-4150

LaDonna Watson · 12121 Richmond Avenue, Suite 115, Houston, TX 77082 · 713-493-2444

Stephen Everett Whitney · Texas Children's Hospital · The Children's Doctors, 1315 Calhoun Avenue, Suite 1003, Houston, TX 77002 · 713-650-0650

Marilyn N. Wilking · Pediatric Medical Group, 4101 Greenbriar Street, Suite 100, Houston, TX 77098-5244 · 713-526-6443

Winnette V. Wimberly · Clear Lake Regional Medical Center (Webster) · 17150 El Camino Real, Houston, TX 77058 · 713-488-6347

Audrey May Winer · (Early Childhood Management, Management of Asthma) · Cypress Fairbanks Medical Center · FM 1960 Pediatric Center, 11301 Fallbrook Drive, Suite 200, Houston, TX 77065 · 713-890-6514

Robert Joseph Yetman · Hermann Hospital · University of Texas Medical School at Houston, 6431 Fannin Street, Room 3.140, Houston, TX 77030 · 713-792-5330

Barry Lewis Zietz · 12121 Richmond Avenue, Suite 124, Houston, TX 77082 · 713-496-1177

Lackland Air Force Base

Brenda Spinney Foley · Wilford Hall Medical Center · Wilford Hall Medical Center, 2200 Bergquist Drive, Suite One, Lackland Air Force Base, TX 78236-5300 · 210-670-7347

Lubbock

Glenn J. Boris · Lubbock Methodist Hospital · Methodist Medical Group, 3606 Twenty-First Street, Suite 307, Lubbock, TX 79410-1225 · 806-796-2136

A. Ray Farmer · St. Mary of the Plains Hospital · St. Mary's Medical Plaza, 4102 Twenty-Fourth Street, Suite 406, Lubbock, TX 79410 · 806-799-8332

Douglas R. Klepper · (Adolescent & Young Adult Medicine) · University Pediatrics, 3502 Ninth Street, Suite 130, Lubbock, TX 79415 · 806-743-1595

Wallace Marsh · (Infectious Disease, Infection Control, Pediatric Advance Life Support) · University Medical Center · Texas Tech University Health Sciences Center, Department of Pediatrics, 3601 Fourth Street, Lubbock, TX 79430 · 806-743-2268

Linda Robins · (Asthma, Adolescent Medicine, General Pediatrics) · 3606 Twenty-First Street, Suite 107, Lubbock, TX 79410 · 806-796-1251

Robert L. Stripling · 3606 Twenty-First Street, Suite 304, Lubbock, TX 79410 806-792-2384

Midland

Ronald P. Boren · Memorial Hospital & Medical Center, Westwood Medical Center · 2002 West Ohio Avenue, Midland, TX 79701-5946 · 915-682-7961

Missouri City

Elissa Atlas · (Preventive Medicine, Development of the Young Child, Adolescent & Young Adult Medicine) · 5819 Highway Six South, Suite 150, Missouri City, TX 77459 · 713-499-6300

Dean Jeffrey Gmoser · Texas Children's Hospital (Houston) · 5819 Highway Six South, Suite 150, Missouri City, TX 77459-4069 · 713-499-6300

Raymond A. Kahn · Texas Children's Hospital (Houston) · 5819 Highway Six South, Suite 150, Missouri City, TX 77459-4069 · 713-499-6300

Plano

Carolyn Dickson Ashworth · Medical Center of Plano · Pediatric Associates of North Texas, 3721 West 15th Street, Suite 603, Plano, TX 75075-7755 · 214-867-6880

Phyllis Ann Davis · Children's Medical Center of Dallas (Dallas), Presbyterian Hospital of Plano, Medical Center of Plano · 6200 West Parker Road, Suite 410, Plano, TX 75093 · 214-608-8380

Richardson

Steven Davis Crow · 1112 North Floyd Road, Richardson, TX 75080 · 214-952-0280

Albert Gerard Karam · Children's Medical Center of Dallas (Dallas), Medical City Dallas Hospital (Dallas), Presbyterian Hospital of Dallas (Dallas) · 1112 North Floyd Road, Richardson, TX 75080 · 214-952-0280

Gary C. Morchower · (General Pediatrics, Pediatric Gastroenterology, Learning Disabilites in Children, Adolescent & Young Adult Medicine) · Children's Medical Center of Dallas (Dallas), Medical City Dallas Hospital (Dallas), Presbyterian Hospital of Dallas (Dallas) · Richardson Professional Park Two, 1112 North Floyd Road, Suite Six, Richardson, TX 75080-4243 · 214-231-2551

John Richard Porter · (Adolescent Medicine, General Pediatrics) · Children's Medical Center of Dallas (Dallas), Medical City Dallas Hospital (Dallas), Presbyterian Hospital of Dallas (Dallas) · 1112 North Floyd Road, Suite 10, Richardson, TX 75080-4243 · 214-235-6911

San Angelo

Karl K. Wehner · Shannon Clinic, Department of Pediatrics, 120 East Beauregard Avenue, San Angelo, TX 76903 · 915-658-1511

San Antonio

Jerri Abrams · 2933 Babcock Road, Suite 300, San Antonio, TX 78229 · 210-616-7304

Maria del Rosario Aguirre · Women's & Children's Hospital, Santa Rosa Children's Hospital, Southwest Texas Methodist Hospital · 1927 Ceralvo Street, San Antonio, TX 78237 · 210-433-0366

Barbara P. Belcher · Santa Rosa Children's Hospital · Child Care Associates, 203 East Evergreen Street, San Antonio, TX 78212 · 210-225-7171

Marshall James Benbow · Southwest Children's Center, 5282 Medical Drive, Suite 310, San Antonio, TX 78229 · 210-614-8687

Joseph Borenstein · 3111 San Pedro Avenue, San Antonio, TX 78212 · 210-732-7141

Dianna Mosley Burns · Santa Rosa Children's Hospital · 1954 East Houston Street, Suite 104, San Antonio, TX 78202 · 210-227-2100

John Thomas Fitch · 7959 Broadway Street, Suite 604, San Antonio, TX 78209 210-826-1891

D. Michael Fouldes · University Hospital-South Texas Medical Center · University of Texas Health Science Center at San Antonio, Department of Pediatrics, 7703 Floyd Curl Drive, San Antonio, TX 78284-7808 · 210-270-3971

Jane Durant Fried · Southwest Texas Methodist Hospital · Northwest Pediatric Associates, 7007 Bandera Road, Suite 19, San Antonio, TX 78238-1265 · 210-680-6000

Wilson Wayne Grant · (Developmental & Behavioral Pediatrics) · Southwest Children's Center, 5282 Medical Drive, Suite 310, San Antonio, TX 78229 · 210-614-8687

William Penniman Groos · Northeast Pediatrics, 8606 Village Drive, Suite A, San Antonio, TX 78217 · 210-657-0220

Fernando Amado Guerra · Santa Rosa Children's Hospital · 401 West Commerce Street, Suite 200, San Antonio, TX 78207 · 210-224-4661

Graham Trevor Hall · 7959 Broadway Street, Suite 600, San Antonio, TX 78209 210-826-7033

Donald M. Hilliard · Santa Rosa Children's Hospital · Child Care Associates, 203 East Evergreen Street, San Antonio, TX 78212 · 210-225-7171

Linda Janet Holley · 1954 East Houston Street, Suite 104, San Antonio, TX 78202 · 210-227-2100

Freeman C. Jardan · Santa Rosa Children's Hospital · 401 West Commerce Street, Suite 200, San Antonio, TX 78207 · 210-224-4661

David Wright Johnson · 3111 San Pedro Avenue, San Antonio, TX 78212 · 210-732-7141

Robert K. Johnson · Santa Rosa Children's Hospital · 401 West Summit Avenue, San Antonio, TX 78212 · 210-736-3126

Jeannine S. Kaufmann · Northwest Pediatric Associates, 7007 Bandera Road, Suite 19, San Antonio, TX 78238-1265 · 210-680-6000

Henry Julius Lipsitt · 3111 San Pedro Avenue, San Antonio, TX 78212 · 210-732-7141

Christine W. Littlefield · Southwest Texas Methodist Hospital · Northwest Pediatric Associates, 7007 Bandera Road, Suite 19, San Antonio, TX 78238-1265 · 210-680-6000

Stephen Allan Maxwell · 3111 San Pedro Avenue, San Antonio, TX 78212 · 210-732-7141

Janet Monier Noll · Northwest Pediatric Associates, 7007 Bandera Road, Suite 19, San Antonio, TX 78238 · 210-680-6000

Rene Michael Ornes, Jr. · Northeast Baptist Hospital · Northeast Pediatrics, 8606 Village Drive, Suite A, San Antonio, TX 78217 · 210-657-0220

Valerie G. Ostrower · 4499 Medical Drive, Suite 347, San Antonio, TX 78229 · 210-614-4499

Michael Ozer · Methodist Healthcare System, Women's & Children's Hospital · Pediatric Medicine, 7922 Ewing Halsell Drive, Suite 440, San Antonio, TX 78229 210-614-2500

Lewis McKinley Purnell · Southwest Texas Methodist Hospital · Southwest Children's Center, 5282 Medical Drive, Suite 310, San Antonio, TX 78229 · 210-614-8687

Frederick Taylor Rhame · Northeast Pediatrics, 8606 Village Drive, Suite A, San Antonio, TX 78217 · 210-657-0220

Katherine Lynn Rodgers · (Neonatal-Perinatal Medicine) · Santa Rosa Children's Hospital, Women's & Children's Hospital, Methodist Healthcare System · Child Care Associates, 203 East Evergreen Street, San Antonio, TX 78212 · 210-225-7171

Jennifer Stone · Child Care Associates, 203 East Evergreen Street, San Antonio, TX 78212 · 210-225-7171

Leslie Gelfer Winakur · (General Pediatrics, Adolescent Medicine) · Southwest Texas Methodist Hospital, Women's & Children's Hospital · 7210 Louis Pasteur Drive, Suite 100, San Antonio, TX 78229 · 210-614-4000

Pamela Runge Wood · University Hospital-South Texas Medical Center · University of Texas Health Science Center at San Antonio, Department of Pediatrics, 7703 Floyd Curl Drive, San Antonio, TX 78284-7808 · 210-270-3971

Seguin

Kathleen Elaine Ethridge · 515 North King Street, Suite 101, Seguin, TX 78155 210-372-3135

Spring

Gary L. Heaton · FM 1960 Pediatric Center, 16740 Champion Forest Drive, Spring, TX 77379 · 713-376-0707

Michael L. Pope · FM 1960 Pediatric Center, 16740 Champion Forest Drive, Spring, TX 77379 · 713-376-0707

Sugar Land

Joan Whitaker Stoerner · Sugar Land Pediatrics, 2121 Williams Trace Boulevard, Suite 100, Sugar Land, TX 77478 · 713-269-2060

Philip S. Zeve · Sugar Land Pediatrics, 2121 Williams Trace Boulevard, Suite 100, Sugar Land, TX 77478 · 713-269-2060

Temple

John K. Blevins · (Pediatric Pulmonology, General Pediatrics) · Scott & White Memorial Hospital · Scott & White Memorial Hospital, Department of Pediatrics, 2401 South 31st Street, Temple, TX 76508-0001 · 817-724-2457

Waco

Lee M. Armstrong · 3115 Pine Avenue, Suite 701, Waco, TX 76708 · 817-757-3133

J. William Ferguson · 3115 Pine Avenue, Suite 304, Waco, TX 76708 · 817-752-4336

Wichita Falls

Karen J. Reed · Wichita General Hospital, Bethania Regional Health Care Center Medical & Surgical Clinic, 1518 Tenth Street, Wichita Falls, TX 76301-4405 · 817-723-5437

Kenneth L. Sultemeier · Medical & Surgical Clinic, 1518 Tenth Street, Wichita Falls, TX 76301-4405 · 817-723-5437

PHYSICAL MEDICINE & REHABILITATION

Amarillo

Grace L. Stringfellow · General Physical Medicine & Rehabilitation · 320 South Polk Street, Suite 600, Amarillo, TX 79101 · 806-373-8983

John A. Tafel · (Sports Medicine, Occupational Injuries, General Orthopaedic Surgery) · Columbia Panhandle Surgical Hospital · Southwest Neuroscience Institute, 3501 Soncy Road, Suite 154, P.O. Box 7688, Amarillo, TX 79114-7688 · 806-356-0264

Neil Roger Veggeberg · General Physical Medicine & Rehabilitation · High Plains Baptist Hospital · High Plains Rehabilitation, 5111 Canyon Drive, Amarillo, TX 79110-3037 · 806-353-7018

Arlington

Robert Ward Prevost, Jr. · General Physical Medicine & Rehabilitation · Arlington Memorial Hospital · Physical Medicine Associates, 901-A Medical Centre Drive, Arlington, TX 76012-4733 · 817-461-8343

Austin

John P. Obermiller · (Sports Medicine) · Healthsouth Rehabilitation Hospital of Austin · Texas Orthopaedics, Sports Medicine & Rehabilitation, 3200 Red River Street, Suite 201, Austin, TX 78705-2655 · 512-476-6846

Joe T. Powell · General Physical Medicine & Rehabilitation · St. David's Healthcare Center, Healthsouth Rehabilitation Hospital of Austin · 3705 Medical Parkway, Suite 440, Austin, TX 78705 · 512-452-5768

Charlotte Hoene Smith · General Physical Medicine & Rehabilitation · St. David's Healthcare Center · 1015 East 32nd Street, Suite 405, Austin, TX 78705 · 512-454-1234

Steven Shelby Tynes · General Physical Medicine & Rehabilitation · Healthsouth Rehabilitation Hospital of Austin · 1215 Red River Street, Suite 442, Austin, TX 78701 · 512-479-3632

Beaumont

Juan E. Davila · General Physical Medicine & Rehabilitation (Electrodiagnostic Medicine) · St. Elizabeth Hospital-Kate Dishman Rehab Center · 2965 Harrison Street, Suite 218, Beaumont, TX 77702 · 409-892-6868

Bedford

Wayne R. English · General Physical Medicine & Rehabilitation · Texas Back Institute, 3201 Airport Freeway, Suite 113, Bedford, TX 76022 · 817-267-6683

College Station

Steve Opersteny · General Physical Medicine & Rehabilitation · Columbia Medical Center · 1602 Rock Prairie Road, Suite 110, College Station, TX 77845 · 409-693-8263

Corpus Christi

Bruce R. McFarland · General Physical Medicine & Rehabilitation · Bay Area Rehabilitation Center, 3857 South Staples Street, Corpus Christi, TX 78411 · 512-854-9596

Dallas

Andrew J. Cole · General Physical Medicine & Rehabilitation · Baylor University Medical Center · Baylor University Medical Center, Department of Physical Medicine & Rehabiltation, 411 North Washington Avenue, Suite 4000, Dallas, TX 75246 · 214-820-2521

Phala Aniece Helm · General Physical Medicine & Rehabilitation (Burns, Diabetic Feet) · Parkland Memorial Hospital · University of Texas-Southwestern Medical Center at Dallas, 5323 Harry Hines Boulevard, Dallas, TX 75235-9055 · 214-648-2288

Karen J. Kowalske · General Physical Medicine & Rehabilitation (Trauma & Burn Rehabilitation, Peripheral Nerve Injuries, Stroke, Electrodiagnostic Medicine) · Parkland Memorial Hospital, Zale Lipshy University Hospital · University of Texas-Southwestern Medical Center at Dallas, Department of Physical Medicine & Rehabilitation, 5323 Harry Hines Boulevard, Dallas, TX 75235-9055 · 214-648-2288

Barry Samuel Smith · General Physical Medicine & Rehabilitation · Baylor University Medical Center · Baylor University Medical Center, Department of Physical Medicine & Rehabiltation, 3500 Gaston Avenue, Dallas, TX 75246-2017 · 214-820-7192

Robert Phillips Wilder · General Physical Medicine & Rehabilitation (Sports Medicine, Electrodiagnostic Medicine) · Baylor University Medical Center · Tom Landry Sports Medicine & Research Center, 411 North Washington Avenue, Suite 4000, Dallas, TX 75246 · 214-820-2521

El Paso

Barry L. Bowser · (Brain Injury, Spinal Cord Injury, Stroke) · Rio Vista Rehabilitation Hospital · Rio Vista Rehabilitation Hospital, 1740 Curie Drive, El Paso, TX 79902-2901 · 915-541-7795

Fort Worth

Victor H. Flores · General Physical Medicine & Rehabilitation · Physical Medicine Associates, 1400 South Main Street, Suite 406, Fort Worth, TX 76104 · 817-336-7422

Wilson J. Garcia · General Physical Medicine & Rehabilitation · All Saints Episcopal Hospital-Fort Worth, Harris Methodist-Fort Worth, Cook Children's Medical Center · 1201 Fifth Avenue, Fort Worth, TX 76104-4304 · 817-332-2784

James Alan Scott · General Physical Medicine & Rehabilitation · Harris Methodist-Fort Worth · 1325 Pennsylvania Avenue, Suite 300, Fort Worth, TX 76104-2110 · 817-878-5690

Jon Nelson Van Deventer · General Physical Medicine & Rehabilitation · Harris Methodist-Fort Worth · 1325 Pennsylvania Avenue, Suite 300, Fort Worth, TX 76104-2110 · 817-878-5690

Houston

R. Edward Carter · General Physical Medicine & Rehabilitation (Spinal Cord Injury, Ventilator Dependent Spinal Cord Injury) · The Institute for Rehabilitation & Research · The Institute for Rehabilitation & Research, 1333 Moursund Avenue, Suite E103, Houston, TX 77030 · 713-797-5910

John C. Cianca · General Physical Medicine & Rehabilitation (Sports Medicine, Musculoskeletal, Myofascial Pain) · Methodist Hospital, The Institute for Rehabilitation & Research · Baylor College of Medicine, Department of Physical Medicine & Rehabilitation, 6550 Fannin Street, Suite 1421, Houston, TX 77030 · 713-627-3156

William H. Donovan · General Physical Medicine & Rehabilitation (Spinal Cord Injury, Amputation) · The Institute for Rehabilitation & Research · The Institute for Rehabilitation & Research, 1333 Moursund Avenue, Houston, TX 77030 · 713-797-5912

Susan J. Garrison · General Physical Medicine & Rehabilitation (Geriatrics, Strokes) · Methodist Hospital · Baylor College of Medicine, Department of Physical Medicine & Rehabilitation, 6550 Fannin Street, Suite 1421, Houston, TX 77030-2720 · 713-798-6198

Theresa Ann Gillis · General Physical Medicine & Rehabilitation (Cancer Rehabilitation) · University of Texas-M. D. Anderson Cancer Center, Department of Neuro-Oncology, 1515 Holcombe Boulevard, Box 100, Houston, TX 77030 · 713-745-2327

Terrence P. Glennon · General Physical Medicine & Rehabilitation (Multiple Sclerosis) · Methodist Hospital · Baylor College of Medicine, Department of Physical Medicine & Rehabilitation, 6550 Fannin Street, Suite 1421, Houston, TX 77030-2720 · 713-798-6198

Martin Grabois · General Physical Medicine & Rehabilitation (Chronic Pain) · Methodist Hospital, The Institute for Rehabilitation & Research · Baylor College of Medicine, Department of Physical Medicine & Rehabilitation, 1333 Moursund Avenue, Room A-221, Houston, TX 77030 · 713-799-5086

Helene K. Henson · General Physical Medicine & Rehabilitation · Methodist Hospital · Baylor College of Medicine, Department of Physical Medicine & Rehabilitation, 6550 Fannin Street, Suite 1421, Houston, TX 77030-2720 · 713-798-6198

Cindy B. Ivanhoe · General Physical Medicine & Rehabilitation (Traumatic Brain Injury) · The Institute for Rehabilitation & Research, 1333 Moursund Avenue, Suite D104, Houston, TX 77030 · 713-797-5246

Zvi Kalisky · General Physical Medicine & Rehabilitation (Traumatic Brain Injury) · Spring Branch Medical Center, Del Oro Institute for Rehabilitation · 7400 Fannin Street, Suite 620, Houston, TX 77054 · 713-799-8672

Charles George Kevorkian · General Physical Medicine & Rehabilitation (Electrodiagnostic Medicine, Musculoskeletal Pain) · St. Luke's Episcopal Hospital · St. Luke's Medical Tower, Suite 2330, 6624 Fannin Street, Houston, TX 77030 713-798-4061

Aaron Martin Levine · General Physical Medicine & Rehabilitation (Neck, Back, Musculoskeletal Pain, Strokes, Orthopaedic Rehabilitation) · Memorial Hospital-Southeast · 11914 Astoria Boulevard, Suite 510, Houston, TX 77089 · 713-484-8123

Ralph M. Mancini · General Physical Medicine & Rehabilitation · West Houston Rehabilitation Associates, 909 Frostwood Drive, Houston, TX 77024 · 713-984-9595

Janusz Markowski · General Physical Medicine & Rehabilitation (Spinal Cord Injury) · VA Medical Center · VA Medical Center, Spinal Cord Injury Service, 2002 Holcombe Boulevard, Mail Code 128, Houston, TX 77030-4211 · 713-794-7128

Maureen R. Nelson · General Physical Medicine & Rehabilitation (Pediatric, Neuromuscular Disease, Electrodiagnostic Medicine) · Texas Children's Hospital · Texas Children's Hospital, 6621 Fannin Street, Houston, TX 77030 · 713-770-5205

Kenneth C. Parsons · General Physical Medicine & Rehabilitation (Spinal Cord Injury, Electromyography, Electrodiagnostic Medicine) · The Institute for Rehabilitation & Research · The Institute for Rehabilitation & Research, 1333 Moursund Avenue, Suite D107, Houston, TX 77030 · 713-797-5252

Michael M. Priebe · General Physical Medicine & Rehabilitation (Spinal Cord Injury) · VA Medical Center · VA Medical Center, Spinal Cord Injury Service, 2002 Holcombe Boulevard, Mail Code 128, Houston, TX 77030-4211 · 713-794-7128

Jonathan Robert Strayer · General Physical Medicine & Rehabilitation (Spinal Cord Injury, Strokes, Electrodiagnostic Medicine, Electromyography) · The Institute for Rehabilitation & Research, The Institute for Rehabilitation & Research Lifebridge Hospital · The Institute for Rehabilitation & Research, 1333 Moursund Avenue, Suite D110, Houston, TX 77030-3405 · 713-797-5724

Michael John Vennix · General Physical Medicine & Rehabilitation (Electrodiagnostic Medicine) · Baylor College of Medicine, Department of Physical Medicine & Rehabilitation, 6550 Fannin Street, Suite 1421, Houston, TX 77030 · 713-798-6198

Stuart A. Yablon · General Physical Medicine & Rehabilitation (Traumatic Brain Injury) · The Institute for Rehabilitation & Research · The Institute for Rehabilitation & Research, 1333 Moursund Avenue, Suite D108, Houston, TX 77030 713-797-5246

Irving

Peter John Rappa · General Physical Medicine & Rehabilitation · Irving Healthcare System · 1906 North Story Road, Irving, TX 75061 · 214-513-2320

Lubbock

Randall Wolcott · General Physical Medicine & Rehabilitation (Electrodiagnostic Medicine) · 2002 Oxford Avenue, Lubbock, TX 79410 · 806-793-8869

Midland

Susan Van de Water · General Physical Medicine & Rehabilitation · Memorial Hospital & Medical Center · Rehabilitation Hospital of Midland Odessa, 1800 Heritage Boulevard, Midland, TX 79703 · 915-520-1600

San Antonio

Douglas Byron Barber · General Physical Medicine & Rehabilitation (Spinal Cord Injury) · Audie L. Murphy Memorial Veterans Hospital, University Health System, HealthSouth Rehabilitation Institute of San Antonio, Santa Rosa Rehabilitation Hospital · University of Texas Health Science Center at San Antonio, Department of Rehabilitation Medicine, 7703 Floyd Curl Drive, San Antonio, TX 78284-7798 · 210-617-5257

Charles E. Cottle II · General Physical Medicine & Rehabilitation (Spinal Cord Injury) · Healthsouth Rehabilitation Institute of San Antonio · South Texas Physical Medicine & Rehabilitation, 4410 Medical Drive, Suite 120, San Antonio, TX 78229 · 210-692-2000

Donald Morgan Currie · General Physical Medicine & Rehabilitation (Pediatric Rehabilitation) · Santa Rosa Children's Hospital · University of Texas Health Science Center at San Antonio, Department of Rehabilitation Medicine, 7703 Floyd Curl Drive, San Antonio, TX 78284-7798 · 210-567-5353

Daniel Dumitru · Electrodiagnostic Medicine · University Health Center—Downtown, University Hospital—South Texas Medical Center, Audie L. Murphy Memorial Veterans Hospital, Warm Springs/Baptist Rehabilitation Network · University of Texas Health Science Center at San Antonio, Department of Rehabilitation Medicine, 7703 Floyd Curl Drive, San Antonio, TX 78284-7798 · 210-567-5347

Diane M. L. Gilbert · General Physical Medicine & Rehabilitation (Total Joint Replacement) · University Hospital-South Texas Medical Center · Reeves Rehabilitation Center, 4502 Medical Drive, San Antonio, TX 78229-4493 · 210-616-2637

John Chandler King · General Physical Medicine & Rehabilitation (Chronic Pain Management, Neurogenic Bowel Management, Botox Therapy) · Reeves Rehabilitation Center—Medical Center Hospital, Audie L. Murphy Memorial Veterans Hospital, Warm Springs/Baptist Rehabilitation Network · University of Texas Health Science Center at San Antonio, Department of Rehabilitation Medicine, 7703 Floyd Curl Drive, San Antonio, TX 78284-7798 · 210-567-5347

Ellen Imber Leonard · General Physical Medicine & Rehabilitation (Pediatric Rehabilitation) · University of Texas Health Science Center at San Antonio, Department of Rehabilitation Medicine, 7703 Floyd Curl Drive, San Antonio, TX 78284-7798 · 210-567-5366

Jose Alfredo Santos · General Physical Medicine & Rehabilitation (Strokes, Post-Total Joint Replacement) · Santa Rosa Rehabilitation Hospital · The Rehabilitation Group, 2829 Babcock Road, Suite 308, San Antonio, TX 78229 · 210-614-3225

Nicolas E. Walsh · General Physical Medicine & Rehabilitation (Industrial Rehabilitation, Musculoskeletal & Pain Medicine) · University Hospital-South Texas Medical Center, Warm Springs/Baptist Rehabilitation Network, Santa Rosa Rehabilitation Hospital, Spring Hill Rehabilitation Network · University of Texas Health Science Center at San Antonio, Department of Rehabilitation Medicine, 7703 Floyd Curl Drive, San Antonio, TX 78284-7798 · 210-567-5350

Alex C. Willingham · (General Rehabilitation, Pediatric, Adult) · Warm Springs/Baptist Rehabilitation Network · Warm Springs Rehabilitation Hospital-San Antonio, 5101 Medical Drive, San Antonio, TX 78229 · 210-616-0100

Temple

John A. Schuchmann · General Physical Medicine & Rehabilitation · Scott & White Memorial Hospital · Scott & White Memorial Hospital, Department of Physical Medicine & Rehabilitation, 2401 South 31st Street, Temple, TX 76508-0001 · 817-724-4875

Tyler

Paul H. Dreyfuss · General Physical Medicine & Rehabilitation (Pain Management) · Neuro-Skeletal Center, 816 South Fleishel Avenue, Tyler, TX 75701 · 903-597-2508

Mark C. Race · General Physical Medicine & Rehabilitation · East Texas Medical Center · 619 South Fleishel Avenue, Suite 203, Tyler, TX 75701 · 903-592-8606

Waco

Brett J. Bolte · General Physical Medicine & Rehabilitation · Hillcrest Baptist Medical Center · Hillcrest Baptist Medical Center, Department of Physical Medicine & Rehabilitation, 3000 Herring Avenue, Waco, TX 76708 · 817-750-7977

PLASTIC SURGERY

Amarillo

Richard Melvin High · General Plastic Surgery (Aesthetic Surgery, Reconstructive Surgery, Hand Surgery, Microsurgery) · High Plains Baptist Hospital, St.

Anthony's Hospital, Columbia Panhandle Surgical Hospital, Amarillo Hospital District-Northwest Texas Hospital · 7120 West Ninth Street, Amarillo, TX 79106 806-376-1188

John C. Kelleher, Jr. · Facial Aesthetic Surgery (Body Contouring, Breast Surgery) · High Plains Baptist Hospital · Panhandle Plastic Surgery, 1810 Coulter Drive, Amarillo, TX 79106-1777 · 806-358-8731

Austin

Robert L. Clement · (Body Contouring, Breast Surgery, Facial Aesthetic Surgery) Seton Medical Center · 3901 Medical Parkway, Suite 100, Austin, TX 78756 · 512-459-3101

Alfred Christian Wilder · Breast Surgery · 3705 Medical Parkway, Suite 460, Austin, TX 78705 · 512-459-1234

Beaumont

Curtis M. Baldwin, Jr. · Facial Aesthetic Surgery · Southeast Texas Plastic Surgery, 2965 Harrison Street, Suite 315, Beaumont, TX 77702-1150 · 409-899-1277

Harold R. Mancusi-Ungaro, Jr. · Facial Aesthetic Surgery (Burns, Facial Trauma, Hand Surgery) · Baptist Hospital Beaumont, St. Elizabeth Hospital, Beaumont Regional Medical Center, Southeast Texas Rehab Hospital · Southeast Texas Plastic Surgery, 2965 Harrison Street, Suite 315, Beaumont, TX 77702-1150 · 409-899-1277

Corpus Christi

Max L. Gouverne · (Facial Aesthetic Surgery, Breast Surgery, Body Contouring) Spohn Hospital, Columbia Surgicare Specialty Hospital · Plastic Surgery Associates, 1102 Ocean Drive, Corpus Christi, TX 78404 · 512-881-9999

Dallas

Fritz E. Barton, Jr. · Facial Aesthetic Surgery (Breast Reconstruction, Augmentation Mammoplasty, Breast Reduction, Body Contouring, Laser Surgery) · Baylor University Medical Center · Dallas Plastic Surgery Institute, 411 North Washington Avenue, Suite 6000, Dallas, TX 75246 · 214-821-9355

H. Steve Byrd · Facial Aesthetic Surgery, Craniofacial Surgery (Craniofacial Contouring, Pediatric) · Children's Medical Center of Dallas · Dallas Plastic Surgery Institute, 411 North Washington Avenue, Suite 6000, Dallas, TX 75246 · 214-821-9662

Jack Pershing Gunter · Facial Aesthetic Surgery (Rhinoplasty) · Presbyterian Hospital of Dallas, Children's Medical Center of Dallas, Parkland Memorial Hospital, Baylor University Medical Center · 8315 Walnut Hill Lane, Suite 125, Dallas, TX 75231 · 214-369-8123

Sam T. Hamra · Facial Aesthetic Surgery (Facelift & Eyelids, Rhinoplasty, Liposuction, Body Contouring, Breast Surgery) · Mary Shiels Hospital, Baylor University Medical Center · 3707 Gaston Avenue, Suite 810, Dallas, TX 75246 · 214-823-9381

Patrick Lynn Hodges · General Plastic Surgery · Presbyterian Hospital of Dallas 8220 Walnut Hill Lane, Suite 206, Dallas, TX 75231-4423 · 214-739-5760

Ian R. Munro · Craniofacial Surgery, Maxillofacial Surgery · Medical City Dallas Hospital · Medical City Dallas Hospital, Building C, Suite 700, 7777 Forest Lane, Dallas, TX 75230-2594 · 214-788-6464

Hamlet T. Newsom · General Plastic Surgery · Presbyterian Hospital of Dallas · 8200 Walnut Hill Lane, Suite 206, Dallas, TX 75231-4423 · 214-739-5760

Harlan Pollock · Facial Aesthetic Surgery (Breast Cosmetic Surgery, Liposuction, Body Contouring, Laser Surgery & Birthmarks) · Presbyterian Hospital of Dallas 8305 Walnut Hill Lane, Suite 210, Dallas, TX 75231 · 214-363-2575

Rod J. Rohrich · Facial Aesthetic Surgery (Breast Surgery, Body Contouring) · Zale Lipshy University Hospital, Baylor University Medical Center · Dallas Plastic Surgery Institute, 411 North Washington Avenue, Suite 6000, Mail Code LB13, Dallas, TX 75246 · 214-821-9114

Kenneth Everett Salyer · Craniofacial Surgery (Maxillofacial Surgery, Facial Aesthetic Surgery, Body Contouring, Head & Neck Surgery, Pediatric Plastic Surgery, Reconstructive Surgery) · Medical City Dallas Hospital · International Craniofacial Institute, 7777 Forest Lane, Suite C-717, Dallas, TX 75230-2594 · 214-788-6555

John B. Tebbetts · Facial Aesthetic Surgery, Breast Surgery (Body Contouring, Rhinoplasty) · Mary Shiels Hospital, Valley View Surgery Center · 2801 Lemmon Avenue West, Suite 300, Dallas, TX 75204 · 214-220-2712

El Paso

Ronald A. Gum · General Plastic Surgery · Providence Memorial Hospital · 125 West Hague Road, Suite 110, El Paso, TX 79902 · 915-532-3056

Herbert J. Nassour · General Plastic Surgery (Reconstructive/Microvascular Surgery, Cosmetic Surgery, General Hand Surgery) · Providence Memorial Hospital, Columbia Medical Center-West, Sierra Medical Center · Providence Medical Plaza, Suite 120, 125 West Hague Road, El Paso, TX 79902 · 915-532-6662

H. Robert Thering · Breast Surgery (Facial Aesthetic Surgery, Pediatric Plastic Surgery) · Providence Memorial Hospital, Sierra Medical Center, Columbia Medical Center-West · Providence Medical Plaza, Suite 120, 125 West Hague Road, El Paso, TX 79902 · 915-532-6662

Fort Worth

Raymond A. Faires · General Plastic Surgery (Hand Surgery, Microsurgery) · Harris Methodist-Southwest, Harris Methodist-Fort Worth, Cook Children's Medical Center, All Saints Episcopal Hospital-Fort Worth, Harris Methodist-HEB (Bedford) · 1325 Pennsylvania Avenue, Suite 325, Fort Worth, TX 76104-2110 · 817-332-9441

Shujaat A. Khan · Breast Surgery (Breast Reconstruction) · Medical Plaza Professional Building, 800 Eighth Avenue, Suite 200, Fort Worth, TX 76104 · 817-335-6363

Larry Earl Reaves · General Plastic Surgery (Facial Aesthetic Surgery, Breast Surgery, Pediatric Plastic Surgery) · Harris Methodist-Fort Worth · 800 Eighth Avenue, Suite 606, Fort Worth, TX 76104-2605 · 817-335-4755

Dennis I. Schuster · General Plastic Surgery · Plaza Medical Center · 747 Eighth Avenue, Fort Worth, TX 76104-2503 · 817-335-6801

Galveston

Steven J. Blackwell · General Plastic Surgery · University of Texas Medical Branch, Department of Surgery, Division of Plastic Surgery, 301 University Boulevard, Galveston, TX 77555-0724 · 409-772-1256

Ted Huang · General Plastic Surgery (Breast Surgery, Facial Aesthetic Surgery) · University of Texas Medical Branch Hospitals, Mainland Center Hospital (Texas City) · 326 Market Street, Galveston, TX 77550 · 409-762-8757

Linda G. Phillips · General Plastic Surgery (Wound Healing, Breast Reconstruction, Body Contouring, Breast Surgery, Microsurgery) · University of Texas Medical Branch, Department of Surgery, Division of Plastic Surgery, 301 University Boulevard, Galveston, TX 77555-0724 · 409-772-1257

Houston

Parviz Arfai · General Plastic Surgery · Methodist Hospital · 7777 Southwest Freeway, Suite 724, Houston, TX 77074 · 713-776-9086

Charles W. Bailey · General Plastic Surgery (Facial Aesthetic Surgery, Breast Reconstruction, Reconstructive Surgery) · Hermann Hospital, Methodist Hospital, Memorial Hospital-Southwest · 7737 Southwest Freeway, Suite 910, Houston, TX 77074 · 713-772-3003

Bonnie Baldwin · Microsurgery (Reconstructive Surgery, Breast Surgery) · University of Texas-M. D. Anderson Cancer Center · University of Texas-M. D. Anderson Cancer Center, Department of Plastic Surgery, 1515 Holcombe Boulevard, Box 62, Houston, TX 77030-4009 · 713-794-1247

Thomas M. Biggs, Jr. · Facial Aesthetic Surgery, Breast Surgery · 1315 Calhoun Avenue, Suite 900, Houston, TX 77002 · 713-650-0800

Keith Eric Brandt · Peripheral Nerve Surgery (Surgery of the Hand, Reconstructive Surgery, General Hand Surgery) · Hermann Hospital · University of Texas Medical School at Houston, 6431 Fannin Street, Room 4.150, Houston, TX 77030 · 713-792-5498

Benjamin E. Cohen · Breast Surgery, Facial Aesthetic Surgery (Aesthetic Surgery of Face and Trunk, General Plastic Surgery) · St. Joseph Hospital · Cohen & Cronin Clinic Association, 1315 Calhoun Street, Suite 920, Houston, TX 77002 · 713-951-0400

Ernest D. Cronin · Breast Surgery, Maxillofacial Surgery (Breast Reconstruction, Cleft Lip & Palate, Cosmetic Surgery) · St. Joseph Hospital · Cohen & Cronin Clinic Association, 1315 Calhoun Street, Suite 920, Houston, TX 77002 · 713-951-0400

Don A. Gard · Head & Neck Surgery · Methodist Hospital · 6560 Fannin Street, Suite 1228, Houston, TX 77030 · 713-790-5555

Stephen Samuel Kroll · Breast Surgery, Head & Neck Surgery (Breast Reconstruction, Microsurgery, Reconstructive Surgery) · University of Texas-M. D. Anderson Cancer Center · University of Texas-M. D. Anderson Cancer Center, 1515 Holcombe Boulevard, Box 62, Houston, TX 77030-4009 · 713-794-1247

Emmanuel G. Melissinos · Microsurgery (Wound Reconstruction, Hand Surgery) · Hermann Hospital · 6410 Fannin Street, Suite 633, Houston, TX 77030 · 713-790-0723

Michael J. Miller · Microsurgery (Reconstructive Surgery, Breast Reconstruction, Cancer Surgery) · University of Texas-M. D. Anderson Cancer Center, St. Luke's Episcopal Hospital, Hermann Hospital · University of Texas-M. D. Anderson Cancer Center, Department of Plastic Surgery, 1515 Holcombe Boulevard, Box 62, Houston, TX 77030-4009 · 713-794-1247

David T. Netscher · Peripheral Nerve Surgery (Hand Surgery) · Methodist Hospital · Baylor College of Medicine, Department of Plastic Surgery, 6560 Fannin Street, Suite 800, Houston, TX 77030 · 713-798-6936

Donald H. Parks · Reconstructive Surgery (Burn Surgery, Acute Burn Care, Skin Tumors, General Plastic Surgery) · Hermann Hospital · University of Texas Medical School at Houston, 6431 Fannin Street, Room 4.156, Houston, TX 77030 · 713-792-5414

Gregory P. Reece · Reconstructive Surgery (Microsurgery, Breast Surgery) · University of Texas-M. D. Anderson Cancer Center · University of Texas-M. D. Anderson Cancer Center, Department of Plastic Surgery, 1515 Holcombe Boulevard, Box 62, Houston, TX 77030-4009 · 713-794-1247

Geoffrey Lawrence Robb · Reconstructive Surgery (Microsurgery, Cancer Reconstructive Surgery, Breast Surgery, General Plastic Surgery) · University of Texas-M. D. Anderson Cancer Center · University of Texas-M. D. Anderson Cancer Center, 1515 Holcombe Boulevard, Box 62, Houston, TX 77030-4009 · 713-794-1247

Mark A. Schusterman · Breast Surgery (Body Contouring, Facial Aesthetic Surgery, Microsurgery) · University of Texas-M. D. Anderson Cancer Center · University of Texas-M. D. Anderson Cancer Center, 1515 Holcombe Boulevard, Box 62, Houston, TX 77030 · 713-794-1247

Saleh Mousa Shenaq · Microsurgery (Reconstructive Surgery, Facial Aesthetic Surgery, Breast Surgery) · Methodist Hospital, Texas Children's Hospital, St. Luke's Hospital, The Institute for Rehabilitation & Research · Texas Medical Center-Baylor College of Medicine, Scurlock Tower, Suite 800, 6560 Fannin Street, Houston, TX 77030 · 713-798-6310

Melvin Spira · General Plastic Surgery (Facial Aesthetic Surgery, Breast Surgery, Body Contouring) · Methodist Hospital, St. Luke's Episcopal Hospital · Baylor College of Medicine, 6560 Fannin Street, Suite 800, Houston, TX 77030-3411 · 713-798-6141

Samuel Stal · Pediatric Plastic Surgery (Cleft Lip & Palate, Craniofacial Surgery, Rhinoplasty, Facial Reconstruction) · Texas Children's Hospital · Clinical Care Center, 6621 Fannin Street, Suite 330, Houston, TX 77030 · 713-770-3185

John Flynn Teichgraeber · Head & Neck Surgery · Hermann Hospital · University of Texas Medical School at Houston, Department of Plastic Surgery, 6431 Fannin Street, Room 4.156, Houston, TX 77030 · 713-792-5454

D. Robert Wiemer · General Plastic Surgery (Facial Aesthetic Surgery, Breast Aesthetic & Reconstructive Surgery) · Methodist Hospital, Diagnostic Center Hospital, St. Luke's Episcopal Hospital · Wiemer Plastic Surgery, 6560 Fannin Street, Suite 1760, Houston, TX 77030-2714 · 713-795-5584

Lubbock

Milton M. Rowley · General Plastic Surgery · St. Mary of the Plains Hospital, Lubbock Methodist Hospital · 3519 Twenty-Second Place, Lubbock, TX 79413 806-792-3715

Midland

Terry D. Tubb · General Plastic Surgery · 1304 West Texas Avenue, Midland, TX 79701 · 915-570-7821

San Antonio

Francis C. Burton, Jr. · General Plastic Surgery · Northeast Baptist Hospital · 8601 Village Drive, Suite 224, San Antonio, TX 78217 · 210-654-9900

Sean Peter Campbell · Craniofacial Surgery (Cleft Lip & Palate Surgery, Pediatric) · 7950 Floyd Curl Drive, Suite 1009, San Antonio, TX 78229 · 210-616-0880

Richard A. Levine · General Plastic Surgery (Facial Aesthetic Surgery) · Northeast Baptist Hospital · 8500 Village Drive, Suite 102, San Antonio, TX 78217 · 210-654-4089

William David McInnis · General Plastic Surgery (Facial Aesthetic Surgery, Reconstructive Surgery, Body Contouring, Breast Surgery) · Southwest Texas Methodist Hospital, South Texas Ambulatory Surgery Hospital · Methodist Plaza, Suite 301, 4499 Medical Drive, San Antonio, TX 78229 · 210-614-3191

William C. Pederson · Reconstructive Surgery (Hand) · Baptist Medical Center The Hand Center of San Antonio, 7940 Floyd Curl Drive, Suite 900, San Antonio, TX 78229-3906 · 210-614-7025

James Martin Smith · General Plastic Surgery (Cleft Lip & Palate Surgery, Burns [Acute and Long-Term Reconstruction], Pediatric Plastic Surgery, Reconstructive Surgery) · Southwest Texas Methodist Hospital, South Texas Ambulatory Surgery Hospital, St. Luke's Baptist Hospital · 4499 Medical Drive, Suite 340, San Antonio, TX 78229-3773 · 210-614-9701

Sugar Land

William B. Riley, Jr. · General Plastic Surgery (Facial Aesthetic Surgery, Breast Surgery, Reconstructive Surgery) · Columbia Fort Bend Medical Center (Missouri City), Memorial Hospital-Southwest, St. Luke's Episcopal Hospital, Hermann Hospital, Texas Children's Hospital · Plastic Surgery Specialists, 4665 Sweetwater Boulevard, Suite 110, Sugar Land, TX 77479 · 713-980-0999

Temple

Peter Grothaus · General Plastic Surgery · Scott & White Memorial Hospital · Scott & White Memorial Hospital, Department of Plastic Surgery, 2401 South 31st Street, Temple, TX 76508-0001 · 817-724-2640

Dennis J. Lynch · General Plastic Surgery · Scott & White Memorial Hospital · Scott & White Memorial Hospital, Department of Plastic Surgery, 2401 South 31st Street, Temple, TX 76508-0001 · 817-724-2640

Charles N. Verheyden · General Plastic Surgery (Laser Surgery & Birthmarks, Reconstructive Surgery) · Scott & White Memorial Hospital · Scott & White Memorial Hospital, Division of Plastic Surgery, 2401 South 31st Street, Temple, TX 76508-0001 · 817-724-4251

Raleigh R. White IV · General Plastic Surgery · Scott & White Memorial Hospital & Clinic · Scott & White Memorial Hospital, Division of Plastic Surgery, 2401 South 31st Street, Temple, TX 76508-0001 · 817-724-2640

Tyler

James T. Clark · General Plastic Surgery (Facial Aesthetic Surgery, Laser Aesthetic Surgery) · East Texas Medical Center, Trinity Mother Frances Health Care Center · East Lake Professional Plaza, Suite 330, 1100 East Lake Street, Tyler, TX 75701 · 903-595-5522

Waco

Eric F. O'Neill · General Plastic Surgery (Breast Reconstruction, Laser Surgery) · Hillcrest Baptist Medical Center, Providence Health Center · 3115 Pine Avenue, Suite 208, Waco, TX 76708 · 817-753-5692

Robert M. Wright, Jr. · General Plastic Surgery · Providence Health Center, Hillcrest Baptist Medical Center · Aesthetic Surgery Center of Waco, 2911 Herring Avenue, Suite 312, Waco, TX 76708-3240 · 817-755-4470

Valerie K. Wright · General Plastic Surgery · Hillcrest Baptist Medical Center · Aesthetic Surgery Center of Waco, 2911 Herring Avenue, Suite 312, Waco, TX 76708-3240 · 817-755-4470

Wichita Falls

Eid B. H. Mustafa · General Plastic Surgery (Cosmetic Surgery, Hand Surgery, Breast Surgery) · 1201 Brook Avenue, Wichita Falls, TX 76301 · 817-322-1122

PSYCHIATRY

Amarillo

Michael D. Jenkins · General Psychiatry · 1901 Medical Park Plaza, Suite 211, Amarillo, TX 79106 · 806-356-2750

Austin

John H. Bannister · Psychoanalysis (Child & Adolescent Psychiatry) · 1301 Capital of Texas Highway South, Suite A-240, Austin, TX 78746 · 512-328-2820

Richard E. Coons · Forensic Psychiatry · Shoal Creek Hospital · 720 West 34th Street, Austin, TX 78705 · 512-454-7741

Virginia M. T. Eubanks · Psychoanalysis · 2200 Parkway, Austin, TX 78703 · 512-477-7676

Tracy Ross Gordy · Mood & Anxiety Disorders, Geriatric Psychiatry (Bi-Polar, Affective Disorders) · Shoal Creek Hospital · Neuropsychiatric Associates of Austin, 1600 West 38th Street, Suite 321, Austin, TX 78731-6406 · 512-454-5716

William Monning Loving · General Psychiatry (Addiction Psychiatry, Addiction Medicine, Medical Treatment of Drug Users, Schizophrenia, Brain Damage, Neuropsychiatry, Psychopharmacology) · Shoal Creek Hospital · Neuropsychiatric Associates of Austin, 1600 West 38th Street, Suite 321, Austin, TX 78731-6406 · 512-454-5716

Jefferson E. Nelson · (Psychopharmacology, Chemical Dependency, Adolescent Psychiatry) · Shoal Creek Hospital, St. David's Pavilion · Neuropsychiatric Associates of Austin, 1600 West 38th Street, Suite 321, Austin, TX 78731-6406 · 512-454-5716

William Howard Reid · Forensic Psychiatry (General Psychiatry, Mental Retardation/Mental Health, Violence) · P.O. Box 49817, Austin, TX 78765-9817 · 512-756-4991

Stephen M. Sonnenberg · Psychoanalysis · 1600 West 38th Street, Suite 403, Austin, TX 78731 · 512-452-1055

Beaumont

Jackson T. Achilles · General Psychiatry · 2497 Liberty Street, Beaumont, TX 77702 · 409-838-1116

Charles F. Adkins · General Psychiatry (Adult, Geriatric Psychiatry) · Behavior Management Center, 3260 Fannin Street, Beaumont, TX 77701-3903 · 409-835-4953

James B. Creed · General Psychiatry (Mood & Anxiety Disorders, Psychopharmacology) · Beaumont Regional Medical Center-Fannin Pavilion · 3560 Delaware Street, Suite 1204, P.O. Box 20217, Beaumont, TX 77720-0217 · 409-899-9265

Edward B. Gripon · General Psychiatry · 3560 Delaware Street, Suite 502, Beaumont, TX 77706-3061 · 409-899-4472

George Edward Groves · General Psychiatry · 3560 Delaware Street, Suite 502, Beaumont, TX 77706-3061 · 409-899-4472

John T. Halbert · General Psychiatry (Geriatric Psychiatry) · Beaumont Regional Medical Center · Behavior Management Center, 3260 Fannin Street, Beaumont, TX 77701-3903 · 409-835-4953

Bellaire

Arthur J. Farley · Psychoanalysis (Child, Adolescent and Adult) · 6300 West Loop, South, Suite 140, Bellaire, TX 77401 · 713-666-6885

Corpus Christi

Carlos R. Estrada · Psychoanalysis (Child & Adult) · 3126 Rodd Field Road, Corpus Christi, TX 78414 · 512-993-8088

James M. May · General Psychiatry · 6625 Wooldridge Road, Suite 402, Corpus Christi, TX 78414 · 512-992-5525

Dallas

Bryon Harlen Adinoff · Addiction Psychiatry (Psychopharmacology, Neuroendocrinology) · VA Medical Center, University of Texas Southwestern Medical Center · VA Medical Center, Chemical Addiction Program, 4500 South Lancaster Road, Dallas, TX 75216 · 214-372-7011

Kenneth Z. Altshuler · General Psychiatry, Psychoanalysis (Early Profound Deafness, Geriatrics, Psychotherapy) · Parkland Memorial Hospital, Zale Lipshy University Hospital, Presbyterian Hospital of Dallas, Children's Medical Center of Dallas · University of Texas-Southwestern Medical Center at Dallas, Department of Psychiatry, 5323 Harry Hines Boulevard, Room F5.400, Dallas, TX 75235-9070 214-648-3856

Jeffry John Andresen · Psychoanalysis (Psychotherapy) · Zale Lipshy University Hospital · University of Texas-Southwestern Medical Center at Dallas, 5323 Harry Hines Boulevard, Dallas, TX 75235-9070 · 214-648-2980

John W. Cain · Mood & Anxiety Disorders (Psychoanalysis, Psychopharmacology) Parkland Memorial Hospital, Zale Lipshy University Hospital · University of Texas-Southwestern Medical Center at Dallas, Department of Psychiatry, 5323 Harry Hines Boulevard, Dallas, TX 75235-8898 · 214-648-3888

Diane Fagelman Birk · Child & Adolescent Psychiatry, Psychoanalysis (General Psychiatry) · Green Oaks Hospital · 12880 Hillcrest Road, Suite 104, Dallas, TX 75230 · 214-387-4747

Joel S. Feiner · Schizophrenia, Violence (Social Community Psychiatry, Public Psychiatry) · Mental Health Connections · Mental Health Connections, 5909 Harry Hines Boulevard, Nine South, Dallas, TX 75235 · 214-879-2826

Ronald Stuart Fleischmann · Psychoanalysis (General Psychiatry) · Green Oaks Hospital · 8117 Preston Road, Suite 685, Dallas, TX 75225 · 214-360-0720

Rhoda S. Frenkel · Child & Adolescent Psychiatry, Psychoanalysis (Child & Adolescent Psychoanalysis) · 8226 Douglas Avenue, Suite 456, Dallas, TX 75225-5926 · 214-363-2836

David L. Garver · Schizophrenia · VA Medical Center · VA Medical Center, 4500 South Lancaster Road, Mail Code 116A, Dallas, TX 75216 · 214-949-0579

Joseph Donald Gaspari · Addiction Psychiatry, Psychoanalysis (Mood & Anxiety Disorders, Sports Psychiatry) · Charter Behavioral Health System of Dallas (Plano) 5956 Sherry Lane, Suite 540, Dallas, TX 75225-8016 · 214-369-6335

Bradford M. Goff · Addiction Psychiatry · 3625 North Hall Street, Suite 680, Dallas, TX 75219 · 214-559-2188

Herbert Leslie Gomberg · Psychoanalysis (Mood & Anxiety Disorders, Neurotic Character Disorders) · Presbyterian Hospital of Dallas · 8226 Douglas Avenue, Suite 430, Dallas, TX 75225 · 214-691-8606

Fred L. Griffin · General Psychiatry (Psychotherapy, Psychoanalysis) · Presbyterian Hospital of Dallas · 8117 Preston Road, Suite 685, Dallas, TX 75225 · 214-360-9260

Irving L. Humphrey · Child & Adolescent Psychiatry, Psychoanalysis (General Psychiatry) · 12880 Hillcrest Road, Suite J-215, Dallas, TX 75230 · 214-404-8677

James L. Knoll III · General Psychiatry · Presbyterian Hospital of Dallas · 8200 Walnut Hill Lane, Dallas, TX 75231 · 214-345-7355

Jerry M. Lewis III · Child & Adolescent Psychiatry, Psychoanalysis (Mood & Anxiety Disorders) · Timberlawn Psychiatric Hospital · 8226 Douglas Avenue, Suite 805, Dallas, TX 75225 · 214-373-6194

Jack Martin · Child & Adolescent Psychiatry (Adult Psychiatry) · Presbyterian Hospital of Dallas, Baylor University Medical Center, Parkland Memorial Hospital, Zale Lipshy University Hospital · 3636 Dickason Avenue, Dallas, TX 75219-4911 · 214-528-3041

Gerald Anthony Melchiode · Psychoanalysis (Psychotherapy, Human Sexuality, General Psychiatry) · 8226 Douglas Avenue, Suite 805, Dallas, TX 75225 · 214-373-6195

Paul C. Mohl · General Psychiatry · Zale Lipshy University Hospital · University of Texas-Southwestern Medical Center at Dallas, 5323 Harry Hines Boulevard, Dallas, TX 75235-9070 · 214-648-2217

Edgar P. Nace · Addiction Psychiatry (Forensic Psychiatry, General Psychiatry, Mood & Anxiety Disorders, Psychopharmacology) · Charter Behavioral Health System of Dallas (Plano), Medical City Dallas Hospital · 7777 Forest Lane, Suite B-413, Dallas, TX 75230 · 214-788-6282

Frederick Petty · Mood & Anxiety Disorders (Post-Traumatic Stress Disorder, Psychopharmacology) · VA Medical Center · VA Medical Center, 4500 South Lancaster Road, Mail Code 116A, Dallas, TX 75216-7191 · 214-376-5451

John H. Reitmann · General Psychiatry (Consult-Liaison Psychiatry) · 3636 Dickason Avenue, Dallas, TX 75219-4911 · 214-521-9660

A. John Rush · Mood & Anxiety Disorders, Psychopharmacology · Parkland Memorial Hospital, St. Paul Medical Center, Presbyterian Hospital of Dallas, Zale Lipshy University Hospital · University of Texas-Southwestern Medical Center at Dallas, 5959 Harry Hines Boulevard, Suite 600, Dallas, TX 75235 · 214-648-8321

Stephen Scherffius · General Psychiatry (Psychoanalysis) · 5950 Berkshire Lane, Suite 1460, Dallas, TX 75225 · 214-373-7442

Larry G. Shadid · Child & Adolescent Psychiatry, Psychoanalysis (Adult Psychotherapy, Family Psychiatry) · 8226 Douglas Avenue, Suite 805, Dallas, TX 75225 214-739-1101

Maxwell H. Soll · Psychoanalysis · Green Oaks Hospital · 12830 Hillcrest Road, Suite 235, Dallas, TX 75230 · 214-233-6507

Kathryn A. Sommerfelt · General Psychiatry (Mood & Anxiety Disorders, Women-Related Illnesses) · 12880 Hillcrest Road, Suite 104, Dallas, TX 75230 · 214-387-4752

Thomas Michael Sonn · Psychoanalysis (Psychotherapy) · 8226 Douglas Avenue, Dallas, TX 75225-5906 · 214-696-8941

Leonora Stephens · General Psychiatry (Marital & Family Therapy, Psychotherapy from a Psychodynamic, Family Systems Perspective, Group Therapy) · 3131 Turtle Creek Boulevard, Suite 1120, Dallas, TX 75219 · 214-522-5120

Rege S. Stewart · Mood & Anxiety Disorders (Psychopharmacology) · Parkland Memorial Hospital, Zale Lipshy University Hospital · University of Texas-Southwestern Medical Center at Dallas, Department of Psychiatry, 5323 Harry Hines Boulevard, Dallas, TX 75235-9070 · 214-648-3300

Patricia Suppes · Mood & Anxiety Disorders (Bi-Polar, Affective Disorders) · University of Texas-Southwestern Medical Center at Dallas, Department of Psychiatry, 5323 Harry Hines Boulevard, Dallas, TX 75235-9070 · 214-648-4211

William Laurence Thornton · General Psychiatry (Psychoanalysis, Inpatient Psychiatry) · Zale Lipshy University Hospital · University of Texas-Southwestern Medical Center at Dallas, Department of Psychiatry, 5161 Harry Hines Boulevard, Dallas, TX 75235-8898 · 214-590-3442

Larry Edward Tripp · General Psychiatry · 3707 Gaston Avenue, Suite 418, Dallas, TX 75246-1521 · 214-824-2273

David L. Tyler · General Psychiatry (Mood Disorders, Psychopharmacology) · Presbyterian Hospital of Dallas · 5445 La Sierra Drive, Suite 202, Dallas, TX 75231 · 214-369-5797

Mark Paul Unterberg · General Psychiatry (Occupational Psychiatry, Psychoanalysis, Sports Psychiatry, Addiction Psychiatry, Mood & Anxiety Disorders, Psychopharmacology, Medical Treatment of Drug Abusers) · Timberlawn Psychiatric Hospital · Timberlawn Hospital, 4600 Samuel Boulevard, Dallas, TX 75228 · 214-373-8990

David A. Waller · Eating Disorders (Child & Adolescent Psychiatry, Behavioral Pediatrics) · Children's Medical Center of Dallas · University of Texas-Southwestern Medical Center at Dallas, Department of Psychiatry, 5323 Harry Hines Boulevard, Dallas, TX 75235-9070 · 214-648-3898

Myron F. Weiner · Geriatric Psychiatry · Zale Lipshy University Hospital · University of Texas-Southwestern Medical Center at Dallas, Department of Psychiatry, 5323 Harry Hines Boulevard, Room F5.400, Dallas, TX 75235-9070 · 214-648-3400

Kimberly A. Yonkers · General Psychiatry (Premenstrual Syndrome, Postpartum Disorders, Mood & Anxiety Disorders, Psychopharmacology) · Zale Lipshy University Hospital, Parkland Memorial Hospital, VA Medical Center · Aston Ambulatory Care Center, Department of Obstetrics & Gynecology, 5323 Harry Hines Boulevard, Dallas, TX 75235-9032 · 214-648-4283

El Paso

Delia M. Gallo · Child & Adolescent Psychiatry (Infant Psychiatry) · Providence Memorial Hospital, Sierra Medical Center, Thomason Hospital · Texas Tech Outpatient Clinic, 424 Executive Center, Suite 101, El Paso, TX 79902 · 915-533-2471; 915-545-6785

J. Raul Jimenez · General Psychiatry · 2311 North Mesa Street, Building I, El Paso, TX 79902 · 915-544-0600

Fort Worth

Norris Duane Purcell · Psychoanalysis · 1814 Eighth Avenue, Suite B-8, Fort Worth, TX 75610-1354 · 817-924-1036

Galveston

Eric N. Avery · General Psychiatry (Consult-Liaison Psychiatry) · University of Texas Medical Branch, Department of Psychiatry, 301 University Boulevard, Galveston, TX 77555-0428 · 409-772-3474

Terrence S. Early · General Psychiatry, Psychopharmacology, Schizophrenia (Mood & Anxiety Disorders, Neuropsychiatry) · University of Texas Medical Branch Hospitals · University of Texas Medical Branch, Department of Psychiatry and Behavioral Sciences, 301 University Boulevard, Galveston, TX 77555-0431 · 409-772-4467

Alan R. Felthous · Forensic Psychiatry · John Sealy Hospital · University of Texas Medical Branch, Department of Psychiatry & Behavioral Sciences, D-28 Graves Building, 301 University Boulevard, Galveston, TX 77555-0428 · 409-772-3984

Jean Patricia Goodwin · Dissociative Disorders, Forensic Psychiatry (Survivors of Childhood Trauma, Psychoanalysis) · University of Texas Medical Branch Hospitals · University of Texas Medical Branch, Department of Psychiatry & Behavioral Sciences, 4.441 Graves Building, 301 University Boulevard, Galveston, TX 77555-0428 · 409-772-9313

Joan R. Hebeler · Child & Adolescent Psychiatry (Mood & Anxiety Disorders, Psychopharmacology) · University of Texas Medical Branch Hospitals · University of Texas Medical Branch, Department of Psychiatry, 3.258 Graves Building, 301 University Boulevard, Galveston, TX 77550 · 409-772-1066

Robert M. A. Hirschfeld · General Psychiatry, Mood & Anxiety Disorders, Psychopharmacology (Depression) · University of Texas Medical Branch, Department of Psychiatry & Behavioral Sciences, 1.200 Graves Building, 301 University Boulevard, Galveston, TX 77555-0429 · 409-772-4956

Joan A. Lang · Psychoanalysis, General Psychiatry (Psychotherapy) · University of Texas Medical Branch Hospitals · University of Texas Medical Branch, Department of Psychiatry, 301 University Boulevard, Galveston, TX 77555-0430 · 409-772-4833

Teresa A. Pigott · Mood & Anxiety Disorders (Depression, Psychopharmacology, Eating Disorders) · University of Texas Medical Branch Hospitals · University of Texas Medical Branch, Department of Psychiatry & Behavioral Sciences, Graves Building, Room 4.442, 301 University Boulevard, Galveston, TX 77555-0428 · 409-747-1322

James M. Russell · Psychopharmacology, Schizophrenia, General Psychiatry · University of Texas Medical Branch Hospitals · University of Texas Medical Branch, Department of Psychiatry, 301 University Boulevard, Galveston, TX 77555-0428 · 409-772-4467

Karen D. Wagner · Child & Adolescent Psychiatry · University of Texas Medical Branch Hospitals · University of Texas Medical Branch, Division of Child & Adolescent Psychiatry, 3.258 Graves Building, 301 University Boulevard, Galveston, TX 77550 · 409-772-9346

Cindy Lou Wigg · Child & Adolescent Psychiatry (Adolescent, Mood & Anxiety Disorders) · University of Texas Medical Branch Hospitals · University of Texas Medical Branch, Department of Psychiatry & Behavioral Sciences, Division of Child & Adolescent Psychiatry, 301 University Boulevard, Galveston, TX 77555-0425 · 409-772-2418

Houston

Roy N. Aruffo · Psychoanalysis (Child, Adolescent & Adult Psychoanalysis) · Houston-Galveston Psychoanalytic Institute · The Houston-Galveston Psychoanalytic Institute, 5300 San Jacinto, Suite 105, Houston, TX 77004-6886 · 713-523-9389

Mariame Aviles · General Psychiatry (Eating Disorders, Obsessive Compulsive Spectrum Disorders) · Methodist Hospital · Baylor College of Medicine, Department of Psychiatry, One Baylor Plaza, Houston, TX 77030 · 713-798-4974

Allan David Axelrad · General Psychiatry, Forensic Psychiatry · 7800 Fannin Street, Suite 400, Houston, TX 77054-2905 · 713-795-5999

Estella Beale · Psychoanalysis (Child Psychiatry) · Houston-Galveston Psychoanalytic Institute · The Houston-Galveston Psychoanalytic Institute, 5300 San Jacinto, Suite 160, Houston, TX 77004-6886 · 713-524-3193

Daniel Michael Brener · Psychoanalysis (General Psychiatry) · Methodist Hospital · 7515 South Main Street, Suite 890, Houston, TX 77030 · 713-796-1460

C. Glenn Cambor · Psychoanalysis (Family Therapy, Group Therapy, General Psychiatry) · 5300 San Jacinto, Suite 110, Houston, TX 77004-6886 · 713-522-3986

Dorothy A. Cato · General Psychiatry · 1215 Barkdull Road, Houston, TX 77006 · 713-522-3133

Ranjit C. Chacko · Geriatric Psychiatry, Mood & Anxiety Disorders (Psychopharmacology, Addiction Psychiatry, General Psychiatry, Neuropsychiatry, Schizophrenia) · Methodist Hospital · 6560 Fannin Street, Suite 832, Houston, TX 77030 · 713-798-4880

Betsy S. Comstock · Suicidology, Psychoanalysis (Adult) · Methodist Hospital · 6560 Fannin Street, Suite 832, Houston, TX 77030 · 713-798-4853

Jorge de la Torre · Psychoanalysis (Short-Term Psychotherapy, Treatment of Character Disorders, Treatment of Exercise Addiction, Mood & Anxiety Disorders) · 5300 San Jacinto, Suite 140, Houston, TX 77004-6886 · 713-528-2819

Herbert I. Dorfan · General Psychiatry (Consult-Liaison Psychiatry) · Methodist Hospital · 6560 Fannin Street, Suite 1616, Houston, TX 77030 · 713-795-0515

William Edwin Fann · Psychopharmacology · Methodist Hospital · Baylor College of Medicine, Department of Pharmacology, 1200 Moursund Avenue, Houston, TX 77030 · 713-798-7919

Francisco Fernandez · General Psychiatry (Consult-Liaison Psychiatry, Neuropsychiatry, Psychopharmacology) · St. Luke's Episcopal Hospital · St. Luke's Episcopal Hospital, 6720 Bertner Avenue, Room Y2439, Houston, TX 77030 · 713-791-2655

David A. Freedman · Psychoanalysis · Methodist Hospital · Baylor College of Medicine, 6560 Fannin Street, Suite 832, Houston, TX 77030 · 713-798-4877

Charles Milton Gaitz · Geriatric Psychiatry (General Psychiatry) · Bellaire Hospital · 6550 Mapleridge, Suite 208, Houston, TX 77081 · 713-512-1559

Bernard Michael Gerber · General Psychiatry · 7800 Fannin Street, Suite 400, Houston, TX 77054 · 713-795-5999

Robert M. Gilliland · Psychoanalysis · Houston-Galveston Psychoanalytic Institute · Houston-Galveston Psychoanalytic Institute, 5300 San Jacinto, Suite 120, Houston, TX 77004 · 713-524-8306

Franklin H. Gittess · Psychoanalysis (Couple and Family Psychotherapy, Eating Disorders) · West Oaks Hospital · 1020 Holcombe Boulevard, Suite 505, Houston, TX 77030 · 713-799-1074

Gregory D. Graham · Psychoanalysis · St. Luke's Episcopal Hospital, Methodist Hospital · 4550 Post Oak Place, Suite 320, Houston, TX 77027 · 713-622-5430

Robert W. Guynn · General Psychiatry · Harris County Psychiatric Center, Hermann Hospital · University of Texas-M. D. Anderson Cancer Center, Department of Psychiatry & Behavioral Sciences, 1300 Moursund Avenue, Room 206, Houston, TX 77030 · 713-792-5531

Sergio E. Henao · Child & Adolescent Psychiatry (Family Therapy) · Memorial Spring Shadows Glen · 902 Frostwood Drive, Suite 135, Houston, TX 77024 · 713-467-2800

David W. Krueger · Psychoanalysis, Eating Disorders (Forensic Psychiatry) · Memorial Spring Shadows Glen · 4550 Post Oak Place, Suite 320, Houston, TX 77027 · 713-622-5430

Mark Edwin Kunik · Geriatric Psychiatry · Methodist Hospital · VA Medical Center, Department of Psychiatry, 2002 Holcombe Boulevard, Houston, TX 77030 · 713-791-1414

James Welton Lomax II · Psychoanalysis (Mood & Anxiety Disorders) · Methodist Hospital · Baylor College of Medicine, One Baylor Plaza, Room 619D, Houston, TX 77030 · 713-798-4878

Jonathan S. Malev · Geriatric Psychiatry · Methodist Hospital · Methodist Hospital, Department of Psychiatry, 6624 Fannin Street, Suite 1530, Houston, TX 77030-2327 · 713-626-3070

Bruce D. Perry · Child & Adolescent Psychiatry (Trauma, Child Abuse and Neglect, Post-Traumatic Stress Disorder, Dissociative Disorders, Mood & Anxiety Disorders, Psychopharmacology, Violence) · Texas Children's Hospital · Texas Children's Hospital, Department of Psychiatry, 6621 Fannin Street, Houston, TX 77030-2399 · 713-770-3750

Richard B. Pesikoff · Child & Adolescent Psychiatry, Forensic Psychiatry · Methodist Hospital · 1020 Holcombe Boulevard, Suite 514, Houston, TX 77030-2213 713-795-5424

Michael L. Pipkin · General Psychiatry, Psychoanalysis (Consult-Liaison Psychiatry) · 7515 South Main Street, Suite 890, Houston, TX 77030 · 713-796-1470

Manuel C. Ramirez · Psychoanalysis (Adult Psychoanalysis, Family Therapy, Child Psychiatry) · The Houston-Galveston Psychoanalytic Institute Center, 5300 San Jacinto, Suite 120, Houston, TX 77004-6886 · 713-524-8306

Priscilla Ray · General Psychiatry, Mood & Anxiety Disorders (Consult-Liaison Psychiatry) · Methodist Hospital · St. Luke's Episcopal Hospital, 6560 Fannin Street, Suite 2120, Houston, TX 77030-2706 · 713-797-0112

James S. Robinson · Psychoanalysis (Adult & Child Psychoanalysis) · 320 Westcott, Suite 103, Houston, TX 77007 · 713-524-2959

Lawrence G. Root · Geriatric Psychiatry · 1315 Calhoun Avenue, Suite 1500, Houston, TX 77002-8232 · 713-757-0894

Mary Louise Scharold · Psychoanalysis · 3400 Bissonnet, Suite 170, Houston, TX 77005 · 713-661-3400

Joseph C. Schoolar · General Psychiatry · Methodist Hospital · Baylor College of Medicine, One Baylor Plaza, Room 311-D, P.O. Box 25302, Houston, TX 77265-5302 · 713-798-7940

Alana R. Spiwak · General Psychiatry, Psychoanalysis (Eating Disorders) · 1020 Holcombe Boulevard, Suite 505, Houston, TX 77030-2213 · 713-799-1074

Alan Craig Swann · Mood & Anxiety Disorders · Hermann Hospital · University of Texas Mental Sciences Institute, 1300 Moursund Avenue, Room 270, Houston, TX 77030 · 713-792-5190

Roy V. Varner · General Psychiatry, Geriatric Psychiatry · Harris County Psychiatric Center · 2800 South MacGregor Way, Houston, TX 77021 · 713-741-7805

Edwin C. Wood · Psychoanalysis · 5300 San Jacinto, Suite 150, Houston, TX 77004-6886 · 713-524-8566

Beth Koster Yudofsky · General Psychiatry, Psychopharmacology (Consult-Liaison Psychiatry) · Baylor College of Medicine, Department of Psychiatry & Behavioral Sciences, One Baylor Plaza, Houston, TX 77030 · 713-798-4882

Stuart C. Yudofsky · Psychopharmacology, Neuropsychiatry, Violence (Aggressive Disorders) · Methodist Hospital · Baylor College of Medicine, One Baylor Plaza, Room 115D, Houston, TX 77030 · 713-798-4945

Lewisville

Nishendu M. Vasavada · General Psychiatry · Lakeside Life Center, 560 West Main Street, Suite 101, Lewisville, TX 75057 · 214-221-1741

Lubbock

Brigitte Curtis · Child & Adolescent Psychiatry (Adult Psychiatry, Eating Disorders) · Lubbock Methodist Hospital, Methodist Children's Hospital, St. Mary of the Plains Hospital, Canyon Lakes Residential Treatment Center · 8008 Slide Road, Suite 35, Lubbock, TX 79424 · 806-794-9661

Elizabeth Davidson · Psychopharmacology (General Psychiatry, Mood & Anxiety Disorders, Schizophrenia) · St. Mary of the Plains Hospital, Charter Plains Behavioral Health System · 8008 Slide Road, Suite 35, Lubbock, TX 79424 · 806-794-9297

Elvira Lim · General Psychiatry (Adult) · 8008 Slide Road, Suite 35, Lubbock, TX 79424 · 806-794-9661

Elizabeth Bradbury Stuyt · Addiction Psychiatry (Dual Disorders) · St. Mary of the Plains Hospital · Texas Tech University Health Sciences Center, Department of Psychiatry, 3601 Fourth Street, Lubbock, TX 79430 · 806-743-2800

Richard L. Weddige · General Psychiatry (Community/Public Psychiatry) · St. Mary of the Plains Hospital, Charter Plains Behavioral Health System, Sunrise Canyon Hospital · Texas Tech University Health Sciences Center, Department of Psychiatry, 3601 Fourth Street, Lubbock, TX 79430 · 806-743-2800

Plano

Baer M. Ackerman · Child & Adolescent Psychiatry (General Psychiatry, Mental Retardation/Mental Health, Mood & Anxiety Disorders) · Seay Behavioral Center, Medical Center of Plano · 1700 Alma Drive, Suite 480, Plano, TX 75075 · 214-422-1814

Richardson

Colin A. Ross · Dissociative Disorders (Dissociative Identity Disorder) · Charter Behavioral Health System of Dallas (Plano) · 1701 Gateway, Suite 349, Richardson, TX 75080 · 214-918-9588; 214-618-3939

San Antonio

Michael P. Arambula · Forensic Psychiatry · 14800 US Highway 281 North, Suite 110, San Antonio, TX 78232 · 210-490-9850

Charles L. Bowden · Mood & Anxiety Disorders, Psychopharmacology (Bi-Polar Disorders) · University of Texas Health Science Center at San Antonio · University of Texas Health Science Center at San Antonio, Department of Psychiatry, 7703 Floyd Curl Drive, San Antonio, TX 78284-7792 · 210-567-5396

Stephen Kyle Brannan · Mood & Anxiety Disorders (Psychopharmacology) · Audie L. Murphy Memorial Veterans Hospital, University Hospital-South Texas Medical Center · University of Texas Health Science Center at San Antonio, Department of Psychiatry, 7703 Floyd Curl Drive, San Antonio, TX 78284-7792 210-567-5396

Claudio Cepeda · Child & Adolescent Psychiatry, Psychoanalysis (General Psychiatry) · Southwest Mental Health Center, University Hospital-South Texas Medical Center · Southwest Mental Health Center, 8535 Tom Slick Drive, San Antonio, TX 78229-3363 · 210-616-0300

John A. Chiles · Schizophrenia (Suicidal Behavior) · University Hospital-South Texas Medical Center · University of Texas Health Science Center at San Antonio, Department of Psychiatry, 7703 Floyd Curl Drive, San Antonio, TX 78284-7792 · 210-567-5470

Melvin Lee Cohen · Child & Adolescent Psychiatry · Laurel Ridge Psychiatric Hospital · 14800 US Highway 281 North, Suite 110, San Antonio, TX 78232 · 210-490-9850

Julia Cunarro · General Psychiatry (Psychotherapy, Psychopharmacology) · Charter Real Behavioral Health System, University Hospital-South Texas Medical Center · 8600 Wurzbach Road, Suite 1002, San Antonio, TX 78240 · 210-614-3338

Patricia Fox · Child & Adolescent Psychiatry · Southwest Mental Health Center Southwest Mental Health Center, 2939 Woodlawn Avenue, San Antonio, TX 78228 · 210-736-4273

Stephen David Gelfond · General Psychiatry (Consult-Liaison Psychiatry) · Santa Rosa Health Care · 2727 Babcock Road, Suite B, San Antonio, TX 78229 · 210-614-9334

Linda Louise Hawkins · General Psychiatry (Geriatric Psychiatry, Addiction Psychiatry, Schizophrenia, Psychopharmacology) · Laurel Ridge Psychiatric Hospital 15600 San Pedro Avenue, Suite 204, San Antonio, TX 78232 · 210-490-0995

Martin Stewart Hirsch · Child & Adolescent Psychiatry · Laurel Ridge Psychiatric Hospital · 11107 Wurzbach Road, Suite 701, San Antonio, TX 78230 · 210-691-2966

Patrick Holden · Child & Adolescent Psychiatry (Mental Retardation/Mental Health) · University Hospital-South Texas Medical Center, Southwest Mental Health Center · University of Texas Health Science Center at San Antonio, Department of Psychiatry, 7703 Floyd Curl Drive, San Antonio, TX 78284-7792 · 210-567-5450

John Houston · Mood & Anxiety Disorders (Affective Disorders) · University of Texas Health Science Center at San Antonio, Department of Psychiatry, 7703 Floyd Curl Drive, San Antonio, TX 78284-7792 · 210-567-5432

Don Duvall Howe · Child & Adolescent Psychiatry (Eating Disorders, Attention Deficit Disorders in Children, Teenage Depression) · Southwest Mental Health Center · 11107 Wurzbach Road, Suite 604, San Antonio, TX 78230 · 210-699-9511

John Barre King · General Psychiatry (Geriatric Psychiatry, Mood & Anxiety Disorders) · 7940 Floyd Curl Drive, Suite 770, San Antonio, TX 78229 · 210-615-8458

Carlos Macedo · Child & Adolescent Psychiatry · Southwest Mental Health Center · Southwest Mental Health Center, 8535 Tom Slick Drive, San Antonio, TX 78229-3363 · 210-616-0300

Thomas A. Martin III · Child & Adolescent Psychiatry · South Texas Behavioral Medicine, 14855 Blanco Road, Suite 220, San Antonio, TX 78216 · 210-493-5230

Diane L. Martinez · Psychoanalysis · University Hospital-South Texas Medical Center · 107 Oakmont Court, San Antonio, TX 78212 · 210-734-4466

Kenneth Lee Matthews · Child & Adolescent Psychiatry (General Psychiatry) · University Hospital-South Texas Medical Center, Southwest Mental Health Center · University of Texas Health Science Center at San Antonio, Department of Psychiatry, 7703 Floyd Curl Drive, San Antonio, TX 78284-7792 · 210-567-5430

William Matuzas · Mood & Anxiety Disorders (Psychopharmacology) · University Hospital-South Texas Medical Center · University of Texas Health Science Center at San Antonio, Department of Psychiatry, 7703 Floyd Curl Drive, San Antonio, TX 78284-7792 · 210-567-5494

Alexander Lewis Miller · Forensic Psychiatry, Mood & Anxiety Disorders, Psychopharmacology, Schizophrenia · University of Texas Health Science Center at San Antonio · University of Texas Health Science Center at San Antonio, Department of Psychiatry, 7703 Floyd Curl Drive, San Antonio, TX 78284-7792 · 210-567-5396

Rene Olvera · Child & Adolescent Psychiatry · Santa Rosa Health Care · Community Guidance Center, 2135 Babcock Road, San Antonio, TX 78229 · 210-614-7070

Steven Ray Pliszka · Child & Adolescent Psychiatry, Psychopharmacology (Attention Deficit Hyperactivity Disorder) · Child Guidance Center of San Antonio, 2135 Babcock Road, San Antonio, TX 78229 · 210-614-7070

Lewis Hilliard Richmond · Child & Adolescent Psychiatry (Adolescents, Group Psychotherapy) · Charter Real Behavioral Health System · 7410 John Smith Drive, Suite 213, San Antonio, TX 78229 · 210-614-3291

Graham Arthur Rogeness · Child & Adolescent Psychiatry · Southwest Mental Health Center · Southwest Mental Health Center, 8535 Tom Slick Drive, San Antonio, TX 78229-3363 · 210-616-0300

Donald R. Royall · Geriatric Psychiatry (Geriatric Medicine) · Audie L. Murphy Memorial Veterans Hospital Geriatric Research Education and Care Center · University of Texas Health Science Center at San Antonio, Department of Psychiatry, 7703 Floyd Curl Drive, San Antonio, TX 78284-7792 · 210-567-8545

Randall Van Sellers · Child & Adolescent Psychiatry (Mood & Anxiety Disorders, Psychopharmacology) · Laurel Ridge Psychiatric Hospital, Charter Real Behavioral Health System · Elm Creek Counseling, 11122 Wurzbach Road, Suite 201, San Antonio, TX 78230 · 210-694-0229

Jose Arturo Silva · Schizophrenia (Violence, Forensic Psychiatry) · Audie L. Murphy Memorial Veterans Hospital · South Texas Veterans Health Care Service-Audie L. Murphy Division, Psychiatry Service, 7400 Merton Minter Boulevard, Mail Code 116A, San Antonio, TX 78284 · 210-617-5300

Lawrence A. Stone · Child & Adolescent Psychiatry, Psychoanalysis · Laurel Ridge Psychiatric Hospital · Laurel Ridge Psychiatric Hospital, 17720 Corporate Woods Drive, San Antonio, TX 78259 · 210-491-9400

Alfredo T. Suescum · Psychoanalysis · 2600 McCullough Street, San Antonio, TX 78212 · 210-733-9091

Christopher Blaine Ticknor · General Psychiatry (Depression, Anxiety Disorders, Forensic Psychiatry, Psychopharmacology) · 7940 Floyd Curl Drive, Suite 770, San Antonio, TX 78229 · 210-692-7775

Kenneth Norman Vogtsberger · Addiction Psychiatry (General Psychiatry) · University Hospital-South Texas Medical Center · University of Texas Health Science Center at San Antonio, Department of Psychiatry, 7703 Floyd Curl Drive, San Antonio, TX 78284-7792 · 210-567-5480

Thomas Roderick Weiss · Addiction Psychiatry · Charter Real Behavioral Health System · 7940 Floyd Curl Drive, Suite 770, San Antonio, TX 78229 · 210-614-5561

Mary Elizabeth Zuelzer · General Psychiatry (Mood & Anxiety Disorders) · 14800 US Highway 281 North, Suite 110, San Antonio, TX 78232 · 210-490-9850

Temple

Greg D. Blaisdell · General Psychiatry (Clinical Psychopharmacology, Mood & Anxiety Disorders) · Scott & White Memorial Hospital & Clinic · Scott & White Memorial Hospital, 2401 South 31st Street, Temple, TX 76508-0001 · 817-724-2456

Jack D. Burke, Jr. · General Psychiatry · Scott & White Memorial Hospital · Scott & White Memorial Hospital, Department of Psychiatry, 2401 South 31st Street, Temple, TX 76508-0001 · 817-724-2111

William J. Meek · General Psychiatry · Scott & White Memorial Hospital · Scott & White Memorial Hospital, Department of Psychiatry, 2401 South 31st Street, Temple, TX 76508-0001 · 817-724-2585

Robert B. Nisbet · Addiction Psychiatry · Scott & White Memorial Hospital & Clinic · Scott & White Memorial Hospital, Department of Psychiatry, 2401 South 31st Street, Temple, TX 76508-0001 · 817-724-2111

Robert R. Rynearson · General Psychiatry · Scott & White Memorial Hospital · Scott & White Memorial Hospital, Department of Psychiatry, 2401 South 31st Street, Temple, TX 76508-0001 · 817-724-2111

Tyler

Joseph P. Arisco · General Psychiatry · Tyler Psychiatry, 3300 South Broadway, Suite 102, Tyler, TX 75701 · 903-593-1786

Waco

J. Clay Sawyer · General Psychiatry · Providence Health Center, Hillcrest Baptist Medical Center · 305 Londonderry Drive, Suite Six, Waco, TX 76712-7906 · 817-776-1421

Wichita Falls

Grant Hulse Wagner · Child & Adolescent Psychiatry · Wichita Falls State Hospital, 6515 Old Lake Road, P.O. Box 300, Wichita Falls, TX 76307 · 817-692-1220 x439

PULMONARY & CRITICAL CARE MEDICINE

Amarillo

T. Bruce Baker · General Pulmonary & Critical Care Medicine (Asthma) · High Plains Baptist Hospital, St. Anthony's Hospital, Amarillo Hospital District-Northwest Texas Hospital · Amarillo Diagnostic Clinic, 6700 West Ninth Street, Amarillo, TX 79106-1701 · 806-358-3171

H. David Bruton · General Pulmonary & Critical Care Medicine · Amarillo Diagnostic Clinic, 6700 West Ninth Street, Amarillo, TX 79106-1701 · 806-358-3171

Gary R. Polk · General Pulmonary & Critical Care Medicine · Amarillo Diagnostic Clinic, 6700 West Ninth Street, Amarillo, TX 79106 · 806-358-3171

Gary Lee Rose · General Pulmonary & Critical Care Medicine · Amarillo Diagnostic Clinic, 6700 West Ninth Street, Amarillo, TX 79106-1701 · 806-358-3171

Austin

Mark C. Clark · (Asbestos-Related Diseases, Bronchology) · Seton Medical Center, St. David's Healthcare Center, Brackenridge Hospital · Pulmonary & Critical Care Consultants of Austin, 1305 West 34th Street, Suite 400, Austin, TX 78705 512-459-6599

William Joel Deaton · General Pulmonary & Critical Care Medicine · Brackenridge Hospital, Seton Medical Center, St. David's Healthcare Center · Pulmonary & Critical Care Consultants of Austin, 1305 West 34th Street, Suite 400, Austin, TX 78705 · 512-459-6599

Frank G. Mazza · General Pulmonary & Critical Care Medicine (Intensive Care Medicine, Diseases of the Chest, Sleep Disorders Medicine) · Seton Medical Center, Seton Northwest Hospital, St. David's Healthcare Center, Brackenridge Hospital · Pulmonary & Critical Care Consultants of Austin, 1305 West 34th Street, Suite 400, Austin, TX 78705 · 512-459-6599

Michael Shapiro · General Pulmonary & Critical Care Medicine · Brackenridge Hospital · Pulmonary & Critical Care Consultants of Austin, 1305 West 34th Street, Suite 400, Austin, TX 78705 · 512-459-6599

Ofelia Utset · General Pulmonary & Critical Care Medicine · Pulmonary & Critical Care Consultants of Austin, 1305 West 34th Street, Suite 400, Austin, TX 78705 · 512-459-6599

Beaumont

Andrew J. Aldrich · General Pulmonary & Critical Care Medicine · Southeast Texas Pulmonary Associates, 810 Hospital Drive, Suite 240, Beaumont, TX 77701-4633 · 409-835-3770

Nathaniel J. Alford, Jr. · General Pulmonary & Critical Care Medicine · Southeast Texas Pulmonary Associates, 810 Hospital Drive, Suite 240, Beaumont, TX 77701-4633 · 409-835-3770

Harold Z. Bencowitz · General Pulmonary & Critical Care Medicine · Southeast Texas Pulmonary Associates, 810 Hospital Drive, Suite 240, Beaumont, TX 77701-4633 · 409-835-3770

Corpus Christi

William W. Burgin · General Pulmonary & Critical Care Medicine · 2601 Hospital Boulevard, Suite 117, Corpus Christi, TX 78405 · 512-884-8209

Mark W. Geneser · General Pulmonary & Critical Care Medicine · Spohn Hospital, Spohn Hospital South, Memorial Medical Center, Doctors Regional Medical Center, Bay Area Medical Center · 613 Elizabeth Street, Suite 406, Corpus Christi, TX 78404 · 512-883-5900

David A. Miller · General Pulmonary & Critical Care Medicine (AIDS, Respiratory Infections) · Spohn Hospital, Doctors Regional Medical Center · Respiratory Associates, 1521 South Staples Street, Suite 503, Corpus Christi, TX 78404 · 512-883-5419

Robert M. C. Wang · General Pulmonary & Critical Care Medicine · 2601 Hospital Boulevard, Suite 105, Corpus Christi, TX 78405 · 512-884-7515

Dallas

Robert D. Black · General Pulmonary & Critical Care Medicine (Acute Respiratory Distress Syndrome, Pulmonary Diseases in Immunocompromised Hosts) · Baylor University Medical Center · Baylor University Medical Center, Division of Pulmonary Medicine, 3500 Gaston Avenue, Dallas, TX 75246-2017 · 214-820-2508

Charles B. Shuey, Jr. · General Pulmonary & Critical Care Medicine (Transplantation) · Baylor University Medical Center · Baylor University Medical Center, 3500 Gaston Avenue, Dallas, TX 75246-2017 · 214-820-2508

Jonathan Charles Weissler · General Pulmonary & Critical Care Medicine (Pulmonary Fibrosis, Immunologic Lung Disease, Critical Care Medicine) · Parkland Memorial Hospital, Zale Lipshy University Hospital · University of Texas-Southwestern Medical Center at Dallas, 5323 Harry Hines Boulevard, Dallas, TX 75235-9034 · 214-648-2534

El Paso

Arthur A. Cohen · General Pulmonary & Critical Care Medicine (Asthma, Bronchology) · Sierra Medical Center, Providence Memorial Hospital, Columbia Medical Center-West · 1733 Curie Drive, Suite 309, El Paso, TX 79902 · 915-533-9388

Gonzalo A. Diaz · General Pulmonary & Critical Care Medicine · El Paso Pulmonary Association, 201 East Blacker Avenue, El Paso, TX 79902 · 915-532-2477

Raul Rivera · General Pulmonary & Critical Care Medicine · Paisalo Medical Plaza, 5301 Alameda Avenue, El Paso, TX 79905 · 915-778-9811

Genaro Vazquez · (Acute Respiratory Failure, Ventilator Management, Bronchology) · Sierra Medical Center, Providence Memorial Hospital, Columbia Medical Center-West, Columbia Medical Center-East, Rio Vista Rehabilitation Hospital · El Paso Pulmonary Association, 201 East Blacker Avenue, El Paso, TX 79902 · 915-532-2477

Fort Worth

Billy M. Eden · General Pulmonary & Critical Care Medicine · Pulmonary Associates, 1201 Fairmount Avenue, Fort Worth, TX 76104 · 817-335-5288

Raleigh R. Gleason III · General Pulmonary & Critical Care Medicine · Harris Methodist-Fort Worth · Pulmonary Associates, 1201 Fairmount Avenue, Fort Worth, TX 76104 · 817-335-5288

John T. Pender, Jr. · General Pulmonary & Critical Care Medicine · Pulmonary Associates, 1201 Fairmount Avenue, Fort Worth, TX 76104 · 817-335-5288

Galveston

Samuel T. Kuna · General Pulmonary & Critical Care Medicine · University of Texas Medical Branch, Department of Internal Medicine, Pulmonary Division, 301 University Boulevard, Galveston, TX 77555-0561 · 409-772-2436

Houston

Kim Bloom · General Pulmonary & Critical Care Medicine · Methodist Hospital, Vencor Hospital-Houston, St. Luke's Episcopal Hospital · Respiratory Consultants of Houston, 6550 Fannin Street, Suite 2403, Houston, TX 77030 · 713-790-6250

Steven Dunning Brown · General Pulmonary & Critical Care Medicine · Lyndon B. Johnson General Hospital, Hermann Hospital · University of Texas Medical School at Houston, 6431 Fannin Street, Room 1.274, Houston, TX 77030 · 713-792-5110

William Eschenbacher · General Pulmonary & Critical Care Medicine (Asthma, Environmental Lung Disease) · Methodist Hospital, St. Luke's Episcopal Hospital · Baylor College of Medicine, Department of Pulmonary Medicine, Smith Tower, Suite 1236, 6550 Fannin Street, Houston, TX 77030 · 713-790-2076

Salah Y. Ghobrial · General Pulmonary & Critical Care Medicine · 17200 Red Oak Drive, Suite 106, Houston, TX 77090 · 713-440-1716

Guillermo Gutierrez · General Pulmonary & Critical Care Medicine (Organ Failure) · Hermann Hospital · University of Texas Medical School at Houston, 6431 Fannin Street, Room 1.274, Houston, TX 77030 · 713-792-5110

Robert Francis Lodato · General Pulmonary & Critical Care Medicine (Respiratory Failure, Septic Shock) · Hermann Hospital · University of Texas Medical School at Houston, 6431 Fannin Street, Room 1.274, Houston, TX 77030 · 713-792-5110 x1110

Rodolfo C. Morice · General Pulmonary & Critical Care Medicine (Chemoprevention, Lung Cancer, Bronchology, Brachytherapy, Stents and Lasers) · University of Texas-M. D. Anderson Cancer Center · University of Texas-M. D. Anderson Cancer Center, 1515 Holcombe Boulevard, Box 76, Houston, TX 77030-4009 713-792-4599

Robert F. Oskenholt · General Pulmonary & Critical Care Medicine · University of Texas Medical School at Houston, Division of Pulmonary & Critical Care Medicine, 6431 Fannin Street, Room 1.274, Houston, TX 77030 · 713-792-5110

Joseph R. Rodarte · General Pulmonary & Critical Care Medicine (Asthma, Chronic Obstructive Pulmonary Disease [COPD]) · Methodist Hospital · Baylor College of Medicine, Department of Pulmonary Medicine, 6550 Fannin Street, Suite 1225, Houston, TX 77030 · 713-790-6218

Edward William Stool · AIDS · 1200 Binz Street, Suite 1260, Houston, TX 77004 713-522-8809

David E. Taylor · General Pulmonary & Critical Care Medicine · Hermann Hospital, Lyndon B. Johnson General Hospital · University of Texas Medical School at Houston, Division of Pulmonary & Critical Care Medicine, 6431 Fannin Street, Room 1.274, Houston, TX 77030 · 713-792-5110

Kenneth L. Toppell · General Pulmonary & Critical Care Medicine (Asthma, Bronchology, Lung Infections) · Park Plaza Hospital, Bellaire Hospital, Hermann Hospital · 1213 Hermann Drive, Suite 570, Houston, TX 77004 · 713-524-3900

Lubbock

Mark William Johnson · General Pulmonary & Critical Care Medicine (Adult Respiratory Distress Syndrome, Sleep-Disordered Breathing) · St. Mary of the Plains Hospital, Lubbock Methodist Hospital · Pulmonary Associates, 3621 Twenty-Second Street, Suite 400, Lubbock, TX 79410-1309 · 806-791-8484

Kenneth Terrell · General Pulmonary & Critical Care Medicine · Pulmonary Associates, 3621 Twenty-Second Street, Suite 400, Lubbock, TX 79410-1309 · 806-791-8484

Pasadena

David Alan Stein · General Pulmonary & Critical Care Medicine · Bayshore Medical Center, Southmore Medical Center · 4003 Woodlawn Street, Pasadena, TX 77504 · 713-941-0088

San Antonio

Charles P. Andrews · General Pulmonary & Critical Care Medicine (Obstructive Lung Disease) · Southwest Texas Methodist Hospital, San Antonio Community Hospital · Pulmonary Physicians, 4410 Medical Drive, Suite 440, San Antonio, TX 78229 · 210-692-9400

Antonio Anzueto · General Pulmonary & Critical Care Medicine (Lung Transplantation, Neuromuscular Disease) · Audie L. Murphy Memorial Veterans Hospital, University Hospital-South Texas Medical Center · Audie L. Murphy Memorial Veterans Hospital, 7400 Merton Minter Boulevard, Mail Code 111E, San Antonio, TX 78284-5700 · 210-617-5256

Charles Leslie Bryan · Lung Infections (Lung Transplantation, Lung Fibrosis) · Audie L. Murphy Memorial Veterans Hospital, University Hospital-South Texas Medical Center, University of Texas Health Science Center · Audie L. Murphy Memorial Veterans Hospital, Division of Pulmonary Diseases, 7400 Merton Minter Boulevard, Mail Code 111E, San Antonio, TX 78284-5700 · 210-617-5256

Charles Alman Duncan · General Pulmonary & Critical Care Medicine · Audie L. Murphy Memorial Veterans Hospital · University of Texas Health Science Center at San Antonio, Division of Pulmonary Diseases and Critical Care Medicine, 7703 Floyd Curl Drive, San Antonio, TX 78284-7885 · 210-567-4820

Pedro G. Fornos · (General Internal Medicine, Pulmonary Medicine) · Baptist Medical Center · Madison Square Medical Building, Suite 201, 311 Camden Street, San Antonio, TX 78215 · 210-227-7293

Peter S. Fornos · General Pulmonary & Critical Care Medicine · Baptist Medical Center · Madison Square Medical Building, Suite 201, 311 Camden Street, San Antonio, TX 78215 · 210-227-7293

Junji Henry Higuchi · General Pulmonary & Critical Care Medicine · 1303 McCullough Avenue, Suite 343, San Antonio, TX 78212 · 210-225-2341

Stephen George Jenkinson · General Pulmonary & Critical Care Medicine (Critical Care) · Audie L. Murphy Memorial Veterans Hospital · University of Texas Health Science Center at San Antonio, Division of Pulmonary Diseases and Critical Care Medicine, 7703 Floyd Curl Drive, San Antonio, TX 78284-7885 · 210-617-5256

Carlos R. Orozco · General Pulmonary & Critical Care Medicine · 343 West Houston Street, Suite 706, San Antonio, TX 78205 · 210-227-0193

Jay I. Peters · General Pulmonary & Critical Care Medicine (Asthma, Lung Transplantation) · Audie L. Murphy Memorial Veterans Hospital · Audie L. Murphy Memorial Veterans Hospital, Division of Pulmonary Diseases, 7400 Merton Minter Boulevard, Mail Code 111E, San Antonio, TX 78284-5700 · 210-617-5256

Temple

Francisco Perez-Guerra · General Pulmonary & Critical Care Medicine · Scott & White Memorial Hospital & Clinic · Scott & White Memorial Hospital, Department of Pulmonary Medicine, 2401 South 31st Street, Temple, TX 76508-0001 · 817-724-2554

Texarkana

Lowell E. Vereen · General Pulmonary & Critical Care Medicine · 1001 Main Street, Suite 110, Texarkana, TX 75501 · 903-792-3660

Tomball

Marque A. Hunter · General Pulmonary & Critical Care Medicine · 425 Holderrieth Street, Suite 109, Tomball, TX 77375 · 713-357-0111

Tyler

George David Gass · General Pulmonary & Critical Care Medicine · Pulmonary Specialists, 619 South Fleishel Avenue, Suite 301, Tyler, TX 75701 · 903-592-6907

William Meshew Girard · General Pulmonary & Critical Care Medicine · University of Texas Health Center-Tyler · University of Texas Health Center-Tyler, US Highway 271 and State Highway 155, P.O. Box 2003, Tyler, TX 75710-2003 903-877-7373

David E. Griffith · General Pulmonary & Critical Care Medicine (Tuberculosis and Mycobacterial Infections, Lung Infections) · University of Texas Health Center-Tyler, Department of Pulmonary Medicine, US Highway 271 and State Highway 155, P.O. Box 2003, Tyler, TX 75710-2003 · 903-877-7267

Steven Idell · General Pulmonary & Critical Care Medicine · University of Texas Health Center-Tyler · University of Texas Health Center-Tyler, US Highway 271 and State Highway 155, P.O. Box 2003, Tyler, TX 75710-2003 · 903-877-7373

J. David Johnson · General Pulmonary & Critical Care Medicine · East Texas Medical Center · Pulmonary Specialists, 619 South Fleishel Avenue, Suite 301, Tyler, TX 75701 · 903-592-6901

Richard S. Kronenberg · General Pulmonary & Critical Care Medicine (Occupational Lung Disease) · University of Texas Health Center-Tyler · University of Texas Health Center-Tyler, US Highway 271 and State Highway 155, P.O. Box 2003, Tyler, TX 75710-2003 · 903-877-7265

Brooke Nicotra · General Pulmonary & Critical Care Medicine · University of Texas Health Center-Tyler · University of Texas Health Center-Tyler, US Highway 271 and State Highway 155, P.O. Box 2003, Tyler, TX 75710-2003 · 903-877-7916

Waco

Rodney C. Richie · General Pulmonary & Critical Care Medicine · Hillcrest Baptist Medical Center, Providence Health Center · Waco Lung Associates, 2911 Herring Avenue, Suite 212, Waco, TX 76708 · 817-755-4444

Philip A. Sanger · General Pulmonary & Critical Care Medicine · Waco Lung Associates, 2911 Herring Avenue, Suite 212, Waco, TX 76708 · 817-755-4444

Robert R. Springer · General Pulmonary & Critical Care Medicine · Hillcrest Baptist Medical Center · Waco Lung Associates, 2911 Herring Avenue, Suite 212, Waco, TX 76708 · 817-755-4444

RADIATION ONCOLOGY

Amarillo

Joseph C. Arko II · General Radiation Oncology · Don & Sybil Harrington Cancer Center, 1500 Wallace Boulevard, Amarillo, TX 79106 · 806-359-4673

Donald G. Pratt · General Radiation Oncology (Lung Cancer, Breast Cancer, Prostate Cancer) · St. Anthony's Hospital, Amarillo Hospital District-Northwest Texas Hospital · Don & Sybil Harrington Cancer Center, 1500 Wallace Boulevard, Amarillo, TX 79106-1745 · 806-354-5880

Arlington

John R. Torrisi · General Radiation Oncology · Columbia Medical Center of Arlington · Texas Cancer Center, 515 West Mayfield Road, Suite 101, Arlington, TX 76017 · 817-467-6092

Austin

George Rhamy Brown · General Radiation Oncology (Brain Cancer, Pediatric Radiation Oncology, Breast Cancer) · St. David's Healthcare Center, Seton Medical Center, Brackenridge Hospital · Texas Radiation Oncology Group, 1305 West 34th Street, Suite 210, Austin, TX 78705 · 512-451-5593

Shannon Douglas Cox · General Radiation Oncology · Texas Radiation Oncology Group, 1305 West 34th Street, Suite 210, Austin, TX 78705 · 512-451-5593

Beaumont

Joseph S. Kong · General Radiation Oncology · University of Texas-M. D. Anderson Cancer Center (Houston) · Julie & Ben Rogers Cancer Institute, 3555 Stagg Drive, Beaumont, TX 77701 · 409-654-5922

Henry O. Williams · General Radiation Oncology · St. Elizabeth Hospital · Cancer Treatment Center, 690 North 14th Street, Beaumont, TX 77702 · 409-899-7181

Corpus Christi

Lalitha Madhav Janaki · General Radiation Oncology (Brachytherapy, Lung Cancer, Brain Cancer, Head & Neck Cancer) · Spohn Hospital, Bay Area Medical Center, Doctors Regional Medical Center, Memorial Medical Center, Driscoll Children's Hospital · Cancer Specialists of South Texas, Corpus Christi Cancer Center, 1625 Rodd Field Road, Corpus Christi, TX 78412 · 512-993-3456

Dallas

Jerry Lee Barker · General Radiation Oncology (Breast Cancer, Lung Cancer, Genito-Urinary Cancer) · Presbyterian Hospital of Dallas · Presbyterian Hospital of Dallas, Radiology Oncology Center, 8200 Walnut Hill Lane, Dallas, TX 75231 214-345-7394

Dan Patrick Garwood · Breast Cancer (Brain Cancer) · Harold C. Simmons Comprehensive Cancer Center · University of Texas-Southwestern Medical Center at Dallas, Department of Radiation Oncology, 5323 Harry Hines Boulevard, Dallas, TX 75235-9122 · 214-648-2296

Eli Glatstein · Lymphomas, Sarcomas, Lung Cancer (Sensitizers, Hodgkin's Disease, Protectors, Photodynamic Therapy) · Harold C. Simmons Comprehensive Cancer Center · University of Texas-Southwestern Medical Center at Dallas, Department of Radiation Oncology, 5323 Harry Hines Boulevard, Dallas, TX 75235-8590 · 214-648-7689

Louis Lee Munoz · General Radiation Oncology (Pediatric Radiation Oncology, Brain Cancer) · St. Paul Medical Center, Medical City Dallas Hospital · St. Paul Medical Center, 5909 Harry Hines Boulevard, Dallas, TX 75235-6209 · 214-879-2696; 214-661-7031

David A. Pistenmaa · General Radiation Oncology, Genito-Urinary Cancer · Medical City Dallas Hospital, The University of Texas-Southwestern Medical Center, Parkland Memorial Hospital, St. Paul Medical Center, Zale Lipshy University Hospital, The Aston Ambulatory Care Center · Medical City Dallas Hospital, Department of Radiation Oncology, Building D, Suite 110, 7777 Forest Lane, Dallas, TX 75230 · 214-788-5662

David Rosenthal · General Radiation Oncology (Head & Neck, Lung, and Gynecologic Cancer) · University of Texas-Southwestern Medical Center at Dallas, 5323 Harry Hines Boulevard, Dallas, TX 75235 · 214-648-2296

Robert Pickett Scruggs III · General Radiation Oncology (Breast Cancer, Head & Neck Cancer, Lymphomas) · Baylor University Medical Center · Charles A. Sammons Cancer Center, Department of Radiation Oncology, 3535 Worth Street, Dallas, TX 75246 · 214-820-3231

Neil Nathan Senzer · General Radiation Oncology (Brachytherapy, Head & Neck Cancer) · Baylor University Medical Center · Charles A. Sammons Cancer Center, Department of Radiation Oncology, 3535 Worth Street, Dallas, TX 75246 · 214-820-3231

Alan A. Slomowitz · General Radiation Oncology (Prostate Cancer, Breast Cancer, Lung Cancer) · Methodist Medical Center · Methodist Medical Center, 1441 North Beckley Avenue, Dallas, TX 75203 · 214-947-1770

El Paso

Ira Andrew Horowitz · (Genito-Urinary Cancer, Lung Cancer, Breast Cancer) · Providence Memorial Hospital, Sierra Medical Center · El Paso Cancer Treatment Center, 1901 Grandview Avenue, El Paso, TX 79902 · 915-545-1600

Fort Worth

Karen Lanette Nielson · Lymphomas, Gynecologic Cancer, Pediatric Radiation Oncology · Harris Methodist-Fort Worth, All Saints Episcopal Hospital-Fort Worth, Plaza Medical Center · M. D. Anderson Moncrief Cancer Center, 1450 Eighth Avenue, Fort Worth, TX 76104 · 817-923-1717

Janice Kelly Tomberlin · Breast Cancer, Head & Neck Cancer · All Saints Episcopal Hospital-Fort Worth, Harris Methodist-Fort Worth, Plaza Medical Center · 1450 Eighth Avenue, Fort Worth, TX 76104 · 817-923-7393

Houston

K. Kian Ang · Head & Neck Cancer · University of Texas-M. D. Anderson Cancer Center · University of Texas-M. D. Anderson Cancer Center, 1515 Holcombe Boulevard, Box 97, Houston, TX 77030-4095 · 713-792-3400

David C. Blackburn · General Radiation Oncology (Genito-Urinary Cancer, Head & Neck Cancer) · Park Plaza Hospital · Park Plaza Hospital, Department of Radiation Oncology, 1313 Hermann Drive, Houston, TX 77004 · 713-527-5043

E. Brian Butler · General Radiation Oncology · Methodist Hospital · Methodist Hospital, 6565 Fannin Street, Suite DB1-37, Houston, TX 77030-2730 · 713-790-2091

James D. Cox · Lung Cancer (Lymphomas, Head & Neck Cancer) · University of Texas-M. D. Anderson Cancer Center · University of Texas-M. D. Anderson Cancer Center, 1515 Holcombe Boulevard, Box 97, Houston, TX 77030-4095 · 713-792-3411

Luis Delclos · Gynecologic Cancer, Brachytherapy · University of Texas-M. D. Anderson Cancer Center · University of Texas-M. D. Anderson Cancer Center, 1515 Holcombe Boulevard, Box 97, Houston, TX 77030-4095 · 713-792-3404

Patricia J. Eifel · Gynecologic Cancer, Pediatric Radiation Oncology · University of Texas-M. D. Anderson Cancer Center · University of Texas-M. D. Anderson Cancer Center, 1515 Holcombe Boulevard, Box 97, Houston, TX 77030-4095 · 713-792-3400

Adam Seth Garden · Head & Neck Cancer · University of Texas-M. D. Anderson Cancer Center · University of Texas-M. D. Anderson Cancer Center, 1515 Holcombe Boulevard, Box 97, Houston, TX 77030-4009 · 713-792-3400

Arthur Donald Hamberger · Breast Cancer (Head & Neck Cancer, Lymphomas, Gynecologic Cancer) · Memorial Hospital-Northwest, Memorial Hospital-Southwest, Memorial Hospital-Memorial City · Memorial Hospital-Northwest, 1631 North Loop, West, Suite 150, Houston, TX 77008 · 713-867-4668

Nora A. Janjan · (Gastroenterologic Cancer, Pain Management, Brachytherapy) · University of Texas-M. D. Anderson Cancer Center · University of Texas-M. D. Anderson Cancer Center, Department of Radiation Oncology, 1515 Holcombe Boulevard, Box 97, Houston, TX 77030-4009 · 713-792-3432

Ritsuko Komaki · Lung Cancer (Thymoma, Esophageal Carcinoma, Brachytherapy) · University of Texas-M. D. Anderson Cancer Center · University of Texas-M. D. Anderson Cancer Center, 1515 Holcombe Boulevard, Box 97, Houston, TX 77030-4095 · 713-792-3420

Gary R. Leach · Genito-Urinary Cancer (Prostate Cancer) · Memorial Hospital-Northwest · Memorial Hospital-Northwest, 1631 North Loop, West, Suite 150, Houston, TX 77008-1529 · 713-867-4668

Moshe H. Maor · Brain Cancer (Central Nervous System) · University of Texas-M. D. Anderson Cancer Center · University of Texas-M. D. Anderson Cancer Center, 1515 Holcombe Boulevard, Box 97, Houston, TX 77030-4009 · 713-792-3400

Marsha Diane McNeese · Breast Cancer (Breast-Preserving Therapy) · University of Texas-M. D. Anderson Cancer Center · University of Texas-M. D. Anderson Cancer Center, 1515 Holcombe Boulevard, Box 97, Houston, TX 77030-4095 · 713-792-3400

Howard Christopher Moench · General Radiation Oncology · Park Plaza Hospital · Park Plaza Hospital, Department of Radiation Oncology, 1313 Hermann Drive, Houston, TX 77004 · 713-527-5043

William H. Morrison · Head & Neck Cancer (Skin Cancer) · University of Texas-M. D. Anderson Cancer Center · University of Texas-M. D. Anderson Cancer Center, 1515 Holcombe Boulevard, Box 97, Houston, TX 77030-4009 · 713-792-3436

Alan Pollack · Genito-Urinary Cancer (Prostate Cancer, Bladder Cancer) · University of Texas-M. D. Anderson Cancer Center · University of Texas-M. D. Anderson Cancer Center, 1515 Holcombe Boulevard, Box 97, Houston, TX 77030-4009 · 713-792-0781

Eric Alan Strom · Breast Cancer · University of Texas-M. D. Anderson Cancer Center · University of Texas-M. D. Anderson Cancer Center, 1515 Holcombe Boulevard, Box 97, Houston, TX 77030-4009 · 713-792-3400

Shiao Y. Woo · Pediatric Radiation Oncology (Tumors of the Central Nervous System, Conformal Radiotherapy, Brain Cancer) · Methodist Hospital · Methodist Hospital, 6565 Fannin Street, Suite DB1-37, Houston, TX 77030-2730 · 713-790-2091

Gunar K. Zagars · Genito-Urinary Cancer, Sarcomas · University of Texas-M. D. Anderson Cancer Center · University of Texas-M. D. Anderson Cancer Center, Department of Radiotherapy, 1515 Holcombe Boulevard, Box 97, Houston, TX 77030-4095 · 713-792-3400

Irving

Gregory Allen Echt · General Radiation Oncology · Irving Cancer Center · Irving Cancer Center, 2001 North MacArthur Boulevard, Suite 120, Irving, TX 75061 · 214-579-4300

Lackland Air Force Base

Bradley Robert Prestidge · General Radiation Oncology · Wilford Hall Medical Center · Wilford Hall Medical Center, Department of Radiation Oncology, 2200 Bergquist Drive, Lackland Air Force Base, TX 78236-5300 · 210-670-7771

Lubbock

Paul Anderson · (Gynecologic Cancer, Genito-Urinary Cancer, Lung Cancer) · University Medical Center, St. Mary of the Plains Hospital · Southwest Cancer Center, 602 Indiana Avenue, Lubbock, TX 79415 · 806-743-1900; 806-796-4700

Jui-Lien Lillian Chou · General Radiation Oncology · University Medical Center Southwest Cancer Center, 602 Indiana Avenue, Lubbock, TX 79415 · 806-743-1900

Midland

James A. Corwin · General Radiation Oncology (Genito-Urinary Cancer, Breast Cancer) · Memorial Hospital & Medical Center · Texas Oncology at the Allison Cancer Center, 301 North N Street, Midland, TX 79701 · 915-685-1559

Plano

Jeffrey Evan Greenberg · General Radiation Oncology (Breast Cancer, Colorectal Cancer, Lymphomas) · Medical Center of Plano · North Texas Cancer Center, 3705 West 15th Street, Plano, TX 75075 · 214-867-3577

San Antonio

Ardow Richard Ameduri · General Radiation Oncology (Pediatric, Adult) · 4450 Medical Drive, San Antonio, TX 78229 · 210-616-5692

Keith Eugene Eyre · General Radiation Oncology · Southwest Texas Methodist Hospital, St. Luke's Baptist Hospital, San Antonio Community Hospital, Santa Rosa Northwest Hospital, Metropolitan Hospital · The Cancer Therapy & Research Center, 4450 Medical Drive, San Antonio, TX 78229 · 210-616-5500

John Edward Freeman · Genito-Urinary Cancer (Prostate Cancer, Pediatric) · St. Luke's Baptist Hospital, Southwest Texas Methodist Hospital · The Cancer Therapy & Research Center, 4450 Medical Drive, San Antonio, TX 78229 · 210-616-5500

Oscar J. Garcia · General Radiation Oncology (Lung Cancer, Gynecologic Cancer) · Grossman Cancer Center, 7979 Wurzbach Boulevard, San Antonio, TX 78229 · 210-616-5648

Terence Spencer Herman · General Radiation Oncology (Pediatric, Combined Modality Therapy for Solid Tumors, Prostate Cancer, Breast Cancer, Sarcomas) · University Health System, Audie L. Murphy Memorial Veterans Hospital · University of Texas Health Science Center at San Antonio, Department of Radiology, 7703 Floyd Curl Drive, San Antonio, TX 78284-7800 · 210-616-5648

J. Carlos Hernandez · General Radiation Oncology (Eye Tumors, Treatment of Cancer While Preserving Organ & Function, Gynecologic Tumors, Pediatric Tumors, Pediatric Radiation Oncology, Brachytherapy) · University of Texas Health Science Center at San Antonio · University of Texas Health Science Center at San Antonio, Department of Radiology, 7703 Floyd Curl Drive, San Antonio, TX 78284-7800 · 210-616-5648

Joaquin Gomez Mira · Lung Cancer · Southwest Texas Methodist Hospital, Nix Health Care System · The Cancer Therapy & Research Center, 4450 Medical Drive, San Antonio, TX 78229 · 210-616-5500

Gary Wayne West · General Radiation Oncology (Breast Cancer, Prostate Cancer) Baptist Medical Center, San Antonio Community Hospital, St. Luke's Baptist Hospital, Santa Rosa Northwest Hospital · 8038 Wurzbach Road, Suite 270, San Antonio, TX 78229 · 210-616-0866

Temple

Gregory P. Swanson · General Radiation Oncology (Prostate Cancer, Breast Cancer) · Scott & White Memorial Hospital & Clinic · Scott & White Memorial Hospital, Department of Radiation Oncology, 2401 South 31st Street, Temple, TX 76508-0001 · 817-724-2417

Waco

Glenn M. Haluska · General Radiation Oncology · Hillcrest Baptist Medical Center · Fentress Cancer Center, 3000 Herring Avenue, Waco, TX 76708 · 817-756-8675

RADIOLOGY

Amarillo

John L. Andrew II · (Neuroradiology) · 1901 Medipark Road, Suite 2058, Amarillo, TX 79106 · 806-355-3352

Ronald Dennis Dillee · General Radiology · Diagnostic Imaging, 1501 Coulter Drive, Amarillo, TX 79175 · 806-354-1700

James A. Guest · General Radiology · Radiological Associates, 7203B I-40 West, Amarillo, TX 79106 · 806-355-9473

Robert L. Pinkston, Jr. · General Radiology · St. Anthony's Hospital · Radiological Associates, 7203B I-40 West, Amarillo, TX 79106 · 806-355-9473

Austin

Thomas B. Fletcher · (Interventional Radiology, Breast) · Seton Medical Center, South Austin Medical Center, St. David's Healthcare Center, Brackenridge Hospital · Austin Radiological Association, 601 West Courtyard Street, Number Five, P.O. Box 4099, Austin, TX 78730 · 512-795-5100

Charles Vincent Wiseman · (Body Imaging, Ultrasound) · Seton Medical Center Austin Radiological Association, 1301 West 38th Street, Suite 113, Austin, TX 78705 · 512-454-5641

Beaumont

Giles J. Andrews · General Radiology · Radiology Associates, 3560 Delaware Street, Suite 207, Beaumont, TX 77706 · 409-899-3682

William K. Cook · General Radiology (Interventional Radiology, Nuclear Medicine, Nuclear Cardiology) · St. Elizabeth Hospital · Radiology Associates, 3560 Delaware Street, Suite 207, Beaumont, TX 77706 · 409-899-3682

James King · General Radiology · Radiology Associates, 2955 Harrison Street, Suite 104, Beaumont, TX 77702-1155 · 409-899-3682

Robert G. McConnell · General Radiology · Radiology Associates, 3560 Delaware Street, Suite 207, Beaumont, TX 77706 · 409-899-3682

Paul W. McCormick · General Radiology · Radiology Associates, 3560 Delaware Street, Suite 207, Beaumont, TX 77706 · 409-899-3682

Daniel Roubin · General Radiology · Radiology Associates, 3560 Delaware Street, Suite 207, Beaumont, TX 77706 · 409-899-3682

Corpus Christi

Richard P. Chepey · General Radiology · Radiology Associates, 2481 Morgan Street, P.O. Box 5608, Corpus Christi, TX 78405 · 512-882-7432

James H. Heslep · General Radiology · Spohn Hospital · Radiology & Imaging of South Texas, 1415 Third Street, Suite 101, Corpus Christi, TX 78404-2101 · 512-881-3005

Chandra S. Katragadda · General Radiology · Spohn Hospital · 1415 Third Street, Suite 101, Corpus Christi, TX 78404-2101 · 512-881-3005

David B. Strong · General Radiology · Radiology Associates, 2481 Morgan Street, P.O. Box 5608, Corpus Christi, TX 78405 · 512-882-7432

Dallas

A. Brooks Chapman · General Radiology (Diagnostic) · Presbyterian Hospital of Dallas · Department of Radiology, 8200 Walnut Hill Lane, Dallas, TX 75231 · 214-345-7770

Guido Currarino · Pediatric Radiology · Children's Medical Center of Dallas · Children's Medical Center of Dallas, Department of Radiology, 1935 Motor Street, Dallas, TX 75235 · 214-640-2305

George C. Curry · General Radiology · Parkland Memorial Hospital · University of Texas-Southwestern Medical Center at Dallas, Department of Radiology, 5323 Harry Hines Boulevard, Dallas, TX 75235-8896 · 214-648-8020

Thomas Sherrod Curry III · General Radiology · Parkland Memorial Hospital · Parkland Memorial Hospital, 5201 Harry Hines Boulevard, Dallas, TX 75235-7793 · 214-590-8000

Norman George Diamond · General Radiology (Vascular & Interventional Radiology, Peripheral Angioplasty, Stents, Biliary Interventions) · Baylor University Medical Center · Baylor University Medical Center, Department of Radiology, 3500 Gaston Avenue, Dallas, TX 75246 · 214-820-3206

Paul Harris Ellenbogen · General Radiology (Ultrasound, Computed Tomography, Magnetic Resonance Imaging, Mammography) · Presbyterian Hospital of Dallas · Southwest Diagnostic Imaging Center, Professional Building Three, Suite 100, 8230 Walnut Hill Lane, Dallas, TX 75231-4496 · 214-345-6905

Walter Philmore Evans III · General Radiology (Mammography) · Baylor University Medical Center · Komen Breast Center, 3535 Worth Street, Dallas, TX 75246 · 214-820-4101

Mark Fulmer · General Radiology · Baylor University Medical Center, Department of Radiology, Roberts Building, First Floor, 3500 Gaston Avenue, Dallas, TX 75246 · 214-820-2310

Steven E. Harms · Magnetic Resonance Imaging (Breast, Musculoskeletal, Temporomandibular Joint) · Baylor University Medical Center · Baylor University Medical Center, Magnetic Resonance Imaging Department, 3500 Gaston Avenue, Dallas, TX 75246 · 214-820-2310

Peter G. Hildenbrand · Neuroradiology · Baylor University Medical Center · Baylor University Medical Center, Department of Radiology, 3500 Gaston Avenue, Dallas, TX 75246 · 214-820-2427

Bassett B. Kilgore · Neuroradiology (Brain, Spine, Head & Neck Radiology) · Southwest Diagnostic Imaging Center, Presbyterian Hospital of Dallas, St. Paul Medical Center · 5430 Glen Lakes Drive, Suite 260, Dallas, TX 75231 · 214-373-8300

Michael Jay Landay · Chest · Parkland Memorial Hospital · Parkland Memorial Hospital, 5201 Harry Hines Boulevard, Dallas, TX 75235-7793 · 214-590-8720

Stephen Paul Lee · General Radiology (Interventional) · Baylor University Medical Center · Baylor University Medical Center, Department of Radiology, 3500 Gaston Avenue, Dallas, TX 75246 · 214-820-3216

Phillip D. Purdy · Neuroradiology (Interventional Neuroradiology, Stroke & Cerebrovascular Disease, Endovascular Aneurysm Therapy) · Zale Lipshy University Hospital, Parkland Memorial Hospital, Children's Medical Center of Dallas, St. Paul Medical Center · University of Texas-Southwestern Medical Center at Dallas, 5323 Harry Hines Boulevard, Dallas, TX 75235-8896 · 214-648-3928

Helen Cornelia Redman · General Radiology (Vascular & Interventional Radiology, Emergency Radiology, Genitourinary Radiology) · Parkland Memorial Hospital, Zale Lipshy University Hospital · University of Texas-Southwestern Medical Center at Dallas, 5323 Harry Hines Boulevard, Dallas, TX 75235-8896 · 214-648-8012

Chet R. Rees · General Radiology (Vascular & Interventional Radiology) · Baylor University Medical Center · Baylor University Medical Center, Department of Radiology, 3500 Gaston Avenue, Dallas, TX 75246 · 214-820-3219

Roger Leland Rian · General Radiology (Urologic Radiology) · Baylor University Medical Center, Department of Radiology, 3600 Gaston Avenue, Dallas, TX 75246 · 214-820-2427

Frank J. Rivera · General Radiology (Vascular & Interventional Radiology, Cardiovascular Disease, Interventional Neuroradiology) · Baylor University Medical Center · Baylor University Medical Center, Department of Vascular Interventional Radiology, 3500 Gaston Avenue, Dallas, TX 75214 · 214-820-3206

Nancy Katherine Rollins · Pediatric Radiology (Invasive) · Children's Medical Center of Dallas · Children's Medical Center of Dallas, Department of Radiology, 1935 Motor Street, Dallas, TX 75235 · 214-640-2305

Paul Timothy Siemers · Neuroradiology · Baylor University Medical Center · Baylor University Medical Center, Department of Radiology, 3500 Gaston Avenue, Dallas, TX 75246 · 214-820-3219

Herbert Louis Steinbach · General Radiology (Diagnostic Ultrasound, Abdominal Computed Tomography, Nuclear Medicine, Nuclear Radiology) · Baylor University Medical Center · Baylor University Medical Center, 3500 Gaston Avenue, Dallas, TX 75246 · 214-820-2196

El Paso

Richard Cohen · General Radiology · Providence Memorial Hospital · Providence Memorial Hospital, Department of Radiology, 2001 North Oregon Street, El Paso, TX 79902 · 915-577-6011

Barbara J. Gainer · General Radiology (Computerized Tomography [CT], Ultrasound, Nuclear Radiology) · Thomason Hospital · Texas Tech University Health Sciences Center, Department of Radiology, 4800 Alberta Avenue, El Paso, TX 79905-2709 · 915-545-6845

R. R. Jauernek · (Neuroradiology, Magnetic Resonance Imaging) · Sierra Medical Center, Department of Radiology, 1625 Medical Center Drive, El Paso, TX 79902 · 915-747-2791

Fort Worth

John L. Coscia, Jr. · General Radiology · Center for Breast Care, 750 Eighth Avenue, Suite 200, Fort Worth, TX 76104 · 817-336-9900

B. J. Gralino, Jr. · General Radiology · Harris Methodist-Fort Worth · Radiology Associates of Tarrant County, 815 Pennsylvania Avenue, Fort Worth, TX 76104 · 817-336-8684

Richard S. Pickering · General Radiology (Interventional Radiology) · Radiology Associates of Tarrant County, 815 Pennsylvania Avenue, Fort Worth, TX 76104 · 817-336-8684

Galveston

Brian W. Goodacre · General Radiology · University of Texas Medical Branch, Department of Radiology, 301 University Boulevard, Galveston, TX 77555-0709 409-772-3481

Sanford A. Rubin · Chest · University of Texas Medical Branch Hospitals · University of Texas Medical Branch, Department of Radiology, UHC Building, Room 2.103, 301 University Boulevard, Galveston, TX 77555-0709 · 409-772-3649

Melvyn H. Schreiber · General Radiology · University of Texas Medical Branch Hospitals · University of Texas Medical Branch, Department of Radiology, 301 University Boulevard, Galveston, TX 77555-0709 · 409-772-9179

Leonard E. Swischuk · Pediatric Radiology · University of Texas Medical Branch, Department of Radiology, UHC Building, Room 2.103, 301 University Boulevard, Galveston, TX 77555-0709 · 409-772-2096

Eric vanSonnenberg · (Interventional Radiology, Cryotherapy, Abdominal Imaging) · University of Texas Medical Branch Hospitals · University of Texas Medical Branch, Department of Radiology, UHC Building, Room 2.103, 301 University Boulevard, Galveston, TX 77555-0709 · 409-772-1823

Eric M. Walser · General Radiology · University of Texas Medical Branch, Department of Radiology, UHC Building, Room 2.103, 301 University Boulevard, Galveston, TX 77555-0709 · 409-772-4880

Gerhard R. Wittich · General Radiology · University of Texas Medical Branch Hospitals · University of Texas Medical Branch, Department of Radiology, UHC Building, Room 2.103, 301 University Boulevard, Galveston, TX 77555-0709 · 409-772-7159

Houston

J. Chuslip Charnsangavej · General Radiology (Abdominal) · University of Texas-M. D. Anderson Cancer Center · University of Texas-M. D. Anderson Cancer Center, 1515 Holcombe Boulevard, Box 57, Houston, TX 77030 · 713-794-1813

Marvin H. Chasen · Chest · University of Texas-M. D. Anderson Cancer Center University of Texas-M. D. Anderson Cancer Center, 1515 Holcombe Boulevard, Box 57, Houston, TX 77030 · 713-792-2708

Lester Paul Gerson · Pediatric Radiology (Neuroradiology) · Texas Children's Hospital, St. Luke's Episcopal Hospital · St. Luke's Episcopal Hospital, Department of Radiology, 6720 Bertner Avenue, Suite P-020, Houston, TX 77030 · 713-791-4095

Stanford Milton Goldman · General Radiology (Genito-Urinary) · Hermann Hospital · University of Texas Medical School at Houston, 6431 Fannin Street, Room 2.132, Houston, TX 77030 · 713-792-5235 x1200

Stanley Fredric Handel · Neuroradiology, Magnetic Resonance Imaging · 6430 Hillcroft Street, Suite 100, Houston, TX 77081 · 713-778-9800

John H. Harris, Jr. · General Radiology (Trauma, Emergency Radiology, Musculoskeletal Radiology) · Hermann Hospital · University of Texas Medical School at Houston, Department of Radiology, 6431 Fannin Street, Suite 2.100, Houston, TX 77030-1501 · 713-704-3539

Yayen Lee · Neuroradiology (Head & Neck Cancer) · University of Texas-M. D. Anderson Cancer Center · University of Texas-M. D. Anderson Cancer Center, Diagnostic Radiology, 1515 Holcombe Boulevard, Box 57, Houston, TX 77030-4009 · 713-792-8634

Norman Edward Leeds · Neuroradiology (Spine, Magnetic Resonance Imaging) University of Texas-M. D. Anderson Cancer Center · University of Texas-M. D. Anderson Cancer Center, 1515 Holcombe Boulevard, Box 57, Houston, TX 77030-4009 · 713-745-0568

Herman I. Libshitz · Chest · University of Texas-M. D. Anderson Cancer Center, Hermann Hospital · University of Texas-M. D. Anderson Cancer Center, 1515 Holcombe Boulevard, Box 57, Houston, TX 77030 · 713-792-2121

M. Nabil Maklad · General Radiology (Ultrasound) · University of Texas Medical School at Houston, Department of Radiology, 6431 Fannin Street, Room 2.100, Houston, TX 77030 · 713-792-5235 x1357

Michel E. Mawad · Neuroradiology (Vascular & Interventional Radiology, Magnetic Resonance Imaging) · Methodist Hospital, 6565 Fannin Street, Mail Stop 033, Houston, TX 77030-2730 · 713-790-4826

William A. Murphy, Jr. · General Radiology (Bone) · University of Texas-M. D. Anderson Cancer Center · University of Texas-M. D. Anderson Cancer Center, 1515 Holcombe Boulevard, Box 57, Houston, TX 77030-4009 · 713-745-1149

Bruce R. Parker · Pediatric Radiology · Texas Children's Hospital · Texas Children's Hospital, Department of Diagnostic Imaging, 6621 Fannin Street, Mail Code 2-2521, Houston, TX 77030 · 713-770-5300

John Roehm · (Interventional & Vascular Radiology) · Methodist Hospital · Methodist Hospital, Department of Radiology, 6565 Fannin Street, Mail Stop F303, Houston, TX 77030 · 713-790-4251

Carol B. Stelling · General Radiology (Mammography, Diagnostic Radiology, Breast Imaging, Breast Cancer Early Diagnosis) · University of Texas-M.D. Anderson Cancer Center, Department of Diagnostic Radiology, 1515 Holcombe Boulevard, Box 57, Houston, TX 77030 · 713-745-1207

Milton Wagner · Pediatric Radiology · Texas Children's Hospital · Texas Children's Hospital, Department of Diagnostic Imaging, 6621 Fannin Street, Mail Code 2-2521, Houston, TX 77030 · 713-770-5300

Sidney Wallace · General Radiology (Vascular & Interventional Radiology, Oncologic Radiology) · University of Texas-M. D. Anderson Cancer Center · University of Texas-M. D. Anderson Cancer Center, 1515 Holcombe Boulevard, Box 57, Houston, TX 77030 · 713-792-2714

Lubbock

Glenn H. Robeson · Neuroradiology · University Medical Center · Texas Tech University Health Sciences Center, 3601 Fourth Street, Room 1B113, Lubbock, TX 79430 · 806-743-3674

Midland

Cheryl W. Hightower · General Radiology (Ultrasound, Nuclear Medicine) · Diagnostic Imaging, 2409 West Illinois Street, Suite C, Midland, TX 79704 · 915-682-9729

Thomas Hinton · General Radiology · Diagnostic Imaging, 2409 West Illinois Street, P.O. Box 5474, Midland, TX 79701 · 915-682-9729

Scott Scheward · General Radiology · Diagnostic Imaging, 2409 West Illinois Street, Suite C, Midland, TX 79704 · 915-682-9729

Roberto R. Spencer · General Radiology · 2202 West Tennessee Avenue, Midland, TX 79701 · 915-686-8684

San Antonio

Carlos Bazan III · Neuroradiology (Central Nervous System Neoplasms, Central Nervous System Infections) · University of Texas Health Science Center at San Antonio, Department of Radiology, 7703 Floyd Curl Drive, San Antonio, TX 78284-7800 · 210-567-6488

Ernesto Blanco · Neuroradiology (Pediatric, Adult) · Santa Rosa Children's Hospital · Santa Rosa Children's Hospital, Department of Radiology, 519 West Houston Street, San Antonio, TX 78207-3108 · 210-704-2371

Robert O. Cone III · General Radiology (Orthopaedic Radiology) · South Texas Radiology Group, 7950 Floyd Curl Drive, Suite SL1-21, San Antonio, TX 78229 210-616-7796

Gerald D. Dodd III · General Radiology (Interventional Ultrasonography) · University of Texas Health Science Center at San Antonio, Department of Radiology, 7703 Floyd Curl Drive, San Antonio, TX 78284-7800 · 210-567-6470

Joel A. Dunlap · Pediatric Radiology · Southwest Texas Methodist Hospital · South Texas Radiology Group, 7950 Floyd Curl Drive, Suite SL1-21, San Antonio, TX 78229 · 210-692-4343

James S. Gilley · General Radiology (Orthopaedic Radiology) · Southwest Texas Methodist Hospital · South Texas Radiology Group, 7950 Floyd Curl Drive, Suite SL1-21, San Antonio, TX 78229 · 210-616-7796

David A. Golden · General Radiology (Vascular & Interventional Radiology) · Southwest Texas Methodist Hospital · South Texas Radiology Group, 7950 Floyd Curl Drive, Suite SL1-21, San Antonio, TX 78229 · 210-692-4343

Harvey Martin Goldstein · General Radiology (Diagnostic, Gastrointestinal, Mammography) · Southwest Texas Methodist Hospital · Southwest Texas Methodist Hospital, Department of Radiology, 7700 Floyd Curl Drive, Sublevel Two, San Antonio, TX 78229 · 210-692-4343

Gerald W. Growcock · General Radiology · Radiology Associates of San Antonio, 343 West Houston Street, Suite 209, San Antonio, TX 78205-2102 · 210-222-2255

Michael Duard Howard · General Radiology (Interventional Radiology) · Baptist Medical Center · Baptist Medical Center, Department of Radiology, 111 Dallas Street, San Antonio, TX 78205-1201 · 210-222-8431

John Randall Jinkins · Neuroradiology (Magnetic Resonance Imaging) · University of Texas Health Science Center at San Antonio, Department of Radiology, 7703 Floyd Curl Drive, San Antonio, TX 78284-7800 · 210-567-6488

Ashwani Kapila · Neuroradiology · Santa Rosa Children's Hospital · Santa Rosa Children's Hospital, Department of Radiology, 519 West Houston Street, San Antonio, TX 78207-3108 · 210-704-2371

James D. Lutz · General Radiology (Vascular & Interventional Radiology) · Metropolitan Hospital, Santa Rosa Children's Hospital, University Hospital-South Texas Medical Center, Audie L. Murphy Memorial Veterans Hospital, Santa Rosa Health Care, Santa Rosa Northwest Hospital, Cancer Therapy & Research Center, Tri-City Community Hospital (Jourdanton) · Santa Rosa Children's Hospital, Department of Radiology, 519 West Houston Street, San Antonio, TX 78207-3108 210-224-1888

Michael J. McCarthy · Chest (Mammography) · University of Texas Health Science Center at San Antonio, Department of Radiology, 7703 Floyd Curl Drive, San Antonio, TX 78284-7800 · 210-567-6488

Darlene Fong Metter · General Radiology (Nuclear Medicine, Nuclear Radiology) · University of Texas Health Science Center at San Antonio, Department of Radiology, 7703 Floyd Curl Drive, San Antonio, TX 78284-7800 · 210-567-6488

Edward Bruce Mewborne · Pediatric Radiology · Santa Rosa Children's Hospital · Santa Rosa Children's Hospital, Department of Radiology, 519 West Houston Street, San Antonio, TX 78207-3108 · 210-228-2011

Vung Duy Nguyen · General Radiology (Orthopaedic Radiology) · Audie L. Murphy Memorial Veterans Hospital · Audie L. Murphy Memorial Veterans Hospital, 7400 Merton Minter Boulevard, Mail Code 114, San Antonio, TX 78284-5700 · 210-617-5300 x5122

Julio C. Palmaz · General Radiology (Interventional Radiology) · University of Texas Health Science Center at San Antonio, Department of Radiology, 7703 Floyd Curl Drive, San Antonio, TX 78284-7800 · 210-567-5564

Rosa Blanes Ramirez · General Radiology (Pediatric, Mammography, Obstetric Ultrasound) · Women's & Children's Hospital · South Texas Radiology Group, 7950 Floyd Curl Drive, Suite SL1-21, San Antonio, TX 78229 · 210-616-7796

Adam Victor Ratner · Magnetic Resonance Imaging (Diagnostic Radiology) · Santa Rosa Health Care, Metropolitan Hospital, Tri-City Community Hospital (Jourdanton), Radiology Network of Texas · Radiology Associates of San Antonio, 343 West Houston Street, Suite 209, San Antonio, TX 78205 · 210-224-1888

Stewart R. Reuter · General Radiology (Vascular & Interventional Radiology) · University Hospital-South Texas Medical Center · University of Texas Health Science Center at San Antonio, Department of Radiology, 7703 Floyd Curl Drive, San Antonio, TX 78284-7800 · 210-567-5558

Kenneth S. Rugh · General Radiology (Pediatric Radiology) · Santa Rosa Children's Hospital · Santa Rosa Children's Hospital, Department of Radiology, 519 West Houston Street, San Antonio, TX 78207-3108 · 210-704-2371

Gladys S. Sepulveda · General Radiology (Mammography) · Women's & Children's Hospital · South Texas Radiology Group, 7950 Floyd Curl Drive, Suite SL1-21, San Antonio, TX 78229 · 210-616-7796

James Richard Stewart · Neuroradiology · Southwest Texas Methodist Hospital South Texas Radiology Group, 7950 Floyd Curl Drive, Suite SL1-21, San Antonio, TX 78229 · 210-616-7796

William T. Sullivan · General Radiology (Musculoskeletal Radiology) · Santa Rosa Children's Hospital · Santa Rosa Children's Hospital, Department of Radiology, 519 West Houston Street, San Antonio, TX 78207-3108 · 210-704-2371

Kenneth D. Williams · Neuroradiology · Santa Rosa Children's Hospital · Santa Rosa Children's Hospital, Department of Radiology, 519 West Houston Street, San Antonio, TX 78207-3108 · 210-704-2371

Robert Gayle Williams · Neuroradiology (Pediatric Radiology) · Southwest Texas Methodist Hospital · South Texas Radiology Group, 7950 Floyd Curl Drive, Suite SL1-21, San Antonio, TX 78229 · 210-616-7796

Tyler

J. Robert Shepherd · General Radiology · University of Texas Health Center-Tyler, US Highway 271 and State Highway 155, P.O. Box 2003, Tyler, TX 75710-2003 · 903-877-7110

John G. Short · General Radiology · East Texas Medical Center · 1020 Clinic Drive, Tyler, TX 75701 · 903-593-2539

Waco

Kerry K. Ford · General Radiology · Hillcrest Baptist Medical Center · Hillcrest Baptist Medical Center, Department of Radiology, 3000 Herring Avenue, Waco, TX 76708 · 817-756-8525

Fred H. Rader, Jr. · General Radiology · Hillcrest Baptist Medical Center · Hillcrest Baptist Medical Center, Department of Radiology, 3000 Herring Avenue, Waco, TX 76708 · 817-756-8525

David O. Risinger · General Radiology · Hillcrest Baptist Medical Center · Hillcrest Baptist Medical Center, Department of Radiology, 3000 Herring Avenue, Waco, TX 76708 · 817-756-8525

Donald L. Risinger · General Radiology · Hillcrest Baptist Medical Center · Hillcrest Baptist Medical Center, Department of Radiology, 3000 Herring Avenue, Waco, TX 76708 · 817-756-8525

Jerry R. Wright · General Radiology · Hillcrest Baptist Medical Center · Hillcrest Baptist Medical Center, Department of Radiology, 3000 Herring Avenue, Waco, TX 76708 · 817-756-8525

RHEUMATOLOGY

Abilene

James T. Halla · General Rheumatology · 1927 Pine Street, Abilene, TX 79601 · 915-673-4751

Amarillo

Gregory D. Middleton · General Rheumatology · Amarillo Diagnostic Clinic, 6700 West Ninth Street, Amarillo, TX 79106 · 806-358-3171

Arlington

Carlos M. Kier · General Rheumatology · 909-B Medical Center Drive, Arlington, TX 76012 · 817-274-0996

Austin

Walter F. Chase · (Clinical Research) · Capitol Medical Clinic, 1301 West 38th Street, Suite 601, Austin, TX 78705 · 512-454-5171

James Everett Crout · General Rheumatology (Lupus, Osteoarthritis, Scleroderma, Vasculitis) · Austin Diagnostic Medical Center · Austin Diagnostic Medical
Center, 12221 MoPac Expressway North, P.O. Box 85075, Austin, TX 78708-5075
512-901-1000

Michael Bowen Pickrell · General Rheumatology · Austin Diagnostic Medical
Center, 12221 MoPac Expressway North, P.O. Box 85075, Austin, TX 78708-5075
512-901-1000

Marshall Rich Sack · General Rheumatology · Austin Diagnostic Medical Center,
12221 MoPac Expressway North, P.O. Box 85075, Austin, TX 78708-5075 · 512-
901-1000

Brian Sam Sayers · General Rheumatology · 1301 West 38th Street, Suite 502,
Austin, TX 78705 · 512-454-3631

Beaumont

Reuben A. Isern · General Rheumatology · Baptist Hospital Beaumont, St. Elizabeth Hospital, Beaumont Regional Medical Center · Rheumatology Associates,
2965 Harrison Street, Suite 214, Beaumont, TX 77702-1149 · 409-898-7172

Mary Louise Olsen · General Rheumatology · Rheumatology Associates, 2965
Harrison Street, Suite 214, Beaumont, TX 77702-1149 · 409-898-7172

Brownwood

Christopher Stephens · General Rheumatology · Scott & White Clinic, 103
South Park Drive, Brownwood, TX 76801 · 915-646-3502

Corpus Christi

James H. Leibfarth · General Rheumatology · Spohn Hospital, Doctors Regional
Medical Center, Bay Area Medical Center · Thomas Spann Clinic, 1533 South
Brownlee, Corpus Christi, TX 78404 · 512-844-6531

Dallas

Alan Lawrence Brodsky · General Rheumatology (Rheumatoid Arthritis, Lupus) · Presbyterian Hospital of Dallas · Arthritis Care & Diagnostic Center, 8230 Walnut Hill Lane, Suite 818, Dallas, TX 75231-4424 · 214-696-1600

Andrew Chubick, Jr. · General Rheumatology (Osteoporosis, Fibromyalgia) · Baylor University Medical Center · Arthritis Centers of Texas, 712 North Washington Avenue, Suite 200, Dallas, TX 75246 · 214-823-6503

Stanley Bruce Cohen · General Rheumatology (Clinical Research, Osteoporosis, Rheumatoid Arthritis, Fibromyalgia) · St. Paul Medical Center · Rheumatology Associates, 5939 Harry Hines Boulevard, Suite 400, Dallas, TX 75235 · 214-879-6705

John Joseph Cush · Rheumatoid Arthritis (Arthritis, Systemic Lupus Erythematosus) · Zale Lipshy University Hospital, Parkland Memorial Hospital, VA Medical Center · University of Texas-Southwestern Medical Center at Dallas, 5323 Harry Hines Boulevard, Dallas, TX 75235-8577 · 214-648-3065

Thomas David Geppert · General Rheumatology (Rheumatoid Arthritis, Gout) · Zale Lipshy University Hospital, Parkland Memorial Hospital · University of Texas-Southwestern Medical Center at Dallas, Department of Internal Medicine, 5323 Harry Hines Boulevard, Dallas, TX 75235 · 214-648-3466

Eric Hurd · General Rheumatology (Rheumatoid Arthritis, Connective Tissue Diseases, Fibromyalgia) · Baylor University Medical Center, Medical Center of Plano (Plano) · Arthritis Center of Texas, 712 North Washington Avenue, Suite 200, Dallas, TX 75246 · 214-823-6503

Sharad Lakhanpal · General Rheumatology (Psoriatic Arthritis, Osteoporosis, Sjogren's Syndrome, Lupus, Vasculitis) · St. Paul Medical Center · Rheumatology Associates, 5939 Harry Hines Boulevard, Suite 400, Dallas, TX 75235 · 214-879-6700

Peter E. Lipsky · General Rheumatology (Immunology) · Parkland Memorial Hospital, Zale Lipshy University Hospital, VA Medical Center · University of Texas-Southwestern Medical Center at Dallas, Department of Internal Medicine, 5323 Harry Hines Boulevard, Dallas, TX 75235-8884 · 214-648-9110

J. Donald Smiley · General Rheumatology (Rheumatoid Arthritis, Systemic Lupus Erythematosus, Scleroderma) · Presbyterian Hospital of Dallas, Parkland Memorial Hospital · Presbyterian Hospital of Dallas, Jackson Building, 8200 Walnut Hill Lane, Dallas, TX 75231 · 214-345-7378

Scott Jeffrey Zashin · General Rheumatology (Lupus, Osteoarthritis, Rheumatoid Arthritis) · Presbyterian Hospital of Dallas, Presbyterian Hospital of Plano (Plano) · Presbyterian Hospital of Dallas, 8230 Walnut Hill Lane, Suite 818, Lockbox 11, Dallas, TX 75231 · 214-363-2812

El Paso

Robert J. Abresch · General Rheumatology · Arthritis Clinic, 1717 North Brown Street, Building 1A, El Paso, TX 79902 · 915-542-2854

Charles Patrick Cavaretta · General Rheumatology · Providence Memorial Hospital · 300 Waymore Drive, El Paso, TX 79902 · 915-577-2624

Raj Marwah · General Rheumatology · 1600 Medical Center Drive, Suite 314, El Paso, TX 79902 · 915-545-1158

Fort Worth

Dan A. Axthelm · General Rheumatology · 6100 Harris Parkway, Suite 230, Fort Worth, TX 76132 · 817-346-5477

Emily Merrell Isaacs · General Rheumatology · Harris Methodist-Fort Worth · 1210 West Presidio, Fort Worth, TX 76102 · 817-336-3951

Claudio Lehmann · General Rheumatology (Rheumatoid Arthritis, Connective Tissue Diseases, Osteoarthritis, Soft Tissue Rheumatism) · Harris Methodist-Fort Worth, All Saints Episcopal Hospital-Fort Worth, Plaza Medical Center · 1350 South Main Street, Suite 2350, Fort Worth, TX 76104 · 817-336-1011

R. Larry Marshall · General Rheumatology · All Saints Episcopal Hospital-Fort Worth, Harris Methodist-Fort Worth · 1650 West Rosedale Street, Suite 302, Fort Worth, TX 76104 · 817-332-9688

Bernard R. Rubin · General Rheumatology (Fibromyalgia, Osteoporosis) · University of North Texas Health Science Center, 3500 Camp Bowie Boulevard, Fort Worth, TX 76107-2699 · 817-735-2661

Galveston

Jerry C. Daniels · General Rheumatology (Lupus, Osteoarthritis) · University of Texas Medical Branch Hospitals · University of Texas Medical Branch, Department of Internal Medicine, Division of Rheumatology, 301 University Boulevard, Galveston, TX 77555-0569 · 409-772-2509

Jeffrey R. Lisse · General Rheumatology · University of Texas Medical Branch, Department of Internal Medicine, Division of Rheumatology, 301 University Boulevard, Galveston, TX 77555-0759 · 409-772-2863

Harlingen

Eugene Nunnery, Jr. · General Rheumatology · Valley Baptist Medical Center · 1713 Treasure Hills Boulevard, Suite 2D, Harlingen, TX 78550-8913 · 210-425-4982

Houston

Joan Appleyard · General Rheumatology · 6410 Fannin Street, Suite 1200, Houston, TX 77030 · 713-704-4028

Frank Couchman Arnett, Jr. · General Rheumatology · Hermann Hospital · University of Texas Medical School at Houston, 6431 Fannin Street, Room 5.270, Houston, TX 77030 · 713-792-5900

Alan W. Friedman · General Rheumatology · University of Texas Medical School at Houston, Division of Immunology & Rheumatology, 6431 Fannin Street, Room MSB 5270, Houston, TX 77030 · 713-704-0986

Martin D. Lidsky · General Rheumatology · VA Medical Center, Department of Rheumatology, 1002 Holcombe Boulevard, Mail Stop 111K, Houston, TX 77030 · 713-664-3598

John D. Reveille · General Rheumatology (AIDS, Lupus, Scleroderma) · Hermann Hospital · University of Texas Medical School at Houston, Department of Rheumatology, 6431 Fannin Street, Room MSB 5.270, Houston, TX 77030 · 713-792-5900

Richard A. Rubin · General Rheumatology · Houston Arthritis Associates, 7515 South Main Street, Houston, TX 77030 · 713-795-0500

Sandra Lee Sessoms · General Rheumatology (Systemic Lupus Erythematosus, Vasculitis) · Methodist Hospital · Baylor College of Medicine, Department of Rheumatology and Oncology, 6550 Fannin Street, Suite 1057, Houston, TX 77030 · 713-798-3750

Carolyn Ann Smith · General Rheumatology · Hermann Hospital · Diagnostic Clinic of Houston, 6448 Fannin Street, Houston, TX 77030 · 713-797-9191

Noranna B. Warner · General Rheumatology · Hermann Hospital · University of Texas Medical School at Houston, Division of Rheumatology, 6655 Travis Street, Suite 880, Houston, TX 77030-1335 · 713-792-5900

Frank R. Wellborne · General Rheumatology (Lupus, Vasculitis) · Memorial Hospital-Southwest, Memorial Hospital-Memorial City · 7737 Southwest Freeway, Suite 980, Houston, TX 77074 · 713-995-9465

Lubbock

Bruce Alex Bartholomew · General Rheumatology · University Medical Center Texas Tech University Health Sciences Center, Department of Internal Medicine, 3601 Fourth Street, Lubbock, TX 79430 · 806-743-3150

Jay Michael Calmes · General Rheumatology · St. Mary of the Plains Hospital, Lubbock Methodist Hospital · 4321 Brownfield Highway, Lubbock, TX 79407-2500 · 806-795-7501

David McConnell Mills · General Rheumatology · St. Mary of the Plains Hospital, Lubbock Methodist Hospital · Lubbock Diagnostic Clinic, 3506 Twenty-First Street, Suite 201, Lubbock, TX 79410-1216 · 806-788-8075

Midland

Bal Krishna Khandelwal · General Rheumatology · 2301 West Michigan Street, Midland, TX 79701-5829 · 915-684-0941

San Antonio

Michael Fischbach · General Rheumatology · Audie L. Murphy Memorial Veterans Hospital · University of Texas Health Science Center at San Antonio, Department of Medicine, Division of Clinical Immunology, Section of Rheumatology, 7703 Floyd Curl Drive, San Antonio, TX 78284-7868 · 210-567-4658

Karl Hans Hempel · General Rheumatology · Nix Health Care System · San Antonio Medical Associates, 703 Nix Professional Building, San Antonio, TX 78205-2522 · 210-224-4811

Rodolpho Molina · General Rheumatology (Osteoporosis) · Methodist Healthcare System, San Antonio Community Hospital, Santa Rosa Northwest Hospital · The Arthritis Diagnostic & Treatment Center, 10130 Huebner Road, San Antonio, TX 78240 · 210-690-8067

I. Jon Russell · Fibromyalgia · University Hospital-South Texas Medical Center University of Texas Health Science Center at San Antonio, Department of Medicine, Division of Clinical Immunology, Section of Rheumatology, 7703 Floyd Curl Drive, San Antonio, TX 78284-7868 · 210-567-4661

Joel Edward Rutstein · General Rheumatology (Osteoporosis, Osteoarthritis, Rheumatoid Arthritis, Fibromyalgia Syndrome) · Santa Rosa Health Care, Methodist Hospital, San Antonio Community Hospital, St. Luke's Baptist Hospital · The Arthritis Diagnostic & Treatment Center, 10130 Huebner Road, San Antonio, TX 78240 · 210-690-8067

James H. Wild · General Rheumatology · 2829 Babcock Road, Suite 110, San Antonio, TX 78229 · 210-616-7309

Sugar Land

Angela McCain · General Rheumatology · West Houston Medical Center, Columbia Fort Bend Medical Center (Missouri City) · 2205 Williams Trace Boulevard, Suite 106, Sugar Land, TX 77478 · 713-980-2717

Temple

Jeffrey William Jundt · General Rheumatology · Scott & White Memorial Hospital & Clinic · Scott & White Memorial Hospital, Division of Rheumatology, 2401 South 31st Street, Temple, TX 76508-0001 · 817-724-2466

Alec Dean Steele · General Rheumatology · Scott & White Memorial Hospital & Clinic · Scott & White Memorial Hospital, Division of Rheumatology, 2401 South 31st Street, Temple, TX 76508-0001 · 817-724-2466

Tyler

William G. Brelsford · General Rheumatology · University of Texas Health Center-Tyler · University of Texas Health Center-Tyler, US Highway 271 and State Highway 155, P.O. Box 2003, Tyler, TX 75710-2003 · 903-877-7328

Roger W. Porter · General Rheumatology · University of Texas Health Center-Tyler · University of Texas Health Center-Tyler, US Highway 271 and State Highway 155, P.O. Box 2003, Tyler, TX 75710-2003 · 903-877-3451

Waco

Eugene Fung · General Rheumatology (Arthritis, Rheumatism, Connective Tissue Disease, Osteoporosis) · Providence Health Center, Hillcrest Baptist Medical Center · Waco Medical Group, 2911 Herring Avenue, Suite 308, Waco, TX 76708 817-755-4582

SURGERY

Amarillo

Richard B. Clarke · General Surgery · Amarillo Surgical Group, Six Medical Drive, Amarillo, TX 79106-4100 · 806-353-6604

Richard D. Dillman, Jr. · General Surgery (General Vascular Surgery, Laparoscopic Surgery) · St. Anthony's Hospital, Amarillo Hospital District-Northwest Texas Hospital, Palo Duro Hospital · 301 Amarillo Boulevard, West, Suite 105, Amarillo, TX 79107 · 806-345-4260

Robert J. Hays · General Surgery · Amarillo Surgical Group, Six Medical Drive, Amarillo, TX 79106 · 806-353-6604

Michael A. Lary · General Vascular Surgery (General Surgery) · High Plains Baptist Hospital, Amarillo Hospital District-Northwest Texas Hospital, St. Anthony's Hospital · Amarillo Surgical Group, Six Medical Drive, Amarillo, TX 79106 · 806-353-6604

John P. McKinley · General Surgery · St. Anthony's Hospital, High Plains Baptist Hospital, Amarillo Hospital District-Northwest Texas Hospital · 301 Amarillo Boulevard, West, Suite 204, Amarillo, TX 79107 · 806-345-2424

William J. Neilson · General Surgery · Amarillo Surgical Group, Six Medical Drive, Amarillo, TX 79106 · 806-353-6604

Arlington

Bohn D. Allen · General Surgery · Arlington Memorial Hospital · 1001 North Waldrop, Suite 701, Arlington, TX 76012-4305 · 817-275-4301

Austin

Robert Edward Askew, Jr. · Breast Surgery (Abdominal) · Seton Medical Center, St. David's Healthcare Center, Seton Northwest Hospital · Askew Surgical Associates, 3901 Medical Parkway, Suite 301, Austin, TX 78756 · 512-454-8725

Robert Edward Askew, Sr. · Breast Surgery · Seton Medical Center · Askew Surgical Associates, 3901 Medical Parkway, Suite 301, Austin, TX 78756 · 512-454-8725

Robert Ashe Bridges · General Vascular Surgery · Seton Medical Center, St. David's Healthcare Center, Brackenridge Hospital, South Austin Medical Center Cardiothoracic & Vascular Surgeons, 1010 West 40th Street, Austin, TX 78756-4079 · 512-459-8753

Phillip J. Church · General Vascular Surgery (Arterial Aneurysm Disease, Arterial Occlusive Disease, Cerebrovascular Occlusive Disease) · Seton Medical Center, St. David's Healthcare Center · Cardiothoracic & Vascular Surgeons, 1010 West 40th Street, Austin, TX 78756-4079 · 512-459-8753

Stephen S. Clark · General Surgery · St. David's Healthcare Center · 3901 Medical Parkway, Suite 202, Austin, TX 78756 · 512-451-7367

Thomas Benton Coopwood · General Surgery · Austin Surgical Clinic, Building Two, 2911 Medical Arts Street, Austin, TX 78705 · 512-478-3402

William Hiatt Hart · General Surgery (Surgical Oncology, Laparoscopic Surgery, Gastrointestinal Surgery) · Brackenridge Hospital, St. David's Healthcare Center, Seton Medical Center · 1111 West 34th Street, Suite 301, Austin, TX 78705 · 512-451-2780

Earl W. Howard III · General Surgery (Breast Surgery, Gastroenterologic Surgery) St. David's Healthcare Center, Seton Medical Center · 1717 West Avenue, Austin, TX 78701 · 512-474-6666

Harry Lamar Jones, Jr. · General Surgery · 3901 Medical Parkway, Suite 201, Austin, TX 78756 · 512-454-5684

Charles Duncan Livingston · General Surgery (Gastroenterologic Surgery, Laparoscopic Surgery, Breast Surgery) · Seton Medical Center · 3901 Medical Parkway, Suite 200, Austin, TX 78756 · 512-467-7151

Mark R. Sherrod · General Surgery (Breast Surgery, Endocrine Surgery) · St. David's Healthcare Center, South Austin Medical Center, Seton Medical Center, Seton Northwest Hospital · 900 East 30th Street, Suite 204, Austin, TX 78705 · 512-476-8312

Mark Thomas Stewart · General Vascular Surgery · Cardiothoracic & Vascular Surgeons, 1010 West 40th Street, Austin, TX 78756-4079 · 512-459-8753

Owen Ewing Winsett · Breast Surgery · Breast Center of Austin, 1301 West 38th Street, Suite 104, Austin, TX 78705 · 512-451-5788

Beaumont

Leon Milton Hicks · Pediatric Surgery (Pediatric Urology) · St. Elizabeth Hospital 2955 Harrison Street, Suite 201, Beaumont, TX 77702-1156 · 409-892-4561

Douglas L. Horton · General Surgery (Breast Surgery, Gastroenterologic Surgery) St. Elizabeth Hospital, Baptist Hospital Beaumont, Beaumont Regional Medical Center, Beaumont Surgery Center · 2929 Calder Avenue, Suite 200, Beaumont, TX 77702 · 409-835-6815

Stuart Scott Kacy · General Surgery · St. Elizabeth Hospital · 2955 Harrison Street, Suite 105, Beaumont, TX 77702-1155 · 409-892-3820

Emmett R. Mackan · General Surgery · St. Elizabeth Hospital · Southeast Texas Surgical Associates, 2929 Calder Avenue, Suite 203, Beaumont, TX 77702-1155 · 409-838-5088

J. Eric Weldon · General Surgery · Southeast Texas Surgical Associates, 2929 Calder Avenue, Suite 203, Beaumont, TX 77702-1155 · 409-838-5088

Corpus Christi

George Y. Alsop · General Surgery · Alsop Surgical Associates, 613 Elizabeth Street, Suite 813, Corpus Christi, TX 78404 · 512-888-7276

John R. Hornung · General Surgery · 1521 South Staples Street, Suite 206, Corpus Christi, TX 78404 · 512-884-1799

Vicente M. Juan · General Surgery (Splenic Surgery, Biliary Surgery) · Spohn Hospital, Memorial Medical Center, Bay Area Medical Center, Doctors Regional Medical Center · 1201 Ocean Drive, Corpus Christi, TX 78404 · 512-887-9995

Malcolm R. Rodger III · General Surgery · Surgical Associates, 613 Elizabeth Street, Suite 601, Corpus Christi, TX 78404-2220 · 512-881-8333

Steven J. Steele · General Vascular Surgery · 3301 South Alameda Street, Suite 304, Corpus Christi, TX 78411 · 512-851-0110

T. Michael Townsend, Jr. · General Vascular Surgery · Spohn Hospital · Surgical Associates, 613 Elizabeth Street, Suite 601, Corpus Christi, TX 78404-2220 · 512-881-8333

Charles T. Volk · General Vascular Surgery · Surgical Associates, 613 Elizabeth Street, Suite 601, Corpus Christi, TX 78404-2220 · 512-881-8333

Dallas

Charles James Carrico · General Surgery (Surgical Critical Care, Trauma) · Parkland Memorial Hospital, Zale Lipshy University Hospital · University of Texas-Southwestern Medical Center at Dallas, 5323 Harry Hines Boulevard, Dallas, TX 75235-9031 · 214-648-3504

G. Patrick Clagett · General Vascular Surgery (Carotid Artery Surgery, Aortic Aneurysms, Infected Vascular Grafts) · The University of Texas-Southwestern Medical Center, Parkland Memorial Hospital, Zale Lipshy University Hospital · University of Texas-Southwestern Medical Center at Dallas, Section of Vascular Surgery, 5323 Harry Hines Boulevard, Dallas, TX 75235-9031 · 214-648-3516

Dale Coln · Pediatric Surgery · Baylor University Medical Center, 3600 Gaston Avenue, Dallas, TX 75246 · 214-828-9040

Wilson V. Garrett · General Vascular Surgery (Carotid Surgery for Stroke Prevention, Treatment of Aortic Aneurysms, Reoperative Vascular Surgery) · Baylor University Medical Center, Doctors Hospital of Dallas · 72 North Washington Avenue, Suite 509, Dallas, TX 75246 · 214-824-7280

Robert M. Goldstein · Transplantation (Hepatobiliary Surgery, Surgical Critical Care, Gastroenterologic Surgery, General Surgery) · Baylor University Medical Center · Baylor University Medical Center, Transplantation Services, 3500 Gaston Avenue, Dallas, TX 75246 · 214-820-2050

Philip C. Guzzetta, Jr. · Pediatric Surgery (Transplantation, General Vascular Surgery) · Children's Medical Center of Dallas, Parkland Memorial Hospital · Children's Medical Center of Dallas, West Tower, Third Floor, 1935 Motor Street, Dallas, TX 75235 · 214-640-6040

John L. Hunt · Trauma (Surgical Critical Care, Burn Surgery) · University of Texas-Southwestern Medical Center at Dallas, Department of Surgery, 5323 Harry Hines Boulevard, Dallas, TX 75235-9060 · 214-648-2152

Ronald C. Jones · General Surgery (Breast Surgery, Endocrine Surgery, Gastroenterologic Surgery) · Baylor University Medical Center · Baylor University Medical Center, Department of Surgery, 3500 Gaston Avenue, Dallas, TX 75246 · 214-820-3250

Goran B. Klintmalm · Transplantation (Liver, Kidney, Pancreas, Small Bowel Transplantation, Immunosuppression, Organ Allocation) · Baylor University Medical Center, Children's Medical Center of Dallas · Baylor University Medical Center, Transplantation Services, 3500 Gaston Avenue, Dallas, TX 75246 · 214-820-2050

Zelig H. Lieberman · Gastroenterologic Surgery (Hepatic Surgery, Biliary Surgery, Oncologic Surgery) · Baylor University Medical Center · Baylor Medical Plaza, Wadley Tower, Suite 958, 3600 Gaston Avenue, Dallas, TX 75246 · 214-826-6276

Robert Nelson McClelland · Gastroenterologic Surgery (Pancreatic, Biliary) · University of Texas-Southwestern Medical Center at Dallas, 5323 Harry Hines Boulevard, Dallas, TX 75235-9031 · 214-648-3540

Gregory John Pearl · General Vascular Surgery · Baylor University Medical Center 712 North Washington Avenue, Suite 509, Dallas, TX 75246-1635 · 214-824-7280

Malcolm O. Perry · General Vascular Surgery (Arterial Trauma, Aortic Surgery) · Parkland Memorial Hospital, St. Paul Medical Center, Zale Lipshy Hospital · St. Paul Medical Center, Department of Surgery, 5909 Harry Hines Boulevard, Dallas, TX 75235 · 214-879-3787

G. Tom Shires III · Gastroenterologic Surgery (General Surgery, Gastrointestinal Cancer) · Parkland Memorial Hospital, Zale Lipshy University Hospital · University of Texas-Southwestern Medical Center at Dallas, 5323 Harry Hines Boulevard, Dallas, TX 75235-9031 · 214-648-3050

Bertram L. Smith · General Vascular Surgery (Abdominal Aneurysm, Carotid/Vertebral Revascularization, Lower Extremity Bypass) · Baylor University Medical Center · 512 North Washington Avenue, Suite 509, Dallas, TX 75246 · 214-824-7280

William Henry Snyder III · Endocrine Surgery · University of Texas-Southwestern Medical Center at Dallas, 5323 Harry Hines Boulevard, Dallas, TX 75235-9031 · 214-648-3510

Clement M. Talkington · General Vascular Surgery · Baylor University Medical Center · 512 North Washington Avenue, Suite 509, Dallas, TX 75246 · 214-824-7280

Erwin R. Thal · Trauma · Parkland Memorial Hospital · University of Texas-Southwestern Medical Center at Dallas, Department of Surgery, 5323 Harry Hines Boulevard, Dallas, TX 75235-7200 · 214-648-3531

Theodore P. Votteler · Pediatric Surgery (Separation of Conjoined Twins, Head & Neck Lesions, Congenital Chest Wall Defects) · Children's Medical Center of Dallas · Pediatric Surgical Associates, 8226 Douglas Avenue, Suite 547, Dallas, TX 75225 · 214-369-6424

El Paso

Steven S. Larson · General Surgery · 1700 Murchison Drive, Suite 202, El Paso, TX 79902 · 915-532-3111

Leo C. Mercer, Jr. · General Surgery · Thomason Hospital · Texas Tech University Health Sciences Center, Department of Surgery, 4800 Alberta Avenue, El Paso, TX 79905-2709 · 915-545-6857

Ruben G. Ramirez · General Surgery · 1250 East Cliff Drive, Suite 3-E, El Paso, TX 79902 · 915-532-4458

Edward Cooper Saltzstein · General Surgery (Breast Surgery, Gastroenterologic Surgery) · Thomason Hospital, Providence Memorial Hospital · Texas Tech University Health Sciences Center, Department of Surgery, 4800 Alberta Avenue, El Paso, TX 79905-2709 · 915-545-6858

Fort Worth

Timothy L. Black · Pediatric Surgery · Cook Children's Medical Center · Pediatric Surgical Associates of Fort Worth, 800 Eighth Avenue, Suite 306, Fort Worth, TX 76104 · 817-336-7881

John L. Crawford · General Vascular Surgery · 800 Fifth Avenue, Suite 408, Fort Worth, TX 76104 · 817-332-2998

Michael Dean Korenman · General Vascular Surgery · 1821 Eighth Avenue, Fort Worth, TX 76110-1351 · 817-927-2329

Douglas D. Lorimer · General Surgery · 757 Eighth Avenue, Suite B, Fort Worth, TX 76104 · 817-336-4200

Charles M. Mann, Jr. · Pediatric Surgery · Pediatric Surgery Associates of Fort Worth, 800 Eighth Avenue, Suite 306, Fort Worth, TX 76104 · 817-336-7881

James P. Miller · Pediatric Surgery · Cook Children's Medical Center · Pediatric Surgical Associates of Fort Worth, 800 Eighth Avenue, Suite 306, Fort Worth, TX 76104 · 817-336-7881

James Lee Norman · General Surgery · 1650 West Magnolia Street, Suite 111, Fort Worth, TX 76104 · 817-924-4464

Peter Lloyd Rutledge · General Surgery · Harris Methodist-Fort Worth · 1050 Fifth Avenue, Suite B, Fort Worth, TX 76104-2903 · 817-332-1144

Galveston

Sally Abston · Trauma (Burn Surgery) · University of Texas Medical Branch Hospitals · University of Texas Medical Branch, Department of General Surgery, 301 University Boulevard, Galveston, TX 77555-0282 · 409-772-2277

B. Mark Evers · Gastroenterologic Surgery · University of Texas Medical Branch Hospitals · University of Texas Medical Branch, Department of Surgery, 301 University Boulevard, Galveston, TX 77555-0533 · 409-772-5254

Jay C. Fish · General Surgery (Renal Transplantation, Endocrine Surgery) · John Sealy Hospital · University of Texas Medical Branch, Department of Surgery, 301 University Boulevard, Room 0536, Galveston, TX 77555-0527 · 409-772-2412

Kristene K. Gugliuzza · Transplantation (General Surgery, Pancreas, Kidney Transplantation, Adult and Pediatric) · University of Texas Medical Branch Hospitals · University of Texas Medical Branch, Department of Surgery, 301 University Boulevard, Route 0542, Galveston, TX 77555-0542 · 409-772-6559

Marilyn Marx · Gastroenterologic Surgery · St. Mary's Hospital · Gulf Coast Medical Group, 200 University Boulevard, Suite 922, Galveston, TX 77550 · 409-762-3778

Kenneth E. McIntyre, Jr. · General Vascular Surgery (Infrainguinal Bypass, Cerebrovascular Disease, Aortic Aneurysm) · University of Texas Medical Branch Hospitals · University of Texas Medical Branch, Department of Surgery, 301 University Boulevard, Galveston, TX 77555-0835 · 409-772-6366

William H. Nealon · General Surgery (Laparoscopy, Surgery of the Pancreas, Bile Ducts and Liver, Therapeutic Endoscopic Retrograde Cholangiopancreatography) · University of Texas Medical Branch Hospitals · University of Texas Medical Branch, Department of Surgery, John Sealy Annex, Room 6.112, 301 University Boulevard, Galveston, TX 77555-0544 · 409-772-6582

James C. Thompson · Gastroenterologic Surgery · John Sealy Hospital · University of Texas Medical Branch, Department of Surgery, 301 University Boulevard, Room 0527, Galveston, TX 77555-0527 · 409-772-1285

Courtney M. Townsend, Jr. · Endocrine Surgery (Surgical Oncology, Breast Surgery) · University of Texas Medical Branch Hospitals · University of Texas Medical Branch, Department of Surgery, 301 University Boulevard, Galveston, TX 77555-0527 · 409-772-1285

Harlingen

Thomas A. Clark · General Surgery (Cardiovascular Surgery, General Vascular Surgery, Surgical Critical Care, Trauma) · Valley Baptist Medical Center · Cardiovascular Associates, 2310 North Ed Carey Drive, Suite 1B, Harlingen, TX 78550 · 210-425-5144

Marion R. Lawler, Jr. · General Surgery · Valley Baptist Medical Center · Cardiovascular Associates, 2310 North Ed Carey Drive, Suite 1B, Harlingen, TX 78550 · 210-425-5144

Houston

Richard John Andrassy · Pediatric Surgery (Cancer Surgery, General Surgery, Trauma, Pediatric Non-Cardiac Thoracic Surgery) · University of Texas-M. D. Anderson Cancer Center, Hermann Hospital · University of Texas Medical School at Houston, 6431 Fannin Street, Room 4.020, Houston, TX 77030 · 713-792-5400

Michael F. Appel · Gastroenterologic Surgery (Endoscopy, Breast Surgery) · St. Luke's Episcopal Hospital · 6624 Fannin Street, Suite 2500, Houston, TX 77030 · 713-795-5600

Robert S. Bloss · Pediatric Surgery · Texas Children's Hospital · Houston Pediatric Surgeons, 6624 Fannin Street, Suite 1590, Houston, TX 77030 · 713-796-1600

Joseph Stapleton Coselli · General Vascular Surgery (Aortic Surgery) · Methodist Hospital · Methodist Hospital, 6560 Fannin Street, Suite 1144, Houston, TX 77030 · 713-790-4313

Joe Ed Dossey · General Surgery · Memorial City Surgical Associates, 920 Frostwood Drive, Suite 740, Houston, TX 77024 · 713-464-1981

James H. Duke, Jr. · General Surgery · Hermann Hospital · University of Texas Medical School at Houston, 6431 Fannin Street, Room 4.168, Houston, TX 77030 713-792-5409

Jose V. Iglesias · General Surgery (Vascular Surgery) · Houston Northwest Medical Center · 17203 Red Oak Drive, Suite 202, Houston, TX 77090 · 713-444-9400

Barry Donald Kahan · Transplantation (Kidney Transplantation) · Hermann Hospital · University of Texas Medical School at Houston, 6431 Fannin Street, Room 6.240, Houston, TX 77030 · 713-792-5670

Richard H. Lynch · General Surgery · Park Plaza Hospital · 1213 Hermann Drive, Suite 850, Houston, TX 77004 · 713-521-9341

Bruce V. MacFadyen, Jr. · Gastroenterologic Surgery, Breast Surgery (Liver Surgery, Pancreatic Surgery, Bile Duct Surgery, Endoscopy, General Surgery) · Hermann Hospital · University of Texas Medical School at Houston, 6431 Fannin Street, Room 4.022, Houston, TX 77030 · 713-792-5408

Kenneth L. Mattox · Trauma, Adult Cardiothoracic Surgery (Cardiovascular Trauma) · Ben Taub General Hospital · Baylor College of Medicine, Department of Surgery, One Baylor Plaza, Houston, TX 77030 · 713-798-4557

Charles H. McCollum · General Vascular Surgery (General Surgery, Vascular Diagnostic Laboratory, General Surgical Oncology, General Thoracic Surgery) · Methodist Hospital · Baylor College of Medicine, Smith Tower, Suite 1609, 6550 Fannin Street, Houston, TX 77030 · 713-798-8400

Frank G. Moody · Gastroenterologic Surgery (General Surgery) · Hermann Hospital · University of Texas Medical School at Houston, 6431 Fannin Street, Room 4.164, Houston, TX 77030 · 713-745-1886

Kelly Steven Oggero · General Surgery (Cancer Surgery, Laparoscopic Surgery) St. Luke's Episcopal Hospital, Hermann Hospital · 6410 Fannin Street, Suite 1220, Houston, TX 77030 · 713-799-1220

John R. Potts III · General Surgery (Endocrine Surgery, Gastroenterologic Surgery) · Lyndon B. Johnson General Hospital, Hermann Hospital · University of

Texas Medical School at Houston, Surgery Clinic, Room 1400, 6410 Fannin Street, Houston, TX 77030 · 713-794-4167

William A. Redwine · General Surgery · St. Luke's Episcopal Hospital · 6624 Fannin Street, Suite 2400, Houston, TX 77030 · 713-790-9151

R. Anders Rosendahl · (Head & Neck Surgery, Tumor Surgery) · 1200 Binz Street, Suite 820, Houston, TX 77004 · 713-520-1230

Phillip Gordon Sutton · General Surgery (Breast Surgery, Gastroenterologic Surgery) · Houston Northwest Medical Center · 17203 Red Oak Drive, Suite 203, Houston, TX 77090 · 713-893-2288

Charles Thomas Van Buren · Transplantation (Kidney Transplantation) · Hermann Hospital · University of Texas Medical School at Houston, 6431 Fannin Street, Room 4.156, Houston, TX 77030 · 713-792-5671

James O. Wallace · General Surgery (Breast Surgery, Gastroenterologic Surgery, General Surgical Oncology) · St. Luke's Episcopal Hospital · 6624 Fannin Street, Suite 2400, Houston, TX 77030 · 713-790-9151

R. Patrick Wood · Transplantation (Liver Transplantation, General Surgery) · Hermann Hospital, Texas Children's Hospital, St. Luke's Episcopal Hospital · University of Texas Medical School at Houston, Department of Surgery, 6431 Fannin Street, Room 6.246, Houston, TX 77030 · 713-704-6801

Humble

Norman Mark Sorgen · General Surgery (Breast Surgery, Gall Bladder Surgery, Hernia Surgery) · Northeast Medical Center Hospital, Columbia Kingwood Medical Center (Kingwood) · 18955 Memorial North, Suite 200, Humble, TX 77338 713-446-1116

Lackland Air Force Base

Henry Wing Cheu · Pediatric Surgery · Wilford Hall Medical Center · Wilford Hall Medical Center, 2200 Bergquist Drive, Suite One, Lackland Air Force Base, TX 78236-5300 · 210-670-7641

Lubbock

David P. Campbell · Pediatric Surgery (Pediatric Non-Cardiac Thoracic Surgery, Pediatric Urology) · Lubbock Methodist Hospital · 3606 Twenty-First Street, Suite 203, Lubbock, TX 79410 · 806-785-1113

Jane F. Goldthorn · Pediatric Surgery · University Medical Center · Medical Office Plaza, Suite G70, 3602 Ninth Street, Lubbock, TX 79415 · 806-743-1613

John A. Griswold, Jr. · Trauma (Burn Surgery) · University Medical Center · University Surgical Associates, Medical Office Plaza, Suite 210, 3502 Ninth Street, Lubbock, TX 79415 · 806-743-1613

George Baird Helfrich · Trauma, Transplantation (Kidney Transplantation) · Lubbock Methodist Hospital · 3606 Twenty-First Street, Suite 104, Lubbock, TX 79410 · 806-792-0595

Stuart R. Lacey · Pediatric Surgery (Pediatric Non-Cardiac Thoracic Surgery) · University Medical Center · Medical Office Plaza, Suite G70, 3602 Ninth Street, Lubbock, TX 79415 · 806-743-2375

William J. Millikan, Jr. · Transplantation, Trauma (Liver Transplantation) · University Medical Center · Texas Tech University Health Sciences Center, Department of Surgery, 3601 Fourth Street, Lubbock, TX 79430 · 806-743-1584

Catherine Ann Ronaghan · Breast Surgery, Trauma · University Medical Center Medical Arts Clinic, 4102 Twenty-Fourth Street, Suite 100, Lubbock, TX 79410 806-788-1111

Robert J. Salem · General Surgery (Breast Surgery, Gastroenterologic Surgery) · Lubbock Methodist Hospital · SWAT Surgical Associates, 3509 Twenty-Second Street, Lubbock, TX 79410-1307 · 806-795-0648

George Thomas Shires · Trauma (General Surgery, Surgical Critical Care) · University Medical Center · Texas Tech University Health Sciences Center, Department of Surgery, 3601 Fourth Street, Room 3A159, Lubbock, TX 79430 · 806-743-1613

Gerald L. Woolam · General Surgery (Breast Surgery, Gastroenterologic Surgery) St. Mary of the Plains Hospital, Lubbock Methodist Hospital · 3702 Twenty-First Street, Suite 203, Lubbock, TX 79410-1230 · 806-792-3303

Midland

Guillermo E. Brachetta · General Surgery · 2300 West Michigan Avenue, Midland, TX 79701-5855 · 915-687-0181

Shelton Viney · General Surgery · 3001 West Illinois Avenue, Midland, TX 79701 915-697-1061

Nacogdoches

Larry L. Walker · General Surgery · 1018 North Mound Street, Suite 105, Nacogdoches, TX 75961 · 409-569-7971

Pasadena

Philip R. Somers · General Surgery · 1112 South Witter Street, Pasadena, TX 77506 · 713-477-1796

San Angelo

John S. Cargile III · General Surgery · 2030 Pulliam Street, Suite Seven, San Angelo, TX 76905 · 915-655-0631

J. Michael Cornell · General Surgery · Shannon Medical Center · 2030 Pulliam Street, Suite Seven, San Angelo, TX 76905-5157 · 915-655-0631

San Antonio

Sabas Fatule Abuabara · Gastroenterologic Surgery (Pancreas) · Baptist Medical Center, Santa Rosa Health Care, Metropolitan Hospital, Southwest Texas Methodist Hospital · 730 North Main Avenue, Suite 704, San Antonio, TX 78205 · 210-271-0264

Anatolio B. Cruz, Jr. · General Surgery · University Hospital-South Texas Medical Center · University of Texas Health Science Center at San Antonio, Department of Surgery, 7703 Floyd Curl Drive, San Antonio, TX 78284-7842 · 210-567-5750

John Edmund Etlinger · Gastroenterologic Surgery · Baptist Medical Center · 4499 Medical Drive, Suite 345, San Antonio, TX 78229 · 210-615-8585

Glenn Alexander Halff · Transplantation (Liver and Kidney Transplantation) · University Hospital-South Texas Medical Center · University of Texas Health Science Center at San Antonio, Department of Surgery, Organ Transplantations Program, 7703 Floyd Curl Drive, San Antonio, TX 78284-7842 · 210-567-5777

Philip Daniel Manfredi · General Surgery (Breast Surgery) · Southwest Texas Methodist Hospital, St. Luke's Baptist Hospital, San Antonio Community Hospital, Women's & Children's Hospital · 7940 Floyd Curl Drive, Suite 520, San Antonio, TX 78229 · 210-614-3964

George Edward Mimari · General Surgery (Laparoscopic Surgery) · Southwest Texas Methodist Hospital · 8042 Wurzbach Road, Suite 630, San Antonio, TX 78229 · 210-614-5067

Boyce B. Oliver · General Surgery · Metropolitan Hospital · 1303 McCullough Avenue, Suite 235, San Antonio, TX 78212 · 210-225-1916

Carey P. Page · General Surgery (Surgical Oncology) · Audie L. Murphy Memorial Veterans Hospital, University of Texas Health Science Center · Audie L. Murphy Memorial Veterans Hospital, 7400 Merton Minter Boulevard, Mail Code 112G, San Antonio, TX 78284 · 210-617-5101

Irving A. Ratner · Pediatric Surgery (Pediatric Surgical Oncology, Pediatric Non-Cardiac Thoracic Surgery) · Santa Rosa Children's Hospital, Southwest Texas Methodist Hospital, Women's & Children's Hospital · 4499 Medical Drive, Suite 350, San Antonio, TX 78229-3713 · 210-614-3856

Jordan Kory Reed · General Surgery (Breast Surgery, Laparoscopic Surgery) · Santa Rosa Children's Hospital · 2829 Babcock Road, Suite 448, San Antonio, TX 78229 · 210-692-7406

Mark Charles Rittenhouse · General Surgery (Gastrointestinal Surgery, Breast Surgery) · St. Luke's Baptist Hospital · 2833 Babcock Road, Suite 425, San Antonio, TX 78229 · 210-614-3349

Arthur Rosenthal · General Surgery (Breast Surgery, Laparoscopic Surgery) · Southwest Texas Methodist Hospital · 8042 Wurzbach Road, Suite 480, San Antonio, TX 78229 · 210-616-0657

Wayne H. Schwesinger · Gastroenterologic Surgery (Laparoscopic Surgery, Biliary Reconstructive Surgery, Laser Endosurgery) · University Hospital-South Texas Medical Center, Audie L. Murphy Memorial Veterans Hospital · University of Texas Health Science Center at San Antonio, Department of Surgery, 7703 Floyd Curl Drive, San Antonio, TX 78284-7842 · 210-567-5730

Kenneth R. Sirinek · Gastroenterologic Surgery (Laparoscopic Surgery) · University Hospital-South Texas Medical Center · University of Texas Health Science Center at San Antonio, Department of Surgery, 7703 Floyd Curl Drive, Room 241-F, San Antonio, TX 78284-7842 · 210-567-5730

Ronald Mack Stewart · Trauma · University of Texas Health Science Center at San Antonio, Department of Surgery, 7703 Floyd Curl Drive, San Antonio, TX 78284-7842 · 210-567-3623

Mellick Tweedy Sykes · General Vascular Surgery (Peripheral Vascular Surgery) · University Hospital-South Texas Medical Center, Baptist Memorial Healthcare System, Methodist Healthcare System, Santa Rosa Health Care · University of Texas Health Science Center at San Antonio, Department of Surgery, 7703 Floyd Curl Drive, San Antonio, TX 78284-7842 · 210-567-5715

Arnold Ira Walder · General Surgery (Breast Surgery, Lymphedema) · St. Luke's Baptist Hospital, Southwest Texas Methodist Hospital · 5282 Medical Drive, Suite 170, San Antonio, TX 78229 · 210-616-0651

Temple

Edward G. Ford · Pediatric Surgery · Scott & White Memorial Hospital & Clinic Scott & White Memorial Hospital, Department of Surgery, 2401 South 31st Street, Temple, TX 76508-0001 · 817-724-2593

John William Roberts · General Surgery · Scott & White Memorial Hospital & Clinic · Scott & White Memorial Hospital, Department of Surgery, 2401 South 31st Street, Temple, TX 76508-0001 · 817-724-2760

Richard E. Symmonds, Jr. · General Surgery · Scott & White Memorial Hospital & Clinic · Scott & White Memorial Hospital, Department of Surgery, 2401 South 31st Street, Temple, TX 76508-0001 · 817-724-2760

Texas City

Beverly Guillory Lewis · Breast Surgery, Gastroenterologic Surgery (General Surgery) · Mainland Center Hospital, University of Texas Medical Branch Hospitals (Galveston) · 1228 North Logan Street, Suite 200, Texas City, TX 77590 · 409-945-0810

Tomball

Jose L. San Luis · General Surgery (Pediatric Surgery, Laparo-Endoscopic Surgery) · Tomball Regional Hospital, Houston Northwest Medical Center (Houston), Cypress Fairbanks Medical Center (Houston) · 425 Holderrieth Street, Suite 110, Tomball, TX 77375 · 713-351-5409

Tyler

Duane Andrews · General Surgery · 910 East Houston Street, Suite 550, Tyler, TX 75702 · 903-592-7393

S. Edwin Duncan · General Vascular Surgery · 1100 South Beckham Avenue, Tyler, TX 75701 · 903-595-2636

Patrick R. Thomas · General Surgery (Vascular Surgery, Breast Surgery) · Trinity Mother Frances Health Care Center, East Texas Medical Center · Trinity Clinic, Department of Surgery, 910 East Houston Street, Suite 550, Tyler, TX 75702 · 903-592-7393

Victoria

Peter P. Rojas · General Surgery · Detar Hospital · Victoria Surgery Associates, 601 East San Antonio Street, Suite 501, Victoria, TX 77901 · 512-575-6396

Waco

Robert W. Crosthwait, Jr. · General Surgery · Providence Health Center, Hillcrest Baptist Medical Center · Cardiovascular Associates, 405 Londonderry Drive, Suite 200, Waco, TX 76712-7996 · 817-772-2300

David Glenn Hoffman · General Surgery (Peripheral Vascular Surgery, Colon & Rectal Cancer, General Colon & Rectal Surgery, General Surgical Oncology) · Providence Health Center, Hillcrest Baptist Medical Center · 2115 North 34th Street, Waco, TX 76708-3114 · 817-752-0303

Webster S. Lowder · General Surgery · Providence Health Center, Hillcrest Baptist Medical Center · 3400 Hillcrest Drive, Waco, TX 76708 · 817-752-2587

Barry F. Oswalt · General Surgery · 2115 North 34th Street, Waco, TX 76708-3114 · 817-752-0303

Ross B. Reagan · General Surgery · 2115 North 34th Street, Waco, TX 76708-3114 · 817-752-0303

Gayland L. Sims · General Surgery · 2115 North 34th Street, Waco, TX 76708-3114 · 817-752-0303

William H. Turney · General Surgery · 2115 North 34th Street, Waco, TX 76708-3114 · 817-752-0303

Wichita Falls

Beth H. Sutton · General Surgery (Breast Surgery, Endocrine Surgery) · Wichita General Hospital, Bethania Regional Health Care Center · 1600 Brook Avenue, Wichita Falls, TX 76301 · 817-723-8465

SURGICAL ONCOLOGY

Austin

Robert Edward Askew, Sr. · Breast Cancer (Endocrine Surgery, General Surgery) Seton Medical Center · Askew Surgical Associates, 3901 Medical Parkway, Suite 301, Austin, TX 78756 · 512-454-8725

Stephen S. Clark · General Surgical Oncology · St. David's Healthcare Center · 3901 Medical Parkway, Suite 202, Austin, TX 78756 · 512-451-7367

Harry Lamar Jones, Jr. · General Surgical Oncology · 3901 Medical Parkway, Suite 201, Austin, TX 78756 · 512-454-5684

Owen Ewing Winsett · Breast Cancer · Breast Center of Austin, 1301 West 38th Street, Suite 104, Austin, TX 78705 · 512-451-5788

Dallas

Janet Hale · Breast Cancer · Medical City Dallas Hospital · Breast Surgeons of North Texas, 7777 Forest Lane, Suite C614, Dallas, TX 75230 · 214-661-7499

Thelma Hurd · General Surgical Oncology (Colon & Rectal Cancer, Gastrointestinal Cancer) · Zale Lipshy University Hospital, Parkland Memorial Hospital, St. Paul Medical Center · University of Texas-Southwestern Medical Center at Dallas, 5323 Harry Hines Boulevard, Dallas, TX 75235-9031 ·

James Frank Huth · General Surgical Oncology (Breast Cancer, Liver Cancer, Melanoma [Soft Tissue Sarcomas]) · Zale Lipshy University Hospital, Parkland Memorial Hospital, Dallas County Hospital District, St. Paul Medical Center, VA Medical Center · University of Texas-Southwestern Medical Center at Dallas, 5323 Harry Hines Boulevard, Dallas, TX 75235-9031 · 214-648-9460

Ronald C. Jones · Breast Cancer (General Surgical Oncology, Melanoma) · Baylor University Medical Center · Baylor University Medical Center, Department of Surgery, 3500 Gaston Avenue, Dallas, TX 75246 · 214-820-3250

Sally Moot Knox · Breast Cancer · Baylor University Medical Center · 3600 Gaston Avenue, Suite 810, Dallas, TX 75246 · 214-826-9797

Joseph Allen Kuhn · General Surgical Oncology (Breast Cancer, Gastrointestinal Cancer, Thyroid Cancer) · Baylor University Medical Center · Sammons Tower, 3409 Worth Street, Suite 420, Dallas, TX 75246-2039 · 214-824-9963

Ann Marilyn Leitch · Breast Cancer (General Surgical Oncology, Melanoma) · Parkland Memorial Hospital, Zale Lipshy University Hospital · University of Texas-Southwestern Medical Center at Dallas, 5323 Harry Hines Boulevard, Dallas, TX 75235-9031 · 214-648-3039

Zelig H. Lieberman · General Surgical Oncology · Baylor University Medical Center · Baylor Medical Plaza, Wadley Tower, Suite 958, 3600 Gaston Avenue, Dallas, TX 75246 · 214-826-6276

John C. O'Brien, Jr. · Melanoma (Head & Neck Surgery, Gastrointestinal Cancer) · Baylor University Medical Center · Baylor University Medical Center, Wadley Tower, Suite 958, 3600 Gaston Avenue, Dallas, TX 75246 · 214-826-6276

George N. Peters · Breast Cancer (Diseases of the Breast, Breast Surgery) · Baylor University Medical Center, Charles A. Sammons Cancer Center · Charles A. Sammons Cancer Center, 3409 Worth Street, Suite 300, Dallas, TX 75246-2039 · 214-821-2962

John T. Preskitt · General Surgical Oncology (Breast Surgery, Gastrointestinal Cancer, Head & Neck Cancer, General Surgery) · Baylor University Medical Center · 3600 Gaston Avenue, Suite 958, Dallas, TX 75246 · 214-826-6276

Fort Worth

John W. Freese · Breast Cancer, Melanoma · All Saints Episcopal, Harris Methodist-Fort Worth, Plaza Medical Center · 1000 Ninth Avenue, Fort Worth, TX 76104-3906 · 817-332-7813

Robert J. Turner III · General Surgical Oncology (Gastrointestinal Cancer, Colon & Rectal Cancer, Melanoma) · All Saints Episcopal Hospital-Fort Worth, Columbia Plaza Medical Center, Harris Methodist-Fort Worth · 1000 Ninth Avenue, Fort Worth, TX 76104-3906 · 817-332-7813

Galveston

Thomas Duke Kimbrough · General Surgical Oncology (Surgical Critical Care, Nutrition in Surgical Patients) · University of Texas Medical Branch Hospitals · University of Texas Medical Branch, Department of Surgery, 301 University Boulevard, Galveston, TX 77555-0542 · 409-772-1201

Courtney M. Townsend, Jr. · General Surgical Oncology · University of Texas Medical Branch Hospitals · University of Texas Medical Branch, Department of Surgery, 301 University Boulevard, Room 0533, Galveston, TX 77555-0533 · 409-772-2490

Houston

Frederick C. Ames · Breast Cancer, Melanoma · University of Texas-M. D. Anderson Cancer Center, 1515 Holcombe Boulevard, Box 106, Houston, TX 77030-4009 · 713-792-6929

Harold Randolph (Randy) Bailey · Colon & Rectal Cancer (Anal Incontinence) Hermann Hospital, Methodist Hospital, St. Luke's Episcopal Hospital, Park Plaza Hospital, The Woman's Hospital of Texas · Colon & Rectal Clinic, Smith Tower, Suite 2307, 6550 Fannin Street, Houston, TX 77030-2717 · 713-790-9250

Charles M. Balch · Breast Cancer, Melanoma · University of Texas-M. D. Anderson Cancer Center · University of Texas-M. D. Anderson Cancer Center, 1515 Holcombe Boulevard, Box 323, Houston, TX 77030-4009 · 713-792-3300

Steven A. Curley · Gastrointestinal Cancer (Liver Cancer, Colon & Rectal Cancer) · University of Texas-M. D. Anderson Cancer Center · University of Texas-M. D. Anderson Cancer Center, Department of Surgical Oncology, 1515 Holcombe Boulevard, Box 106, Houston, TX 77030-4009 · 713-794-4957

Douglas Brian Evans · Gastrointestinal Cancer (Pancreatic Cancer, Endocrine Cancer) · University of Texas-M. D. Anderson Cancer Center · University of Texas-M. D. Anderson Cancer Center, Department of Surgery, 1515 Holcombe Boulevard, Box 106, Houston, TX 77030-4009 · 713-794-4324

Gilchrist L. Jackson · General Surgical Oncology (Head & Neck Surgery, Endocrine Surgery, Colon & Rectal Cancer) · St. Luke's Episcopal Hospital, Methodist Hospital · 6624 Fannin Street, Suite 1700, Houston, TX 77030-2329 · 713-791-8700

Jeffrey E. Lee · Melanoma (Endocrine Surgery, Pancreatic Cancer) · University of Texas-M. D. Anderson Cancer Center · University of Texas-M. D. Anderson Cancer Center, Department of Surgical Oncology, 1515 Holcombe Boulevard, Box 106, Houston, TX 77030 · 713-792-7218

Paul F. Mansfield · Gastrointestinal Cancer, Melanoma (Intraperitoneal Therapy for Carcinomatosis, General Surgical Oncology) · University of Texas-M. D. Anderson Cancer Center · University of Texas-M. D. Anderson Cancer Center, Department of Surgical Oncology, 1515 Holcombe Boulevard, Box 106, Houston, TX 77030-4009 · 713-794-5499

Peter W. T. Pisters · Gastrointestinal Cancer (Pancreatic Cancers, Soft Tissue Sarcomas, General Surgical Oncology) · University of Texas-M. D. Anderson Cancer Center · University of Texas-M. D. Anderson Cancer Center, Department of Surgical Oncology, 1515 Holcombe Boulevard, Box 106, Houston, TX 77030-4009 · 713-794-1572

Rafael Etomar Pollock · General Surgical Oncology (Sarcomas) · University of Texas-M. D. Anderson Cancer Center · University of Texas-M. D. Anderson Cancer Center, 1515 Holcombe Boulevard, Box 106, Houston, TX 77030 · 713-794-4324

Mark S. Roh · Gastrointestinal Cancer (Liver Cancer) · University of Texas-M. D. Anderson Cancer Center · University of Texas-M. D. Anderson Cancer Center, 1515 Holcombe Boulevard, Box 106, Houston, TX 77030-4009 · 713-792-7961

Merrick Ira Ross · Melanoma, Breast Cancer · University of Texas-M. D. Anderson Cancer Center · University of Texas-M. D. Anderson Cancer Center, 1515 Holcombe Boulevard, Box 106, Houston, TX 77030 · 713-792-7217

S. Eva Singletary · Breast Cancer · University of Texas-M. D. Anderson Cancer Center · University of Texas-M. D. Anderson Cancer Center, 1515 Holcombe Boulevard, Box 106, Houston, TX 77030-4009 · 713-792-6937

John Michael Skibber · Colon & Rectal Cancer · University of Texas-M. D. Anderson Cancer Center · University of Texas-M. D. Anderson Cancer Center, 1515 Holcombe Boulevard, Box 106, Houston, TX 77030-4009 · 713-792-5165

Lubbock

Annabel E. Barber · General Surgical Oncology (Surgical Critical Care, Gastroenterologic Surgery, Endocrine Surgery, General Surgery) · University Medical Center · Texas Tech University Health Sciences Center, Department of Surgery, 3601 Fourth Street, Lubbock, TX 79430 · 806-743-1584

Catherine Ann Ronaghan · Breast Cancer · University Medical Center · Medical Arts Clinic, 4102 Twenty-Fourth Street, Suite 100, Lubbock, TX 79410 · 806-788-1111

Gerald L. Woolam · (Breast Surgery, Gastrointestinal Cancer) · St. Mary of the Plains Hospital, Lubbock Methodist Hospital · 3702 Twenty-First Street, Suite 203, Lubbock, TX 79410-1230 · 806-792-3303

San Antonio

William E. Bode · Colon & Rectal Cancer · St. Luke's Baptist Hospital, Southwest Texas Methodist Hospital, Santa Rosa Northwest Hospital, Baptist Medical Center · Colon and Rectal Surgical Associates of San Antonio, Medical Center Tower One, Suite 101, 7950 Floyd Curl Drive, San Antonio, TX 78229 · 210-614-0880

Anatolio B. Cruz, Jr. · General Surgical Oncology · University Hospital-South Texas Medical Center · University of Texas Health Science Center at San Antonio, Department of Surgery, 7703 Floyd Curl Drive, San Antonio, TX 78284-7842 210-567-5750

George Richard Holt · General Surgical Oncology (Head & Neck Cancer) · North Central Baptist Hospital, University Hospital-South Texas Medical Center · 540 Madison Oak Drive, Suite 450, San Antonio, TX 78258 · 210-490-6371

George Edward Mimari · General Surgical Oncology · Southwest Texas Methodist Hospital · 8042 Wurzbach Road, Suite 630, San Antonio, TX 78229 · 210-614-5067

Boyce B. Oliver, Jr. · General Surgical Oncology · Metropolitan Hospital · 1303 McCullough Avenue, Suite 235, San Antonio, TX 78212 · 210-225-1916

Randal Allen Otto · General Surgical Oncology (Head & Neck Cancer) · University Hospital-South Texas Medical Center · University of Texas Health Science Center at San Antonio, Department of Otolaryngology-Head & Neck Surgery, 7703 Floyd Curl Drive, San Antonio, TX 78284-7777 · 210-567-5669

Carey P. Page · General Surgical Oncology · University Hospital-South Texas Medical Center, Audie L. Murphy Memorial Veterans Hospital · Audie L. Murphy Memorial Veterans Hospital, 7400 Merton Minter Boulevard, Mail Code 112G, San Antonio, TX 78284 · 210-617-5101

Raul Ramos · Colon & Rectal Cancer · Baptist Medical Center, Santa Rosa Health Care, Santa Rosa Northwest, San Antonio Community Hospital · Colon and Rectal Surgical Associates of San Antonio, Medical Center Tower One, Suite 101, 7950 Floyd Curl Drive, San Antonio, TX 78229-3916 · 210-614-0880

Mark Charles Rittenhouse · General Surgical Oncology (Gastrointestinal Cancer, Breast Cancer, Melanoma, Soft Tissue) · St. Luke's Baptist Hospital · 2833 Babcock Road, Suite 425, San Antonio, TX 78212 · 210-227-7367

Arthur Rosenthal · General Surgical Oncology (Breast Surgery, Laparoscopic Surgery) · Southwest Texas Methodist Hospital · 8042 Wurzbach Road, Suite 480, San Antonio, TX 78229 · 210-616-0657

Jonathan O. Tramer · General Surgical Oncology · Southwest Texas Methodist Hospital, University Hospital-South Texas Medical Center · General Surgery Associates, 8042 Wurzbach Road, Suite 310, San Antonio, TX 78229 · 210-614-5113

Arnold Ira Walder · General Surgical Oncology (Breast Cancer) · St. Luke's Baptist Hospital, Southwest Texas Methodist Hospital · 5282 Medical Drive, Suite 170, San Antonio, TX 78229 · 210-616-0651

Ronald Paul Williams · General Surgical Oncology (Orthopaedic Oncology) · University Hospital-South Texas Medical Center, Audie L. Murphy Memorial Veterans Hospital, St. Luke's Baptist Hospital, Santa Rosa Health Care · University of Texas Health Science Center at San Antonio, Department of Orthopaedics, 7703 Floyd Curl Drive, San Antonio, TX 78264-7774 · 210-567-6446

Temple

John C. Hendricks · General Surgical Oncology (Gastroenterological Surgery, Endocrine Surgery) · Scott & White Memorial Hospital · Scott & White Memorial Hospital, Department of Surgery, 2401 South 31st Street, Temple, TX 76508-0001 · 817-724-2448

Waco

William H. Turney · General Surgical Oncology · 2115 North 34th Street, Waco, TX 76708-3114 · 817-752-0303

THORACIC SURGERY

Amarillo

Deborah Burge McCollum · Adult Cardiothoracic Surgery · Amarillo Surgical Group, Six Medical Drive, Amarillo, TX 79106-4100 · 806-353-6604

Robert Duncan Sutherland · Adult Cardiothoracic Surgery · St. Anthony's Hospital · Amarillo Surgical Group, Six Medical Drive, Amarillo, TX 79106-4100 · 806-353-6604

Austin

Homer Stuart Arnold · General Thoracic Surgery · Seton Medical Center · Cardiothoracic & Vascular Surgeons, 1010 West 40th Street, Austin, TX 78756-4079 · 512-459-8753

Stephen James Dewan · General Thoracic Surgery · Seton Medical Center · Cardiothoracic & Vascular Surgeons, 1010 West 40th Street, Austin, TX 78756-4079 · 512-459-8753

Emery Walter Dilling · General Thoracic Surgery · Seton Medical Center · Cardiothoracic & Vascular Surgeons, 1010 West 40th Street, Austin, TX 78756-4079 512-459-8753

Lewis George King · General Thoracic Surgery · Cardiothoracic & Vascular Surgeons, 1010 West 40th Street, Austin, TX 78756-4079 · 512-459-8753

John Dawson Oswalt · Adult Cardiothoracic Surgery · Brackenridge Hospital · Cardiothoracic & Vascular Surgeons, 1010 West 40th Street, Austin, TX 78756-4079 · 512-459-8753

Beaumont

James A. Allums · Adult Cardiothoracic Surgery (General Thoracic Surgery, General Vascular Surgery) · St. Elizabeth Hospital, Baptist Hospital Beaumont, Park Place Hospital (Port Arthur) · Thoracic & Cardiovascular Surgical Associates, 2955 Harrison Street, Suite 204, Beaumont, TX 77702 · 409-899-4747

John T. Kirchmer, Jr. · Adult Cardiothoracic Surgery (Cardiac Surgery, Vascular Surgery) · St. Elizabeth Hospital, Baptist Hospital Beaumont, Park Place Hospital (Port Arthur) · Thoracic & Cardiovascular Surgical Associates, 2955 Harrison Street, Suite 204, Beaumont, TX 77702 · 409-899-4747

Corpus Christi

Sergio Taveres · General Thoracic Surgery · Spohn Hospital · Cardiovascular Associates, 613 Elizabeth Street, Suite 302, Corpus Christi, TX 78404-2222 · 512-884-1635

Dallas

Peter A. Alivizatos · Transplantation (Heart & Lung Transplantation) · Baylor University Medical Center · Baylor University Medical Center, Barnett Tower, Suite 404, 3600 Gaston Avenue, Dallas, TX 75246 · 214-824-6718

Robert F. Hebeler, Jr. · Adult Cardiothoracic Surgery · Baylor University Medical Center · 3409 Worth Street, Suite 720, Dallas, TX 75246-2091 · 214-821-3603

Albert Carl Henry III · Adult Cardiothoracic Surgery · Baylor University Medical Center · 3409 Worth Street, Suite 720, Dallas, TX 75246 · 214-821-3603

Steven Roy Leonard · Pediatric Cardiac Surgery · 2730 North Stemmons Freeway, Suite 104, P.O. Box 36306, Dallas, TX 75235 · 214-631-2557

Hisashi Nikaidoh · Pediatric Cardiac Surgery (Pediatric Non-Cardiac Thoracic Surgery) · Children's Medical Center of Dallas, Parkland Memorial Hospital · P.O. Box 36306, Dallas, TX 75235 · 214-640-7280

Melvin Ray Platt · General Thoracic Surgery (Coronary Artery Bypass Surgery, Mitral Valve Repair, Adult Cardiothoracic Surgery, Thoracic Oncological Surgery) Presbyterian Hospital of Dallas · Cardiothoracic Surgical Associates of North Texas, 8230 Walnut Hill Lane, Suite 208, Dallas, TX 75231-8230 · 214-692-6135

Maruf A. Razzuk · Adult Cardiothoracic Surgery (Thoracic Outlet Disorders) · Baylor University Medical Center · Baylor University Medical Center, Wadley Tower, Suite 561, 3600 Gaston Avenue, Dallas, TX 75246-1905 · 214-823-7795

William Steves Ring · Transplantation (Adult Cardiothoracic Surgery, Pediatric Cardiac Surgery, Adult and Pediatric Heart & Lung Transplantation, General Thoracic Surgery) · Zale Lipshy University Hospital, St. Paul Medical Center, Children's Medical Center of Dallas, Parkland Memorial Hospital · University of Texas-Southwestern Medical Center at Dallas, 5323 Harry Hines Boulevard, Dallas, TX 75235-8879 · 214-648-3568

William Henry Snyder III · General Thoracic Surgery · University of Texas-Southwestern Medical Center at Dallas, Department of Surgery, 5323 Harry Hines Boulevard, Dallas, TX 75235-9060 · 214-648-3510

Harold C. Urschel, Jr. · General Thoracic Surgery (Thoracic Outlet Syndrome, Lung Volume Reduction, Lung Cancer) · The University of Texas-Southwestern Medical Center, Baylor University Medical Center · Baylor University Medical Center, Barnett Tower, Suite 1201, 3600 Gaston Avenue, Dallas, TX 75246-1905 214-824-2503

Lonnie L. Whiddon · General Thoracic Surgery (Adult Cardiothoracic Surgery, Transplantation) · Methodist Medical Center, Baylor University Medical Center, Doctors Hospital, The Medical Center of Mesquite · Texas Cardiothoracic Surgery Associates, 221 West Colorado Boulevard, Suite 825, Dallas, TX 75208 · 214-942-5222

Richard E. Wood · General Thoracic Surgery (Cardiovascular Surgery, Peripheral Vascular Surgery, Heart & Lung Transplant Surgery, Pacemakers, Gastrointestinal Cancer, Thoracic Oncological Surgery) · Baylor University Medical Center · Baylor Medical Plaza, Barnett Tower, Suite 404, 3600 Gaston Avenue, Dallas, TX 75246-1804 · 214-827-3890

El Paso

Felice Bruno · General Thoracic Surgery · El Paso Southwest Cardiovascular Associates, 1600 Medical Center Drive, Suite 212, El Paso, TX 79902 · 915-532-3977

Charles A. Dow · General Thoracic Surgery · West Texas Heart Associates, 1812 North Oregon Street, El Paso, TX 79902 · 915-545-1082

Joseph Neil Kidd · Adult Cardiothoracic Surgery · Sierra Medical Center · El Paso Southwest Cardiovascular Associates, 1600 Medical Center Drive, Suite 212, El Paso, TX 79902 · 915-532-3977

John E. Liddicoat · General Thoracic Surgery (General Vascular Surgery, Adult Cardiothoracic Surgery) · Columbia Medical Center-West, Columbia Medical Center-East, Providence Memorial Hospital, Sierra Medical Center · Rio Grande Cardiovascular Associates, 1201 North Mesa Street, Suite A, El Paso, TX 79902 · 915-533-9207

Fort Worth

Karamat Ullah Choudhry · General Thoracic Surgery (Cardiac Surgery, Vascular Surgery) · Columbia Plaza Medical Center · 1650 West Rosedale Street, Suite 300, Fort Worth, TX 76104-7400 · 817-335-1131

Lawrence S. Fox · Pediatric Cardiac Surgery (Repair of Congenital Heart Defects Early in Life) · Cook Children's Medical Center · Cook Children's Medical Center, Department of Cardiovascular Surgery, 801 Seventh Avenue, Fort Worth, TX 76104-2796 · 817-885-4124

Manucher Nazarian · Adult Cardiothoracic Surgery (Vascular Surgery) · Harris Methodist-Fort Worth, All Saints Episcopal Hospital-Fort Worth · 757 Eighth Avenue, Suite A, Fort Worth, TX 76104-2503 · 817-336-4454

Robert W. Sloane, Jr. · Adult Cardiothoracic Surgery · Harris Methodist-Fort Worth · 901 South Lake Street, Fort Worth, TX 76104 · 817-336-5005

Galveston

Vincent R. Conti · (Adult Cardiothoracic Surgery) · University of Texas Medical Branch Hospitals · University of Texas Medical Branch, Department of Surgery, 301 University Boulevard, Galveston, TX 77555-0528 · 409-772-1203

Scott Lick · Transplantation (Adult Cardiothoracic Surgery) · University of Texas Medical Branch Hospitals · University of Texas Medical Branch, Department of Surgery, 301 University Boulevard, Galveston, TX 77555-0528 · 409-772-1203

Joseph B. Zwischenberger · Adult Cardiothoracic Surgery (General Thoracic Surgery, Extracorporeal and Intracorporeal Gas Exchange for Severe Respiratory Failure, Minimally Invasive Thoracic Surgery) · University of Texas Medical Branch Hospitals, John Sealy Hospital · University of Texas Medical Branch, Department of Surgery, Cardiothoracic Division, 301 University Boulevard, Galveston, TX 77555-0528 · 409-772-1739

Harlingen

Marion R. Lawler, Jr. · Adult Cardiothoracic Surgery · Valley Baptist Medical Center · Cardiovascular Associates, 2310 North Ed Carey Drive, Suite 1B, Harlingen, TX 78550 · 210-425-5144

Houston

John Charles Baldwin · Adult Cardiothoracic Surgery, Transplantation (Heart & Lung Transplantation, General Cardiovascular Disease, Heart Failure, Pacemakers, General Internal Medicine, General Vascular Surgery, General Thoracic Surgery, Thoracic Oncological Surgery) · Methodist Hospital, St. Joseph Hospital, Ben Taub General Hospital · Baylor College of Medicine, Department of Surgery, One Baylor Plaza, Houston, TX 77030 · 713-798-8100

Demetrio G. Boulafendis · Adult Cardiothoracic Surgery · 8830 Long Point Road, Suite 606, Houston, TX 77055-3026 · 713-464-1922

Denton A. Cooley · Adult Cardiothoracic Surgery (General Vascular Surgery, General Thoracic Surgery, Pediatric Cardiac Surgery) · Texas Heart Institute, St. Luke's Episcopal Hospital, Texas Children's Hospital · Texas Heart Institute, 1101 Bates Street, Suite P-514, P.O. Box 20345, Houston, TX 77225-0345 · 713-791-4900

Joseph Stapleton Coselli · Adult Cardiothoracic Surgery (Coronary Artery Surgery, Cardiac Valvular Surgery) · Methodist Hospital · Methodist Hospital, 6560 Fannin Street, Suite 1144, Houston, TX 77030 · 713-790-4313

J. Michael Duncan · Adult Cardiothoracic Surgery (General Vascular Surgery) · St. Luke's Episcopal Hospital · Texas Heart Institute, 1101 Bates Street, Suite P-514, P.O. Box 20345, Houston, TX 77225-0345 · 713-791-4900

Rafael Espada · Adult Cardiothoracic Surgery (General Vascular Surgery, Thoracic Oncological Surgery) · Methodist Hospital · Methodist Hospital, 6535 Fannin Street, Room A-886, Houston, TX 77030 · 713-790-4556

O.H. Frazier · Adult Cardiothoracic Surgery, Transplantation (Heart Transplantation, Cardiac Surgery) · Texas Heart Institute, St. Luke's Episcopal Hospital · Texas Heart Institute, 1101 Bates Street, Suite P-357, P.O. Box 20345, Houston, TX 77225-0345 · 713-791-3000

Grady L. Hallman, Jr. · Pediatric Cardiac Surgery · St. Luke's Episcopal Hospital, Texas Heart Institute · Texas Heart Institute, 1101 Bates Street, Suite P-514, Houston, TX 77030 · 713-791-4129

J. F. Howell · Adult Cardiothoracic Surgery (General Thoracic Surgery, General Vascular Surgery) · Methodist Hospital · Methodist Hospital, 6535 Fannin Street, Room A-802, Houston, TX 77030-2705 · 713-797-1724

James J. Livesay · General Thoracic Surgery (Adult Cardiothoracic Surgery) · St. Luke's Episcopal Hospital, Texas Heart Institute · Texas Heart Institute, 1101 Bates Street, Suite P-514, Houston, TX 77030 · 713-791-4976

Jonathan C. Nesbitt · General Thoracic Surgery (Lung Surgery, Lung Cancer, Esophageal Cancer, Benign Diseases of the Esophagus and Lung, Pediatric Non-Cardiac Thoracic Surgery) · University of Texas-M. D. Anderson Cancer Center University of Texas-M. D. Anderson Cancer Center, Department of Thoracic and Cardiovascular Surgery, 1515 Holcombe Boulevard, Box 109, Houston, TX 77030-4095 · 713-792-6932

George P. Noon · Adult Cardiothoracic Surgery (Transplantation) · Methodist Hospital, St. Luke's Episcopal Hospital, Hermann Hospital, Texas Children's Hospital · Baylor College of Medicine, 6550 Fannin Street, Suite 1619, Houston, TX 77030 · 713-790-3155

David A. Ott · Adult Cardiothoracic Surgery, Pediatric Cardiac Surgery · Texas Heart Institute, St. Luke's Episcopal Hospital, Texas Children's Hospital · Texas Heart Institute, 1101 Bates Street, Suite P-514, P.O. Box 20345, Houston, TX 77225-0345 · 713-791-4917

Joe B. Putnam, Jr. · General Thoracic Surgery (Thoracic Oncological Surgery, Esophageal Diseases) · University of Texas-M. D. Anderson Cancer Center, Hermann Hospital · University of Texas-M. D. Anderson Cancer Center, Department of Thoracic Surgery and Cardiovascular Surgery, 1515 Holcombe Boulevard, Box 109, Houston, TX 77030-4095 · 713-792-6932

Michael J. Reardon · Adult Cardiothoracic Surgery (General Thoracic Surgery, Thoracic Oncological Surgery) · Methodist Hospital · Baylor College of Medicine, 6550 Fannin Street, Suite 2435, Houston, TX 77030 · 713-798-6633

George J. Reul · Adult Cardiothoracic Surgery (Pediatric Cardiac Surgery, General Vascular Surgery) · Texas Heart Institute, St. Luke's Episcopal Hospital, Texas Children's Hospital · Texas Heart Institute, 1101 Bates Street, Suite 0298H, P.O. Box 20345, Houston, TX 77225-0345 · 713-791-4929

Jack A. Roth · General Thoracic Surgery, Thoracic Oncological Surgery · University of Texas-M. D. Anderson Cancer Center · University of Texas-M. D. Anderson Cancer Center, Department of Thoracic Surgery and Cardiovascular Surgery, 1515 Holcombe Boulevard, Box 109, Houston, TX 77030 · 713-792-6932

Hazim Jawad Safi · Adult Cardiothoracic Surgery (Aortic Aneurysm) · Methodist Hospital · Baylor College of Medicine, 6550 Fannin Street, Suite 1603, Houston, TX 77030 · 713-790-4597

Michael S. Sweeney · Adult Cardiothoracic Surgery · 6431 Fannin Street, Suite 1.220, Houston, TX 77030 · 713-796-1121

Lubbock

Donald L. Bricker · Adult Cardiothoracic Surgery (General Thoracic Surgery, Thoracic Oncological Surgery) · St. Mary of the Plains Hospital, Lubbock Methodist Hospital · Southwestern Cardiovascular Surgery Associates, 3420 Twenty-Second Place, Lubbock, TX 79410 · 806-792-8185

San Antonio

John H. Calhoon · Pediatric Cardiac Surgery, Transplantation (Heart & Lung Transplantation, Adult Cardiac Surgery) · University Hospital-South Texas Medical Center, Audie L. Murphy Memorial Veterans Hospital · University of Texas Health Science Center at San Antonio, Department of Surgery, Division of Cardiothoracic Surgery, 7703 Floyd Curl Drive, San Antonio, TX 78284-7841 · 210-567-5615

Lawrence R. Hamner III · Adult Cardiothoracic Surgery (General Vascular Surgery, Thoracoscopic Surgery) · Methodist Healthcare System, St. Luke's Baptist Hospital, Baptist Memorial Healthcare System, San Antonio Community Hospital, Santa Rosa Health Care, Nix Health Care System, Metropolitan Hospital · 4330 Medical Drive, Suite 300, San Antonio, TX 78229-3324 · 210-616-0008

Javier J. Marcos · Adult Cardiothoracic Surgery · South Texas Cardiovascular Center, 4330 Medical Drive, Suite 275, San Antonio, TX 78229-3324 · 210-615-6626

James Bruce McGovern · Pediatric Non-Cardiac Thoracic Surgery (Pediatric Surgery) · Southwest Texas Methodist Hospital · 7711 Louis Pasteur Drive, Suite 311, San Antonio, TX 78229 · 210-616-0693

Otto LaWayne Miller, Jr. · Adult Cardiothoracic Surgery · University Hospital-South Texas Medical Center · University of Texas Health Science Center at San Antonio, Department of Surgery, Division of Cardiothoracic Surgery, 7703 Floyd Curl Drive, San Antonio, TX 78284-7841 · 210-567-5615

Charles H. Moore III · Adult Cardiothoracic Surgery (Heart Transplantation, Adult Cardiovascular Surgery) · San Antonio Community Hospital, Southwest Texas Methodist Hospital · 8201 Ewing Halsell Drive, Suite 210, San Antonio, TX 78229 · 210-616-0837

Edward Yoshiaki Sako · Adult Cardiothoracic Surgery (Heart and Lung Transplantation, Lung Preservation [Research]) · University Hospital-South Texas Medical Center, Audie L. Murphy Memorial Veterans Hospital · University of Texas Health Science Center at San Antonio, Department of Surgery, Division of Cardiothoracic Surgery, 7703 Floyd Curl Drive, San Antonio, TX 78284-7841 · 210-567-5615

John Marvin Smith III · Adult Cardiothoracic Surgery (General Vascular Surgery) Southwest Texas Methodist Hospital · CardioThoracic Surgical Associates, South Texas Cardiovascular Center, Suite 300, 4330 Medical Drive, San Antonio, TX 78229-3326 · 210-616-0008

Melvin Douglas Smith · Pediatric Non-Cardiac Thoracic Surgery (Thoracic, Abdominal, Neonatal Surgery, Congenital Anomalies of the Thorax [Ribs and Vertebrae], General Surgery, General Surgical Oncology) · Southwest Texas Methodist Hospital, Santa Rosa Health Care, Santa Rosa Children's Hospital, Women's & Children's Hospital · Diagnostic Clinic of San Antonio MedPlex, 5282 Medical Drive, Suite 450, San Antonio, TX 78229-6024 · 210-692-7337

Venkatesan Srinivasan · Adult Cardiothoracic Surgery, Pediatric Cardiac Surgery · Northeast Baptist Hospital · 1303 McCullough Avenue, Suite 429, San Antonio, TX 78212 · 210-226-1334

J. Kent Trinkle · General Thoracic Surgery, Transplantation (Lung Transplantation) · University Hospital-South Texas Medical Center · University of Texas Health Science Center at San Antonio, Department of Surgery, Division of Cardiothoracic Surgery, 7703 Floyd Curl Drive, San Antonio, TX 78284-7841 · 210-567-5617

Leopoldo Zorrilla · Adult Cardiothoracic Surgery (Heart Transplantation) · Southwest Texas Methodist Hospital, Metropolitan Hospital, St. Luke's Baptist Hospital, San Antonio Community Hospital, Baptist Medical Center · 4330 Medical Drive, Suite 325, San Antonio, TX 78229 · 210-615-1777

Tyler

Charles H. Lee · General Thoracic Surgery · Cardiovascular Surgery, 800 East Dawson Street, P.O. Box 150, Tyler, TX 75710 · 903-595-6680

Peter M. Sanfelippo · General Thoracic Surgery (Cardiac Surgery, Peripheral Vascular Surgery) · University of Texas Health Center-Tyler · University of Texas Health Center-Tyler, Department of Surgery, US Highway 271 and State Highway 155, P.O. Box 2003, Tyler, TX 75710-2003 · 903-877-7457

William F. Turner, Jr. · General Thoracic Surgery (Adult Cardiothoracic Surgery) · Trinity Mother Frances Health Care Center, East Texas Medical Center · Cardiovascular Surgery, 800 East Dawson Street, P.O. Box 150, Tyler, TX 75710 · 903-595-6680

Waco

Robert W. Crosthwait, Jr. · Adult Cardiothoracic Surgery · Providence Health Center, Hillcrest Baptist Medical Center · Cardiovascular Associates, 405 Londonderry Drive, Suite 200, Waco, TX 76712-7996 · 817-772-2300

Philip H. Croyle · General Thoracic Surgery (Adult Cardiothoracic Surgery) · Providence Health Center, Hillcrest Baptist Medical Center · Cardiovascular Associates, 405 Londonderry Drive, Suite 200, Waco, TX 76712 · 817-772-2300

William A. Peper · General Thoracic Surgery (Adult Cardiothoracic Surgery, Surgical Critical Care) · Providence Health Center, Hillcrest Baptist Medical Center · Cardiovascular Associates, Providence Medical Plaza, Suite 200, 405 Londonderry Drive, Waco, TX 76712 · 817-772-2300

UROLOGY

Abilene

William D. Davis · General Urology · 1149 Ambler Street, Abilene, TX 79601 · 915-673-7871

T. Harrop Miller · General Urology (Pediatric Urology, Urologic Oncology) · Abilene Regional Medical Center, Hendrick Medical Center · 6250 Regional Plaza, Suite 1000, Abilene, TX 79606 · 915-695-5000

Amarillo

Richard G. Kibbey III · General Urology · Amarillo Urology, 1901 Medical Park Drive, Amarillo, TX 79106 · 806-355-9447

Virgil A. Pate III · General Urology · St. Anthony's Hospital · Amarillo Urology, 1901 Medical Park Drive, Amarillo, TX 79106 · 806-355-9447

Austin

Richard T. Chopp · Urologic Oncology · Austin Diagnostic Medical Center, 12221 MoPac Expressway North, P.O. Box 85075, Austin, TX 78708-5075 · 512-901-4021

Stephen Walter Hardeman · General Urology · Austin Diagnostic Medical Center, 12221 MoPac Expressway North, P.O. Box 85075, Austin, TX 78708-5075 · 512-901-4021

David L. McCarron · General Urology · Seton Medical Center · 3100 Red River Street, Austin, TX 78705 · 512-477-5905

Jan N. Ogletree · General Urology (Pediatric Urology, Impotence) · Seton Medical Center, Children's Hospital of Austin · Austin Genito-Urinary Associates, 3705 Medical Parkway, Suite 515, Austin, TX 78705 · 512-450-1111

Larry E. Phillips · General Urology (Endourology, Urologic Oncology) · Seton Medical Center · 3100 Red River Street, Austin, TX 78705-3214 · 512-477-5905

John P. Schneider · General Urology (Bladder Cancer, Prostate Cancer, Stone Disease, Incontinence, Urologic Oncology) · St. David's Healthcare Center, Seton Medical Center, Brackenridge Hospital · Park Saint David's, 900 East 30th Street, Suite 215, Austin, TX 78705 · 512-478-1727

Beaumont

Joseph Denton Harris IV · General Urology (Prostatic Surgery) · St. Elizabeth Hospital, Baptist Hospital Beaumont, Beaumont Regional Medical Center · 2900 North Street, Suite 204, Beaumont, TX 77702 · 409-899-4111

John A. Henderson IV · General Urology · St. Elizabeth Hospital · 2900 North Street, Suite 204, Beaumont, TX 77702 · 409-899-4111

George S. Hoffman · General Urology · St. Elizabeth Hospital · 2955 Harrison Street, Suite 307, Beaumont, TX 77702-1157 · 409-892-2000

Brownsville

John Jaderlund · General Urology · 844 Central Boulevard, Suite 430, Brownsville, TX 78520 · 210-544-7833

Bryan

Alan K. Young, Jr. · General Urology · St. Joseph Regional Health Center · 1404 Bristol Street, Bryan, TX 77802 · 409-779-6615

Ralph R. Young, Jr. · General Urology · St. Joseph Regional Health Center · 1404 Bristol Street, Bryan, TX 77802 · 409-779-6615

Corpus Christi

John F. Cram · General Urology · Urology Associates, 613 Elizabeth Street, Suite 608, Corpus Christi, TX 78404-2227 · 512-888-5318

Martin E. Hanisch · General Urology (Impotence, Endourology) · Spohn Hospital, Doctors Regional Medical Center, Bay Area Medical Center, Driscoll Children's Hospital · 1521 South Staples Street, Suite 803, Corpus Christi, TX 78404-3152 · 512-884-6381

F. James McCutchon · General Urology (Endourology, Urologic Oncology) · Spohn Hospital, Spohn Hospital South, Spohn Kleberg Memorial Hospital (Kingsville), Doctors Regional Medical Center, Bay Area Medical Center · Urology Associates, 613 Elizabeth Street, Suite 608, Corpus Christi, TX 78404-2227 · 512-888-5318

Gordon R. Welch, Jr. · General Urology (Impotence, Endourology) · Spohn Hospital, Doctors Regional Medical Center, Bay Area Medical Center · Urology Group, 1521 South Staples Street, Suite 803, Corpus Christi, TX 78404 · 512-884-6381

Dallas

Terry D. Allen · Pediatric Urology · Children's Medical Center of Dallas · Children's Medical Center of Dallas, Bank One Building, 14th Floor, 6300 Harry Hines Boulevard, Dallas, TX 75235 · 214-640-2480

James S. Cochran · General Urology · Urology Specialists, 8210 Walnut Hill Lane, Suite 208, Dallas, TX 75231 · 214-691-1902

David H. Ewalt · Pediatric Urology (Neuro-Urology & Voiding Dysfunction [Pediatric only]) · Children's Medical Center of Dallas, Baylor University Medical Center, Medical City Dallas Hospital, Presbyterian Hospital of Dallas, Presbyterian Hospital of Plano (Plano) · Baylor University Medical Center, Barnett Tower, Suite 1205, 3600 Gaston Avenue, Dallas, TX 75246 · 214-826-6021; 214-368-8163

Steven M. Frost · General Urology (Urologic Oncology) · Baylor University Medical Center · Baylor University Medical Center, Barnett Tower, Suite 1205, 3600 Gaston Avenue, Dallas, TX 75246-1812 · 214-826-6021

Pat Fox Fulgham · General Urology (Urologic Oncology, Laparoscopic Surgery, Imaging, Endourology, Impotence) · Presbyterian Hospital of Dallas · Urology Specialists, Presbyterian Professional Building, Suite 208, 8210 Walnut Hill Lane, Dallas, TX 75231 · 214-691-1902

Lon Michael Goldstein · Pediatric Urology (Urologic Oncology) · Children's Medical Center of Dallas, Baylor University Medical Center, Presbyterian Hospital of Dallas, Medical City Dallas Hospital · Baylor University Medical Center, Barnett Tower, Suite 1205, 3600 Gaston Avenue, Dallas, TX 75246-1812 · 214-826-6021

George E. Hurt, Jr. · General Urology (Pediatric, Adult) · Presbyterian Hospital of Dallas, Baylor University Medical Center · Baylor University Medical Center, Barnett Tower, Suite 1205, 3600 Gaston Avenue, Dallas, TX 75246-1812 · 214-826-6021

John Dowling McConnell · General Urology (Prostate Disease) · Zale Lipshy University Hospital, Parkland Memorial Hospital · University of Texas-Southwestern Medical Center at Dallas, Division of Urology, 5323 Harry Hines Boulevard, Dallas, TX 75235-9110 · 214-648-4765

Donald L. McKay, Jr. · General Urology (Female Incontinence, Impotence, Urologic Oncology, Pediatric Urology) · Medical City Dallas Hospital, St. Paul Medical Center · Medical City Dallas Hospital, Building A, Suite 230, 7777 Forest Lane, Dallas, TX 75230 · 214-661-7765; 214-879-8541

Arthur I. Sagalowsky · Urologic Oncology, Transplantation · Zale Lipshy University Hospital · University of Texas-Southwestern Medical Center at Dallas, 5323 Harry Hines Boulevard, Dallas, TX 75235-9110 · 214-648-3976

Robert C. Schoenvogel · General Urology · Baylor University Medical Center · Charles A. Sammons Cancer Center, 3409 Worth Street, Suite 540, Dallas, TX 75246 · 214-827-1602

Key H. Stage · General Urology (Urologic Oncology, Endourology) · Baylor University Medical Center · Baylor University Medical Center, Barnett Tower, Suite 907, 3600 Gaston Avenue, Dallas, TX 75246 · 214-826-8844

Philippe E. Zimmern · Neuro-Urology & Voiding Dysfunction · University of Texas-Southwestern Medical Center at Dallas, 5323 Harry Hines Boulevard, Room J8112, Dallas, TX 75235-9110 · 214-648-9395

El Paso

Fernando Diaz-Ball · General Urology · Texas Tech University Health Sciences Center, Department of Surgery, 4800 Alberta Avenue, El Paso, TX 79905 · 915-545-6880

David O. Taber · General Urology (Infertility-Sterility, Renal Calculus Disease, Prostate Diseases) · Providence Memorial Hospital · 125 West Hague Road, Suite 170, El Paso, TX 79902 · 915-533-0800

Fort Sam Houston

Ian M. Thompson, Jr. · Urologic Oncology · Brooke Army Medical Center · Brooke Army Medical Center, Urology Service, Department of Surgery, 2450 Stanley Road, Fort Sam Houston, TX 78234-6219 · 210-916-6163

Fort Worth

J. Daniel Johnson · General Urology (Incontinence, Vaginal Urology) · Fort Worth Urology Clinic, 1415 Pennsylvania Avenue, Fort Worth, TX 76104-2113 · 817-336-5711

Robert J. Murchison · General Urology · All Saints Episcopal Hospital-Fort Worth · Associates in Urology, 1650 West Magnolia Street, Suite 204, Fort Worth, TX 76104 · 817-921-5131

V. Gary Price · General Urology · Harris Methodist-Fort Worth · Associates in Urology, 1821 Eighth Avenue, Fort Worth, TX 76110-1351 · 817-923-7353

Addison E. Thurman · General Urology (Urologic Oncology, Impotence) · Harris Methodist-Fort Worth, Plaza Medical Center, All Saints Episcopal Hospital-Fort Worth, All Saints Hospital-City View · Fort Worth Urology Clinic, 1415 Pennsylvania Avenue, Fort Worth, TX 76104-2113 · 817-336-5711

Sidney A. Worsham III · General Urology · 800 Eighth Avenue, Suite 626, Fort Worth, TX 76104-2605 · 817-877-1288

Galveston

Durwood E. Neal, Jr. · General Urology (Kidney Stones) · University of Texas Medical Branch, Department of Surgery, Division of Urology, 301 University Boulevard, Galveston, TX 77555-0540 · 409-772-2091

Eduardo Orihuela · Urologic Oncology · University of Texas Medical Branch, Department of Surgery, Division of Urology, 301 University Boulevard, Galveston, TX 77555-0540 · 409-772-2091

Michael M. Warren · General Urology · University of Texas Medical Branch Hospitals · University of Texas Medical Branch, Department of Urology, 301 University Boulevard, Galveston, TX 77555-0540 · 409-772-2091

Houston

Richard J. Babaian · Urologic Oncology (Prostate) · University of Texas-M. D. Anderson Cancer Center · University of Texas-M. D. Anderson Cancer Center, 1515 Holcombe Boulevard, Box 110, Houston, TX 77030 · 713-792-3250

George S. Benson · Impotence, Neuro-Urology & Voiding Dysfunction (Implants) · Lyndon B. Johnson General Hospital, Hermann Hospital · University of Texas Medical School at Houston, 6431 Fannin Street, Room 6.018, Houston, TX 77030 · 713-792-5640

Timothy Boone · Neuro-Urology & Voiding Dysfunction (Urodynamics, Incontinence) · Methodist Hospital · Baylor College of Medicine, Scott Department of Urology, 6560 Fannin Street, Suite 1002, Houston, TX 77030 · 713-798-4001

C. David Cawood · General Urology (Prostate Cancer, Urinary Stones, Endourology, Urologic Oncology) · Methodist Hospital, St. Luke's Episcopal Hospital, Texas Children's Hospital · Houston Urologic Associates, 6560 Fannin Street, Suite 1270, Houston, TX 77030 · 713-790-9779

Joseph N. Corriere, Jr. · General Urology (Reconstructive Urology) · Hermann Hospital · University of Texas Medical School at Houston, 6431 Fannin Street, Room 6.018, Houston, TX 77030 · 713-792-5640

Irving J. Fishman · Impotence (Implants) · St. Luke's Episcopal Hospital, Methodist Hospital, Texas Children's Hospital · Baylor College of Medicine, 6624 Fannin Street, Suite 1280, Houston, TX 77030 · 713-798-5150

Edmond T. Gonzales · Pediatric Urology · Texas Children's Hospital · Texas Children's Hospital, 6621 Fannin Street, Suite 270, Houston, TX 77030 · 713-770-3160

Donald P. Griffith · Endourology (Stone Disease, Ureteroscopy, Prostate Cancer, Renal Cancer, Interstitial Cystitis) · Methodist Hospital, St. Luke's Episcopal Hospital, Memorial Hospital-Memorial City, Spring Branch Medical Center · Uro-Center of Houston, 6624 Fannin Street, Suite 2280, Houston, TX 77030 · 713-799-8899

H. Barton Grossman · Urologic Oncology · University of Texas-M. D. Anderson Cancer Center · University of Texas-M. D. Anderson Cancer Center, 1515 Holcombe Boulevard, Box 110, Houston, TX 77030-4095 · 713-792-3250

Paul B. Handel · General Urology · Hermann Hospital · 1213 Hermann Drive, Suite 675, Houston, TX 77004 · 713-522-1118

Seth Paul Lerner · Urologic Oncology (Urinary Tract Reconstruction) · Methodist Hospital, Texas Children's Hospital, St. Luke's Episcopal Hospital, Ben Taub General Hospital, VA Medical Center, Diagnostic Clinic · Baylor College of Medicine, 6560 Fannin Street, Suite 2100, Houston, TX 77030 · 713-798-6841

Larry I. Lipshultz · Impotence (Male Infertility) · Methodist Hospital, St. Luke's Episcopal Hospital · Baylor College of Medicine, 6560 Fannin Street, Suite 2100, Houston, TX 77030 · 713-798-6163

Edward J. McGuire · Neuro-Urology & Voiding Dysfunction (Incontinence) · University of Texas Health Science Center, Hermann Hospital, University of Texas-M. D. Anderson Cancer Center, Methodist Hospital · University of Texas Medical School at Houston, 6431 Fannin Street, Room 6.018, Houston, TX 77030 713-792-5640

Ronald A. Morton, Jr. · General Urology (Urologic Oncology, Prostate Cancer) · Methodist Hospital, St. Luke's Episcopal Hospital · Baylor College of Medicine, Department of Urology, 6550 Fannin Street, Suite 2100, Houston, TX 77030 · 713-798-8820

Michael L. Ritchey · Pediatric Urology · Hermann Hospital, Texas Children's Hospital · 6410 Fannin Street, Suite 622, Houston, TX 77030 · 713-704-5869

David R. Roth · Pediatric Urology · Texas Children's Hospital · Texas Children's Hospital, 6621 Fannin Street, Suite 270, Houston, TX 77030 · 713-770-3160

Peter T. Scardino · Urologic Oncology · Methodist Hospital · Baylor College of Medicine, 6560 Fannin Street, Suite 1035, Houston, TX 77030 · 713-798-6153

Kevin Slawin · Urologic Oncology (Benign Prostatic Hypertrophy) · Baylor College of Medicine, Department of Urology, 6550 Fannin Street, Suite 2100, Houston, TX 77030 · 713-798-4001

David A. Swanson · (Urologic Oncology) · University of Texas-M. D. Anderson Cancer Center · University of Texas-M. D. Anderson Cancer Center, Department of Urology, 1515 Holcombe Boulevard, Box 110, Houston, TX 77030 · 713-792-3250

Andrew C. von Eschenbach · Urologic Oncology · University of Texas-M. D. Anderson Cancer Center · University of Texas-M. D. Anderson Cancer Center, 1515 Holcombe Boulevard, Box 110, Houston, TX 77030-4095 · 713-792-3250

Kerrville

Randolph C. Zuber · General Urology (Prostate Cancer) · Sid Peterson Memorial Hospital · Sid Peterson Memorial Hospital, Department of Urology, 710 Water Street, Suite 300, Kerrville, TX 78028 · 210-257-7533

Laredo

Carlos H. Mata · General Urology · Doctors Hospital of Laredo, Mercy Regional Health Center · Doctors Hospital of Laredo, Department of Urology, 500 East Mann Road, Suite E, Laredo, TX 78041 · 210-722-5262

Longview

John M. Ferrell · General Urology · Good Shepherd Medical Center, Longview Regional Hospital · 806 Medical Circle Drive, Suite 400, Longview, TX 75601 · 903-757-2502

Lubbock

Odis Lynn Avant · General Urology (Neuro-Urology & Voiding Dysfunction, Urologic Oncology) · Lubbock Methodist Hospital, St. Mary of the Plains Hospital Lubbock Urology Clinic, 4102 Twenty-Second Place, Lubbock, TX 79410 · 806-795-9384

Jonathan S. Vordermark II · Pediatric Urology · University Medical Center · Texas Tech University Health Sciences Center, Department of Urology University Associates, Medical Office Plaza, Suite 260, 3502 Ninth Street, Lubbock, TX 79415 · 806-743-1810

Midland

Michael J. Dragun · General Urology · West Texas Urology, 2203 West Tennessee Avenue, Midland, TX 79701 · 915-687-0311

John B. Staub · General Urology · Memorial Hospital & Medical Center · West Texas Urology, 2203 West Tennessee Avenue, Midland, TX 79701 · 915-687-0311

San Angelo

John S. Ballard III · General Urology · Angelo Community Hospital · West Texas Medical Associates, 3555 Knickerbocker Road, San Angelo, TX 76904-7610 · 915-949-9555

John P. Coughlin · General Urology · 2030 Pulliam Street, Suite One, San Angelo, TX 76905 · 915-653-4206

Jack S. Rice, Jr. · General Urology · Angelo Community Hospital · West Texas Medical Associates, 3555 Knickerbocker Road, San Angelo, TX 76904-7610 · 915-949-9555

San Antonio

Thomas P. Ball, Jr. · General Urology (Impotence, Incontinence, Reconstructive Surgery) · University Hospital-South Texas Medical Center, Audie L. Murphy Memorial Veterans Hospital · University of Texas Health Science Center at San Antonio, Department of Urology, 7703 Floyd Curl Drive, San Antonio, TX 78284-7845 · 210-567-5640

Lynn H. Banowsky · General Urology (Renal Transplantation) · Urology Consultants, 8038 Wurzbach Road, Suite 430, San Antonio, TX 78229 · 210-616-0410

Thomas H. Bartholomew · Pediatric Urology · Southwest Texas Methodist Hospital · 4499 Medical Drive, Suite 101, San Antonio, TX 78229 · 210-692-0368

George V. Burkholder · General Urology (Urologic Oncology, Kidney Stones) · Urology Clinic of San Antonio, 4410 Medical Drive, Suite 300, San Antonio, TX 78229 · 210-614-4544

George D. Case · General Urology · Nix Health Care System · 914 Nix Professional Building, 414 Navarro Street, San Antonio, TX 78205-2562 · 210-225-7191

Arthur Santana Centeno · General Urology · Santa Rosa Health Care · Urologic Surgical Associates, Santa Rosa Professional Pavilion, Suite 990, 315 North San Saba, San Antonio, TX 78207 · 210-226-7020

William P. Fitch III · Impotence (Penile Revascularization, Penile Prosthetics, Prostate Cancer) · San Antonio Community Hospital · Urology Consultants, 8038 Wurzbach Road, Suite 430, San Antonio, TX 78229 · 210-616-0410

Clayton Howard Hudnall · General Urology · Urologic Surgical Associates, Santa Rosa Professional Pavilion, Suite 990, 315 North San Saba, San Antonio, TX 78207 · 210-226-7020

Jerry E. Kruse · General Urology · Metropolitan Hospital · Urology Associates, 1303 McCullough Avenue, Suite 561, San Antonio, TX 78212 · 210-227-9376

Edward James Mueller · General Urology (Contact Laser Prostatectomy, Stress Urinary Incontinence in Females, Impotence) · Baptist Medical Center, San Antonio Community Hospital, Santa Rosa Northwest Hospital, Southwest Texas Methodist Hospital · Methodist Plaza, Suite 261, 4499 Medical Drive, San Antonio, TX 78229 · 210-614-0222

Michael E. Newell · General Urology · Southwest Texas Methodist Hospital · Urology Clinic of San Antonio, 4410 Medical Drive, Suite 300, San Antonio, TX 78229 · 210-614-4544

Thomas Kevin O'Neill · General Urology · Southwest Texas Methodist Hospital · Urology Clinic of San Antonio, 4410 Medical Drive, Suite 300, San Antonio, TX 78229 · 210-614-4544

Juan A. Reyna · General Urology (Female Urology, Urologic Oncology, Endourology, Neuro-Urology & Voiding Dysfunction) · Santa Rosa Health Care · Urologic Surgical Associates, Santa Rosa Professional Pavilion, Suite 990, 315 North San Saba, San Antonio, TX 78207 · 210-226-7020

Elizabeth Lipscombe Ritchie · Pediatric Urology · Women's & Children's Hospital, Southwest Texas Methodist Hospital, Santa Rosa Children's Hospital · 8211 Fredericksburg Road, San Antonio, TX 78229 · 210-616-0895

Lewis F. Russell, Jr. · General Urology (Prostate Disease) · Baptist Medical Center, Nix Health Care System · 8500 Village Drive, Suite 300, San Antonio, TX 78217 · 210-655-2411

Michael F. Sarosdy · Urologic Oncology · University of Texas Health Science Center at San Antonio · University of Texas Health Science Center at San Antonio, Division of Urology, 7703 Floyd Curl Drive, San Antonio, TX 78284-7845 · 210-567-5643

William W. Schuessler · Endourology (Laparoscopy, Stones, Incontinence, Prostate Cancer) · Southeast Baptist Hospital · 4242 East Southcross Boulevard, Suite 11, San Antonio, TX 78222 · 210-333-9010

Rene A. Sepulveda · General Urology · Urologic Surgical Associates, Santa Rosa Professional Pavilion, Suite 990, 315 North San Saba, San Antonio, TX 78207 · 210-226-7020

Randall P. Singleton · General Urology (Endourology, Urologic Oncology) · St. Luke's Baptist Hospital, Southwest Texas Methodist Hospital, San Antonio Community Hospital, Santa Rosa Health Care · Urology Clinic of San Antonio, 4410 Medical Drive, Suite 300, San Antonio, TX 78229 · 210-614-4544

C. Ritchie Spence · General Urology (Impotence, Urologic Oncology) · Southwest Texas Methodist Hospital · Urology Clinic of San Antonio, 4410 Medical Drive, Suite 300, San Antonio, TX 78229 · 210-614-4544

Sherman

Roberto L. Oliveras, Jr. · General Urology · 1117 Gallagher Road, Suite 20, P.O. Box 1337, Sherman, TX 75091 · 903-892-5577

Temple

K. Scott Coffield · General Urology · Scott & White Memorial Hospital · Scott & White Memorial Hospital, Department of Urology, 2401 South 31st Street, Temple, TX 76508-0001 · 817-724-4178

T. Philip Reilly · General Urology (Urologic Oncology) · Scott & White Memorial Hospital · Scott & White Memorial Hospital, Department of Urology, 2401 South 31st Street, Temple, TX 76508-0001 · 817-724-1773

Tyler

Stanton P. Champion · General Urology · Trinity Mother Frances Health Care Center, East Texas Medical Center · Urology Tyler, 910 East Houston Street, Suite 470, Tyler, TX 75702 · 903-597-4424

R. Stephen Hillis · General Urology · East Texas Medical Center, Trinity Mother Frances Health Care Center · Urology Tyler, 910 East Houston Street, Suite 470, Tyler, TX 75702 · 903-597-4424

James F. McAndrews · General Urology · Urology Tyler, 910 East Houston Street, Suite 470, Tyler, TX 75702 · 903-597-4424

Waco

Robert F. Corwin · General Urology (Pediatric Urology, Endourology) · Hillcrest Baptist Medical Center, Providence Health Center · 2911 Herring Drive, Suite 310, Waco, TX 76708-3244 · 817-755-4500

Stephen H. Corwin · General Urology (Pediatric Urology, Endourology) · Hillcrest Baptist Medical Center, Providence Health Center · 2911 Herring Drive, Suite 310, Waco, TX 76708-3244 · 817-755-4500

Donald A. Stewart · General Urology · Central Texas Urologic Associates, 3408 Hillcrest Drive, Waco, TX 76708 · 817-752-1611

Mark W. Story · General Urology · Hillcrest Baptist Medical Center, Providence Health Center · Central Texas Urologic Associates, 3408 Hillcrest Drive, Waco, TX 76708 · 817-752-1611

Wichita Falls

John S. Dryden · General Urology · Wichita General Hospital · Urology Clinic, 1630 Eleventh Street, Wichita Falls, TX 76301 · 817-723-8195

WYOMING

ADDICTION MEDICINE

Casper

Berton Toews · General Addiction Medicine · 2417 East 15th Street, Casper, WY 82609 · 307-265-3791

ALLERGY & IMMUNOLOGY

Cheyenne

Russell I. Williams, Jr. · General Allergy & Immunology (Pediatric Allergy & Immunology) · Cheyenne Allergy and Asthma Clinic, 414 East 23rd Street, Cheyenne, WY 82001 · 307-634-7905

ANESTHESIOLOGY

Casper

Todd Witzeling · General Anesthesiology · Wyoming Medical Center, 1233 East Second Street, Casper, WY 82601 · 307-577-2123

Cheyenne

J. Sloan Hales · General Anesthesiology · Cheyenne Anesthesia Center, 1920 Evans Avenue, Cheyenne, WY 82001 · 307-635-4255

CARDIOVASCULAR DISEASE

Casper

Wesley W. Hiser · General Cardiovascular Disease · Wyoming Cardio-Pulmonary Services, 1230 East First Street, Casper, WY 82601 · 307-266-3174

Cheyenne

Robert J. Davis · General Cardiovascular Disease · Internal Medicine Group, 1200 East 20th Street, Cheyenne, WY 82001 · 307-635-4141

Michael A. Demos · General Cardiovascular Disease (Cardiac Catheterization, Nuclear Cardiology) · United Medical Center · Cheyenne Internal Medicine & Neurology, 5050 Powderhouse Road, Cheyenne, WY 82009 · 307-634-1311

Lawrence Hattel · General Cardiovascular Disease · Internal Medicine Group, 1200 East 20th Street, Cheyenne, WY 82001 · 307-635-4141

CLINICAL PHARMACOLOGY

Casper

Joseph Steiner · University of Wyoming Family Practice, 1522 East A Street, Casper, WY 82601 · 307-266-3076

DERMATOLOGY

Casper

Rowan E. Tichenor · Clinical Dermatology (Dermatopathology, Skin Cancer Surgery & Reconstruction) · Wyoming Medical Center · 424 South Melrose Street, Casper, WY 82601 · 307-266-2772

Cheyenne

Larry E. Seitz · Clinical Dermatology · United Medical Center · Cheyenne Skin Clinic, 2112 Seymour Avenue, Cheyenne, WY 82001 · 307-635-0226

Sandra K. Surbrugg · Clinical Dermatology · Cheyenne Skin Clinic, 2112 Seymour Avenue, Cheyenne, WY 82001 · 307-635-0226

ENDOCRINOLOGY & METABOLISM

Cheyenne

Eric J. Wedell · General Endocrinology & Metabolism · Internal Medicine Group, 1200 East 20th Street, Cheyenne, WY 82001 · 307-635-4141

FAMILY MEDICINE

Cheyenne

John C. Carmen II · Frontier Family Medicine, 2029 Bluegrass Circle, Suite 200, Cheyenne, WY 82009 · 307-632-1957

Michael C. Herber · (Sports Medicine, Preventive Care/Health Maintenance, Geriatric Medicine) · United Medical Center · 3001 Henderson Drive, Suite F, Cheyenne, WY 82001 · 307-778-2577

GASTROENTEROLOGY

Casper

Charles L. Lyford · General Gastroenterology · Internal Medicine and Gastroenterology Associates, 167 South Conwell Street, Suite Four, Casper, WY 82601 · 307-265-1792

Cheyenne

Kenneth Kranz · General Gastroenterology · Internal Medicine Group, 1200 East 20th Street, Cheyenne, WY 82001 · 307-635-4141 .

Thomas G. Tietjen · General Gastroenterology · Internal Medicine Group, 1200 East 20th Street, Cheyenne, WY 82001 · 307-635-4141

HAND SURGERY

Cheyenne

John E. Winter · General Hand Surgery · 6020 Yellowstone Road, Cheyenne, WY 82009 · 307-634-0872

INFECTIOUS DISEASE

Casper

Mark E. Dowell · General Infectious Disease (Respiratory Infections, AIDS) · Wyoming Medical Center · Wyoming Infectious Diseases, 940 East Third Street, Suite 201, Casper, WY 82601 · 307-577-0454

Cheyenne

Philip M. Sharp · General Infectious Disease · Cheyenne Internal Medicine & Neurology, 5050 Powderhouse Road, Cheyenne, WY 82009 · 307-634-1311

INTERNAL MEDICINE (GENERAL)

Casper

Thomas Burke · 940 East Third Street, Casper, WY 82601 · 307-577-4230

Cheyenne

Darryl D. Bindschadler · Internal Medicine Group, 1200 East 20th Street, Cheyenne, WY 82001 · 307-635-4141

Philip M. Sharp · Cheyenne Internal Medicine & Neurology, 5050 Powderhouse Road, Cheyenne, WY 82009 · 307-634-1311

Jackson

Dennis L. Butcher · Teton Internal Medicine, 555 East Broadway, Suite 220, Box 3009, Jackson, WY 83001-3009 · 307-733-7222

Laramie

W. Jean Coates · Laramie Clinic, 1303 East Grand Avenue, Laramie, WY 82070-4137 · 307-745-4884

Daniel S. Klein · (General Internal Medicine, Cancer Prevention) · Ivinson Memorial Hospital · Intermountain Internal Medicine, 3116 Willet Drive, Laramie, WY 82070 · 307-745-8800

Kenneth L. Robertson · Intermountain Internal Medicine, 3116 Willet Drive, Laramie, WY 82070 · 307-745-8800

Riverton

Roger L. Gose · Internal Medicine Associates, 511 North 12th Street, East, Riverton, WY 82501-3805 · 307-856-4176

Sheridan

Christopher C. Brown · (General Internal Medicine, General Infectious Disease, General Allergy & Immunology) · Memorial Hospital of Sheridan County · 1058 Kentucky, Sheridan, WY 82801 · 307-674-5366

NEPHROLOGY

Cheyenne

Jean A. Halpern · General Nephrology (General Internal Medicine) · United Medical Center · Associates in Internal Medicine, 1111 Logan Avenue, Cheyenne, WY 82001 · 307-635-9131

NEUROLOGICAL SURGERY

Cheyenne

George J. Guidry · General Neurological Surgery · 800 East 20th Street, Suite 205, Cheyenne, WY 82007 · 307-778-2860

NEUROLOGY

Casper

Malvin Cole · General Neurology (Behavioral Neurology, Epilepsy) · Wyoming Medical Center · Cole Neurological Associates, 246 South Washington Street, Casper, WY 82601-2921 · 307-234-5004

Kathy Gardner · General Neurology · 1032 East First Street, Casper, WY 82601 307-234-9037

Cheyenne

Daniel G. Johnson · General Neurology · Cheyenne Internal Medicine & Neurology, 5050 Powderhouse Road, Cheyenne, WY 82009 · 307-634-1311

Roy Kanter · General Neurology · Cheyenne Internal Medicine & Neurology, 5050 Powderhouse Road, Cheyenne, WY 82009 · 307-634-1311

Reed C. Shafer · General Neurology (Electrodiagnosis, Electromyography, Headache, Electroencephalography) · United Medical Center · Cheyenne Internal Medicine & Neurology, 5050 Powderhouse Road, Cheyenne, WY 82009 · 307-634-1311

OBSTETRICS & GYNECOLOGY

Casper

Samuel T. Scaling · General Obstetrics & Gynecology (Infertility, Reproductive Surgery) · Wyoming Medical Center · Casper Clinic, 940 East Third Street, Suite 211, Casper, WY 82601 · 307-577-4225

Cheyenne

Robert L. McGuire · General Obstetrics & Gynecology · Cheyenne Obstetrics & Gynecology, 421 East 17th Street, Cheyenne, WY 82001 · 307-634-5216

OPHTHALMOLOGY

Casper

Matthew T. Dodds · General Ophthalmology (Anterior Segment—Cataract) · Wyoming Medical Center · Wyoming Center for Sight, 111 South Jefferson Street, Suite 105, Casper, WY 82601 · 307-237-2511

Cheyenne

Rodney A. Anderson · General Ophthalmology · United Medical Center, Yellowstone Surgery Center · Eye Care Clinic, 6252 Yellowstone Road, Cheyenne, WY 82009-3432 · 307-778-2771

Randolph L. Johnston · Vitreo-Retinal Surgery (Retinal Diseases) · United Medical Center · Cheyenne Eye Clinic, 1300 East 20th Street, Cheyenne, WY 82001 307-634-7765

Sheridan

Jonathan Herschler · Glaucoma (General Ophthalmology) · Memorial Hospital of Sheridan County · Eye Clinic of Northern Wyoming, 350 South Brooks Street, Sheridan, WY 82801 · 307-674-4449

ORTHOPAEDIC SURGERY

Cheyenne

Richard E. Torkelson · General Orthopaedic Surgery · United Medical Center · 800 East 20th Street, Suite 100, Cheyenne, WY 82001 · 307-632-9261

John E. Winter · General Orthopaedic Surgery · 6020 Yellowstone Road, Cheyenne, WY 82009 · 307-634-0872

Jackson

Kenneth L. Lambert · Trauma · Orthopaedics of Jackson Hole, St. John's Hospital, Truman Medical Center (Kansas City, MO) · Orthopaedics of Jackson Hole, 555 East Broadway, P.O. Box 7434, Jackson, WY 83001 · 307-733-3900

Laramie

Robert Curnow · General Orthopaedic Surgery · Gem City Bone and Joint Clinic, 1909 Vista Drive, Laramie, WY 82070-5530 · 307-745-8851

David Kieffer · Sports Medicine/Arthroscopy · Gem City Bone and Joint Clinic, 1909 Vista Drive, Laramie, WY 82070-5539 · 307-745-8851

Richard B. Southwell · Sports Medicine/Arthroscopy · Gem City Bone and Joint Clinic, 1909 Vista Drive, Laramie, WY 82070-5530 · 307-745-8851

OTOLARYNGOLOGY

Casper

Kent T. Christensen · General Otolaryngology (Head & Neck Surgery, Pediatric Otolaryngology, Sinus & Nasal Surgery) · Wyoming Medical Center · Wyoming Otolaryngology, 940 East Third Street, Casper, WY 82601-3237 · 307-577-4240

Cheyenne

William P. Gibbens · General Otolaryngology · United Medical Center · The Southeast Wyoming Ear, Nose and Throat Clinic, 5320 Education Drive, Cheyenne, WY 82009 · 307-632-5589

Joseph M. Vigneri · General Otolaryngology · Wyoming Otolaryngology, 940 East Third Street, Cheyenne, WY 82601-3237 · 307-577-4240

PATHOLOGY

Casper

Gregory A. Brondos · General Pathology · Wyoming Medical Center, 1233 East Second Street, Casper, WY 82601 · 307-577-2365

Cheyenne

Thomas V. Toft · General Pathology · Anapath Diagnostics, 800 East 20th Street, Suite 206, Cheyenne, WY 82001 · 307-635-7931

Ronald W. Waeckerlin · General Pathology · Clinical Laboratories, Anapath Diagnostics, 800 East 20th Street, Suite 105, Cheyenne, WY 82001 · 307-635-7931

Gary L. Yordy · General Pathology · Anapath Diagnostics, 800 East 20th Street, Suite 206, Cheyenne, WY 82001 · 307-635-7931

PEDIATRICS

Cheyenne

Russell I. Williams, Jr. · (Pediatric Allergy & Immunology) · Cheyenne Children's Clinic, 433 East 19th Street, Cheyenne, WY 82001 · 307-635-7961; 307-634-7905

PEDIATRICS (GENERAL)

Casper

Michael Grannum · 940 East Third Street, Casper, WY 82601 · 307-577-4260

Richard D. Green · 940 East Third Street, Casper, WY 82601 · 307-577-4280

Cheyenne

Robert W. Leland · Cheyenne Children's Clinic, 433 East 19th Street, Cheyenne, WY 82001 · 307-635-7961

Gary Melinkovich · Cheyenne Children's Clinic, 433 East 19th Street, Cheyenne, WY 82001 · 307-635-7961

Robert R. Prentice · Cheyenne Children's Clinic, 433 East 19th Street, Cheyenne, WY 82001 · 307-635-7961

Jackson

James R. Little · Jackson Pediatrics, 557 East Broadway, Box 1029, Jackson, WY 83001-1029 · 307-733-4627

PLASTIC SURGERY

Casper

Donald M. Greer · General Plastic Surgery · Wyoming Medical Center, Casper Surgery Center · 1300 East A Street, Suite 209, Casper, WY 82601 · 307-265-1212

Cheyenne

Paul V. Slater · General Plastic Surgery · 2232 Del Range Boulevard, Suite 206, Cheyenne, WY 82009 · 307-638-8987

PSYCHIATRY

Casper

Stephen L. Brown · Child & Adolescent Psychiatry · 2417 East 15th Street, Casper, WY 82609 · 307-234-3638

William L. Clapp · General Psychiatry · 2417 East 15th Street, Casper, WY 82609 307-237-1702

Cheyenne

Arthur N. Merrell · General Psychiatry · Southeast Wyoming Mental Health Center, 2526 Seymour Avenue, P.O. Box 1005, Cheyenne, WY 82003 · 307-634-9653

PULMONARY & CRITICAL CARE MEDICINE

Casper

Wesley W. Hiser · General Pulmonary & Critical Care Medicine · Wyoming Cardio-Pulmonary Services, 1230 East First Street, Casper, WY 82601 · 307-266-3174

Donald D. Smith · General Pulmonary & Critical Care Medicine · Casper Clinic, 940 East Third Street, Suite 201, Casper, WY 82601 · 307-577-0477

Cheyenne

Darryl D. Bindschadler · General Pulmonary & Critical Care Medicine · Internal Medicine Group, 1200 East 20th Street, Cheyenne, WY 82001 · 307-635-4141

RADIOLOGY

Cheyenne

D. Michael Kellam · General Radiology · Cheyenne Radiology, 800 East 20th Street, Suite 11, Cheyenne, WY 82001 · 307-634-7711

RHEUMATOLOGY

Casper

Anne M. MacGuire · General Rheumatology (Osteoarthritis, Scleroderma, Rheumatoid Arthritis) · Wyoming Medical Center · 940 East Third Street, Suite 206, Casper, WY 82601 · 307-577-0445

SURGERY

Casper

James A. Anderson · General Vascular Surgery (General Surgery, General Thoracic Surgery, General Surgical Oncology) · Wyoming Medical Center · Casper Clinic, 940 East Third Street, Suite 202, Casper, WY 82601-3251 · 307-577-4220

Cheyenne

Take G. Pullos · General Surgery · Consultants in Surgery, 5201 Yellowstone Road, Cheyenne, WY 82009 · 307-632-1114

THORACIC SURGERY

Casper

Gary D. Weiss · General Thoracic Surgery · Wyoming Cardiac and Thoracic Surgery, 301 South Fenway Street, Suite 101, Casper, WY 82601 · 307-265-0070

Cheyenne

David G. Silver · General Thoracic Surgery (Cardiovascular Surgery) · United Medical Center · 2232 Del Range Boulevard, Suite 100, Cheyenne, WY 82009 · 307-638-6624

UROLOGY

Casper

Tarver B. Bailey · General Urology · Central Wyoming Urologicals, 301 South Fenway Street, Suite 202, Casper, WY 82601-3053 · 307-577-8600

James B. Haden · General Urology · Central Wyoming Urologicals, 301 South Fenway Street, Suite 202, Casper, WY 82601-3053 · 307-577-8600

Cheyenne

Taylor H. Haynes II · General Urology · 3100 Henderson Drive, Suite 16, Cheyenne, WY 82001 · 307-637-7278

Jackson

Roland Fleck · General Urology · 555 East Broadway, P.O. Box 1766, Jackson, WY 83001 · 307-733-7677

Laramie

Lyman R. Brothers III · General Urology (Urologic Oncology, Pediatric Urology) Ivinson Memorial Hospital, Routt Memorial Hospital (Steamboat Springs, CO) · Urology Clinic, 204 McCollum Drive, Laramie, WY 82070 · 307-745-3097

APPENDIX

Some health problems may be addressed by physicians in more than one specialty. To help the reader better use The Best Doctors in America® regional guides, we have included this guideline for finding various doctors who treat the same diseases or disorders.

Asthma, Allergy
Allergy & Immunology
  General Allergy & Immunology
  Immunodeficiency
Pediatrics
  Pediatric Pulmonology
Pulmonary & Critical Care Medicine
  Asthma
  General Pulmonary & Critical Care
    Medicine

Breast
Endocrinology & Metabolism
  Paget's Disease
Medical Oncology/Hematology
  Breast Cancer
  Lymphomas
Pathology
  Breast Pathology
Plastic Surgery
  Breast Surgery
  Microsurgery
  Reconstructive Surgery
Radiation Oncology
  Breast Cancer
Surgery
  Breast Surgery
  Endocrine Surgery
Surgical Oncology
  Breast Cancer

Cancer
Anesthesiology
  Pain
Clinical Pharmacology
Colon & Rectal Surgery
  Colon & Rectal Cancer
Dermatology
  Aesthetic Surgery

Cutaneous Lymphomas
Melanoma
Skin Cancer Surgery & Reconstruction
Gastroenterology
  Endoscopy
  Gastrointestinal Cancer
  Inflammatory Bowel Disease
Geriatric Medicine
Infectious Disease
  Cancer & Infections
  Transplantation Infections
Medical Oncology/Hematology
  AIDS
  Bone Marrow Transplantation
  Breast Cancer
  Clinical Pharmacology
  Disorders of Bleeding, Thrombosis
  Gastrointestinal Cancer
  General Medical Oncology/Hematology
  Genito-Urinary Cancer
  Prostate Cancer
  Head & Neck Cancer
  Immunotherapy, Cancer Biotherapy
  Leukemia
  Lung Cancer
  Lymphomas
  Myeloma
  Neuro-Oncology
  Solid Tumors
Nephrology
  Cancer of the Kidney
  Kidney Disease
  Kidney Transplantation
Neurology
  General Adult Neurology
  Neuro-Oncology
  Neuro-Rehabilitation
Neurology, Child
  Neuro-Oncology

Neurological Surgery
  Stereotactic Radiosurgery
  Tumor Surgery
Nuclear Medicine
  General Nuclear Medicine
  Oncology
  Radiation Accidents & Injury
Obstetrics & Gynecology
  Gynecologic Cancer
Ophthalmology
  Neuro-Ophthalmology
  Ocular Oncology
Orthopaedic Surgery
  Tumor Surgery
Otolaryngology
  Facial Plastic Surgery
  Head & Neck Surgery
  Laryngology
  Otology/Neurotology
Pediatrics
  Metabolic Diseases
  Pediatric Endocrinology
  Pediatric Hematology-Oncology
  Pediatric Infectious Disease
Psychiatry
  General Psychiatry
Pulmonary & Critical Care Medicine
Radiation Oncology
  Brachytherapy
  Brain Cancer
  Breast Cancer
  Gastrointestinal Cancer
  General Radiation Oncology
  Genito-Urinary Cancer
  Prostate Cancer
  Gynecologic Cancer
  Head & Neck Cancer
  Hypothermia
  Lung Cancer
  Lymphomas
  Particle Beam Radiation
  Pediatric Radiation Oncology
  Radiosurgery
  Sarcomas
Surgery
  Breast Surgery
  Endocrine Surgery
  Gastroenterologic Surgery
  Pediatric Surgery
Surgical Oncology
  Breast Cancer
  Colon & Rectal Cancer
  Gastrointestinal Cancer
  Immunotherapy, Cancer Biotherapy
  Melanoma
Thoracic Surgery
  General Thoracic Surgery
  Pediatric Non-Cardiac Thoracic Surgery
  Thoracic Oncological Surgery

Urology
  Neuro-Urology & Voiding Dysfunction
  Urologic Oncology
  Prostate Cancer

Cardiac/Heart
Anesthesiology
  Adult Cardiovascular
  Cardiothoracic Anesthesiology
  Critical Care Medicine
  General Anesthesiology
  Pain
  Pediatric Cardiovascular
Cardiovascular Disease
  Cardiac Catheterization
  Cardiac Positron Emission Tomography
    (PET)
  Cardiac Rehabilitation
  Clinical Exercise Testing
  Echocardiography
  Electrophysiology
  General Cardiovascular Disease
  Heart Failure
  Magnetic Resonance Imaging
  Nuclear Cardiology
  Pacemakers
  Transplantation Medicine
  Vaso-Spastic Diseases
Clinical Pharmacology
Geriatric Medicine
Infectious Disease
  Endocarditis
  Transplantation Infections
  Vasculitis
Nuclear Medicine
  General Nuclear Medicine
  Nuclear Cardiology
Pediatrics
  Pediatric Cardiology
  Pediatric Critical Care
  Pediatric Pulmonology
Pulmonary & Critical Care Medicine
  General Pulmonary & Critical Care
    Medicine
Radiology
  Cardiovascular Disease
  Magnetic Resonance Imaging
Rheumatology
  Rheumatic Fever
Surgery
  General Vascular Surgery
Thoracic Surgery
  Adult Cardiothoracic Surgery
  Pediatric Cardiac Surgery
  Transplantation

Children & Adolescents
Addiction Medicine
  Addicted Pregnant Women

Allergy & Immunology
  General Allergy & Immunology
  Immunodeficiency
Anesthesiology
  Critical Care Medicine
  Pain
  Pediatric Anesthesiology
  Pediatric Cardiovascular
Cardiovascular Disease
  Echocardiography
Clinical Pharmacology
Dermatology
  Acne
  Clinical Dermatology
  Laser Surgery
  Pediatric Dermatology
Eating Disorders
  Pediatric Obesity
Endocrinology
  Diabetes
Gastroenterology
  Inflammatory Bowel Disease
Hand Surgery
  Pediatric Orthopaedic Surgery
  Reconstructive Surgery
Infectious Disease
  Diarrhea
  Endocarditis
  Hospital-Acquired Infections
  Lyme Disease
  Respiratory Infections
Medical Oncology/Hematology
  Leukemia
  Neuro-Oncology
Neurological Surgery
  Pediatric Neurological Surgery
  Tumor Surgery
Neurology
  Epilepsy
  Neuro-Oncology
Neurology, Child
  AIDS
  Central Nervous System Infections
  Child Development
  Epilepsy
  General Child Neurology
  Inherited Biochemical Disorders
  Metabolic Diseases
  Movement Disorders
  Neonatal Neurology
  Neuro-Oncology
  Neuromuscular Disease
  Neurovirology
Nuclear Medicine
  General Nuclear Medicine
  Pediatric
Obstetrics & Gynecology
  Pediatric & Adolescent Gynecology

Ophthalmology
  Optics & Refraction
  Pediatric Ophthalmology
  Vitreo-Retinal Surgery
Orthopaedic Surgery
  Pediatric Orthopaedic Surgery
  Spinal Surgery
Otolaryngology
  Otology
  Otology/Neurotology
  Pediatric Otolaryngology
  Sinus & Nasal Surgery
Pathology
  Neuropathology
  Surgical Pathology
Pediatrics
  Abused Children
  Adolescent & Young Adult Medicine
  Metabolic Diseases
  Neonatal-Perinatal Medicine
  Pediatric & Adolescent Gynecology
  Pediatric Cardiology
  Pediatric Critical Care
  Pediatric Endocrinology
  Pediatric Gastroenterology
  Pediatric Hematology-Oncology
  Pediatric Infectious Disease
  Pediatric Nephrology
  Pediatric Pulmonology
Plastic Surgery
  Pediatric Plastic Surgery
  Reconstructive Surgery
Psychiatry
  Addiction Psychiatry
  Child & Adolescent Psychiatry
  Dissociative Disorders
  Eating Disorders
  Forensic Psychiatry
  General Psychiatry
  Mental Retardation/Mental Health
  Mood & Anxiety Disorders
  Psychoanalysis
  Psychopharmacology
  Schizophrenia
  Suicidology
  Violence
Pulmonary & Critical Care Medicine
  Asthma
  Bronchology
  Cystic Fibrosis
Radiation Oncology
  General Radiation Oncology
  Pediatric Radiation Oncology
Radiology
  Neuroradiology
Surgery
  Pediatric Surgery
  TransplantationThoracic Surgery

Pediatric Cardiac Surgery
Pediatric Non-Cardiac Thoracic Surgery
Urology
Pediatric Urology
Transplantation

Colon & Rectal
Anesthesiology
Pain
Colon & Rectal Surgery
Colon & Rectal Cancer
General Colon & Rectal Surgery
Gastroenterology
Endoscopy
Gastrointestinal Cancer
Gastrointestinal Motility
Medical Oncology/Hematology
Clinical Pharmacology
Gastrointestinal Cancer
Pediatrics
Pediatric Gastroenterology
Radiation Oncology
Gastrointestinal Cancer
Surgery
Gastroenterologic Surgery
Pediatric Surgery
Surgical Oncology
Colon & Rectal Cancer
Gastrointestinal Cancer

Critical Care Medicine
Anesthesiology
Adult Cardiovascular
Critical Care Medicine
Pain
Pediatric Anesthesiology
Pediatric Cardiovascular
Infectious Disease
Hospital-Acquired Infections
Neurology
Critical Care Medicine
Obstetrics & Gynecology
Maternal & Fetal Medicine
Pediatrics
Neonatal-Perinatal Medicine
Pediatric Critical Care
Pediatric Pulmonology
Pulmonary & Critical Care Medicine
AIDS
Asthma
Bronchology
Cystic Fibrosis
General Pulmonary & Critical Care
Medicine
Lung Infections
Surgery
Endocrine Surgery
Gastroenterologic Surgery
Pediatric Surgery

Diabetes
Eating Disorders
Obesity
Endocrinology & Metabolism
Diabetes
Geriatric Medicine
Infectious Disease
Transplantation Infections
Urinary Tract Infections
Nephrology
Dialysis
General Nephrology
Glomerular Diseases
Hypertension
Kidney Disease
Nuclear Medicine
Kidney
Obstetrics & Gynecology
Maternal & Fetal Medicine
Ophthalmology
Medical Retinal Diseases
Ophthalmic Genetics
Vitreo-Retinal Surgery
Pediatrics
Pediatric Endocrinology
Pediatric Nephrology
Pathology
Hematopathology
Surgery
Endocrine Surgery
Transplantation
Urology
Urologic Infections

Endocrine & Thyroid
Clinical Pharmacology
Eating Disorders
Obesity
Endocrinology & Metabolism
Diabetes
Neuroendocrinology
Paget's Disease
Thyroid
Gastroenterology
Endoscopy
Gastrointestinal Cancer
General Gastroenterology
Pancreatic Disease
Geriatric Medicine
Medical Oncology/Hematology
Gynecologic Cancer
Nephrology
General Nephrology
Hypertension
Neurological Surgery
Vascular Neurological Surgery
Nuclear Medicine
General Nuclear Medicine
Thyroid

Obstetrics & Gynecology
  Pediatric & Adolescent Gynecology
  Reproductive Endocrinology
  Reproductive Surgery
Ophthalmology
  Ocular Oncology
  Oculoplastic & Orbital Surgery
Otolaryngology
  Otology/Neurotology
  Pediatric Otolaryngology
  Sinus & Nasal Surgery
Pathology
  ENT Pathology
Pediatrics
  Pediatric Endocrinology
Radiation Oncology
  Gastroenterologic Cancer
Surgery
  Endocrine Surgery
  Gastroenterologic Surgery
Urology
  Endourology

Gastrointestinal
Anesthesiology
  Pain
Clinical Pharmacology
Colon & Rectal Surgery
  Colon & Rectal Cancer
  General Colon & Rectal Surgery
Eating Disorders
Gastroenterology
  Endoscopy
  Esophageal Disease
  Functional Gastrointestinal Disorders
  Gastrointestinal Bleeding
  Gastrointestinal Cancer
  Gastrointestinal Motility
  General Gastroenterology
  Hepatology
  Inflammatory Bowel Disease
  Pancreatic Disease
  Peptic Disorders
Infectious Disease
  Diarrhea
  Tropical Disease & Travel Medicine
Medical Oncology/Hematology
  Clinical Pharmacology
  Gastrointestinal Cancer
Pathology
  Liver Pathology
  Surgical Pathology
Pediatrics
  Pediatric Gastroenterology
Radiation Oncology
  Colon & Rectal Cancer
  Gastrointestinal Cancer
  General Radiation Oncology

Surgery
  Gastroenterologic Surgery
Surgical Oncology
  Colon & Rectal Cancer
  Gastrointestinal Cancer

Hematology
Geriatric Medicine
Medical Oncology/Hematology
  Disorders of Bleeding/Thrombosis
  General Medical Oncology/Hematology
  Leukemia
  Lymphomas
Nephrology
  Dialysis
Pathology
  Hematopathology
Pediatrics
  Pediatric Hematology-Oncology
Radiation Oncology
  Lymphomas

Gynecology
Clinical Pharmacology
Dermatology
  Genital Dermatological Disease
  Herpes Virus Infections
  Mucous Membrane Disease
Infectious Disease
  Anaerobic Infections
  General Infectious Disease
  Herpes Virus Infections
  Sexually Transmitted Disease
  Urinary Tract Infections
Medical Oncology/Hematology
  Clinical Pharmacology
  Gynecologic Cancer
Obstetrics & Gynecology
  Genetics
  Genital Dermatological Disease
  Gynecologic Cancer
  Infectious Disease
  Maternal & Fetal Medicine
  Pediatric & Adolescent Gynecology
  Reproductive Endocrinology
  Reproductive Surgery
Pathology
  Gynecologic Pathology
Pediatrics
  Adolescent & Young Adult Medicine
  Pediatric & Adolescent Gynecology
Radiation Oncology
  General Radiation Oncology
  Gynecologic Cancer

Hand
Hand Surgery
  Elbow Surgery

General Hand Surgery
Microsurgery
Paralytic Disorders
Pediatric Orthopaedic Surgery
Peripheral Nerve Surgery
Reconstructive Surgery
Neurological Surgery
Peripheral Nerve Surgery
Orthopaedic Surgery
Pediatric Orthopaedic Surgery
Peripheral Nerve Surgery
Reconstructive Surgery
Rheumatoid Arthritis
Trauma
Plastic Surgery
Microsurgery
Peripheral Nerve Surgery
Reconstructive Surgery

Head & Neck
Medical Oncology/Hematology
Head & Neck Cancer
Neurological Surgery
Cranial Nerve Surgery
Epilepsy Surgery
Neurology
Headache
Neuro-Ophthalmology
Strokes
Epilepsy
Neurology, Child
Epilepsy
Neuro-Oncology
Nuclear Medicine
Brain
Ophthalmology
Otolaryngology
Facial Plastic Surgery
Head & Neck Surgery
Laryngology
Otology/Neurotology
Pediatric Otolaryngology
Skull-Base Surgery
Pathology
ENT Pathology
Plastic Surgery
Craniofacial Surgery
Facial Aesthetic Surgery
Head & Neck Surgery
Maxillofacial Surgery
Reconstructive Surgery
Radiation Oncology
Brain Cancer
General Radiation Oncology
Head & Neck Cancer
Radiology
Neuroradiology

Immunodeficiency, AIDS
Addiction Medicine
General Addiction Medicine
Allergy & Immunology
General Allergy & Immunology
Immunodeficiency
Clinical Pharmacology
Dermatology
Herpes Virus Infections
Pediatric Dermatology
Gastroenterology
Endoscopy
Inflammatory Bowel Disease
Infectious Disease
AIDS
Diarrhea
Fungal Infections
General Infectious Disease
Herpes Virus Infections
Hospital-Acquired Infections
Sexually Transmitted Disease
Toxoplasmosis
Transplantation Infections
Medical Oncology/Hematology
AIDS
Lymphomas
Neurological Surgery
General Neurological Surgery
Neurology
Infectious & Demyelinating Diseases
Neurology, Child
AIDS
Pathology
Hematopathology
Pediatrics
Pediatric Gastroenterology
Pediatric Hematology-Oncology
Pediatric Infectious Disease
Pediatric Nephrology
Pulmonary & Critical Care Medicine
AIDS
General Pulmonary & Critical Care
Medicine
Lung Infections
Radiation Oncology
General Radiation Oncology

Infections
Addiction Medicine
Addicted Pregnant Women
Allergy & Immunology
General Allergy & Immunology
Immunodeficiency
Clinical Pharmacology
Dermatology
Acne
Cutaneous Immunology

Genital Dermatological Disease
Hansen's Disease
Herpes Virus Infections
Gastroenterology
Endoscopy
Inflammatory Bowel Disease
Geriatric Medicine
Infectious Disease
AIDS
Anaerobic Infections
Antibiotic Pharmacology
Bone Infections
Cancer & Infections
Diarrhea
Endocarditis
Fungal Infections
General Infectious Disease
Herpes Virus Infections
Hospital-Acquired Infections
Lyme Disease
Respiratory Infections
Sexually Transmitted Disease
Toxoplasmosis
Transplantation Infections
Tropical Diseases & Travel Medicine
Urinary Tract Infections
Vasculitis
Virology
Medical Oncology/Hematology
Clinical Pharmacology
Immunotherapy
Nephrology
Kidney Transplantation
Neurology
Infectious & Demyelinating Diseases
Neurology, Child
Central Nervous System Infections
Child Development
Neurovirology
Obstetrics & Gynecology
Genital Dermatological Disease
Infectious Disease
Maternal & Fetal Medicine
Ophthalmology
Corneal Diseases & Transplantation
Uveitis
Pediatrics
Pediatric Hematology-Oncology
Pediatric Infectious Disease
Pediatric Pulmonology
Plastic Surgery
Wound Healing
Pulmonary & Critical Care Medicine
AIDS
Bronchology
General Pulmonary & Critical Care
Medicine
Lung Infections

Rheumatology
Infectious Arthritis
Rheumatic Fever
Vasculitis
Surgery
General Vascular Surgery
Wound Healing
Urology
Urological Infections

Liver/ Hepatic
Anesthesiology
Hepatic Disease
Colon & Rectal Surgery
Colon & Rectal Cancer
Gastroenterology
Endoscopy
Functional Gastrointestinal Disorders
Gastrointestinal Bleeding
Hepatology
Infectious Disease
Transplantation Infections
Pathology
Liver Pathology
Pediatrics
Pediatric Gastroenterology
Surgery
Gastroenterologic Surgery
Pediatric Surgery
Transplantation
Surgical Oncology
Gastrointestinal Cancer
Melanoma

Magnetic Resonance Imaging
Cardiovascular Disease
Neurology
Radiology

Neuro
Anesthesiology
Complications of Anesthesia
Neuroanesthesia
Pain
Pediatric Anesthesiology
Cardiovascular Disease
Clinical Exercise Testing
Echocardiography
Pacemakers
Vaso-spastic Diseases
Endocrinology & Metabolism
Neuroendocrinology
Geriatric Medicine
Hand Surgery
Microsurgery
Peripheral Nerve Surgery
Medical Oncology/Hematology

Gastrointestinal Cancer
Neuro-Oncology
Neurological Surgery
  Cranial Nerve Surgery
  Epilepsy Surgery
  General Neurological Surgery
  Pediatric Neurological Surgery
  Peripheral Nerve Surgery
  Spinal Surgery
  Stereotactic Radiosurgery
  Trauma
  Tumor Surgery
  Vascular Neurological Surgery
Neurology
  Behavioral Neurology
  Critical Care Medicine
  Degenerative Diseases
  Electromyography
  Epilepsy
  General Adult Neurology
  Geriatric Neurology
  Headache
  Infectious & Demyelinating Diseases
  Magnetic Resonance Imaging
  Movement Disorders
  Neuro-Rehabilitiation
  Neuro-Oncology
  Neuro-Ophthalmology
  Neurogenetics
  Neuromuscular Disease
  Neuropsychiatry
  Stroke
Neurology, Child
  AIDS
  Central Nervous System Infections
  Child Development
  Epilepsy
  General Child Neurology
  Inherited Biochemical Disorders
  Metabolic Diseases
  Movement Disorders
  Neonatal Neurology
  Neuro-Oncology
  Neuromuscular Disease
  Neurovirology
Ophthalmology
  Glaucoma
  Neuro-Ophthalmology
  Pediatric Ophthalmology
Orthopaedic Surgery
  Peripheral Nerve Surgery
  Reconstructive Surgery
  Spinal Surgery
  Trauma
Otolaryngology
  Laryngology
  Otology/Neurotology

Pathology
  ENT Pathology
  Neuropathology
Pediatrics
  Metabolic Diseases
  Pediatric Endocrinology
  Pediatric Infectious Disease
Physical Medicine & Rehabilitation
Plastic Surgery
  Head & Neck Surgery
  Microsurgery
  Peripheral Nerve Surgery
  Reconstructive Surgery
Psychiatry
  Geriatric Psychiatry
  Mood & Anxiety Disorders
  Neuropsychiatry
Pulmonary & Critical Care Medicine
  General Pulmonary & Critical Care
    Medicine
Radiation Oncology
  Pediatric Radiation Oncology
  Sarcomas
Radiology
  Neuroradiology
Surgery
  Endocrine Surgery
  Trauma
Urology
  Neuro-Urology & Voiding Dysfunction
  Pediatric Urology

Obstetrics
Addiction Medicine
  Addicted Pregnant Women
Anesthesiology
  Obstetric Anesthesia
Infectious Disease
  Anaerobic Infections
  General Infectious Disease
  Herpes Virus Infections
  Hospital-Acquired Infections
  Sexually Transmitted Disease
  Toxoplasmosis
Obstetrics & Gynecology
  Genetics
  Genital Dermatological Disease
  Gynecologic Cancer
  Infectious Disease
  Maternal & Fetal Medicine
  Pediatric & Adolescent Gynecology
  Reproductive Endocrinology
  Reproductive Surgery
Pathology
  Gynecological Pathology
Pediatrics
  Neonatal-Perinatal Medicine

Psychiatry
  Mood & Anxiety Disorders
Surgery
  Endocrine Surgery

Orthopaedic/ Bone
Allergy & Immunology
  General Allergy & Immunology
  Immunodeficiency
Anesthesiology
  Orthopaedic Procedures
  Pain
Endocrinology & Metabolism
  Paget's Disease
Geriatric Medicine
Hand Surgery
  Elbow Surgery
  General Hand Surgery
  Microsurgery
  Paralytic Disorders
  Pediatric Orthopaedic Surgery
  Peripheral Nerve Surgery
  Reconstructive Surgery
Infectious Disease
  Anaerobic Infections
  Bone Infections
  Cancer & Infections
Medical Oncology/Hematology
  Bone Marrow Transplantation
  Breast Cancer
  Leukemia
  Myeloma
Neurological Surgery
  Spinal Surgery
  Trauma
Nephrology
  Kidney Disease
Nuclear Medicine
  Bone
Orthopaedic Surgery
  Foot & Ankle Surgery
  Hip Surgery
  Knee Surgery
  Pediatric Orthopaedic Surgery
  Peripheral Nerve Surgery
  Reconstructive Surgery
  Rheumatoid Arthritis
  Shoulder Surgery
  Spinal Surgery
  Sports Medicine/Arthroscopy
  Trauma
  Tumor Surgery
Otolaryngology
  Facial Plastic Surgery
  Sinus & Nasal Surgery
Pathology
  Bone Pathology
  Hematopathology

Pediatrics
  Pediatric Hematology-Oncology
Plastic Surgery
  Craniofacial Surgery
  Facial Aesthetic Surgery
  Head & Neck Surgery
  Maxillofacial Surgery
  Reconstructive Surgery
Radiation Oncology
  Pediatric Radiation Oncology
  Sarcomas
Rheumatology
  Osteoarthritis
  Osteoporosis
  Lupus
  Rheumatoid Arthritis

Pain
Anesthesiology
  Ambulatory Anesthesia
  Complications of Anesthesia
  Neuroanesthesia
  Obstetric Anesthesia
  Orthopaedic Procedures
  Pain
  Pediatric Anesthesiology
Medical Oncology/Hematology
  Neuro-Oncology
Neurological Surgery
  Peripheral Nerve Surgery
  Spinal Surgery
  Tumor Surgery
Neurology
  Behavioral Neurology
  Headache
  Neuro-Oncology
Otolaryngology
  Otology/Neurotology
Physical Medicine & Rehabilitation
  General Physical Medicine &
    Rehabilitation
Plastic Surgery
  Peripheral Nerve Surgery
Psychiatry
  General Psychiatry
Rheumatology
  Infectious Arthritis
  Rheumatoid Arthritis

Plastic & Aesthetic Surgery
Dermatology
  Aesthetic Surgery
  Laser Surgery
  Wound Healing
Hand Surgery
  Reconstructive Surgery
Ophthalmology
  Oculoplastic & Orbital Surgery

Otolaryngology
  Facial Plastic Surgery
  Head & Neck Surgery
  Otology/Neurotology
  Skull-Base Surgery
Plastic Surgery
  Body Contouring
  Breast Surgery
  Craniofacial Surgery
  Facial Aesthetic Surgery
  Head & Neck Surgery
  Laser Surgery & Birthmarks
  Maxillofacial Surgery
  Microsurgery
  Pediatric Plastic Surgery
  Peripheral Nerve Surgery
  Reconstructive Surgery
  Wound Healing
Surgery
  Breast Surgery
  Wound Healing

Pulmonary/ Lung
Anesthesiology
  Cardiothoracic Anesthesiology
Infectious Disease
  Respiratory Infections
  Fungal Infections
  Toxoplasmosis
  Transplantation Infections
  Virology
Geriatric Medicine
Medical Oncology/Hematology
  Lung Cancer
Nuclear Medicine
  General Nuclear Medicine
  Pulmonary
Otolaryngology
  Head & Neck Surgery
  Laryngology
  Pediatric Otolaryngology
Sinus & Nasal Surgery
Pediatrics
  Neonatal-Perinatal Medicine
  Pediatric Cardiology
  Pediatric Pulmonology
Physical Medicine & Rehabilitation
  General Physical Medicine &
    Rehabilitation
Pulmonary & Critical Care Medicine
  AIDS
  Asthma
  Bronchology
  Cystic Fibrosis
  General Pulmonary & Critical Care
    Medicine
  Lung Infections

Radiation Oncology
  General Radiation Oncology
  Lung Cancer
Surgery
  Gastroenterologic Surgery
Thoracic Surgery
  Adult Cardiothoracic Surgery
  General Thoracic Surgery
  Pediatric Cardiac Surgery
  Pediatric Non-Cardiac Thoracic Surgery
  Thoracic Oncological Surgery
  Transplantation

Reconstruction
Dermatology
  Skin Cancer Surgery & Reconstruction
Hand Surgery
  Elbow Surgery
  Microsurgery
  Paralytic Disorders
  Peripheral Nerve Surgery
  Reconstructive Surgery
Ophthalmology
  Oculoplastic & Orbital Surgery
Orthopaedic Surgery
  Reconstructive Surgery
  Sports Medicine/Arthroscopy
  Trauma
  Tumor Surgery
Otolaryngology
  Facial Plastic Surgery
  Head & Neck Surgery
  Laryngology
  Pediatric Otolaryngology
  Skull-Base Surgery
Neurological Surgery
  Peripheral Nerve Surgery
Plastic Surgery
  Breast Surgery
  Facial Aesthetic Surgery
  Head & Neck Surgery
  Laser Surgery & Birthmarks
  Microsurgery
  Peripheral Nerve Surgery
  Reconstructive Surgery
Surgery
  Breast Surgery
  Wound Healing
Urology
  Endourology
  Neuro-Urology & Voiding Dysfunction
  Pediatric Urology
  Urologic Oncology

Seizure Disorders
Neurological Surgery
  Epilepsy Surgery
  Pediatric Neurological Surgery

Neurology
  Epilepsy
  General Adult Neurology
Neurology, Child
  Epilepsy

Trauma
  Hand Surgery
    Reconstructive Surgery
  Neurological Surgery
    Pediatric Neurological Surgery
    Trauma
  Orthopaedic Surgery
    Reconstructive Surgery
    Trauma
  Otolaryngology
    Head & Neck Surgery
  Plastic Surgery
    Craniofacial Surgery
    Head & Neck Surgery
    Maxillofacial Surgery
  Psychiatry
    Child & Adolescent Psychiatry
    Dissociative Disorders
    Geriatric Psychiatry
    Mood & Anxiety Disorders
    Neuropsychiatry
    Psychopharmacology
    Suicidology
    Violence
  Surgery
    General Vascular Surgery
    Trauma Surgery

Urology/ Nephrology
  Cardiovascular Disease
    Heart Failure/ Kidney Failure
  Clinical Pharmacology
  Geriatric Medicine
  Infectious Disease
    Hospital-Acquired Infections
    Urinary Tract Infections
  Medical Oncology & Hematology
    Genito-Urinary Cancer
  Nephrology
    Dialysis
    General Nephrology
    Glomerular Diseases
    Hypertension
    Kidney Disease
    Kidney Transplantation
  Nuclear Medicine
    Kidney
  Pediatrics
    Pediatric Nephrology
  Radiation Oncology
    Genito-Urinary Cancer

Rheumatology
  Lupus
Surgery
  Pediatric Surgery
  Transplantation
Urology
  Endourology
  General Urology
  Impotence
  Neuro-Urology & Voiding Dysfunction
  Pediatric Urology
  Renal Hypertension
  Transplantation
  Urologic Oncology
  Urological Infections

Vascular
  Allergy & Immunology
    General Allergy & Immunology
  Anesthesiology
    Adult Cardiovascular
    Critical Care Anesthesiology
    Pediatric Cardiovascular
  Cardiovascular Disease
    Cardiac Catheterization
    Cardiac Rehabilitation
    General Cardiovascular Disease
    Vaso-Spastic Diseases
  Dermatology
    Clinical Dermatology
    Cutaneous Immunology
    Laser Surgery
    Skin Cancer Surgery & Reconstruction
    Wound Healing
  Gastroenterology
    Inflammatory Bowel Disease
  Hand Surgery
    Reconstructive Surgery
  Infectious Disease
    Vasculitis
  Medical Oncology & Hematology
    Disorders of Bleeding, Thrombosis
  Nephrology
    General Nephrology
    Glomerular Diseases
    Hypertension
    Kidney Disease
  Neurological Surgery
    General Neurological Surgery
    Pediatric Neurological Surgery
    Trauma
    Tumor Surgery
    Vascular Neurological Surgery
  Neurology
    Headache
    Strokes

Neurology, Child
  Child Development
  General Child Neurology
Ophthalmology
  Medical Retinal Diseases
  Vitreo-Retinal Surgery
Otolaryngology
  Head & Neck Surgery
Plastic Surgery
  Pediatric Plastic Surgery
  Reconstructive Surgery

Rheumatology
  Vasculitis
Surgery
  General Vascular Surgery
  Trauma Surgery
  Wound Healing
Urology
  Endourology
  Impotence
Renal Hypertension

INDEX

A

Aas, Johannes, 179
Aase, Jon M., 392
Abbott, Oscar D., 693
Abboud, Charles, 176
Abboud, Hanna Emile, 600
Abbruzzese, James Lewis, 588
Abel, Martin D., 166
Abernathy, Robert Shields, 7
Abman, Steven H., 67
Abrahams, Lisa Ann, 410
Abrams, David Saul, 504
Abrams, Jerri, 737
Abrams, Richard S., 47
Abramson, Lawrence Jack, 5
Abresch, Robert J., 800
Abston, Sally, 810
Abuabara, Sabas Fatule, 815
Accurso, Frank Joseph, 67
Acebo, Francisco A., 536
Aceto, Thomas, Jr., 291
Achilles, Jackson T., 484, 757
Ackerman, Baer M., 767
Aclin, Richard R., 19
Acosta, Daniel, 544
Adair, Richard, 186
Adam, Karolina, 632
Adams, Elton J., 348
Adams, George L., 208
Adams, Harold P., Jr., 106
Adams, James Mervyn, 708
Adams, Mark A., 283
Adams, Richard O., 232
Adamson, Steven C., 179
Addo, Ferdinand E. K., 417
Adducci, Christopher J., 433
Adinoff, Allen D., 33
Adinoff, Bryon Harlen, 758
Adkins, Charles F., 757
Adkison, H. William, 378
Adler, Susan K., 557
Adrogue, Horacio Jose, 599
Aeling, John L., 37
Agerter, David C., 178
Aggarwal, Rahul, 211
Agnew, Hewes D., 350
Agnew, Samuel G., 14
Agrawal, Remedios Ching, 721
Aguirre, Gilberto, 656
Aguirre, Maria del Rosario, 738

Ahlin, Thomas D., 418
Ahlquist, David A., 181
Ahmann, David L., 192
Ahmed, Iftikar, 174
Ahrens, Richard C., 91, 115
Aiello, Leslie Franklin, 726
Ajani, Jaffer A., 588
Akright, Bruce Donald, 639
Akright, Laura Sand, 532
Aksamit, Allen J., Jr., 196
Alam, Rafeul, 487
Albers, Robert C., 139
Albin, Glen, 167
Albores-Saavedra, Jorge, 685
Albrecht, Bruce H., 58
Aldinger, Keith, 577
Aldrich, Andrew J., 773
Aldridge, John L., 436
Alexander, Randell C., 115
Alexander, Samuel E., 58
Alexander, Steven Roy, 698
Alexander, William Allan, 497
Alexanian, Raymond, 588
Alford, Bobby R., 678
Alford, Nathaniel J., Jr., 773
Alfrey, Allen C., 52
Algren, John Travis, 497
Aliperti, Giuseppe, 255
Alivizatos, Peter A., 826
Allen, Bohn D., 805
Allen, Brent T., 314
Allen, Jerry H., 294
Allen, John, 180
Allen, Mark J., 254
Allen, Mark S., 236
Allen, Rhea J., 100
Allen, Robert, 464
Allen, Steven J., 497
Allen, Steven R., 641
Allen, Terry D., 835
Allen, William R., 704
Allender, James Hudson, 704
Allgood, Steven C., 127
Allison, David, 394
Allison, James Eblen III, 731
Allred, Craig D., 693
Allums, James A., 825
Al-Mefty, Ossama, 11
Almquist, Adrian K., 168
Alpern, Robert J., 597
Alpers, David H., 255
Alpert, Jack Nathaniel, 613
Alsop, George Y., 806

Alsup, Ace Hill III, 569
Alt, Thomas H., 173
Alter, Blanche P., 706
Altman, Denis I., 271
Altshuler, Kenneth Z., 758
Alverson, Dale C., 392
Alward, Wallace L. M., 110
Amadio, Peter C., 183
Amand, Pamela A. St., 628
Amar, Meera, 533
Amar, N. J., 492
Amato, Anthony Arnold, 615
Ameduri, Ardow Richard, 785
Ameln, Richard T., 97
Amer, Jules, 70
Ames, Frederick C., 821
Amin, Bipin R., 417
Ampuero, Francisco, 388
Amstutz, Samuel W., 148
Anand, Rajiv, 646
Andersen, Arnold E., 121
Andersen, John Milton, 699
Anderson, Barrie, 109
Anderson, Charles B., 335
Anderson, Charles W., 398
Anderson, D. Claire, 309
Anderson, Dale R., 474
Anderson, David C., 195, 234
Anderson, Edward F., 465
Anderson, Eric J., 323
Anderson, Garland D., 632
Anderson, James A., 856
Anderson, James T., 87
Anderson, John V., 290
Anderson, Judith R., 46
Anderson, Kenneth W., 118
Anderson, Lee Stewart, 650
Anderson, Paul, 784
Anderson, Paul N., 50
Anderson, Philip C., 248
Anderson, Rebecca S., 331
Anderson, Renner S., 218
Anderson, Robert, 595
Anderson, Robert F., Jr., 118
Anderson, Robert J., 53
Anderson, Rodney A., 852
Anderson, Ross E., 179
Andrassy, Richard John, 811
Andreasen, Nancy C., 121
Andres, Robert L., 632
Andresen, Jeffry John, 758
Andrew, Christopher R., 269
Andrew, John L. II, 786

Bissett, Joseph K., 4
Bitter, Mitchell, 66
Bitzer, Lon G., 26
Bjerregaard, Preben, 245
Bjork, Randall, 56
Black, David, 283
Black, Donald W., 121
Black, James, 150
Black, James Nelson, 504
Black, Karen Shipp, 532
Black, Katheryn, 131
Black, Robert D., 774
Black, Timothy L., 809
Blackburn, David C., 782
Blackett, Piers R., 454
Blackwell, Steven J., 751
Blackwell, Thomas A., 575
Blahey, Maria S., 535
Blaine, James, 253
Blaisdell, Greg D., 771
Blake, Jerome, 476
Blake, Robert L., Jr., 251
Blakely, Richard W., 577
Blakeman, Gordon J., 72
Blakes, Albert L., 730
Blanchett, Michael Gerard, 540
Blanco, Ernesto, 794
Blanco, Jorge D., 633
Bland, Wiley R., 347
Blaney, Susan M., 709
Blankenship, Jerry B., 462
Blanton, Joseph C., 296
Blatchford, Garnet J., 356
Bleicher, Bob J., 371
Blevins, Field, 389
Blevins, John K., 741
Blevins, Richard Dyer, 345
Blevins, Thomas Craig, 528
Bleyer, W. Archie, 709
Bligard, Carey A., 96
Bligard, Eric W., 110
Blinder, Morey, 264
Block, Frank E., Jr., 3
Blodgett, John T., 343
Blodi, Christopher F., 113
Bloedel, Carla, 394
Blond, Carl Joseph, 600
Bloom, Kenneth, 721
Bloom, Kim, 775
Bloomberg, Gordon R., 294
Bloome, Michael A., 651
Blum, Robert W., 217
Blumenschein, George, 585
Blumenschein, Sarah, 699
Blumenthal, Harvey J., 448
Blumenthal, Malcolm N., 164
Blumhardt, Ralph, 625
Blute, Michael L., 237

Blyth, Bruce, 67
Boardman, Dennis Richard, 731
Boatman, Dennis L., 128
Bocanegra, Javier Cerda, 540
Bocell, James R., Jr., 667
Bock, S. Allan, 31
Boddicker, Marc E., 466
Bode, William E., 517, 823
Bodey, Gerald P., 564
Boesch, Karen R., 300
Boesen, Peter V., 114
Bogdanovich, Michael Bruce, 534
Bogenschutz, Michael, 399
Bohigian, George M., 280
Bohmfalk, George L., 608
Boisaubin, Eugene, 575
Boldt, David H., 592
Boldt, H. Culver, 110
Bolger, Michael, 264
Bolivar-Briceno, Ricardo, 564
Bolline, Stephen C., 731
Bollinger, Barbara J., 417
Bollinger, John W., 430
Bollinger, Steven H., 414
Bolman, R. Morton III, 235
Bolte, Brett J., 748
Boman, Darius A., 687
Bomer, Donald L., 683
Bond, John H., 180
Bond, Russell R., Jr., 298
Bonebrake, Alfred J., 275
Bonelli, Andres, 554
Bonilla, Juan Alfredo, 681
Bonilla-Felix, Melvin A., 709
Boniuk, Isaac, 280
Boniuk, Milton, 651
Bonner, Timothy C., 202
Bonte, Frederick J., 623
Book, Earl E., 327
Boone, Timothy, 838
Boop, Frederick, 11
Booth, A. Michael, 432
Bootin, Debra Mucasey, 732
Borchardt, Carrie M., 221
Borden, Thomas A., 405
Boren, Ronald P., 736
Borenstein, Joseph, 738
Borg, Robert, 15
Borgardus, Carl R., 458
Borgstede, James P., 82
Boris, Glenn J., 736
Borowsky, Benjamin, 261
Boss, James W., 553
Bost, Brent W., 628
Boucek, Mark M., 67
Boudreau, Robert J., 199
Boulafendis, Demetrio G., 828

Bourgeois, Blaise F. D., 271
Bourgeois, Michael J., 719
Bourne, Cecil Martindale, 571
Bourne, William M., 204
Bovenmyer, Dan Allen, 96
Bovenmyer, John A., 96
Bowden, Charles L., 768
Bower, Charles Michael, 15
Bower, James S., 304
Bower, Thomas C., 233
Bowes, Anita King, 681
Bowes, Harrison N., 656
Bowling, John R., 582
Bowman, Bradley, 647
Bowman, Robert Wayne, 647
Bowman, William Paul, 704
Bowser, Barry L., 743
Boyce, Mark W., 178
Boyd, Charles Marion, 12
Boyd, Gary D., 553
Boyd, James H., 285
Boyd, Robert Allen, 732
Boydston, Teresa W., 574
Boylan, Thomas, 34
Bozalis, John R., 436
Braby, Daniel E., 339
Bracey, Arthur W., 688
Brachetta, Guillermo E., 517, 814
Brackett, Fred B., 515
Braddock, Suzanne W., 357
Braden, David, 577
Bradford, John W., 323
Bradford, Reagan H., Jr., 450
Bradley, Vincent H., 495
Bradshaw, Karen D., 629
Bradshaw, Major William, 564
Bradsher, Robert W., 8
Brady, Alfred Bernard, Jr., 505
Brandt, Keith Eric, 752
Brandt, Thomas R., 355
Branham, Gregory H., 286
Brannan, Stephen Kyle, 768
Brantigan, Charles O., 85
Brasher, George W., 492
Braun, Robert, 137
Braverman, Alan C., 245
Braverman, Sheldon P., 656
Braxton, Frank W., 265
Bray, John D., 490, 721
Breckbill, David, 157
Breed, David R., 696
Breeze, Robert E., 54
Bregman, Richard M., 458
Brehm, G. Scott, 319
Breitwieser, Wayne R., 429
Brelsford, William G., 804
Brener, Daniel Michael, 763
Brennan, Brian Alfred, 92

Brennan, Daniel C., 267
Brennan, James Patrick, 598
Brennan, Michael D., 176
Brenton, Randall S., 112
Bressinick, Rene Edward, 5
Bressler, Robert Burgess, 488
Brewer, L. Eileen Doyle, 709
Brewer, Marshall L., 479
Brice, Sylvia, 37
Bricker, Donald L., 830
Bricker, John Timothy, 710
Bridges, Ben F., 583
Bridges, Robert Ashe, 805
Bridwell, Keith H., 283
Brier, Arnold M., 182
Briggs, Brian T., 423
Brindle, Jeffrey S., 429
Brindley, George W., 672
Brindley, Glen O., 659
Brindley, Hanes H., Jr., 672
Brindley, Mace L., 683
Briney, Walter G., 84
Bringewald, Peter Robert, 647
Brinker, Karl Robert, 597
Brinson, Cynthia C., 534
Briseno, Charles George, 580
Bristow, Michael R., 34
Britton, B. Hill, Jr., 452
Britton, Howard A., 721
Broadwater, J. Ralph, 4, 27
Broberg, Peter H., 643
Brodine, William N., 244
Brodland, David G., 174
Brodsky, Alan Lawrence, 799
Brodsky, James W., 663
Brondos, Gregory A., 853
Bronson, Michael A., 217
Brook, Charles J., 305
Brookens, Bruce R., 34
Brooker, Andrew F., 660
Brookhouser, Patrick E., 366
Brooks, Charles L., 137
Brooks, Michael S., 124
Brooks, Robert S., 88
Brosseau, James D., 417
Brotherman, Donald P., 647
Brothers, Lyman R. III, 858
Broughton, Daniel D., 218
Broun, Goronwy O., Jr., 265
Browder, J. Bond, 583
Brown, Addison W., 112
Brown, Bertron Travis, 570
Brown, Bruce W., 570
Brown, Byron L., 499
Brown, Carl A., 208
Brown, Charles E. L., 627
Brown, Christopher C., 850
Brown, Dale, Jr., 633
Brown, David L., 166

Brown, David R., 391
Brown, Dennistoun, 348
Brown, George Rhamy, 780
Brown, Henry S., 248
Brown, James C. N., 121
Brown, Lawrence Randolph, 230
Brown, Lewis A., 491
Brown, Michael Edwin, 728
Brown, Orval E., 675
Brown, Raeford E., 3
Brown, Richard W., 688
Brown, Robert S., 110
Brown, Ronald, 136
Brown, Sandra M., 654
Brown, Spencer H., Jr., 461
Brown, Stephen L., 855
Brown, Steven Dunning, 775
Brown, Thomas J., 613
Brown, William C., 76
Browne, Kevin Brian, 681
Brownfield, Elisha L., 575
Broze, George J., Jr., 265
Brubaker, Richard, 204
Bruce, Derek A., 603
Bruce, Robert R., 462
Bruhl, Daniel Edward, 650
Bruner, Janet M., 689
Bruneteau, Richard John, 370
Brunning, Richard D., 210
Bruno, Felice, 827
Brunsvold, Robert A., 409
Brunt, Michael, 315
Bruschwein, Dean A., 347
Brutinel, W. Mark, 225
Bruton, H. David, 772
Bryan, Bruce, 276
Bryan, Charles Leslie, 777
Bryan, Gary W., 673
Bryan, William J., 667
Bryan, Wilson Werber, 611
Bryer, Mark, 306
Bublitz, Deborah K., 73
Buchanan, George R., 699
Buchanan, Robert T., 457
Buchman, Mark T., 558
Bucholz, Robert W., 663
Bucknam, Robert C., 74
Buehler, Bruce A., 368
Buell, James C., 511
Buell, Walter F., 616
Bugay, Glenn Lamar, 571
Buja, Louis Maximilian, 689
Bukstein, Michael J., 313
Bull, James C., 351
Bullen, Michael Glen, 561
Bullock, Arnold D., 319
Buls, John G., 173
Bunata, Robert E., 558

Bunch, George P., 396
Bunke, Martin, 10
Bunker, Thomas G., 475
Bunn, Paul A., Jr., 51
Bunn, Simon Milford, Jr., 695
Burd, Ronald M., 428
Burford, Duncan D., Sr., 343
Burg, John R., 324
Burgin, William W., 773
Burke, Jack D., Jr., 771
Burke, M. Shannon, 60
Burke, Thomas, 849
Burke, Thomas W., 633
Burke, William J., 370
Burkett, Robert J., 677
Burkhead, Wayne Z., Jr., 663
Burkholder, George V., 841
Burks, A. Wesley, Jr., 2
Burks, James K., 532
Burleigh, Peter L., 336
Burnbaum, Mitchell D., 57
Burnett, Hugh F., 26
Burnett, Raymond G., 473
Burns, Debra Lou, 728
Burns, Dennis K., 685
Burns, Dianna Mosley, 738
Burns, George Paul, 673
Burns, Linda J., 190
Burns, Richard, 259
Burns, Terry R., 692
Burnside, John Wayne, 571
Buroker, Thomas R., 104
Burris, Howard A. III, 592
Burrow, Maida L., 38
Burton, Francis C., Jr., 754
Bury, Jan, 420
Bury, Robert J., 420
Busby, Stephen P., 612
Busch, Lyndon John, 496
Bush, Mickey V., 542
Bushnell, David L., 108
Buster, John E., 633
Buswell, Richard S., 322
Butcher, Dennis L., 850
Butler, David F., 522
Butler, E. Brian, 782
Butler, Ian J., 620
Butler, Steven A., 339
Butler, Thomas C., 567
Butterfield, Donald G., 42
Butts, Donald R., 517
Butz, Gerald W., 482
Buxton, Lawrence F., 616
Buzdar, Aman U., 589
Bybee, Joseph David, 577
Byers, Norman T., 420
Byrd, Bill F., 622
Byrd, H. Steve, 750

Cvetkovich, Lorna L., 146
Czaja, Albert J., 181

D

Dabaghi, Rashad E., 543
Dabezies, Eugene Jean, 559, 668
Dacey, Ralph G., Jr., 269
Dacso, Clifford Clark, 577
Dagg, Kathy K., 445
Dahl, C. Robert, 43
Dahl, Charles P., 423
Dahl, Mark V., 173
Dale, Lowell C., 188
Dallas, John S., 707
Dalrymple, Glenn V., 364
Dalton, John Howard, 730
Dalton, Robert J., 190
Daly, Peter J., 207
Damasio, Antonio, 106
Damasio, Hanna, 106
Dambro, Mark R., 537
Dambro, Nancy N., 705
Damle, Jayant S., 409
Dandridge, W. C., Jr., 313
Danes, David T., 323
Danford, David A., 368
Daniel, James F., 725
Daniel, M. Scott, 572
Daniels, Jerry C., 801
Daniels, John S., 261
Daniels, Wheeler T., 338
Danielson, Gordon K., 236
Danney, Mark Maxwell, 721
Darby, Byron G., 627
Darouiche, Rabih, 564
Dart, Richard C., 36
Daube, Jasper R., 197
Dauber, Ira, 34
Daugherty, Marylin A., 60
Daugird, Allen J., 252
Dauser, Robert C., 606
Davenport, James Albert, 501
Davenport, N. Alan, 574
David, Jeffrey J., 369
Davidson, Allan B., 80
Davidson, Craig L., 186
Davidson, Elizabeth, 767
Davidson, James E., 574
Davidson, Joyce, 154
Davidson, Susan A., 58
Davies, Scott F., 224
Davila, Juan E., 742
Davis, Carolyn T., 152
Davis, Donald Robert, 661
Davis, Glenn Raymond, 6

Davis, Karlotta M., 58
Davis, Kathleen, 83
Davis, Kathleen Cecilia, 322
Davis, Larry E., 387
Davis, Phyllis Ann, 737
Davis, R. Craig, 19
Davis, R. Douglas, 659
Davis, Richard C., 536
Davis, Robert E., 548
Davis, Robert J., 847
Davis, Thomas D., 410
Davis, William A., 97
Davis, William D., 833
Davison, James A., 112
Dawood, Mohamed Yusoff, 633
Daws, William R., 118
Dawson, Donald L., 66
Dawson, George, 534
Dawson, Mark C., 535
Dawson, Thomas Britton, 727
Day, Daniel K., 202
Day, Howard A., 143
Day, James L., 343
Day, John W., 195
De Angelis, Anthony Joseph, 342
De Behnke, Richard Davis, 569
De Fronzo, Ralph Anthony, 532
de la Garza, Christine, 639
de la Torre, Jorge, 764
de Larios, Michael Steven, 536
De Noia, Emanuel P., 581
De Staffany, Nelson D., 504
Dean, Joseph, 397
Dean, Thurston E., 669
Dearborn, Shirley Ella, 456
Dearden, Craig Lee, 574
Deaton, William Joel, 773
Decker, John T., 67
Deckert, Gordon H., 458
DeCoster, Thomas, 390
Deer, David A., 156
DeFrance, Lori L., 217
Dehan, Christopher Paul, 674
Dehdashti, Farrokh, 272
Dehner, Louis P., 288
Delaney, B. Peyton, 617
Delaney, John P., 232
Delclos, Luis, 783
Delee, Jesse C., 670
Delgado-Ayala, Mauricio R., 618
Dell'Aglio, Mark J., 327
Dellinger, R. Phillip, 304
Delmez, James A., 267

Delwood, Donald M., 260
DeMarco, Daniel Carl, 545
Demarest, Gerald B. III, 404
DeMiranda, Federico C., 19
Demmler, Gail J., 711
Demmy, Todd L., 317
DeMonte, Franco, 606
Demos, Michael A., 847
Deneke, James, 25
Denfield, Susan Warren, 711
Dennis, Douglas A., 63
Denson, Susan E., 711
Depenbusch, S. L. Francis, 147
DePompolo, Robert W., 220
Derderian, Raymond, 596
DeRemee, Richard A., 225
Dernbach, Timothy A., 350
Dernovsek, Kim, 38
Dertkash, Robert S., 64
Deschamps, Claude, 236
Deskin, Ronald W., 678
Des Rosiers, Joseph L., 627
DeVere, Ronald, 613
Devig, Patrick M., 433
DeVillez, Richard L., 525
Devineni, Venkata, 306
Dewald, Paul A., 300
Dewan, Stephen James, 825
Dewey, Richard B., Jr., 611
Dewey, Richard C., 334
Dewitt, Barbara, 156
DeWitt, Robert D., 569
Di Donna, George J., 507
Di Pette, Donald J., 514, 576
Diamond, Lynne Marie, 541
Diamond, Norman George, 788
Diaz, Gonzalo A., 774
Diaz, Joseph David, 491
Diaz, Laura K., 496
Diaz-Ball, Fernando, 836
DiBisceglie, Adrian M., 255
Dick, Fred R., 115
Dick, M. Marga, 300
Dicken, Charles H., 174
Dickey, J. Rayner, 678
Dickey, Nancy W., 536
Dickins, John Roddey Edwards, 16
Dickson, Bryan A., 699
Dickson, E. Rolland, 181
Dickson, Jesse H., 667
Dieckert, J. Paul, 659
Diederich, Dennis A., 142
Diehl, Andrew Kemper, 581
Dieperink, Willem, 223
Dietrich, Dennis W., 335

Dietz, Mark A., 55
Dignan, R. D., 515
Dildy, Dale W., Jr., 20
Dillee, Ronald Dennis, 786
Dilling, Emery Walter, 825
Dillman, Richard D., Jr., 804
DiMagno, Eugene P., 181
Dinehart, Scott M., 5
Dinh, Ha, 4
Dinn, James R., 662
DiStefano, Alfred, 585
Diven, Steven C., 707
Dobie, Robert A., 681
Dobyns, James Harold, 560
Dobyns, Richard C., 99
Doce, Conrad D., 434
Dodd, Gerald D. III, 794
Dodds, Matthew T., 852
Doddy, Karyn R., 398
Dodge, Philip R., 271
Dodson, Leonard E., 528
Dodson, Mark A., 536
Dodson, W. Edwin, 271
Doebbeling, Bradley N., 102
Doherty, Gerard M., 316
Doherty, Mark Gerard, 639
Doka, David S., 650
Dolan, Eugen J., 333
Dolen, S. Ender, 639
Doll, Donald, 263
Dollahite, Harry Anderson, 665
Domet, Mark J., 369
Domina, Alan H., 375
Domingues, Charles C., 662
Dominguez, Edward A., 360
Dominguez, Roland J., 731
Dominick, Jerome, 378
Donadio, James V., 193
Donalson, Ronald J., 608
Donley, Robert F., 194
Donohoue, Patricia A., 116
Donohue, John H., 234
Donohue, Robert E., 89
Donovan, Donald Thomas, 678
Donovan, Thomas K., 286
Donovan, William H., 744
Donowho, Everett M., Jr., 693
Doody, Dian L., 295
Doody, Kevin J., 631
Doody, Rachelle S., 613
Dooley, Cornelius P., 382
Doran, Terence I., 721
Dorfan, Herbert I., 764
Dorin, Maxine, 388
Dorsen, Michael, 603
Doss, Noble W., Jr., 627

Dosser, G. Pete, 439
Dossey, Joe Ed, 812
Doubleday, C. William, 523
Dougherty, Charles H., 296
Dougherty, Sarsfield P., 347
Doughman, Donald J., 202
Douglas, Gary L., 666
Douglas, John M., Jr., 45
Douthit, Douglas D., 146
Dow, Charles A., 827
Dowell, Duane L., 699, 728
Dowell, Mark E., 849
Dowton, S. Bruce, 291
Doyle, Marilyn, 711
Dozois, Roger R., 172, 233, 235
Drage, Charles W., 225
Dragun, Michael J., 840
Drazek, Jane K., 153
Draznin, Boris, 40
Draznin, Elena, 75
Dreessen, Philip R., 732
Drennan, James C., 390
Drevetz, Wayne C., 301
Dreyer, Charles F., 621
Dreyer, Zoann Eckert, 711
Dreyfuss, Paul H., 748
Driks, Michael R., 258
Driscoll, Charles E., 99
Driscoll, David J., 215
Driver, M. Coleman, Jr., 644
Droge, Molly, 728
Drummond, Alonzo John, 551
Drummond, Ronald G., 479
Drutz, Jan Edwin, 732
Dryden, John S., 844
DuBose, Thomas Durward, Jr., 599
Dubovsky, Steven L., 77
Duda, Ralph J., Jr., 250
Dudgeon, Maureen, 140
Duginsky, Thomas, 615
Duick, Daniel S., 249
Duick, Gregory F., 133
Duke, Daniel Gist, 656
Duke, James H., Jr., 812
Dukinfield, Michael P., 178
Dull, William Lister, 123
Dumitru, Daniel, 747
Dunbar, Burdett S., 498
Duncan, Charles Alman, 777
Duncan, J. Michael, 829
Duncan, Kenneth H., 45
Duncan, Kim F., 374
Duncan, Marilyn H., 393
Duncan, Newton Oran III, 678
Duncan, S. Edwin, 818
Duncan, Scott C., 526

Dungy, Claibourne I., 119
Dunkel, Thomas B., 228
Dunlap, Joel A., 794
Dunlap, John L., 140
Dunn, Dale M., 692
Dunn, David L., 232
Dunn, Marvin, 132
Dunn, Randall Clifford, 634
Dunn, William F., 226
Dunnigan, Ann C., 212
Dunnigan, Earl J., 418
Dunnigan, Ralph T., Jr., 419
DuPont, Herbert L., 564
Duran, Jose M., 545
Durand, John L., 508
Duriex, Dennis Efren, 567
Durr, Samuel J., 465
Durrie, Daniel S., 279
Dusenberry, Kathryn Ellen, 228
Duthie, Susan E., 290
Duvic, Madeleine, 523
Dyck, Peter J., 197
Dyck, Walter P., 553
Dyke, David R., 359
Dykman, Thomas R., 24
Dysert, Peter A., 685
Dysken, Maurice William, 222
Dyson, Maynard C., 705

E

Eades, Brian J., 626
Eales, Frazier, 235
Eames, Gretchen M., 705
Earle, John D., 229
Early, Terrence S., 762
Easley, Thomas D., 493
Eastwood, M. Robin, 301
Eastwood, Thomas F., 554
Eaton, R. Philip, 379
Ebbert, Larry P., 471
Ebeling, John D., 143
Eberle, Catherine M., 359
Ebers, Douglas D., 369
Ebersold, Michael J., 194
Eccarius, Scott G., 474
Echt, Gregory Allen, 784
Eck, Jack, 50
Eck, Marci J., 336
Eckard, Donald, 157
Eckel, Robert H., 39, 40
Eckenrode, James F., 257
Eckert, Elke D., 222
Eckhoff, P. James, Jr., 480
Ecklund, Steven Richard, 84
Eckman, Mark, 184

Hardy, David Ray, 725
Harford, Antonia, 385
Hargreaves, James, 415
Harik, Sami I., 11
Harken, Alden H., 85
Harkey, Michael R., 453
Harlass, Frederick E., 631
Harle, Brian, 640
Harle, Mark A., 501
Harley, John B., 460
Harman, Thomas R., 179
Harmon, Daniel James, 571
Harmon, Keith R., 224
Harmon, Mark K., 645
Harmon, Robert J., 77
Harmon, Susan, 444
Harms, Steven E., 789
Harner, Stephen G., 209
Harper, Daniel A., 341
Harper, Edwin Leeth, 15
Harper, James D., 496
Harper, Randall C., 694
Harper, Richard L., 606
Harper, William F., 583
Harrer, Grant W., 332
Harrington, Brian Boru, 501
Harrington, Jeffrey V., 660
Harrington, John Norris, 648
Harrington, Stephen C., 178
Harris, Brent R., 695
Harris, Jack R., 492
Harris, James R., 336
Harris, John H., Jr., 792
Harris, Joseph Denton IV, 834
Harris, Paul C., 609
Harris, Richard L., 565
Harris, Robert J., 295
Harris, T. Stuart, 22
Harris, W. Turner, 13
Harrison, Garth F., 305
Harrison, Gunyon M., 713
Harrison, Mark N., 52
Harrison, Paul B., 159
Harrison, Phil W., 254
Harrison, Preston E., Jr., 618
Harrison, V. Lee, 329
Harrod, Charles Scott, 46
Hart, Blaine L., 402
Hart, Denise, 601
Hart, Mark B., 423
Hart, Robert G., 617
Hart, William Hiatt, 805
Hart, William M., Jr., 280
Hartenbach, David E., 296
Hartford, C. Edward, 85
Hartley, Guilford G., 187
Hartley, James M., 136
Hartley, Roy W., 135
Hartshorn, Denzel F., 66

Hartshorne, Michael F., 388
Hartstein, Jack, 278
Harvey, William C., 623
Hashimoto, Frederick, 383
Hassenbusch, Samuel J., 607
Hastings, John D., 448
Hatch, Mark William, 681
Hatcher, Robert L., 532
Hatlelid, J. Michael, 270
Hatlelid, R. Robert, 266
Hattel, Lawrence, 847
Hauer-Jensen, Martin, 27
Haufrect, Eric J., 634
Hauge, Chris W., 45
Haughey, Bruce H., 286
Hauser, Mary F., 199
Hausinger, Sheryl Ann, 733
Hausner, Richard J., 689
Haut, Arthur, 9
Hawes, Michael J., 61
Hawkins, Linda Louise, 768
Hawkins, Richard J., 64
Haws, Robert M., 718
Hawtrey, Charles E., 129
Hay, Donald P., 301
Hay, Ian D., 177
Haycraft, Gordon L., 243
Hayes, David L., 169
Hayes, David M., 350
Hayes, Marshall W., 662
Haynes, Taylor H. II, 857
Haynes, W. Ducote, 23
Haynie, Thomas Powell III, 624
Hayreh, Sohan F., 107
Hays, Robert J., 804
Hays, Taru, 68
Hazuka, Mark Bernard, 82
Head, William C., 669
Headinger, Michael E., 148
Headley, Roxanne, 71
Heaney, Robert M., 262
Heard, Jeanne K., 8
Hearne, Steven Eric, 551
Heath, Paul W., 506
Heaton, Gary L., 740
Heaton, Steuart L., 682
Hebeler, Joan R., 707, 762
Hebeler, Robert F., Jr., 826
Hebert, Adelaide A., 523
Heck, Heidi Rebecca, 640
Heckman, James Donald, 670
Heckman, Michael M., 663
Hector, David A., 513
Hedemark, Linda L., 224
Hedges, Parke Joseph, 640
Heggeness, Michael H., 667
Heiken, Jay P., 309
Heinrich, George Ronald, 499

Heiser, David P., 366
Heitsman, Jay C., 120
Heitzman, Martin, 612
Held, Beverly L., 519
Held, Kristin Story, 656
Helfrich, George Baird, 814
Helikson, Mary Alice, 312
Heller, Kimberly Koester, 541
Hellman, Richard N., 192
Helm, Phala Aniece, 743
Helms, Thomas P., 494
Helseth, Hovald K., Jr., 235
Heltemes, Bradley, 188
Heltne, Carl E., 167
Helzberg, John H., 254
Hempel, Karl Hans, 803
Hemsell, David L., 630
Henao, Sergio E., 765
Henderson, John A. IV, 834
Henderson, Mark, 581
Henderson, Robert C., 626
Henderson, Ronald E., Jr., 695
Henderson, Thomas T., 644
Hendricks, John C., 824
Hendrickson, Jon R., 19
Henkes, David N., 694
Henneford, Gordon E., 339
Henneford, John R., 340
Henry, Albert Carl III, 826
Henry, George Morrison, 11
Henry, John, 379
Henry, Rodney L., 511
Henson, Helene K., 745
Henthorn, Daniel R., 139
Herber, Michael C., 848
Herbert, Lawrence L., 347
Herbert, R. Wayne, 20
Hered, John, 143
Herlihy, John J., 474
Herlihy, Richard E., 462
Herman, David C., 204
Herman, Gail E., 713
Herman, James Jay, 488
Herman, Paul S., 733
Herman, Peter S., 522
Herman, Terence Spencer, 785
Hermreck, Arlo S., 158
Hernandez, Alfred Joe, Jr., 548
Hernandez, J. Carlos, 786
Hernandez, Jesus Antonio, 547
Hernandez, Jose Alberto, 686
Herndon, James H., Jr., 520
Herring, John A., 663
Herrington, Preston B., 396
Herschler, Jonathan, 852

Houston, John, 769
Hoverman, Isabel Vreeland, 570
Hoverson, David, 382
Hovland, Kenneth R., 61
Howard, Ben J., 464
Howard, Campbell P., 290
Howard, Earl W. III, 805
Howard, Lillian G., 555
Howard, Michael Duard, 794
Howard, Robert Lee, 501
Howard, Todd K., 314
Howard, William J., 478
Howarth, Cathryn B., 698
Howe, Don Duvall, 769
Howe, Robert B., 187
Howell, J. F., 829
Howerton, Ernest E., 644
Howland, William Charles III, 485
Hruska, Keith A., 267
Hsi, Andrew, 393
Huang, Ted, 751
Huber, Philip J., Jr., 516
Hubmayr, Rolf D., 226
Hucaby, Deborah Susan, 730
Huddleston, Charles B., 318
Hudgens, Richard W., 301
Hudnall, Clayton Howard, 842
Hudson, M'liss A., 320
Huff, J. Clark, 37
Huff, Kalai, 242
Huff, Robert W., 640
Huffman, David H., 50
Hughens, H. Kennon, 496
Hughes, James A., 429
Hughes, Jane B. L., 657
Hughes, Ronald Dallas, 11
Hughson, H. Eric, 331
Hulbert, John C., 237
Hummell, Paul R., 494
Humphrey, Irving L., 759
Humphrey, Paul W., 312
Hunder, Gene G., 231
Hunkeler, John D., 279
Hunnicutt, Robert W., 666
Hunsicker, Lawrence G., 105
Hunt, John L., 808
Hunt, Judson Mark, 597
Hunt, Lyn I., 705
Hunt, Robert S., 311, 315
Hunter, David M., 657
Hunter, David W., 230
Hunter, M. Brooke, 339
Hunter, Marque A., 778
Hunter, Rosemary S., 399
Hunter, Verda, 264
Hura, Claudia E., 601
Hurd, Eric, 799

Hurd, Howard Perrin II, 511
Hurd, Paul W., 616
Hurd, Robert N., 325
Hurd, Thelma, 819
Hurewitz, David S., 436
Hurley, Brian, 479
Hurley, Cathy A., 584
Hurley, Donna Schroeder, 627
Hurley, Douglas Lee, 568
Hurley, Joseph J., 314
Hurst, Bradley S., 59
Hurst, Daniel L., 621
Hurst, David M., 78
Hurst, Paul G., 35
Hurt, Bruce A., 684
Hurt, George E., Jr., 836
Hurt, Richard D., 189
Hurwitz, Richard L., 713
Husby, Lucinda Mae, 330
Huska, Michael J., 186
Husmann, Douglas A., 237
Hussain, Nasir, 576
Hussey, David H., 123
Huston, David Paul, 488
Hutchens, Curt H., 236
Hutchens, Thomas, 421
Hutchins, Laura F., 9
Hutchinson, Lewis R., 682
Huth, James Frank, 819
Hutton, William L., 648
Huycke, Mark M., 443
Hyde, William Harold, 697
Hyder, Jace W., 133
Hyers, Thomas Morgan, 305
Hyland, Glen, 430
Hyland, John Walton, 506
Hyland, Lowell J., 464

I

Iannacone, Susan Theresa, 619
Ibarguen, Eduardo, 722
Iber, Conrad, 225
Idell, Steven, 779
Iglesias, Jose V., 812
Ihde, Daniel C., 265
Illig, William P., 454
Illige-Sauicier, Martha, 41
Imber, Richard, 37
Imray, Thomas J., 372
Infante, Ernesto, 614
Ingle, James N., 192
Ingraham, Daniel M., 520
Ingram, Ronald W., 655
Inhofe, Perry D., 442
Ippen, Gregory A., 47

Ipson, Merle A., 703
Irvine, Patrick W., 182
Isaacs, Emily Merrell, 800
Isaacson, Richard N., 162
Iseman, Michael D., 80
Isenberg, Keith E., 301
Isensee, Christopher H., 663
Isern, Reuben A., 798
Ivanhoe, Cindy B., 745

J

Jack, William D. II, 506
Jackman, Warren M., 437
Jackson, Carlayne Elizabeth, 617
Jackson, Charles David, 18
Jackson, Gilchrist L., 821
Jackson, John Richard, 542
Jackson, Mary Anne, 290
Jackson, Oscar Branche, Jr., 644
Jackson, Rhett Kern, 444
Jackson, Richard A., 578
Jackson, Richard Henry, 603
Jackson, Richard J., 27
Jackson, Robert W., 664
Jackson, Thomas Henry, Jr., 527
Jacobs, Lawrence A., 460
Jacobs, Richard F., 17
Jacobs, Robert Lee, 491
Jacobs, Steven J., 110
Jacobson, Jacob G., 76
Jacobson, Robert Morris, 516
Jacocks, M. Alex, 461
Jaderlund, John, 834
Jaeckle, Kurt A., 614
Jafek, Bruce W., 65
Jaffe, Norman, 713
Jagannath, Sundar, 9
Jahn, Paul B., 431
Jahnigen, Dennis W., 44
Jahnke, Robert W., 402
James, David H., Jr., 20
James, Elizabeth, 289
James, John, 2
Jamieson, Michael, 514
Janaki, Lalitha Madhav, 780
Janes, Robert H., Jr., 26
Janjan, Nora A., 783
Jankovic, Joseph, 614
Janney, Christine G., 288
Janusz, Alvin J., 480
Jaranson, James M., 223
Jardan, Freeman C., 739
Jarratt, Michael Taylor, 518

Reid, William Howard, 757
Reidy, Robert W., 389
Reilly, T. Philip, 843
Reinarz, James Allen, 563
Reineck, Henry John, 601
Reinert, Charles Marshall, 664
Reiter, Alex A., 636
Reiter, John Henry, 333
Reiter, Peter Joseph, 103
Reitmann, John H., 760
Reitz, Rolfe D., 447
Remmers, August Ray, Jr., 599
Remmers, Paul A., 576
Rennard, Stephen I., 371
Rettenmaier, Lawrence J., 125
Reuben, Jeffrey D., 668
Reul, George J., 830
Reuter, S. Harold, 679
Reuter, Stewart R., 796
Reveille, John D., 801
Reves, Randall, 46
Rex, John H., 566
Reyerson, Donald Harvey, 119
Reymond, Ralph, 156
Reyna, Juan A., 842
Reyna, Richard S., 582
Reyna, Rowland Sanchez, 556, 582
Reynaud, Albert C., 325
Reynolds, George E. S. III, 734
Reynolds, James R., 481
Reynolds, John A., 341
Reynolds, Teresa A., 157
Reynolds, Tommy Ray, 481
Rezai, Karim, 108
Rhame, Frank S., 185
Rhame, Frederick Taylor, 739
Rhead, William J., 117
Rhinehart, Donald F., 447
Rhodes, Ray N., Jr., 730
Rhodes, Rollie E., 453
Rian, Roger Leland, 789
Rice, Jack S., Jr., 841
Rice, Stuart G., 419
Rich, Joseph D., 343
Richard, James M., 451
Richards, B. Stephens III, 664
Richards, Dallas L., 139
Richards, John A., 666
Richardson, Carol Joan, 708
Richardson, Charles T., 546
Richardson, John M., 730
Richardson, John S., 502
Richardson, Ronald Lee, 192
Richardson, Thomas F., 303
Richenbacher, Wayne E., 128
Richerson, Hal B., 92

Richie, Rodney C., 779
Richmond, Cliff M., 694
Richmond, George Merritt, Jr., 542
Richmond, Lewis Hilliard, 770
Richmond, Ronald, 312
Rickard, Thomas R., 329
Rickman, Michael Z., 443
Ridgway, E. C., 40
Riecke, William B., 408
Riela, Anthony Richard, 619
Rier, Kevin, 129
Riggs, Patrick K., 655
Riggs, Thomas E., 443
Rikkers, Layton F., 373
Riley, Charles, 401
Riley, Fred Whitcomb, Jr., 626
Riley, William B., Jr., 755
Riley, William J., 716
Rimer, Bobby Alan, 626
Ring, William Steves, 826
Ringdahl, Erika N., 252
Ringel, Steven P., 56
Rinker, Charles F., 349
Rinner, Steven Eric, 598
Rios, Miguel A., 595
Risi, George F., 330
Risinger, David O., 797
Risinger, Donald L., 797
Ritchey, Michael L., 839
Ritchie, Elizabeth Lipscombe, 842
Rittenhouse, Mark Charles, 816, 824
Ritter, Frank J., 198
Ritterbusch, John F., 390
Ritvo, Joanne H., 78
Rivera, Frank J., 790
Rivera, Raul, 774
Rivero, Dennis, 390
Rizza, Robert A., 177
Ro, Jay Y., 691
Roach, Ewell S., 619
Roach, James William, 666
Roaten, Shelley, Jr., 537
Robb, Geoffrey Lawrence, 753
Robbins, Laurence J., 44
Roberge, Natalie A., 680
Roberts, Albert Dee, Jr., 573
Roberts, Charles C., 290
Roberts, Howard H., 275
Roberts, Jesse A., 264
Roberts, John William, 817
Roberts, Larry C., 518
Roberts, Laura W., 400
Roberts, Lynne Jeanine, 521
Roberts, Robert, 510
Roberts, Robin A., 522

Roberts, Scott, 146
Roberts, W. Mark, 716
Robertson, Dennis M., 204
Robertson, Kenneth L., 850
Robertson, R. Paul, 176
Robertson, William G. III, 515
Robeson, Glenn H., 793
Robeson, Steven C., 406
Robillard, Jean E., 117
Robinow, Jay S., 307
Robinowitz, Bernard N., 439
Robins, Linda, 736
Robins, N. Scott, 580
Robins, Patrick R., 339
Robinson, David, 146
Robinson, Frank E., 570
Robinson, James S., 766
Robinson, Joe T., 18
Robinson, Robert G., 122
Robinson, Sally Sue, 731
Robinson, Thomas A., 323
Robinson, William A., 51
Robinson, William A., Jr., 505
Robison, Leon R., 257
Rocchini, Albert P., 214
Roche, Richard J., 382
Rock, Robert L., 644
Rockefeller, John D., 141
Rockwood, Charles A., Jr., 671
Rodarte, Joseph R., 776
Rodemyer, Carol R., 120
Rodenbiker, Harold T., Jr., 422
Rodger, Malcolm R. III, 807
Rodgers, George Piper, 505
Rodgers, Katherine Lynn, 740
Rodgers, Louis D., 127
Rodgers, Roger William, 595
Rodnitzky, Robert L., 107
Rodriguez, Abelardo, 542
Rodriguez, Moses, 197
Rodriguez, Victorio, 593
Roe, Charles R., 701
Roeder, Robert E., 132
Roehm, John, 793
Roenigk, Randall K., 175
Rogeness, Graham Arthur, 770
Rogers, J. Drew, 307
Rogers, James Henry, Jr., 724
Rogers, James N., 502
Rogers, James T., 261
Rogers, John C., 540
Rogers, Randall David, 517
Rogers, Robert Jean, 487
Rogers, Roy S. III, 175
Rogers, Tom, Jr., 730
Rogers, William F., 83
Roh, Mark S., 822

Van Sickle, Mary L., 637
Van Stiegmann, Gregory, 86
Van Stone, John C., 266
Van Tassel, Robert A., 169
Van Wyk, William J., 558
Vancaillie, Thierry G., 641
Vance, William S., Jr., 508
Vandenberg, Byron F., 94
Vander Ark, Gary, 55
Vanderhoof, Jon A., 369
Vandermeer, Robert D., 665
VanderSchilden, John L., 14
Vandersteen, Paul R., 411
Vandivort, Monica R., 359
VanEtta, Linda L., 184
VanGilder, John C., 105
Vanhooser, Jonathan Ross, 459
Vannatta, Gerald B., 444
Vanover, Marilyn Jean, 641
Vanover, Randall Mark, 582
vanSonnenberg, Eric, 791
Vanzant, Robert C., 540
Vardaman, Arnold, 608
Varecka, Thomas F., 184
Varenhorst, Michael P., 149
Varghese, George, 153
Varma, Surendra Kumar, 720
Varner, Roy V., 766
Varnum, Robert, 80
Vartian, Carl Victor, 566
Varvares, Mark A., 287
Vasavada, Nishendu M., 766
Vaughan, Thurman Ray, 485
Vaughn, Gary E., 519
Vaughn, Thomas C., 628
Vaurio, Carl E., 188
Vazquez, Genaro, 774
Veach, Lisa A., 101
Veggeberg, Neil Roger, 741
Veitch, John M., 257
Vela, B. Sylvia, 380
Velez, Ruben L., 598
Velosa, Jorge A., 193
Vennix, Michael John, 746
Ventura, Gerard J., 592
Verani, Mario S., 511
Vereen, Lowell E., 778
Verfeillie, Catherine M., 191
Verghese, Abraham C., 563
Vergne-Marini, Pedro J., 598
Verheyden, Charles N., 755
Verm, Ray Alan, 549
Vermillion, C. Dale, 351
Vernava, Anthony M. III, 247,
    316
Verner, E. Farley, 568
Vesole, David H., 10
Vickstrom, Douglas E., 102
Viere, Robert G., 665

Vietti, Teresa J., 293
Vigil, Deborah A., 388
Vigil, Luis F., 496
Vigneri, Joseph M., 853
Villamaria, Frank J., 503
Villasenor, Hector Raul, 513
Viney, Shelton, 814
Virgilio, Joanne F., 52
Viswanathan, Baluswamy, 720
Vogel, Albert V., 400
Vogel, Curt M., 313
Vogel, Stanley J., 142
Vogel, Susan M., 579
Vogtsberger, Kenneth
    Norman, 771
Volk, Charles R., 422
Volk, Charles T., 807
Vollers, J. Michael, 3
Volpe, Joseph Anthony, 623
von Eschenbach, Andrew C.,
    840
Von Hoff, Daniel D., 594
von Minden, Milton C., 52
von Noorden, Gunter K., 653
Vordermark, Jonathan S. II,
    840
Vosburgh, John B., 452
Vose, Julie M., 362
Voss, Carolyn, 384
Votteler, Theodore P., 809
Vrabec, Jeffrey T., 678
Vriesendorp, Francine Joanna,
    615
Vuitch, Milan F., 687

W

Waagner, David C., 720
Waber, Lewis J., 702
Wade, Paul Douglas, 574
Waeckerlin, Ronald W., 854
Wagener, Jeffrey Scott, 70
Wagner, Charles W., 27
Wagner, Clyde W., Jr., 582
Wagner, Grant Hulse, 772
Wagner, Karen D., 763
Wagner, Milton, 793
Wagner, Stanley C., 508
Wagoner, Jack, Jr., 9
Wagonfeld, Samuel, 79
Wahl, Timothy O., 357
Wakefield, Peggy L., 728
Walburn, John Norman, 369
Walden, H. Douglas, 263
Walder, Arnold Ira, 817, 824
Waldman, J. Deane, 394
Waldman, Steven D., 132

Waldron, C. Milton, 62
Walgren, Kenneth L., 574
Walker, Daniel R., 324
Walker, David H., 688
Walker, John F., 672
Walker, Larry L., 815
Walker, Melvin O., Jr., 261
Walker, Sara E., 310
Wall, Donna A., 293
Wall, Michael, 107
Wall, Robert E., 59
Wall, Terry J., 156
Wallace, Darryl, 315
Wallace, James O., 813
Wallace, Richard James, Jr.,
    568
Wallace, Sidney, 793
Waller, David A., 761
Waller, Jack Douglas, 518
Wallfisch, Harry K., 497
Walser, Eric M., 791
Walsh, James W., 230
Walsh, Nicolas E., 748
Walsh, Peter, 43
Walters, Robert M., 557
Waltman, Steven E., 467
Walton, Jerry L., 468
Walton, Martha A., 658
Waner, Milton, 16
Wang, Robert C., 680
Wang, Robert M. C., 774
Warady, Bradley A., 290
Ward, Albert R., 347
Ward, Clark Anderson, 459
Ward, J. Perry, 456
Ward, Kent E., 455
Ward, Patrick C. J., 209
Ward, Robert L., 575
Warder, Daryl E., 605
Warmann, Jeffrey R., 672
Warner, David O., 167
Warner, Mark A., 167
Warner, Noranna B., 802
Warner, Richard, 76
Warnes, Carole A., 170
Warren, Marvin, 323
Warren, Michael M., 838
Warren, Robert Wells, 717
Warwick, Warren, 214
Wascher, Daniel, 390
Washburn, Daniel Dean, 439
Wasserman, Richard L., 486
Wasserman, Todd H., 308
Waters, Jeffrey A., 296
Watkins, John B., 294
Watkins, Michael G., 505
Watson, Kathleen V., 188
Watson, Keith C., 666
Watson, LaDonna, 735

Z